American Cancer Society
Atlas of
Clinical Oncology

Published

Blumgart, Fong, Jarnagin	*Hepatobiliary Cancer (2001)*
Cameron	*Pancreatic Cancer (2001)*
Char	*Tumors of the Eye and Ocular Adnexa (2001)*
Eifel, Levenback	*Cancer of the Female Lower Genital Tract (2001)*
Grossbard	*Malignant Lymphomas (2001)*
Pollock	*Soft Tissue Sarcomas (2001)*
Posner, Vokes, Weichselbaum	*Cancer of the Upper Gastrointestinal Tract (2001)*
Prados	*Brain Cancer (2001)*
Shah	*Cancer of the Head and Neck (2001)*
Silverman	*Oral Cancer (1998)*
Sober, Haluska	*Skin Cancer (2001)*
Wiernik	*Adult Leukemias (2001)*
Willett	*Cancer of the Lower Gastrointestinal Tract (2001)*
Winchester, Winchester	*Breast Cancer (2000)*

Forthcoming

Carroll, Grossfeld	*Prostate Cancer (2002)*
Clark, Duh, Jahan, Perrier	*Endocrine Tumors (2002)*
Droller	*Urothelial Cancer (2002)*
Fuller, Seiden, Young	*Uterine and Endometrial Cancer (2003)*
Ginsberg	*Lung Cancer (2002)*
Ozols	*Ovarian Cancer (2002)*
Raghavan	*Germ Cell Tumors (2002)*
Richie, Steele	*Kidney Tumors (2003)*
Volberding	*Viral and Immunological Malignancies (2003)*
Yasko	*Bone Tumors (2002)*

American Cancer Society
Atlas of
Clinical Oncology

Editors

GLENN D. STEELE JR, MD
Geisinger Health System

THEODORE L. PHILLIPS, MD
University of California

BRUCE A. CHABNER, MD
Harvard Medical School

Managing Editor

TED S. GANSLER, MD, MBA
Director of Health Content, American Cancer Society

American Cancer Society
Atlas of
Clinical Oncology

Cancer of the Upper Gastrointestinal Tract

Mitchell C. Posner, MD

Associate Professor of Surgery
Chief, Surgical Oncology
University of Chicago
Chicago, Illinois

Everett E. Vokes, MD

Director, Section of Hematology/Oncology
John E. Ultmann Professor of Medicine
and Radiation and Cellular Oncology
University of Chicago
Chicago, Illinois

Ralph R. Weichselbaum, MD

Daniel K. Ludwig Professor
Chairman, Radiation and Cellular Oncology
Head, Molecular Oncology
University of Chicago
Chicago, Illinois

2002
BC Decker Inc
Hamilton • London

BC Decker Inc
20 Hughson Street South
P.O. Box 620, LCD 1
Hamilton, Ontario L8N 3K7
Tel: 905-522-7017; 1-800-568-7281
Fax: 905-522-7839; 1-888-311-4987
E-mail: info@bcdecker.com
Website: www.bcdecker.com

ISBN 1–55009–101-8
Printed in Canada

Cover figure (top left) courtesy of Dr. Hart, from Chapter 4, Barrett's Esophagus with High-Grade Dysplasia and/or Esophageal Adenocarcinoma.

Cover figure (top right) courtesy of Dr. Posner, from Chapter 7, Techniques of Esophageal Resection.

Cover figure (bottom) courtesy of Drs. Lew and Posner, Chapter 13, Surgical Treatment of Localized Gastric Cancer. The figure was drawn by Lydia Johns, Department of Surgery, University of Chicago.

Sales and Distribution

United States
BC Decker Inc
P.O. Box 785
Lewiston, NY 14092-0785
Tel: 905-522-7017; 1-800-568-7281
Fax: 905-522-7839; 1-888-311-4987
E-mail: info@bcdecker.com
Website: www.bcdecker.com

Canada
BC Decker Inc
20 Hughson Street South
P.O. Box 620, LCD 1
Hamilton, Ontario L8N 3K7
Tel: 905-522-7017; 1-800-568-7281
Fax: 905-522-7839; 1-888-311-4987
E-mail: info@bcdecker.com
Website: www.bcdecker.com

Foreign Rights
John Scott & Company
International Publishers' Agency
P.O. Box 878
Kimberton, PA 19442
Tel: 610-827-1640
Fax: 610-827-1671
E-mail: jsco@voicenet.com

U.K., Europe, Scandinavia, Middle East
Elsevier Science
Customer Service Department
Foots Cray High Street
Sidcup, Kent
DA14 5HP, UK
Tel: 44 208 308 5760
Fax: 44 181 308 5702
E-mail: cservice@harcourt.com

Australia, New Zealand
Elsevier Science Australia
Customer Service Department
STM Division
Locked Bag 16
St. Peters, New South Wales, 2044
Australia
Tel: 61 02 9517-8999
Fax: 61 02 9517-2249
E-mail: stmp@harcourt.com.au
Website: www.harcourt.com.au

Japan
Igaku-Shoin Ltd.
Foreign Publications Department
3-24-17 Hongo
Bunkyo-ku, Tokyo, Japan 113-8719
Tel: 81 3 3817 5680
Fax: 81 3 3815 6776
E-mail: fd@igaku-shoin.co.jp

Singapore, Malaysia, Thailand, Philippines, Indonesia, Vietnam, Pacific Rim, Korea
Elsevier Science Asia
583 Orchard Road
#09/01, Forum
Singapore 238884
Tel: 65-737-3593
Fax: 65-753-2145

Notice: The authors and publisher have made every effort to ensure that the patient care recommended herein, including choice of drugs and drug dosages, is in accord with the accepted standard and practice at the time of publication. However, since research and regulation constantly change clinical standards, the reader is urged to check the product information sheet included in the package of each drug, which includes recommended doses, warnings, and contraindications. This is particularly important with new or infrequently used drugs.

Dedication

In memory of Michael Burt, MD, PhD, friend, colleague, and mentor who by his extraordinary example continues to inspire me

and

to Janice, Sara and Alexa who bring joy and meaning to each and every day.

Mitchell C. Posner

To my wife Tamara, and my children Natalie and Katherine.

Everett E. Vokes

To my wife Donna and my children Matt, Chuck and Ben.

Ralph R. Weichselbaum

Contents

III   SMALL BOWEL

Preface

Collectively, cancer of the esophagus, stomach, and small intestine represents the second most common site and cause of death among the digestive system cancers. These disparate malignancies have one thing in common: that consistently effective treatment remains elusive. This volume of the *Atlas of Clinical Oncology* series published by the American Cancer Society brings together a talented and experiences group of contributors to provide, through prose and pictures, a current and thorough review of upper gastrointestinal cancer. Epidemiologic factors, molecular and biologic determinants, diagnostic/staging methods, and treatment modalities are described for each organ site. Advances in imaging, interventional gastroenterology, surgical technique, and combined-modality therapy are emphasized since they have had a substantial impact on the management of this challenging group of cancers. The future is bright and promising as the genetic events that dictate the malignant process are further elucidated, allowing therapy to be better tailored to both the patient and the tumor target.

The editors would like to thank all of the authors for their commitment in both time and scholarship to *Cancer of the Upper Gastrointestinal Tract* and for creating what we believe is a significant contribution to the literature. We would also like to acknowledge Charmaine Sherlock and Kimmy Rolfe at BC Decker Inc for their expertise and assistance in preparing this volume and thank Brian Decker for his invaluable suggestions and guidance in bringing this endeavor to completion.

MCP
EEV
RRW

November 2001

Contributors

EDDIE K. ABDALLA, MD
Department of Surgical Oncology
University of Texas M.D. Anderson Cancer
    Center
Houston, Texas
Invasive Techniques for Palliation of
    Advanced Gastric Cancer

RICHARD B. ARENAS, MD
Department of Surgery
Tufts University School of Medicine
Baystate Health Systems
Springfield, Massachusetts
Gastric Lymphoma

LINDA MORRIS BROWN, DrPH
Division of Cancer Epidemiology and Genetics
National Cancer Institute
Bethesda, Maryland
Epidemiology of Esophageal Cancer

EZRA E.W. COHEN, MD
Department of Medicine
University of Chicago
Chicago, Illinois
Molecular Biology of Esophageal Cancer

KEVIN C. CONLON, MD, MBA
Department of Surgery
Memorial Sloan-Kettering Cancer Center
New York, New York
Diagnosis and Staging of Gastric Cancer

SUSAN S. DEVESA, PhD
Division of Cancer Epidemiology and Genetics
National Cancer Institute
Bethesda, Maryland
Epidemiology of Esophageal Cancer

TOMISLAV DRAGOVICH, MD, PhD
Department of Medicine
University of Arizona
Arizona Cancer Center
Tucson, Arizona
Nonsurgical Palliative Therapy of Advanced
    Gastric Cancer

MARK K. FERGUSON, MD
Department of Surgery
University of Chicago
University of Chicago Medical Center
Chicago, Illinois
Squamous Cell Carcinoma of the Esophagus
Palliation of Esophageal Cancer

JOSEPH F. FRAUMENI, JR, MD
Division of Cancer Epidemiology and Genetics
National Cancer Institute
Bethesda, Maryland
Epidemiology of Esophageal Cancer

ARUNAS E. GASPARAITIS, MD
Division of Biological Science Division
University of Chicago
Department of Diagnostic Radiology
University of Chicago Hospitals and Medical Center
Chicago, Illinois
Diagnosis of Small-Bowel Tumors

HANS GERDES, MD
Department of Internal Medicine
Joan and Sanford I. Weill Medical College of
    Cornell University
Memorial Sloan-Kettering Cancer Center
New York, New York
Diagnosis and Preoperative Staging of
    Esophageal Cancer
Palliation of Esophageal Cancer

DANIEL G. HALLER, MD
Department of Medicine
University of Pennsylvania
Philadelphia, Pennsylvania
Adjuvant Therapy for Gastric Cancer

JOHN HART, MD
Department of Pathology
University of Chicago
University of Chicago Hospitals
Chicago, Illinois
Barrett's Esophagus with High-Grade Dysplasia and/or Esophageal Adenocarcinoma
Pathology of Small-Bowel Tumors

ROGER D. HURST, MD, FRCS (ED), FACS
Department of Surgery
University of Chicago
Chicago, Illinois
Epidemiology of Small-Bowel Tumors

NORA T. JASKOWIAK, MD
Department of Surgery
University of Chicago
Chicago, Illinois
Adenocarcinoma of the Esophagus and Gastroesophageal Junction

MADHUKAR KAW, MD
Department of GI Medicine and Nutrition
University of Texas M.D. Anderson Cancer Center
Houston, Texas
Invasive Techniques for Palliation of Advanced Gastric Cancer

HEDY LEE KINDLER, MD
Section of Hematology/Oncology
University of Chicago
Chicago, Illinois
Nonsurgical Palliative Therapy of Advanced Gastric Cancer

SHIH-FAN KUAN, MD, PhD
Department of Pathology
University of Chicago
University of Chicago Hospitals
Chicago, Illinois
Pathology of Gastric Neoplasms

JOHN I. LEW, MD
Department of Surgery
University of Chicago
Chicago, Illinois
Surgical Treatment of Localized Gastric Cancer

PETER M. MACENEANEY, MB, FRCR
Department of Radiology
University of Chicago
Chicago, Illinois
Diagnosis of Small-Bowel Tumors

ARNOLD J. MARKOWITZ, MD
Department of Medicine
Joan and Sanford I. Weill Medical College of Cornell University
Memorial Sloan-Kettering Cancer Center
New York, New York
Diagnosis and Preoperative Staging of Esophageal Cancer

ANN M. MAUER, MD
Department of Medicine
University of Chicago
Chicago, Illinois
Multimodality Therapy for Carcinoma of the Esophagus

FABRIZIO MICHELASSI, MD
Department of Surgery
University of Chicago
Chicago, Illinois
Management of Benign and Malignant Small-Bowel Neoplasms

NUBIA MUÑOZ, MD, MPH
Unit of Field and Intervention Studies
International Agency for Research on Cancer
Lyon, France
Epidemiology of Gastric Cancer

PETER W.T. PISTERS, MD, FACS
Department of Surgical Oncology
University of Texas M.D. Anderson
    Cancer Center
Houston, Texas
*Invasive Techniques for Palliation of
    Advanced Gastric Cancer*

MITCHELL C. POSNER, MD
Department of Surgery
University of *Chicago*
Chicago, Illinois
*Adenocarcinoma of the Esophagus and
    Gastroesophageal Junction*
Techniques of Esophageal Resection
Surgical Treatment of Localized Gastric Cancer

CHARLES M. RUDIN, MD, PhD
Department of Medicine and Committee
    on Cancer Biology
University of Chicago
Chicago, Illinois
Molecular Biology of Esophageal Cancer

DANNY M. TAKANISHI, JR, MD
Department of Surgery
University of Hawaii
Honolulu, Hawaii
*Management of Benign and Malignant
    Small-Bowel Neoplasms*

RALPH R. WEICHSELBAUM, MD
Daniel K. Ludwig Professor
Chairman, Department of Radiation and
    Cellular Oncology
University of Chicago
Chicago, Illinois
*Multimodality Therapy for Carcinoma of
    the Esophagus*

MARTIN R. WEISER, MD
Department of Surgery
Joan and Sanford I. Weill Medical College
    of Cornell University
Memorial Sloan-Kettering Cancer Center
New York, New York
Diagnosis and Staging of Gastric Cancer

SHU-YUAN XIAO, MD
Department of Pathology
University of Texas Medical Branch
Galveston, Texas
Pathology of Small-Bowel Tumors

Epidemiology of Esophageal Cancer

LINDA MORRIS BROWN, DrPh

SUSAN S. DEVESA, PhD

JOSEPH F. FRAUMENI, JR., MD

This chapter reviews the epidemiology of esophageal cancer and its two major histologic types, squamous cell carcinoma of the esophagus (SCE) and adenocarcinoma of the esophagus (ACE). Although the tumors share a poor prognosis, they have rather distinct histopathologic and epidemiologic profiles. Squamous cell carcinoma of the esophagus arises from squamous epithelium that undergoes inflammatory, atrophic, and dysplastic changes whereas ACE arises through metaplastic intestinal-type changes that replace the squamous epithelium. This chapter reviews the descriptive patterns of both tumors, along with known and suspected risk or protective factors. Because ACE made up only a small fraction of esophageal cancers until recently, results from most epidemiologic studies of esophageal cancer that did not distinguish histologic types largely reflect the risk factors for SCE. Although most of the epidemiologic studies in the past have referred to SCE, special attention has recently centered on ACE in view of the rising incidence rates of this tumor.

DEMOGRAPHIC CHARACTERISTICS

Esophageal cancer is known for its marked variation by geographic region, ethnicity, and gender. In the United States, esophageal cancer accounts for only 1 percent of all diagnosed cancers; however, it is the seventh leading cause of death from cancer among men.[1] According to estimates provided by the American Cancer Society, approximately 9,200 men and 2,900 women are expected to die from esophageal cancer in the United States during 2000.[1] The lifetime risk of being diagnosed with esophageal cancer in the United States is 0.99 percent for African American men, 0.67 percent for white men, 0.43 percent for African American women, and 0.25 percent for white women.[2]

United States Mortality Patterns

Based on data from the National Center for Health Statistics, mortality rates for esophageal cancer almost doubled in the nonwhite population between 1950 and 1984, reaching a high of 14.1 per 100,000 among nonwhite men and 3.6 per 100,000 among nonwhite women (Figure 1–1). Since 1985, however, there has been a steady decrease, with rates for nonwhite men and women falling to 9.8 per 100,000 and 2.5 per 100,000, respectively, in 1995 to 1996. Mortality rates in the white population changed little during the period of 1950 to 1984, but a striking increase in rates among men occurred during the period of 1985 to 1996. Mortality rates for white men and women in 1995 to 1996 were 5.9 per 100,000 and 1.3 per 100,000, respectively. Rates specifically for African Americans (available since the early 1970s) are higher than rates for all nonwhite populations combined.

Maps showing age-adjusted mortality rates by state economic area for white Americans and African Americans during the period of 1970 to 1994 are presented in Figures 1–2 and 1–3. There were striking differences by geographic area that are more pronounced among white Americans than African Americans and among men than women. Elevated rates for white Americans were primarily in the northeastern and mid-Atlantic states, in scattered Midwestern areas, and (females only) in the Far West. Low rates were seen among white men in the southern and Rocky Mountain states and among white women in the central portion of the country. Data for African Americans were sparse in most areas since this American population is concentrated primarily in the South and in urban areas of the East. Although patterns for African Americans are less clear than among white Americans, elevated rates for both males and females were seen in the mid-Atlantic states (including Washington, D.C.) and in coastal Georgia. From 1992 to 1996, Washington, D.C. had the highest rates for esophageal cancer among men (16.6 per 100,000) and women (3.4 per 100,000), and Utah had the lowest rates (3.4 per 100,000 among men and 0.6 per 100,000 among women).[3]

United States Survival Patterns

Survival data based on follow-up of newly diagnosed cases since the 1970s are available from the Surveillance, Epidemiology, and End Results (SEER) program. Presented in this chapter are data from nine SEER population-based cancer registries surveying approximately 10 percent of the US population. Although survival among patients diagnosed with esophageal cancer is poor for all race and gender groups, significant improvements in the 5-year relative survival rates have occurred over the past two decades (Table 1–1).[2] The 5-year relative survival rates for those diagnosed during 1989 to 1995 were higher for white Americans than for African Americans (13.3% vs 8.9%) and higher for females than for males (13.1% vs 12.1%). Survival rates for those with SCE and those with ACE are similar (Table 1–2). There is a strong decreasing gradient in survival with increasing extent of disease for all esophageal cancer patients and for both SCE and ACE patients. Recent 5-year patient survival rates for all esophageal cancers have ranged from 24.9 percent (for localized disease at diagnosis) to 12.7 percent (for regional disease at diagnosis) to 1.9 percent (for distant disease at diagnosis). Although the percentage of all esophageal tumors is distributed evenly among localized, regional, distant, and unstaged tumors, a higher percentage of SCE has been localized (28%), compared with ACE (23%). A decreasing trend in survival is also observed with increasing age at diagnosis (not shown in table). For all esophageal cancer patients combined, the recent 5-year survival rates have ranged from 17.3 percent for patients < 45 years of age to 9.8 percent for patients ≥ 75 years of age.

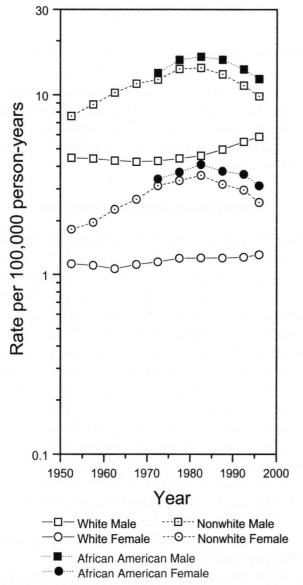

Figure 1–1. Trends in esophageal cancer mortality rates (per 100,000 person-years, age-standardized to the 1970 US population) in the United States by race and sex, 1950 to 1996. (Data from Surveillance, Epidemiology, and End Results [SEER] program, National Cancer Institute.)

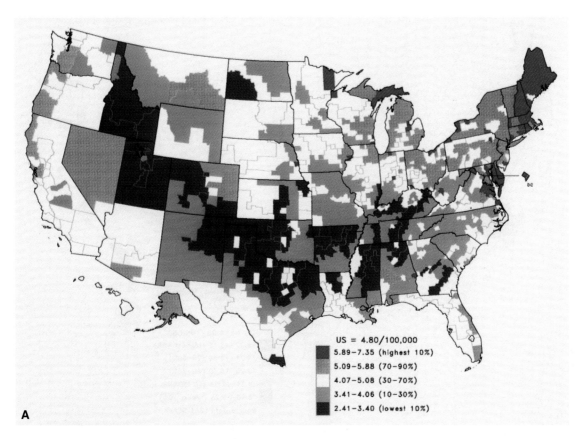

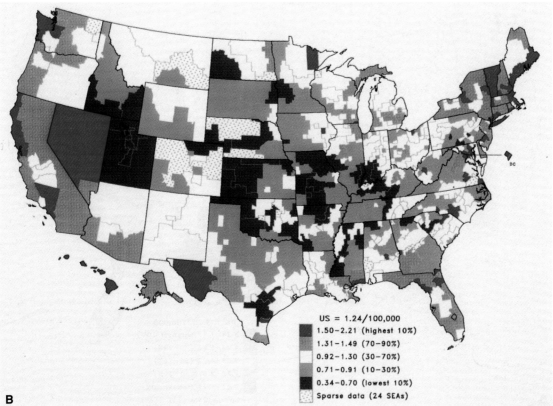

Figure 1–2.   Cancer mortality rates for esophageal cancer by state economic area (SEA) (per 100,000 person-years, age-standardized to the 1970 US population) for white males (*A*) and females (*B*), from 1970 to 1994. (Data from the National Center for Health Statistics.)

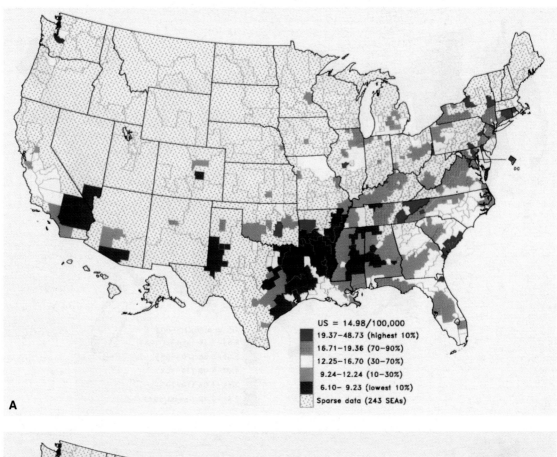

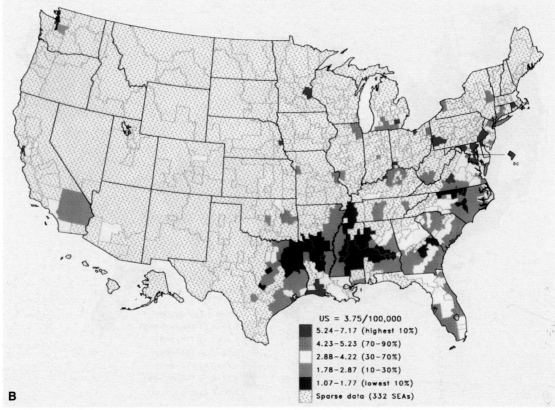

Figure 1–3.   Cancer mortality rates for esophageal cancer by state economic area (SEA) (per 100,000 person-years, age-standardized to the 1970 US population) for African American males (*A*) and females (*B*), from 1970 to 1994. (Data from the National Center for Health Statistics.)

Table 1–1. ESOPHAGEAL CANCER 5-YEAR RELATIVE SURVIVAL RATES* BY DIAGNOSIS YEAR, GENDER, AND RACE

Year of Diagnosis	All Races			White			Blacks		
	Total	Males	Females	Total	Males	Females	Total	Males	Females
1974–76	4.6	3.7	6.8	5.1	4.4	6.6	4.0	2.1	9.0
1977–79	5.0	4.7	5.8	5.6	5.6	5.6	2.8	2.4	4.3
1980–82	6.8	6.1	8.5	7.4	6.6	9.2	5.4	4.6	7.2
1983–85	8.3	7.0	11.8	9.3	7.8	13.1	6.3	5.2	9.5
1986–88	9.9	10.0	9.7	10.8	11.4	9.6	7.3	7.1	8.0
1989–95	12.3	12.1	13.1	13.3	13.2	13.6	8.9	8.0	10.7

*per 100,000.
Data from Surveillance, Epidemiology, and End Results (SEER), National Cancer Institute. Based on data from population-based registries in Connecticut, New Mexico, Utah, Iowa, Hawaii, Atlanta, Detroit, Seattle-Puget Sound, and San Francisco–Oakland. Rates are based on follow-up of patients through 1996.

United States Incidence Patterns

As suggested by the relatively unfavorable survival rates, the incidence and mortality patterns for esophageal cancer are quite similar. Age-adjusted incidence rates for esophageal cancer among African American men peaked at 19.9 per 100,000 in 1985 to 1987 and then began a marked decline, reaching 13.3 per 100,000 in 1994 to 1996, whereas rates among white men increased steadily during the period of 1976 to 1996 with rates approaching 6.1 per 100,000 in 1994 to 1996 (Figure 1–4). Rates among white women changed little, but rates have declined among African American women since the mid-1980s. The dramatic decrease in total esophageal cancer rates for African American males was driven by the concurrent drop in rates for SCE. However, the SCE rate decreased after 1987 for all race and gender groups. Among white males, the incidence of ACE rose from 0.76 per 100,000 in 1976 to 1978 to 3.6 per 100,000 in 1994 to 1996, an increase of more than 350 percent. With the decrease in SCE and the increase in ACE, rates for ACE among white men have recently surpassed those for SCE. Rates of ACE among white females, although much lower than among white males, also increased more than 350 percent, from 0.12 per 100,000 in 1976 to 1978 to 0.44 per 100,000 in 1994 to 1996. In addition, ACE increased almost 200 percent among African American males, from 0.29 per 100,000 in 1976 to 1978 to 0.83 per 100,000 in 1994 to 1996; however, the rates of SCE remained considerably higher. Rates of ACE over the 21-year period varied more for African American females since the rates were based on only 34 cases. Decreases in the reported incidence of esophageal cancers not attributed to SCE or ACE were also seen over the 21-year time period. Even if some cases of ACE were previously misclassified as other or undefined histology, the small difference (0.25 per 100,000) between the rates for 1976 to 1978 and 1994 to 1996 could not account for the large increase among white males (2.8 per 100,000) observed between these two periods.

Table 1–2. ESOPHAGEAL CANCER SURVIVAL RATES BY STAGE CELL TYPE, AND STAGE DISTRIBUTION PERCENT, 1989 TO 1995

Stage	All Esophagus		Squamous Cell		Adenocarcinoma	
	Rate	Percent	Rate	Percent	Rate	Percent
All stages	12.3	100	11.7	100	13.5	100
Localized	24.9	24	20.1	28	34.1	23
Regional	12.7	25	12.6	26	12.1	27
Distant	1.9	25	2.3	22	1.6	30
Unstaged	10.5	25	10.2	25	10.1	19

Data from Surveillance, Epidemiology, and End Results (SEER), National Cancer Institute. Based on data from population-based registries in Connecticut, New Mexico, Utah, Iowa, Hawaii, Atlanta, Detroit, Seattle-Puget Sound, and San Francisco–Oakland. Rates are based on follow-up of patients through 1996.
*per 100,000.

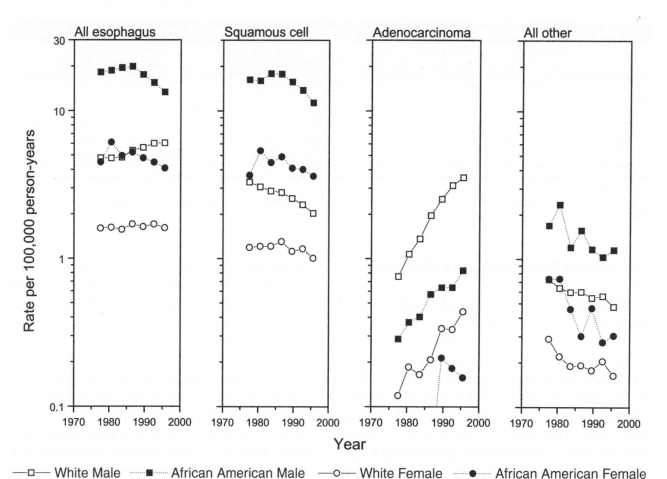

—□— White Male   ····■···· African American Male   —○— White Female   ····●···· African American Female

Figure 1–4.   Trends in esophageal cancer incidence rates (per 100,000 person-years, age-standardized to the 1970 US population) in nine Surveillance, Epidemiology, and End Results (SEER) areas in the United States by cell type, race, and sex, 1976 to 1996. (Data from SEER program, National Cancer Institute.)

Figure 1–5 shows age-specific incidence rates for all esophageal cancers and for esophageal cancer by cell type, for 1990 to 1996. For all esophageal cancers among adults (age ≥ 25 years), rates were highest among African American males and lowest for white females at all but the highest ages. At ages 35 to 54 years, rates for African American females exceeded those for white males, but among individuals 55 years of age and older, the rates for white males surpassed those for African American females. Among white Americans, incidence rates rose steadily with age for females whereas they increased and then plateaued for men aged 75 years or more. Among African Americans, incidence rose until age 74 years and then decreased for both men and women. The rates of SCE were considerably higher among African American than among white men at all ages whereas rates for African American females exceeded those for white men, except for

the oldest age group. For ACE, rates at all ages were highest among white males and generally lowest among African American females although the rates among African American females were less stable due to the small number of cases. Rates for African American males surpassed those for white females of all ages except those aged 85 years and older. Rates rose with age for white females and for African American and white men except for the most elderly. Rates for esophageal cancer of other cell types (including the unspecified category) rose consistently with age, were substantially higher at all ages in men than in women, and were generally higher in African American men than in white men.

Based on incidence data from the SEER program, 1990 to 1996, the overall rates for esophageal cancer varied from a high of 4.8 per 100,000 in Detroit to a low of 2.0 per 100,000 in Utah (Table 1–3). There was also considerable variation in the African American

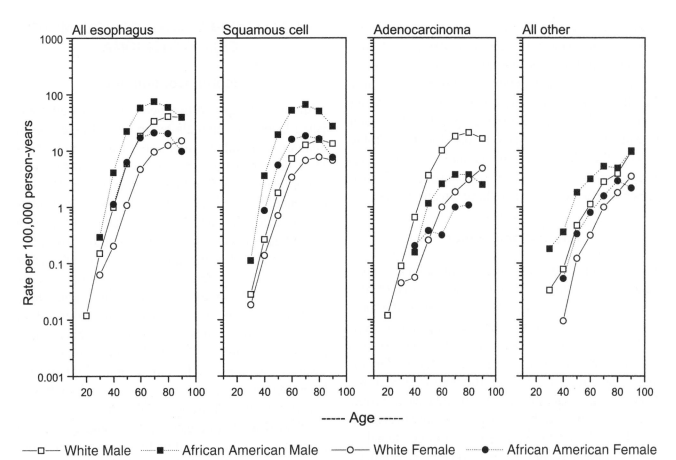

—□— White Male   ·····■····· African American Male   —○— White Female   ·····●····· African American Female

Figure 1–5. Age-specific esophageal cancer incidence rates in nine Surveillance, Epidemiology, and End Results (SEER) program areas in the United States by cell type, race, and sex, 1990 to 1996. (Data from SEER program, National Cancer Institute.)

rate/white rate ratio, ranging from 3.2 in Detroit and Atlanta to only 1.1 in Hawaii. (No cases among African Americans were reported in Utah.) Dramatic differences were seen, according to cell type. For SCE, the rates were highest among African Americans in

Connecticut (11.2 per 100,000) and lowest among whites in Utah (0.7 per 100,000). For ACE, the highest rate was 2.1 per 100,000, among whites in Seattle, whereas the lowest was 0.3 per 100,000, among African Americans in San Francisco–Oakland and in

Table 1–3. AGE-ADJUSTED ESOPHAGEAL CANCER INCIDENCE RATES,* 1990 TO 1996, BY RACE AND CELL TYPE								
	All Esophagus			Squamous Cell			Adenocarcinoma		
Registry	Total	White	Afr Am	Total	White	Afr Am	Total	White	Afr Am
All 9 SEER registries	4.0	3.6	9.0	2.2	1.6	7.9	1.5	1.7	0.4
San Francisco–Oakland	4.0	3.8	7.3	2.2	1.7	6.6	1.4	1.8	0.3
Connecticut	4.5	4.0	12.8	2.5	2.0	11.2	1.7	1.7	0.7
Detroit (Metropolitan)	4.8	3.8	9.1	3.0	1.7	7.8	1.4	1.6	0.5
Hawaii	3.1	4.0	4.4	2.4	2.9	4.4	0.5	0.7	0.0
Iowa	3.4	4.0	6.1	1.3	1.3	5.2	1.8	1.8	0.9
New Mexico	2.9	3.0	5.0	1.3	1.2	3.9	1.2	1.3	0.0
Seattle (Puget Sound)	4.3	4.4	5.4	2.0	1.9	4.8	2.0	2.1	0.3
Utah	2.0	2.0	0.0	0.7	0.7	0.0	1.1	1.1	0.0
Atlanta (Metropolitan)	4.6	3.1	9.9	3.1	1.4	8.9	1.1	1.3	0.4

Afr Am = African American; SEER = Surveillance, Epidemiology, and End Results.
*Rates per 100,000 person-years, age-adjusted using 1970 US standard, from nine Surveillance, Epidemiology, and End Results (SEER) program areas.
Data from SEER, National Cancer Institute.

Seattle. (No cases of ACE were reported among African Americans in Hawaii, New Mexico, or Utah.)

The overall incidence rates for esophageal cancer among males and females combined in the nine SEER registries were more than two times greater among African Americans (8.2 per 100,000) than among white Americans (3.5 per 100,000) (Table 1–4). Although based on small numbers, rates among Hispanics, Asians and Pacific Islanders, and Native Americans were lower than those among whites.

International Patterns

International differences in esophageal cancer incidence rates from 1988 to 1992 are dramatic[4] and largely reflect the geographic variations in the incidence of SCE. Published rates among males were highest in Calvados, France (22.3 per 100,000, followed by rates in Hong Kong and in Miyagi, Japan), and lowest in Israel (1.7 per 100,000) (Figure 1–6). However, the highest rates in the world have occurred in parts of China and Iran, which are not covered by population-based tumor registries. Among females, the rates ranged from 8.3 per 100,000 in Bombay, India, to 0.2 per 100,000 in Tarragona, Spain. Rates for African Americans ranked among the highest whereas those for white Americans were among the lowest. Internationally, the male/female rate ratio has varied from less than 1.4 to more than 20. The upward trend in ACE incidence seen in the United States has been reported in several countries in Europe.[5–13]

Table 1–4. AGE-ADJUSTED ESOPHAGEAL CANCER INCIDENCE RATES,* 1990–1996, BY RACE/ETHNICITY AND GENDER

Race/Ethnicity	Rate per 100,000 Persons		
	Total	Males	Females
All races	3.8	6.3	1.8
White	3.5	5.7	1.6
White Hispanic	2.5	4.7	—
White non-Hispanic	3.6	5.8	1.7
African American	8.2	13.5	4.2
Asian/Pacific Islander	2.5	4.5	0.8
Native American	1.3	2.5	0.4
Hispanic	2.4	4.4	—

*Rates per 100,000 person-years, age-adjusted using 1970 US standard. Data from Surveillance, Epidemiology, and End Results (SEER), National Cancer Institute. Based on data from population-based registries in Connecticut, New Mexico, Utah, Iowa, Hawaii, Atlanta, Detroit, Seattle-Puget Sound, and San Francisco–Oakland.

ETIOLOGIC FACTORS FOR SQUAMOUS CELL CARCINOMA

Alcohol Consumption

Although attempts to produce cancer in well-nourished laboratory animals by prolonged ingestion of ethanol have failed,[14] there are clear-cut epidemiologic data indicating that alcoholic beverages are a major cause of SCE in Western populations.[15,16] The evidence is based on a number of cohort studies among alcoholics and heavy consumers of alcohol as well as case-control studies around the world.[15,17] For example, the incidence of esophageal cancer was significantly elevated among a cohort of alcoholic men and women attending an outpatient clinic in Denmark[18] and among a population-based cohort of Swedish men and women with a discharge diagnosis of alcoholism.[19] Furthermore, strong dose-response relationships for ethanol consumption have been demonstrated in many case-control studies in the United States, Europe, South America, Asia, and South Africa, after adjustment for smoking.[20–36] The percentage of SCE attributable to intake of more than one drink of alcohol a day in the United States has recently been estimated at 77 percent for white men and 82 percent for African American men.[37]

In some developing countries with exceptionally high rates of SCE, including rural parts of Africa, Iran, and China, alcohol drinking has not been shown to be a risk factor.[38–45] However, a strong dose-response relationship has been reported among Hong Kong Chinese,[31] in Shanghai, China (an urban area with high rates of esophageal cancer), and in Heilongjiang Province, a low-risk area in northern China.[30,46] Alcohol also recently emerged as a risk factor in southern India although only 36 percent of the cases and 14 percent of the controls reported drinking alcoholic beverages.[47]

Only a few studies of alcohol-related esophageal cancer have investigated covariables such as risk in nonsmokers and duration of use. In Italy, Hong Kong, and South America, the dose-response gradients for alcohol consumption remained strong when analyses were restricted to lifelong nonsmokers.[28,48–50] Other measures of exposure, such as duration and the age at which an individual started drinking alcohol, have not shown significant risk gradients in case-control studies in France, Hong Kong, Paraguay, and Argentina.[29,32,35,51] Years elapsed since cessation of drinking alcohol did not affect the risk of esophageal cancer in France or Argentina[35,51] but did in Hong Kong and Paraguay, after investigators excluded an elevated risk among those who had recently quit drinking (probably due to early symptoms of cancer).[29,32]

Risk variability by type of alcoholic beverage may reflect culturally or economically determined drinking habits. Generally, the beverage most strongly associated with the risk of esophageal cancer has been the one most frequently consumed by the study population.[25,26,52] In most studies, the risk was greatest among users of "hard" liquor[20,21,23,24] although one study suggested a reduced risk in three regions of France.[26] Beer consumption was a key determinant of risk in several studies[26,53,54] whereas wine consumption was most strongly implicated in a region of Italy where wine is the major contributor to ethanol intake.[52] A study of esophageal cancer in a high-risk area of coastal South Carolina revealed an elevated risk associated with use of moonshine (home-brewed whiskey), particularly among African Americans,[20] further suggesting that regional variation in the type of alcoholic beverage consumed may contribute to the excess risk in some areas. Consumption of apple brandy in France, home-brewed rum in

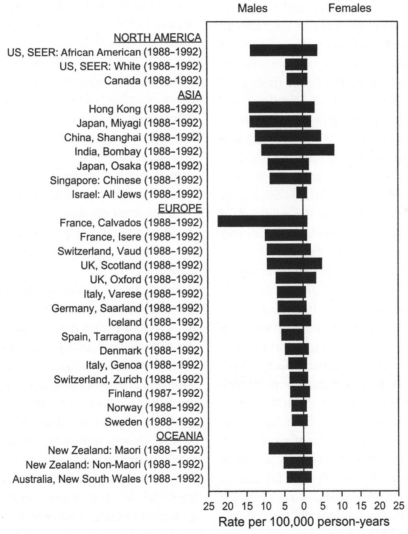

Figure 1–6. International variation in esophageal cancer incidence rates (per 100,000 person-years, age-standardized to the world population) by continent, registry, and sex, circa 1988 to 1992. (SEER = Surveillance, Epidemiology, and End Results.) (Adapted from Parkin DM, Whelan SL, Ferlay J, et al. Cancer incidence in five continents. Vol. VII. Lyon: International Agency for Research on Cancer; 2000.)

Puerto Rico, and aguardiente (a local spirit) in Paraguay has been associated with an excess risk of esophageal cancer in these countries, where these beverages are commonly used.[32,55,56] In Japan, shochu (the beverage with the highest alcohol content) was associated with the greatest risk of esophageal cancer.[27] Consumption of hot alcoholic beverages, especially hot calvados, was associated with elevated risks of esophageal cancer in France whereas the intake of cold calvados was not, suggesting a role for thermal injury to the esophagus.[26] It was suggested that the formerly widespread habit of drinking hot calvados contributed to the geographic variation of esophageal cancer and to the recent downward trend in incidence in western France.[26,57]

Although alcohol is strongly related to risk of esophageal cancer, the components or mechanisms responsible for its carcinogenicity have not been identified. Some studies have reported an excess risk for men who drink undiluted liquor (instead of liquor diluted with water, ice, or a mixer)[16,21,58] and have reported drinking dark liquor poses no more risk than drinking light liquor.[16] While certain kinds of alcoholic beverages, including beer and whiskey, may contain compounds that are carcinogenic, such findings suggest that the risk of SCE is associated with alcohol per se rather than to the presence of contaminants, flavoring compounds, or additives that may vary among types of beverages.[15] Alcohol itself may enhance cancer development by acting as a chronic irritant or by promoting dietary deficiencies.[26,59,60] It may also enhance an individual's susceptibility to tobacco or other carcinogens through a variety of mechanisms (eg, by interfering with deoxyribonucleic acid [DNA] repair mechanisms, altering the immune system or metabolic pathways, increasing absorption, or enhancing the activation of procarcinogens).[59,60] A recent study from Japan suggests that acetaldehyde, a metabolite of alcohol and a recognized animal carcinogen, may play a critical role in the mechanism by which alcohol causes esophageal cancer.[61] In this study, a significantly higher frequency of the mutant acetaldehyde dehydrogenase 2 (ALDH2*2) allele that blocks the metabolism of acetaldehyde to acetate was found in cancer patients than in controls with similar levels of alcohol consumption.[61]

Tobacco Consumption

Tobacco use, regardless of form, is a major risk factor for esophageal cancer in most parts of the world.[16,20,23,28,31,33,38,40,51,62–64] In the United States, the percentage of SCE attributable to the smoking of any form of tobacco (in cigarettes, cigars, or pipes) for 6 months or longer has recently been estimated at 65 percent for white men and 57 percent for African American men.[37] A case-control study in a high-risk area of Shanxi Province, China, did not find a significant association with tobacco use, but the amount of tobacco used (< one cigarette per day, on average) was too small to show consistent results.[44] However, in urban Shanghai, where 70 percent of the male patients smoked 20 or more cigarettes per day, there was a strong and significant association with cigarette smoking.[46] Significant positive trends in risk were associated with the intensity, duration, and number of packs per year times number of years smoked.[46] A significant association between esophageal cancer and the intensity of cigarette smoking was also noted in an area in northeast China with a relatively low incidence[30] but not in southern India, where only 4 percent of the case patients and 8 percent of the controls reported smoking only cigarettes.[47]

In some studies, pipe smokers have shown a higher risk of esophageal cancer than smokers of commercial cigarettes,[20,23,24,36,62] perhaps because pipe tobacco condensates are swallowed, allowing tobacco carcinogens direct contact with the esophagus.[62] A number of known or suspected carcinogens such as nitrosamines, 2-naphthylamine, benzo[a]pyrene, and benzene have been identified in tobacco smoke condensate,[65] but the specific agents responsible for esophageal cancer and mechanisms of action are unclear.[66]

Several case-control studies have reported strong positive dose-response effects with both duration and intensity of cigarette smoking[20,25,32,34] although duration of use seemed more important in some studies.[28,34,51] In most studies evaluating the effect of quitting smoking, a 50 percent reduction in risk has been seen for ex-smokers compared to current smokers,[20,23,28,33,34,51] along with an inverse effect with time elapsed since cessation of smoking.[20,25,32,34] The risk for those who quit smoking for 10 or more years was similar to the risk for nonsmokers in South Carolina[20] whereas the risk for ex-smokers in Paraguay and California remained elevated even among smokers who had quit for 20 or more years. Smoking was also significantly related to esophageal cancer risk among nondrinkers in Italy, France, and Hong Kong,[49,50,64] supporting an independent effect of tobacco smoke on the esophageal epithelium.[64]

In several studies from South America, the risks of esophageal cancer from the use of black (air-cured) tobacco were two or more times higher than those for blond (flue-cured) tobacco.[25,35,67] Laboratory studies have indicated that the smoke of black tobacco contains higher levels of aromatic amines and tobacco-specific nitrosamines than the smoke of blond tobacco.[67] In addition, the urine of smokers of black tobacco shows twice the mutagenic activity of the urine of smokers of blond tobacco.[68] In several studies, risks were higher with hand-rolled cigarettes than with commercial cigarettes.[25,30,36,62,67] Although the carcinogenic ingredients are not clearly known, hand-rolled cigarettes have a high tar content and usually contain black tobacco.[67]

A case-control study in Bombay, India, identified the smoking of bidi (native cigarettes of coarse tobacco in a dry termburni leaf), the chewing of pan (a mixture of betel leaf, sliced areca nut, and aqueous shell lime), and the chewing of pan-tobacco (pan plus natively cured dry tobacco) as major risk factors for esophageal cancer.[69] A study in southern India found elevated risks for bidi and for bidi plus cigarettes but not for pan plus chewing tobacco, possibly due to the local habit of spitting out the quid and its extracts with the saliva rather than swallowing it.[47]

Alcohol-Tobacco Interaction

In western Europe and North America, 80 to 90 percent of the risk of SCE has been attributed to alcohol and tobacco use.[70] Alcohol and tobacco appear to act independently, with the importance of each factor depending on the baseline characteristics of the population under study.[71] In a population with a high percentage of heavy drinkers, the major factor appears to be alcohol[72] whereas tobacco seems more important in a population with many heavy smokers.[24,71] In most studies, heavy consumers of both alcohol and tobacco have the highest risk of esophageal cancer, often consistent with multiplicative interaction.[25,28,30,33–35,46,46,73]

Socioeconomic Status

The highest rates of SCE are generally found in areas of the world where the population is impoverished.[74] Within various populations, the risk of esophageal cancer is greatest among those with the lowest socioeconomic status (SES).[30,38,45,75–81] The measures of SES that are assessed most often in case-control studies are income, education, and occupation.

Income was the social-class variable most strongly associated with SCE in a case-control study conducted among African American and white men in three areas of the United States.[37] Significantly elevated risks of 4.3 for whites and 8.0 for African Americans were observed for the lowest versus the highest level of annual income, after adjusting for potential confounding factors such as smoking and drinking.[37] An association with low income has been noted in other studies in the United States and China,[39,76,82,83] risks are especially high for subjects whose incomes are at or below the poverty level.[37,79] Elevated risks of esophageal cancer have also been associated with low levels of education[21,26,45,75,77,81,84–86] and low-status occupations.[38,77,81] In addition, increased risks have been reported for single men in comparison to married men,[26,36,77,78,81,83,87] a finding that was stronger in the United States for African American than for white men.[37]

Low SES is obviously a surrogate for a set of lifestyle and other environmental factors, such as poor housing, unemployment, workplace hazards, limited access to medical care, stress, poor nutrition, and exposure to infectious agents.[82] Some of these factors, such as nutritional status, may affect an individual's susceptibility to environmental carcinogens.[88,89] For example, the number of esophageal cancers among male residents of hostels for single homeless people in Glasgow, Scotland, was considerably higher than expected. The finding is probably related not solely to alcohol abuse or smoking but also to the complex social problems of poverty, nutritional deficiencies, poor living conditions, and homelessness.[90]

Diet and Nutrition

Food Groups and Nutrients

A number of studies have indicated that dietary insufficiencies contribute to the varying incidence of SCE around the world.[91–94] Populations at high risk for this tumor are generally malnourished, and risk tends to increase as body mass index (BMI) decreases.[20,72,95–97] Until recently, esophageal cancer was unusually common in women from the rural northern areas of Sweden, many of whom had Plummer-Vinson syndrome, which is associated with vitamin and iron deficiencies.[98] Esophageal cancer has also been reported as a sequel of celiac disease, a malabsorption syndrome characterized by malnutrition.[99,100]

A protective effect of fruits and vegetables, especially those eaten raw, is supported by a large quantity of data, including data from case-control studies of esophageal cancer in Europe,[63,101–103] Asia,[30,31,33,39,49,84] North America,[20,22,23,53,72,97] and South America.[25,104] Fruits and vegetables contain a variety of micronutrients and other dietary components (eg, carotenoids; vitamins A, C, and E; selenium; fiber; indoles; and isothiocyanates) with potential anticarcinogenic effects.[105–107] A number of case-control studies have suggested a protective effect of vitamin C from supplements and food sources[20,30,72,84,97,108–110] and especially from fruits and citrus fruits. Vitamin C blocks the endogenous formation of N-nitroso compounds, which are suspected in the etiology of esophageal cancer in some high-risk areas of the world.[111–114]

Case-control studies have attempted to evaluate other food groups and nutrients, but the evidence is less convincing.[92] Although early studies examined the risk associated with total vitamin A intake, recent case-control studies suggested that an elevated risk is associated with high consumption of retinol-containing foods such as liver[20,101,102] whereas carotene appears to be either protective or unrelated to risk.[20,53,63,101,102,115]

Elevated risks associated with other animal sources of food (especially barbecued or fried meats) have been noted in some case-control studies of esophageal cancer.[20,23,25,32,35,53,72,101,103,116] Heterocyclic amines are potent mutagens and carcinogens formed during the cooking of meat, and their levels increase with rising temperature and duration of cooking (particularly with red meats), with the highest mutagenic activity being produced by pan frying, broiling, and barbecuing.[117] In addition, the higher risks associated with red meat (especially cured or processed meat) as well as with moldy breads and cereals, pickled vegetables, and salted fish suggest an effect of N-nitroso compounds or their precursors (nitrates and amines).[31,39,44,49,85,111–113,116,118] Furthermore, the endogenous formation of N-nitroso compounds may contribute to the development of esophageal tumors, particularly when accompanied by low intake of vitamins C and E, which interfere with the nitrosation process.[114]

A protective effect of the frequent consumption of fresh fish has been reported in two European case-control studies.[103,119] Fish and fish oils contain polyunsaturated omega-3 essential fatty acids that may reduce cancer risk by suppressing cell growth and proliferation or by enhancing apoptosis.[120]

It has been difficult to disentangle the influence of dietary and nutritional factors from the potent effects of alcohol and tobacco on the risk of esophageal cancer. In particular, heavy consumption of alcoholic beverages can interfere with the consumption and use of a variety of nutrients, including the B vitamins, zinc, protein, and vitamins A, C, and D.[59,60] Also, because poor nutrition is a risk factor for esophageal cancer, it is conceivable that alcohol increases risk partly by reducing nutrient intake. Beer, wine, and hard liquor provide a share of the daily caloric needs and consequently reduce appetite, but they provide almost none of the daily requirements for micronutrients and protein. Not only do smokers appear to have a lower intake of several nutrients (including vitamin C) than do nonsmokers,[121,122] but the amount of vitamin C needed to achieve steady-state plasma concentrations is approximately 40 percent greater in smokers than in nonsmokers.[123] In addition, tobacco products and some alcoholic beverages are sources of N-nitroso compounds that may elevate the risk of esophageal cancer.[111]

Hot Food and Beverages

It has been hypothesized that the consumption of herbal teas that are high in tannin, safrole, or other agents might be responsible for the elevated rates of esophageal cancer in residents of coastal South Carolina.[124] While a study in South Carolina found that several herbal teas were commonly used, intake was generally not more frequent in case subjects than in controls,[20] so that consumption of herbal teas or local plant products is unlikely to explain the high rates in this area. Several studies have suggested that drinking tea at normal temperatures does not increase risk.[20,125–127] In fact, consumption of green tea at normal temperatures was associated with a reduced risk of esophageal cancer in a large case-control study in Shanghai and in a high-risk area in Jiangsu Province, China.[39,126]

However, drinking tea at exceptionally high temperatures (including green tea, as found in a Japanese study[33]) has long been suggested as a risk factor in several populations.[92,128] The findings are consistent with the excess risks associated with the consumption of burning hot soup, gruel, porridge, or other beverages in various populations.[27,30,31,42,44,84,104] In high-risk areas of South America, chronic thermal injury from maté, a local tea prepared as an infusion of the herb *Ilex paraguayenis* and usually drunk very hot, has been linked to esophageal cancer.[25,32,35,104] Because most people either drink hot maté or drink both hot and cold maté,[32] it has been difficult to determine whether the effects are due to specific components of maté, to the elevated temperature, or to both factors.[32,92] However, a study in Paraguay revealed a significant twofold risk for the consumption of very hot maté compared to hot or warm maté,[32] and a study in Argentina found an elevated risk for the consumption of hot or very hot maté compared to warm maté.[35] Based on the South American data, a working group of the International Agency for Research on Cancer concluded in 1991 that "hot maté drinking is probably carcinogenic to humans."[129]

Occupation and Industry

Esophageal cancer is not usually viewed as an occupational disease although elevated risks have been reported for several exposures. Most findings have come from occupational cohort studies although some findings have emerged from case-control studies. Because most studies were unable to adjust for the confounding effects of smoking and drinking, the results of occupational analyses are often equivocal. Presented below are some of the more consistent findings.

Occupational Risks Due to Lifestyle Factors

Farmers are usually considered to have a healthier lifestyle than the general population.[130] The lower risks of esophageal cancer reported among farmers in Sweden and Denmark seemed related to their lower intake of alcohol[130–133] although the elevated risks among Italian farmers may have resulted from a higher consumption of alcohol compared to that of the general population.[132] Excess risks reported among Swedish brewery workers[133,134] and among Norwegian and Swedish waiters[133,135] appeared to be due to a higher intake of alcohol in these groups.

Perchloroethylene

The most consistent occupational association with esophageal cancer has been the excess risk among dry cleaners and other occupational groups (eg, metal polishers and platers) exposed to perchloroethylene (PCE),[136–139] a substance used by the dry cleaning industry as a cleaner and by other industries as a degreaser and solvent.[138] Cohort studies among dry cleaning union members by the National Cancer Institute and the National Institute for Occupational Safety and Health have revealed twofold excesses in esophageal cancer mortality. In addition, a modest excess of esophageal cancer, which could not be explained by the use of alcohol or cigarettes, was observed among dry cleaning workers in a case-control study in Washington state.[137] An excess of esophageal cancer mortality has also been noted among metal polishers and platers.[139]

Combustion Products and Fossil Fuels

Esophageal cancer may be caused by exposure to fumes from incomplete combustion of organic material; increased risks have been observed for chimney sweeps, printers, gas station attendants, vulcanization workers, asphalt workers, and metal workers exposed to metalworking fluids.[140] An excess risk was observed in a Swedish cohort of chimney sweeps exposed to a mixture of polycyclic aromatic hydrocarbons (PAHs), nitrogen compounds, arsenic, asbestos, and sulfur dioxide.[141] Although a proportionate mortality study among workers at the US Government Printing Office observed no excess risk of esophageal cancer,[142] elevated risks have been reported in the printing industry in Russia and France, notably among bookbinders potentially exposed to benzene and among pressmen exposed to PAHs.[143,144] An excess risk of esophageal cancer was also reported among automobile manufacturing workers exposed to metalworking fluid.[145] In a cohort of filling station managers, the number of esophageal cancers was greater than expected for managers of small stations, possibly due to greater exposure to gasoline vapors and exhausts.[146] Elevated risks also have been observed in the rubber industry,[147,148] particularly among vulcanization workers[133,149] who are potentially exposed to PAHs, styrene, toluene, ethylbenzene, acrylonitrile, and vinyl chloride.[150,151] In addition, a significantly high risk of esophageal cancers was observed in a cohort of mastic asphalt workers heavily exposed to bitumen fumes.[152]

Silica and Metal Dust

Ingested silica and metal dust particles cleared from the lungs may damage the esophageal mucosa and promote cell proliferation.[23,153] Occupational exposure to silica dust at a large iron-steel complex in China was associated with a significant 2.8-fold risk and a strong positive gradient in risk with increasing duration of exposure.[153] This finding confirms the results of an earlier study that reported an elevated proportionate mortality ratio among workers at the iron-steel complex who made fire-resistant silica bricks.[154] An association with silica exposure was also noted in a recent study based on death-certificate data on occupation and industry from 24 US states.[155] In addition, a population-based case-control study of esophageal cancer in the United States found a significant association with occupational exposure to metal dust, especially from beryllium.[23] However, a nested case-control study among US automobile-manufacturing workers exposed to metal dust from iron and steel operations reported no excess risks.[145]

Asbestos

Increased risks of esophageal cancer have been reported among asbestos insulation workers in the United States and Canada.[156] However, no excess risk was reported among workers who had potential exposure to asbestos at Texas refineries and at a petrochemical plant.[157,158] Because of the inconsistent results, the relationship between asbestos exposure and esophageal cancer remains unclear.

Meat Packing and Slaughtering: Viral Exposure

Butchers and other workers employed in meat packing and meat slaughtering have shown elevated risks of esophageal cancer, suggesting a possible effect of exposure to bovine and human papillomaviruses.[133]

Other Risk Factors

A number of studies have linked ionizing radiation to esophageal cancer, particularly among patients irradiated for ankylosing spondylitis and for breast cancer.[159,160] In addition, significant excesses of risk have been reported among atomic-bomb survivors in Japan.[161]

Constituents of drinking water have been suspected in some studies of esophageal cancer. In Shanghai, China, excess risks have been related to the drinking of river water found to be mutagenic by the Ames test.[85] Similarly, water contaminated with petroleum and its by-products has been suspected in a high-risk area of Saudi Arabia.[162] On the other hand, high nitrate levels in drinking water were not related to esophageal cancer risk in northern England.[163]

Elevated risks of esophageal cancer have been reported with certain medical conditions (such as pernicious anemia,[164] achalasia,[165,166] some autoimmune diseases,[167] and chemical injuries to the esophagus)[168] and following gastrectomy.[169] In addition, aspirin use appeared to reduce the risk of esophageal cancer in cohort and case-control studies.[170,171] The ingestion of opium, either by smoking or eating, was linked to esophageal cancer in high-risk areas of Iran.[172]

The role of human papillomavirus (HPV) infection in the etiology of SCE is not entirely clear. Human papillomaviruses, especially types 16 and 18,[173] appear to play an etiologic role in some geographic areas, particularly regions with an exceptionally high incidence of esophageal cancer, such as China and South Africa,[3,174] but study results have not been consistent.[175,176]

Several studies in high-risk areas of Iran and China have indicated a familial tendency for esophageal cancer although it is difficult to distinguish genetic from environmental factors.[44,177,178] In clinical studies, a high risk of SCE has been reported in association with tylosis, a dominantly inherited disorder characterized by palmar and plantar keratoses.[173,179,180]

There is evidence that genetic polymorphisms (eg, ADH3, ADH2, CYP2E1) may increase susceptibility to SCE through interactions with alcohol, tobacco, and certain dietary components,[181,182] but more work is needed to confirm this. Several somatic mutations have been reported, including mutation of p53, a tumor-suppressor gene that promotes DNA repair, stimulates apoptosis, and inhibits cell proliferation.[183,184]

A striking excess risk of SCE has been demonstrated following the development of other tumors of the upper aerodigestive tract, including the oral cavity, pharynx, and larynx.[185,186] This constellation of multiple primary cancers is not surprising since alcohol and tobacco are the major risk factors for these tumors and since genetic mechanisms may also be shared.

Impact of Risk Factors in the United States

In a recent case-control study of SCE patients in three areas of the United States, moderate and heavy levels of alcohol intake, the use of tobacco, the infrequent consumption of raw fruits and vegetables, and low income were found to account for over 98 percent of the SCE among both African American and white men and for 99 percent of the excess incidence among African Americans compared to whites.[37] The higher incidence rates observed among African Americans after exposure to the same risk factors as whites may reflect a susceptibility state conditioned by genetic traits or by nutritional, viral, or other factors associated with low social class. Whatever the mechanism, it is clear that lifestyle modifications that include a reduction in the consumption of alcoholic beverages (especially among heavy drinkers) and in the use of tobacco, as well as improvements in diet and living conditions, would markedly lower the incidence of SCE in all racial and ethnic groups. Thus, it is likely that declines in the prevalence of smoking since the 1960s, especially among men, may have contributed to the downward trends reported for this cancer. However, recent increases in cigar smoking could negatively impact these trends.[187]

ETIOLOGIC FACTORS FOR ESOPHAGEAL ADENOCARCINOMAS

Tobacco Consumption

In the United States, cigarette smoking is a significant risk factor for ACE, with a doubling of risk for smokers of more than one pack a day.[96,188–190] Risks have been significantly elevated also for heavy smokers in China, Greece, and France[46,170,191] although smoking is a less potent cause of ACE than SCE. Unlike findings for SCE, being an ex-smoker does not appear to attenuate risks; instead, the risks remain elevated for more than 30 years after smoking cessation.[96,188,189,191] This finding suggests that smoking may affect an early stage of esophageal carcinogenesis and may thus still contribute to the rising incidence of ACE in the face of recent downward trends in smoking prevalence in the United States.[188]

Gastroesophageal Reflux Disease

A major risk factor is gastroesophageal reflux disease (GERD), which predisposes to the metaplastic columnar epithelium characteristic of Barrett's esophagus, a precursor lesion for ACE.[192,193] Significant twofold or greater risks of ACE have been associated with the presence of GERD symptoms.[189,194–196] It has been hypothesized that the use of drugs such as anticholinergic agents that relax the lower esophageal sphincter may promote GERD and thus contribute to the risk of ACE.[197] However, in two US case-control studies, the use of anticholinergic drugs was not associated with risk of ACE.[194,198] Questions have also emerged about histamine H_2 receptor antagonists for treatment of GERD, but no clear relationship to ACE risk has been demonstrated. In evaluating the possible role of *Helicobacter pylori* infection, a case-control study in the United States found that infection with cagA+ strains was actually associated with a reduced risk of ACE.[199] Further investigations are needed to determine whether the decreasing prevalence of *H. pylori* infection in the population may contribute in some way to the upward trend of ACE.

Alcohol Consumption

While several case-control studies have suggested an association between alcohol intake and the risk of ACE, the risks are much lower than those seen with SCE.[96,189,190] In fact, no association with any measure of alcohol intake or type of beverage was noted in a large population-based case-control study in the United States.[188]

Socioeconomic Status

Low income has been related to excess risk of ACE in two US studies[188,189] although the effect is less pronounced than for SCE. This differential is consistent with studies reporting a higher percentage of ACE cases in people working in professional and skilled occupations, as compared with the percentage of SCE cases in such workers.[96,200,201]

Diet and Nutrition

In contrast to SCE, for which high-risk populations are generally poorly nourished, risks for ACE tend to increase as BMI increases:[95,96,190,194,202–204] subjects in the upper quartile of BMI have three to seven times the risk of subjects in the lowest quartile.[202–204] The mechanism by which obesity affects the risk of ACE is unclear although it may be linked to the predisposition of obese individuals to GERD.[190,202] Whatever the process, it seems likely that obesity contributes to the upward trend in ACE, in view of the sharply increasing prevalence of individuals classified as overweight in the United States.[205]

Various foods, food groups, and nutrients have been related to the risk of ACE, but the most consistent finding is a protective effect of fruits, vegetables, and fiber.[96,202,206] Fruits and vegetables contain various substances with potential anticarcinogenic effects,[106,109] and dietary fiber may have a mechanical cleansing or clearance action that removes or dilutes carcinogens from epithelial surfaces of the upper digestive tract.[207]

Genetic Susceptibility

Some case reports have suggested a familial tendency to Barrett's esophagus and ACE, [208,209] but further studies are needed to clarify the possible role of susceptibility genes.

Impact of Risk Factors in the United States

The incidence of ACE in the United States has been rising over the past couple of decades, especially among white men. Data emerging from recent studies suggest that the relationship with obesity and (possibly) smoking may account for part of the upward trend. Both smoking and obesity increase the incidence of GERD and its progression to Barrett's esophagus, the main precursor of ACE. The protective effects of fruits and vegetables and the modest effects of low SES are interesting but do not appear to explain the upward trends. In a case-control study in Seattle, only about half of the cases could be explained by known or suspected risk factors,[190] indicating the need for further epidemiologic and interdisciplinary research into the origins of this increasingly common cancer.

REFERENCES

1. American Cancer Society. Cancer facts and figures—2000. Atlanta (GA): American Cancer Society; 2000.
2. Ries L, Kosary C, Hankey B, et al., editors. SEER cancer statistics review, 1973–1996. Bethesda (MD): National Cancer Institute; 1999.
3. Cooper K, Taylor L, Govind S. Human papillomavirus DNA in oesophageal carcinomas in South Africa. J Pathol 1995;175:273–7.
4. Parkin DM, Whelan SL, Ferlay J, et al., editors. Cancer incidence in five continents. Vol. VII. Lyon: International Agency for Research on Cancer; 2000.
5. McKinney A, Sharp L, Macfarlane GJ, Muir CS.

Oesophageal and gastric cancer in Scotland 1960–90. Br J Cancer 1995;71:411–5.

6. Hansen S, Wiig JN, Giercksky KE, Tretli S. Esophageal and gastric carcinoma in Norway 1958–1992: incidence time trend variability according to morphological subtypes and organ subsites. Int J Cancer 1997;71:340–4.

7. Armstrong RW, Borman B. Trends in incidence rates of adenocarcinoma of the oesophagus and gastric cardia in New Zealand, 1978–1992. Int J Epidemiol 1996;25:941–7.

8. Thomas RJ, Lade S, Giles GG, Thursfield V. Incidence trends in oesophageal and proximal gastric carcinoma in Victoria. Aust N Z J Surg 1996;66:271–5.

9. Harrison SL, Goldacre MJ, Seagroatt V. Trends in registered incidence of oesophageal and stomach cancer in the Oxford region, 1974–88. Eur J Cancer Prev 1992;1:271–4.

10. Tuyns AJ. Oesophageal cancer in France and Switzerland: recent time trends. Eur J Cancer Prev 1992;1:275–8.

11. Moller H. Incidence of cancer of oesophagus, cardia and stomach in Denmark. Eur J Cancer Prev 1992;1:159–64.

12. Levi F, Randimbsion L, La Vecchia C. Esophageal and gastric carcinoma in Vaud, Switzerland, 1976–1994 [letter]. Int J Cancer 1998;75:160–1.

13. Hansson LE, Sparen P, Nyren O. Increasing incidence of both major histological types of esophageal carcinomas among men in Sweden. Int J Cancer 1993;54:402–7.

14. Schottenfeld D. Alcohol as a co-factor in the etiology of cancer. Cancer 1979;43:1962–6.

15. International Agency for Research on Cancer. Alcohol drinking. Vol. 44. Lyon, France: International Agency for Research on Cancer; 1988.

16. Brown LM, Hoover R, Gridley G, et al. Drinking practices and risk of squamous-cell esophageal cancer among black and white men in the United States. Cancer Causes Control 1997;8:605–9.

17. Thomas DB. Alcohol as a cause of cancer. Environ Health Perspect 1995;103 Suppl 8:153–60.

18. Tonnesen H, Moller H, Andersen JR, et al. Cancer morbidity in alcohol abusers. Br J Cancer 1994;69:327–32.

19. Adami HO, McLaughlin JK, Hsing AW, et al. Alcoholism and cancer risk: a population-based cohort study. Cancer Causes Control 1992;3:419–25.

20. Brown LM, Blot WJ, Schuman SH, et al. Environmental factors and high risk of esophageal cancer among men in coastal South Carolina. J Natl Cancer Inst 1988;80:1620–5.

21. Pottern LM, Morris LE, Blot WJ, et al. Esophageal cancer among black men in Washington, D.C. I. Alcohol, tobacco, and other risk factors. J Natl Cancer Inst 1981; 67:777–83.

22. Mettlin C, Graham S, Priore R, et al. Diet and cancer of the esophagus. Nutr Cancer 1981;2:143–7.

23. Yu MC, Garabrant DH, Peters JM, Mack TM. Tobacco, alcohol, diet, occupation, and carcinoma of the esophagus. Cancer Res 1988;48:3843–8.

24. Wynder EL, Bross IJ. A study of etiological factors in cancer of the esophagus. Cancer 1961;14:389–413.

25. De Stefani E, Munoz N, Esteve J, et al. Mate drinking, alcohol, tobacco, diet, and esophageal cancer in Uruguay. Cancer Res 1990;50:426–31.

26. Launoy G, Milan C, Day NE, et al. Oesophageal cancer in France: potential importance of hot alcoholic drinks. Int J Cancer 1997;71:917–23.

27. Hanaoka T, Tsugane S, Ando N, et al. Alcohol consumption and risk of esophageal cancer in Japan: a case-control study in seven hospitals. Jpn J Clin Oncol 1994;24:241–6.

28. Castellsague X, Munoz N, De Stefani E, et al. Independent and joint effects of tobacco smoking and alcohol drinking on the risk of esophageal cancer in men and women. Int J Cancer 1999;82:657–64.

29. Cheng KK, Duffy SW, Day NE, et al. Stopping drinking and risk of oesophageal cancer. BMJ 1995;310:1094–7.

30. Hu J, Nyren O, Wolk A, et al. Risk factors for oesophageal cancer in northeast China. Int J Cancer 1994;57:38–46.

31. Cheng KK, Day NE, Duffy SW, et al. Pickled vegetables in the aetiology of oesophageal cancer in Hong Kong Chinese. Lancet 1992;339:1314–8.

32. Rolon PA, Castellsague X, Benz M, Munoz N. Hot and cold mate drinking and esophageal cancer in Paraguay. Cancer Epidemiol Biomarkers Prev 1995;4:595–605.

33. Kinjo Y, Cui Y, Akiba S, et al. Mortality risks of oesophageal cancer associated with hot tea, alcohol, tobacco and diet in Japan. J Epidemiol 1998;8:235–43.

34. Brown LM, Hoover RN, Greenberg RS, et al. Are racial differences in squamous cell esophageal cancer explained by alcohol and tobacco use? J Natl Cancer Inst 1994;86: 1340–5.

35. Castelletto R, Castellsague X, Munoz N, et al. Alcohol, tobacco, diet, mate drinking, and esophageal cancer in Argentina. Cancer Epidemiol Biomarkers Prev 1994;3: 557–64.

36. Segal I, Reinach SG, de Beer M. Factors associated with oesophageal cancer in Soweto, South Africa. Br J Cancer 1988;58:681–6.

37. Brown LM, Hoover R, Silverman D, et al. The excess incidence of squamous cell esophageal cancer among US black men: role of social class and other risk factors. Am J Epidemiol 2001;153:114–22.

38. Vizcaino AP, Parkin DM, Skinner ME. Risk factors associated with oesophageal cancer in Bulawayo, Zimbabwe. Br J Cancer 1995;72:769–73.

39. Gao CM, Takezaki T, Ding JH, et al. Protective effect of allium vegetables against both esophageal and stomach cancer: a simultaneous case-referent study of a high-epidemic area in Jiangsu Province, China. Jpn J Cancer Res 1999;90:614–21.

40. Sammon AM. A case-control study of diet and social factors in cancer of the esophagus in Transkei. Cancer 1992; 69:860–5.

41. Cook-Mozaffari PJ, Azordegan F, Day NE, et al. Oesophageal cancer studies in the Caspian littoral of Iran: results of a case-control study. Br J Cancer 1979;39:293–309.

42. De Jong UW, Breslow N, Hong JG, et al. Aetiological factors in oesophageal cancer in Singapore Chinese. Int J Cancer 1974;13:291–303.

43. Chen F, Cole P, Mi Z, Xing LY. Corn and wheat-flour consumption and mortality from esophageal cancer in Shanxi, China. Int J Cancer 1993;53:902–6.

44. Wang YP, Han XY, Su W, et al. Esophageal cancer in Shanxi Province, People's Republic of China: a case-control study in high and moderate risk areas. Cancer Causes Control 1992;3:107–13.

45. Yu Y, Taylor PR, Li JY, et al. Retrospective cohort study of risk-

factors for esophageal cancer in Linxian, People's Republic of China. Cancer Causes Control 1993;4:195–202.

46. Gao YT, McLaughlin JK, Blot WJ, et al. Risk factors for esophageal cancer in Shanghai, China. I. Role of cigarette smoking and alcohol drinking. Int J Cancer 1994;58:192–6.

47. Sankaranarayanan R, Duffy SW, Padmakumary G, et al. Risk factors for cancer of the oesophagus in Kerala, India. Int J Cancer 1991;49:485–9.

48. Tavani A, Negri E, Franceschi S, La Vecchia C. Risk factors for esophageal cancer in lifelong nonsmokers. Cancer Epidemiol Biomarkers Prev 1994;3:387–92.

49. Cheng KK, Duffy SW, Day NE, Lam TH. Oesophageal cancer in never-smokers and never-drinkers. Int J Cancer 1995;60:820–2.

50. La Vecchia C, Negri E. The role of alcohol in oesophageal cancer in non-smokers, and of tobacco in non-drinkers. Int J Cancer 1989;43:784–5.

51. Launoy G, Milan CH, Faivre J, et al. Alcohol, tobacco and oesophageal cancer: effects of the duration of consumption, mean intake and current and former consumption. Br J Cancer 1997;75:1389–96.

52. Barra S, Franceschi S, Negri E, et al. Type of alcoholic beverage and cancer of the oral cavity, pharynx and oesophagus in an Italian area with high wine consumption. Int J Cancer 1990;46:1017–20.

53. Graham S, Marshall J, Haughey B, et al. Nutritional epidemiology of cancer of the esophagus. Am J Epidemiol 1990;131:454–67.

54. Jensen OM. Cancer morbidity and causes of death among Danish brewery workers. Int J Cancer 1979;23:454–63.

55. Tuyns AJ, Pequignot G, Abbatucci JS. Oesophageal cancer and alcohol consumption; importance of type of beverage. Int J Cancer 1979;23:443–7.

56. Martinez I. Factors associated with cancer of the esophagus, mouth, and pharynx in Puerto Rico. J Natl Cancer Inst 1969;42:1069–94.

57. Launoy G, Faivre J, Pienkowski P, et al. Changing pattern of oesophageal cancer incidence in France. Int J Epidemiol 1994;23:246–51.

58. Boyland E. Water could reduce the hazard of cancer from spirits. Br J Ind Med 1988;46:423–4.

59. Garro AJ, Lieber CS. Alcohol and cancer. Annu Rev Pharmacol Toxicol 1990;30:219–49.

60. Blot WJ. Alcohol and cancer. Cancer Res 1992;52:2119s–23s.

61. Yokoyama A, Muramatsu T, Ohmori T, et al. Esophageal cancer and aldehyde dehydrogenase-2 genotypes in Japanese males. Cancer Epidemiol Biomarkers Prev 1996;5:99–102.

62. Tuyns AJ, Esteve J. Pipe, commercial and hand-rolled cigarette smoking in oesophageal cancer. Int J Epidemiol 1983;12:110–3.

63. Tavani A, Negri E, Franceschi S, La Vecchia C. Risk factors for esophageal cancer in women in northern Italy. Cancer 1993;72:2531–6.

64. Tavani A, Negri E, Franceschi S, La Vecchia C. Tobacco and other risk factors for oesophageal cancer in alcohol non-drinkers. Eur J Cancer Prev 1996;5:313–8.

65. National Research Council. Environmental tobacco smoke, measuring exposures and assessing health effects. Washington (DC): National Academy Press; 1986. p. 30–1.

66. International Agency for Research on Cancer. Tobacco smoking. Vol. 38. Lyon, France: International Agency for Research on Cancer; 1986.

67. De Stefani E, Barrios E, Fierro L. Black (air-cured) and blond (flue-cured) tobacco and cancer risk. III: Oesophageal cancer. Eur J Cancer 1993;29A:763–6.

68. Malaveille C, Vineis P, Esteve J, et al. Levels of mutagens in the urine of smokers of black and blond tobacco correlate with their risk of bladder cancer. Carcinogenesis 1989;10:577–86.

69. Jussawalla DJ, Deshpande VA. Evaluation of cancer risk in tobacco chewers and smokers: an epidemiologic assessment. Cancer 1971;28:244–52.

70. Schottenfeld D. Epidemiology of cancer of the esophagus. Semin Oncol 1984;11:92–100.

71. Tuyns AJ. Oesophageal cancer in non-smoking drinkers and in non-drinking smokers. Int J Cancer 1983;32:443–4.

72. Ziegler RG, Morris LE, Blot WJ, et al. Esophageal cancer among black men in Washington, D.C. II. Role of nutrition. J Natl Cancer Inst 1981;67:1199–206.

73. Kato I, Nomura AM, Stemmermann GN, Chyou PH. Prospective study of the association of alcohol with cancer of the upper aerodigestive tract and other sites. Cancer Causes Control 1992;3:145–51.

74. Day NE. Some aspects of the epidemiology of esophageal cancer. Cancer Res 1975;35:3304–7.

75. Faggiano F, Partanen T, Kogevinas M, Boffetta P. Socioeconomic differences in cancer incidence and mortality. IARC Sci Publ 1997;(138)65–176.

76. Ernster VL, Selvin S, Sacks ST, et al. Major histologic types of cancers of the gum and mouth, esophagus, larynx, and lung by sex and by income level. J Natl Cancer Inst 1982;69:773–6.

77. Pukkala E, Teppo L. Socioeconomic status and education as risk determinants of gastrointestinal cancer. Prev Med 1986;15:127–38.

78. Kato I, Tominaga S, Terao C. An epidemiological study on marital status and cancer incidence. Jpn J Cancer Res 1989;80:306–11.

79. McWhorter WP, Schatzkin AG, Horm JW, Brown CC. Contribution of socioeconomic status to black/white differences in cancer incidence. Cancer 1989;63:982–7.

80. Bouchardy C, Parkin DM, Khlat M, et al. Education and mortality from cancer in Sao Paulo, Brazil. Ann Epidemiol 1993;3:64–70.

81. Ferraroni M, Negri E, La Vecchia C, et al. Socioeconomic indicators, tobacco and alcohol in the aetiology of digestive tract neoplasms. Int J Epidemiol 1989;18:556–62.

82. Gorey KM, Vena JE. Cancer differentials among US blacks and whites: quantitative estimates of socioeconomic-related risks. J Natl Med Assoc 1994;86:209–15.

83. Swanson GM, Belle SH, Satariano WA. Marital status and cancer incidence: differences in the black and white populations. Cancer Res 1985;45:5883–9.

84. Gao YT, McLaughlin JK, Gridley G, et al. Risk factors for esophageal cancer in Shanghai, China. II. Role of diet and nutrients. Int J Cancer 1994;58:197–202.

85. Tao X, Zhu H, Matanoski GM. Mutagenic drinking water and risk of male esophageal cancer: a population-based case-control study. Am J Epidemiol 1999;150:443–52.

86. Faggiano F, Lemma P, Costa G, et al. Cancer mortality by

educational level in Italy. Cancer Causes Control 1995;6: 311–20.

87. Ernster VL, Sacks ST, Selvin S, Petrakis NL. Cancer incidence by marital status: U.S. Third National Cancer Survey. J Natl Cancer Inst 1979;63:567–85.

88. Cassel J. The contribution of the social environment to host resistance: the Fourth Wade Hampton Frost Lecture. Am J Epidemiol 1976;104:107–23.

89. Tollefson L. The use of epidemiology, scientific data, and regulatory authority to determine risk factors in cancer of some organs of the digestive system. 2. Esophageal cancer. Regul Toxicol Pharmacol 1985;5:255–75.

90. Lamont DW, Toal FM, Crawford M. Socioeconomic deprivation and health in Glasgow and the west of Scotland—a study of cancer incidence among male residents of hostels for the single homeless. J Epidemiol Community Health 1997;51:668–71.

91. Sasaki R, Aoki K, Takeda S. Contribution of dietary habits to esophageal cancer in Japan. Prog Clin Biol Res 1990; 346:83–92.

92. Cheng KK, Day NE. Nutrition and esophageal cancer. Cancer Causes Control 1996;7:33–40.

93. Esophageal cancer studies in the Caspian littoral of Iran: results of population studies—a prodrome. Joint Iran-International Agency for Research on Cancer Study Group. J Natl Cancer Inst 1977;59:1127–38.

94. Franceschi S. Role of nutrition in the aetiology of oesophageal cancer in developed countries. Endoscopy 1993;25:613–6.

95. Tretli S, Robsahm TE. Height, weight and cancer of the oesophagus and stomach: a follow-up study in Norway. Eur J Cancer Prev 1999;8:115–22.

96. Kabat GC, Ng SK, Wynder EL. Tobacco, alcohol intake, and diet in relation to adenocarcinoma of the esophagus and gastric cardia. Cancer Causes Control 1993;4:123–32.

97. Brown LM, Swanson CA, Gridley G, et al. Dietary factors and the risk of squamous cell esophageal cancer among black and white men in the United States. Cancer Causes Control 1998;9:467–74.

98. Larsson LG, Sandstrom A, Westling P. Relationship of Plummer-Vinson disease to cancer of the upper alimentary tract in Sweden. Cancer Res 1975;35:3308–16.

99. Holmes GK, Stokes PL, Sorahan TM, et al. Coeliac disease, gluten-free diet, and malignancy. Gut 1976;17:612–9.

100. Harris OD, Cooke WT, Thompson H, Waterhouse JA. Malignancy in adult coeliac disease and idiopathic steatorrhoea. Am J Med 1967;42:899–912.

101. Tuyns AJ, Riboli E, Doornbos G, Pequignot G. Diet and esophageal cancer in Calvados (France). Nutr Cancer 1987;9:81–92.

102. Decarli A, Liati P, Negri E, et al. Vitamin A and other dietary factors in the etiology of esophageal cancer. Nutr Cancer 1987;10:29–37.

103. Launoy G, Milan C, Day NE, et al. Diet and squamous-cell cancer of the oesophagus: a French multicentre case-control study. Int J Cancer 1998;76:7–12.

104. Victora CG, Munoz N, Day NE, et al. Hot beverages and oesophageal cancer in southern Brazil: a case-control study. Int J Cancer 1987;39:710–6.

105. Steinmetz KA, Potter JD. Vegetables, fruit, and cancer. I. Epidemiology. Cancer Causes Control 1991;2:325–57.

106. Steinmetz KA, Potter JD. Vegetables, fruit, and cancer prevention: a review. J Am Diet Assoc 1996;96:1027–39.

107. Combs GFJ, Clark LC, Turnbull BW. Reduction of cancer mortality and incidence by selenium supplementation. Med Klin 1997;92 Suppl 3:42–5.

108. Barone J, Taioli E, Hebert JR, Wynder EL. Vitamin supplement use and risk for oral and esophageal cancer. Nutr Cancer 1992;18:31–41.

109. Block G. Vitamin C and cancer prevention: the epidemiologic evidence. Am J Clin Nutr 1991;53:270S–82S.

110. Tuyns AJ. Protective effect of citrus fruit on esophageal cancer. Nutr Cancer 1983;5:195–200.

111. Mirvish SS. Role of N-nitroso compounds (NOC) and N-nitrosation in etiology of gastric, esophageal, nasopharyngeal and bladder cancer and contribution to cancer of known exposures to NOC [published erratum appears in Cancer Lett 1995;97(2):271]. Cancer Lett 1995;93:17–48.

112. Lu SH, Chui SX, Yang WX, et al. Relevance of N-nitrosamines to oesophageal cancer in China. IARC Sci Publ 1991;(105):11–7.

113. Siddiqi MA, Tricker AR, Kumar R, et al. Dietary sources of N-nitrosamines in a high-risk area for oesophageal cancer—Kashmir, India. IARC Sci Publ 1991;(105):210–3.

114. Lu SH, Ohshima H, Fu HM, et al. Urinary excretion of N-nitrosamino acids and nitrate by inhabitants of high- and low-risk areas for esophageal cancer in Northern China: endogenous formation of nitrosoproline and its inhibition by vitamin C. Cancer Res 1986;46:1485–91.

115. Nomura AM, Ziegler RG, Stemmermann GN, et al. Serum micronutrients and upper aerodigestive tract cancer. Cancer Epidemiol Biomarkers Prev 1997;6:407–12.

116. De Stefani E, Deneo-Pellegrini H, Boffetta P, Mendilaharsu M. Meat intake and risk of squamous cell esophageal cancer: a case-control study in Uruguay. Int J Cancer 1999;82:33–7.

117. Layton DW, Bogen KT, Knize MG, et al. Cancer risk of heterocyclic amines in cooked foods: an analysis and implications for research. Carcinogenesis 1995;16:39–52.

118. Hietanen E, Bartsch H. Gastrointestinal cancers: role of nitrosamines and free radicals. Eur J Cancer Prev 1992;1 Suppl 3:51–4.

119. Fernandez E, Chatenoud L, La Vecchia C, et al. Fish consumption and cancer risk. Am J Clin Nutr 1999;70:85–90.

120. Rose DP, Connolly JM. Omega-3 fatty acids as cancer chemopreventive agents. Pharmacol Ther 1999;83:217–44.

121. Schectman G, Byrd JC, Gruchow HW. The influence of smoking on vitamin C status in adults. Am J Public Health 1989;79:158–62.

122. Gridley G, McLaughlin JK, Blot WJ. Dietary vitamin C intake and cigarette smoking [letter]. Am J Public Health 1990;80:1526.

123. Kallner AB, Hartmann D, Hornig DH. On the requirements of ascorbic acid in man: steady-state turnover and body pool in smokers. Am J Clin Nutr 1981;34:1347–55.

124. Morton JF. Tannin and oesophageal cancer [letter]. Lancet 1987;2:327–8.

125. La Vecchia C, Negri E, Franceschi S, et al. Tea consumption and cancer risk. Nutr Cancer 1992;17:27–31.

126. Gao YT, McLaughlin JK, Blot WJ, et al. Reduced risk of esophageal cancer associated with green tea consumption. J Natl Cancer Inst 1994;86:855–8.

127. Li JY, Ershow AG, Chen ZJ, et al. A case-control study of cancer of the esophagus and gastric cardia in Linxian. Int J Cancer 1989;43:755–61.

128. Ghadirian P. Thermal irritation and esophageal cancer in northern Iran. Cancer 1987;60:1909–14.

129. International Agency for Research on Cancer. Coffee, tea, mate, methylxanthines and methylglyoxal. Vol. 51. Lyon, France: International Agency for Research on Cancer; 1991. p. 273–87.

130. Blair A, Zahm SH. Cancer among farmers. Occup Med 1991;6:335–54.

131. Wiklund K, Dich J. Cancer risks among male farmers in Sweden. Eur J Cancer Prev 1995;4:81–90.

132. Ronco G, Costa G, Lynge E. Cancer risk among Danish and Italian farmers. Br J Ind Med 1992;49:220–5.

133. Chow WH, McLaughlin JK, Malker HS, et al. Esophageal cancer and occupation in a cohort of Swedish men. Am J Ind Med 1995;27:749–57.

134. Carstensen JM, Bygren LO, Hatschek T. Cancer incidence among Swedish brewery workers. Int J Cancer 1990; 45:393–6.

135. Kjaerheim K, Andersen A. Incidence of cancer among male waiters and cooks: two Norwegian cohorts. Cancer Causes Control 1993;4:419–26.

136. Blair A, Stewart PA, Tolbert PE, et al. Cancer and other causes of death among a cohort of dry cleaners. Br J Ind Med 1990;47:162–8.

137. Vaughan TL, Stewart PA, Davis S, Thomas DB. Work in dry cleaning and the incidence of cancer of the oral cavity, larynx, and oesophagus. Occup Environ Med 1997;54: 692–5.

138. Ruder AM, Ward EM, Brown DP. Cancer mortality in female and male dry-cleaning workers. J Occup Med 1994;36: 867–74.

139. Blair A. Mortality among workers in the metal polishing and plating industry, 1951–1969. J Occup Med 1980;22: 158–62.

140. Gustavsson P, Evanoff B, Hogstedt C. Increased risk of esophageal cancer among workers exposed to combustion products. Arch Environ Health 1993;48:243–5.

141. Hogstedt C, Andersson K, Frenning B, Gustavsson A. A cohort study on mortality among long-time employed Swedish chimney sweeps. Scand J Work Environ Health 1982;8 Suppl 1:72–8.

142. Greene MH, Hoover RN, Eck RL, Fraumeni JFJ. Cancer mortality among printing plant workers. Environ Res 1979;20:66–73.

143. Bulbulyan MA, Ilychova SA, Zahm SH, et al. Cancer mortality among women in the Russian printing industry. Am J Ind Med 1999;36:166–71.

144. Luce D, Landre MF, Clavel T, et al. Cancer mortality among magazine printing workers. Occup Environ Med 1997;54:264–7.

145. Sullivan PA, Eisen EA, Woskie SR, et al. Mortality studies of metalworking fluid exposure in the automobile industry: VI. A case-control study of esophageal cancer. Am J Ind Med 1998;34:36–48.

146. Lagorio S, Forastiere F, Iavarone I, et al. Mortality of filling station attendants. Scand J Work Environ Health 1994;20: 331–8.

147. Parkes HG, Veys CA, Waterhouse JA, Peters A. Cancer mortality in the British rubber industry. Br J Ind Med 1982; 39:209–20.

148. Sorahan T, Parkes HG, Veys CA, et al. Mortality in the British rubber industry 1946–85. Br J Ind Med 1989;46:1–10.

149. Norell S, Ahlbom A, Lipping H, Osterblom L. Oesophageal cancer and vulcanisation work. Lancet 1983;1:462–3.

150. Rappaport SM, Fraser DA. Air sampling and analysis in a rubber vulcanization area. Am Ind Hyg Assoc J 1977;38: 205–10.

151. Solionova LG, Smulevich VB, Turbin EV, et al. Carcinogens in rubber production in the Soviet Union. Scand J Work Environ Health 1992;18:120–3.

152. Hansen ES. Cancer incidence in an occupational cohort exposed to bitumen fumes. Scand J Work Environ Health 1989;15:101–5.

153. Pan G, Takahashi K, Feng Y, et al. Nested case-control study of esophageal cancer in relation to occupational exposure to silica and other dusts. Am J Ind Med 1999;35:272–80.

154. Xu Z, Pan GW, Liu LM, et al. Cancer risks among iron and steel workers in Anshan, China. Part I: proportional mortality ratio analysis. Am J Ind Med 1996;30:1–6.

155. Fillmore CM, Petralia SA, Dosemeci M. Cancer mortality in women with probable exposure to silica: a death certificate study in 24 states of the U.S. Am J Ind Med 1999; 36:122–8.

156. Selikoff IJ, Hammond EC, Seidman H. Mortality experience of insulation workers in the United States and Canada, 1943–1976. Ann N Y Acad Sci 1979;330:91–116.

157. Dement JM, Hensley L, Kieding S, Lipscomb H. Proportionate mortality among union members employed at three Texas refineries. Am J Ind Med 1998;33:327–40.

158. Tsai SP, Waddell LC, Gilstrap EL, et al. Mortality among maintenance employees potentially exposed to asbestos in a refinery and petrochemical plant. Am J Ind Med 1996;29:89–98.

159. Weiss HA, Darby SC, Doll R. Cancer mortality following x-ray treatment for ankylosing spondylitis. Int J Cancer 1994;59:327–38.

160. Ahsan H, Neugut AI. Radiation therapy for breast cancer and increased risk for esophageal carcinoma. Ann Intern Med 1998;128:114–7.

161. Shimizu Y, Kato H, Schull WJ. Studies of the mortality of A-bomb survivors. 9. Mortality, 1950–1985. Part 2. Cancer mortality based on the recently revised doses (DS86). Radiat Res 1990;121:120–41.

162. Amer MH, El-Yazigi A, Hannan MA, Mohamed ME. Water contamination and esophageal cancer at Gassim Region, Saudi Arabia. Gastroenterology 1990;98:1141–7.

163. Barrett JH, Parslow RC, McKinney PA, et al. Nitrate in drinking water and the incidence of gastric, esophageal, and brain cancer in Yorkshire, England. Cancer Causes Control 1998;9:153–9.

164. Hsing AW, Hansson LE, McLaughlin JK, et al. Pernicious anemia and subsequent cancer. A population-based cohort study. Cancer 1993;71:745–50.

165. Aggestrup S, Holm JC, Sorensen HR. Does achalasia predispose to cancer of the esophagus? Chest 1992;102:1013–6.

166. Sandler RS, Nyren O, Ekbom A, et al. The risk of esophageal cancer in patients with achalasia. A population-based study. JAMA 1995;274:1359–62.

167. Dai Q, Zheng W, Ji BT, et al. Prior immunity-related medical conditions and oesophageal cancer risk: a population-based case-control study in Shanghai. Eur J Cancer Prev 1997;6:152–7.

168. Schettini ST, Ganc A, Saba L. Esophageal carcinoma secondary to a chemical injury in a child. Pediatr Surg Int 1998;13:519–20.

169. La Vecchia C, D'Avanzo B, Negri E, et al. Gastrectomy and subsequent risk of oesophageal cancer in Milan. J Epidemiol Community Health 1994;48:310–2.

170. Garidou A, Tzonou A, Lipworth L, et al. Lifestyle factors and medical conditions in relation to esophageal cancer by histologic type in a low-risk population. Int J Cancer 1996;68:295–9.

171. Farrow DC, Vaughan TL, Hansten PD, et al. Use of aspirin and other nonsteroidal anti-inflammatory drugs and risk of esophageal and gastric cancer. Cancer Epidemiol Biomarkers Prev 1998;7:97–102.

172. Ghadirian P, Stein GF, Gorodetzky C, et al. Oesophageal cancer studies in the Caspian littoral of Iran: some residual results, including opium use as a risk factor. Int J Cancer 1985;35:593–7.

173. Sur M, Cooper K. The role of the human papilloma virus in esophageal cancer. Pathology 1998;30:348–54.

174. Han C, Qiao G, Hubbert NL, et al. Serologic association between human papillomavirus type 16 infection and esophageal cancer in Shaanxi Province, China. J Natl Cancer Inst 1996;88:1467–71.

175. Lagergren J, Wang Z, Bergstrom R, et al. Human papillomavirus infection and esophageal cancer: a nationwide seroepidemiologic case-control study in Sweden. J Natl Cancer Inst 1999;91:156–62.

176. Rugge M, Bovo D, Busatto G, et al. p53 alterations but no human papillomavirus infection in preinvasive and advanced squamous esophageal cancer in Italy. Cancer Epidemiol Biomarkers Prev 1997;6:171–6.

177. Hu N, Dawsey SM, Wu M, et al. Familial aggregation of oesophageal cancer in Yangcheng County, Shanxi Province, China. Int J Epidemiol 1992;21:877–82.

178. Ghadirian P. Familial history of esophageal cancer. Cancer 1985;56:2112–6.

179. Ashworth MT, McDicken IW, Southern SA, Nash JR. Human papillomavirus in squamous cell carcinoma of the oesophagus associated with tylosis. J Clin Pathol 1993;46:573–5.

180. Howel-Evans W, McConnel RB, Clarke CA, Shepherd PM. Carcinoma of the oesphagus with keratosis palmariz et plantassis (tylosis). Quant J Med 1958;27:413–31.

181. Lin DX, Tang YM, Peng Q, et al. Susceptibility to esophageal cancer and genetic polymorphisms in glutathione S-transferases T1, P1, and M1 and cytochrome P450 2E1. Cancer Epidemiol Biomarkers Prev 1998;7:1013–8.

182. Harty LC, Caporaso NE, Hayes RB, et al. Alcohol dehydrogenase 3 genotype and risk of oral cavity and pharyngeal cancers. J Natl Cancer Inst 1997;89:1698–705.

183. Montesano R, Hainaut P. Molecular precursor lesions in oesophageal cancer. Cancer Surv 1998;32:53–68.

184. Xing EP, Yang GY, Wang LD, et al. Loss of heterozygosity of the Rb gene correlates with pRb protein expression and associates with p53 alteration in human esophageal cancer. Clin Cancer Res 1999;5:1231–40.

185. Shapshay SM, Hong WK, Fried MP, et al. Simultaneous carcinomas of the esophagus and upper aerodigestive tract. Otolaryngol Head Neck Surg 1980;88:373–7.

186. Kuwano H, Morita M, Tsutsui S, et al. Comparison of characteristics of esophageal squamous cell carcinoma associated with head and neck cancer and those with gastric cancer. J Surg Oncol 1991;46:107–9.

187. Iribarren C, Tekawa IS, Sidney S, Friedman GD. Effect of cigar smoking on the risk of cardiovascular disease, chronic obstructive pulmonary disease, and cancer in men. N Engl J Med 1999;340:1773–80.

188. Gammon MD, Schoenberg JB, Ahsan H, et al. Tobacco, alcohol, and socioeconomic status and adenocarcinomas of the esophagus and gastric cardia. J Natl Cancer Inst 1997;89:1277–84.

189. Brown LM, Silverman DT, Pottern LM, et al. Adenocarcinoma of the esophagus and esophagogastric junction in white men in the United States: alcohol, tobacco, and socioeconomic factors. Cancer Causes Control 1994;5:333–40.

190. Vaughan TL, Davis S, Kristal A, Thomas DB. Obesity, alcohol, and tobacco as risk factors for cancers of the esophagus and gastric cardia: adenocarcinoma versus squamous cell carcinoma. Cancer Epidemiol Biomarkers Prev 1995;4:85–92.

191. Lagergren J, Bergstrom R, Lindgren A, Nyren O. The role of tobacco, snuff, and alcohol use in the aetiology of cancer of the oesophagus and gastric cardia. Int J Cancer 2000;85:340–6.

192. Garewal HS, Sampliner R. Barrett's esophagus: a model premalignant lesion for adenocarcinoma. Prev Med 1989;18:749–56.

193. Spechler SJ, Goyal RK. Barrett's esophagus. N Engl J Med 1986;315:362–71.

194. Chow WH, Finkle WD, McLaughlin JK, et al. The relation of gastroesophageal reflux disease and its treatment to adenocarcinomas of the esophagus and gastric cardia. JAMA 1995;274:474–7.

195. MacDonald WC, MacDonald JB. Adenocarcinoma of the esophagus and/or gastric cardia. Cancer 1987;60:1094–8.

196. Lagergren J, Bergstrom R, Lindgren A, Nyren O. Symptomatic gastroesophageal reflux as a risk factor for esophageal adenocarcinoma. N Engl J Med 1999;340:825–31.

197. Wang HH, Hsieh CC, Antonioli DA. Rising incidence rate of esophageal adenocarcinoma and use of pharmaceutical agents that relax the lower esophageal sphincter (United States). Cancer Causes Control 1994;5:573–8.

198. Vaughan TL, Farrow DC, Hansten PD, et al. Risk of esophageal and gastric adenocarcinomas in relation to use of calcium channel blockers, asthma drugs, and other medications that promote gastroesophageal reflux. Cancer Epidemiol Biomarkers Prev 1998;7:749–56.

199. Chow WH, Blaser MJ, Blot WJ, et al. An inverse relation between cagA+ strains of *Helicobacter pylori* infection and risk of esophageal and gastric cardia adenocarcinoma. Cancer Res 1998;58:588–90.

200. Powell J, McConkey CC. The rising trend in oesophageal adenocarcinoma and gastric cardia. Eur J Cancer Prev 1992;1:265–9.

201. Ward MH, Dosemeci M, Cocco P. Mortality from gastric cardia and lower esophagus cancer and occupation. J Occup Med 1994;36:1222–7.

202. Brown LM, Swanson CA, Gridley G, et al. Adenocarcinoma of the esophagus: role of obesity and diet. J Natl Cancer Inst 1995;87:104–9.

203. Lagergren J, Bergstrom R, Nyren O. Association between body mass and adenocarcinoma of the esophagus and gastric cardia. Ann Intern Med 1999;130:883–90.

204. Chow WH, Blot WJ, Vaughan TL, et al. Body mass index and risk of adenocarcinomas of the esophagus and gastric cardia. J Natl Cancer Inst 1998;90:150–55.

205. Kuczmarski RJ, Flegal KM, Campbell SM, Johnson CL. Increasing prevalence of overweight among US adults. The National Health and Nutrition Examination Surveys, 1960 to 1991. JAMA 1994;272:205–11.

206. Tzonou A, Lipworth L, Garidou A, et al. Diet and risk of esophageal cancer by histologic type in a low-risk population. Int J Cancer 1996;68:300–4.

207. McLaughlin JK, Gridley G, Block G, et al. Dietary factors in oral and pharyngeal cancer. J Natl Cancer Inst 1988;80:1237–43.

208. Romero Y, Cameron AJ, Locke GR, et al. Familial aggregation of gastroesophageal reflux in patients with Barrett's esophagus and esophageal adenocarcinoma. Gastroenterology 1997;113:1449–56.

209. Eng C, Spechler SJ, Ruben R, Li FP. Familial Barrett esophagus and adenocarcinoma of the gastroesophageal junction [published erratum appears in Cancer Epidemiol Biomarkers Prev 1993;2(5):505]. Cancer Epidemiol Biomarkers Prev 1993;2:397–9.

2

Diagnosis and Preoperative Staging of Esophageal Cancer

ARNOLD J. MARKOWITZ, MD
HANS GERDES, MD

The clinical presentation of esophageal cancer in the United States and Europe has been changing, but unfortunately, esophageal cancer remains a dreadful disease. Patients with esophageal cancer commonly present (after a prolonged asymptomatic preclinical period) with advanced inoperable disease and a very poor prognosis. As described in Chapter 1, the majority of cases of esophageal cancer are of the squamous cell or adenocarcinoma types. Squamous cell carcinomas typically arise in the proximal to midesophagus, whereas adenocarcinomas are most commonly found in the distal esophagus.

Whereas historically, esophageal squamous cell carcinoma was the most common histologic type of esophageal cancer, more recent reports have shown that over the past few decades, there has been a marked increase in the incidence of adenocarcinomas of the distal esophagus, esophagogastric junction, and gastric cardia.[1,2] This has had an important impact on the development of new approaches to screening, diagnosis, and prevention for this disease. As the predominant cell type of esophageal cancer is changing, so is the location of the tumor, from the upper and midesophagus more distally toward the esophagogastric junction. This may also play an important role in patterns of growth and spread and in the choice of the most appropriate and accurate staging modalities.

Patients with esophageal cancer most often present with symptoms of dysphagia, weight loss, and chest pain with or without swallowing. The diagnostic assessment usually begins with an upper-gastrointestinal barium radiographic study (barium swallow) or endoscopy. Once a diagnosis of esophageal cancer has been made, the patient should then undergo a complete staging assessment to evaluate the initial stage and extent of disease. Reliable and precise pretreatment clinical staging information is crucial to providing the patient with an accurate prediction of survival and to determining appropriate management options. Determination of extent of disease at initial presentation can identify those unfortunate patients who present with advanced unresectable stage IV disease and thus spare them potential additional morbidity and the cost of unnecessary surgery.

Given the recent significant increase in the incidence of adenocarcinomas of the esophagogastric junction, precise localization of tumors detected in or around this area may be helpful in better characterizing this entity and may be useful in developing better approaches to managing these tumors. These lesions may be more accurately defined as distal esophageal tumors, "true" esophagogastric-junction tumors, or proximal gastric tumors.

Precise pretreatment staging of esophageal cancer is very important in the initial evaluation and assessment of these patients. Since prognosis and management options are highly dependent on accurate staging, optimal pretreatment assessment and stratification by stage will allow these patients to be offered the most appropriate stage-specific treatment options. In addition, precise determination of extent of disease is essential for those patients who are being considered for an investigational treatment protocol.

This chapter will discuss approaches to the diagnosis and staging of esophageal cancer as practiced in the United States and specifically at a comprehensive cancer center. The various staging modalities that have been evaluated will be discussed, and we will present what we feel represents the state-of-the-art approach to the pretreatment staging of esophageal cancer. Both diagnosis and staging will be addressed together under each modality heading. Some of the methods presented have been shown to be highly sensitive and specific but are not yet widely available and thus cannot be considered the standard of care.

STAGING

Over the past century, esophageal cancer staging has evolved with the development of the international classification system of cancer staging. This system permits the accurate description of tumors to facilitate communication between clinicians caring for patients, to guide therapy, to predict prognosis, and to help standardize subject enrollment and evaluate results in investigative research.

The Tumor-Node-Metastasis System

The American Joint Committee on Cancer (AJCC) Staging and End Result Reporting was originally organized in 1959 with the support of medical, surgical, radiologic, and pathologic societies, the American Cancer Society, and the National Cancer Institute. Through the creation of task forces appointed to consider malignant neoplasms at different locations, the AJCC published the first comprehensive manual on cancer staging in 1977. Based on published data, the manual's emphasis was on simplicity, practicality, and credibility.

These guidelines were originally created in parallel to those published by the International Union Against Cancer (Union Internationale Contre le Cancer [UICC]), which is a consortium of multiple national committees on tumor-node-metastasis (TNM) staging, including American, British, Canadian, French, German, Italian, and Japanese groups. The AJCC manual and the UICC guidelines have since been revised several times and have together

become an internationally recognized system of cancer staging. The most recent edition of the AJCC cancer staging manual was published in 1997.[3]

According to the AJCC, esophageal cancer is classified according to the extent of the primary tumor (T) and the presence and extent of lymph node metastases (N) and distant organ metastases (M) (Table 2–1).

The primary tumor (T) stage is based on the depth of tumor invasion into and through the wall of the esophagus. Histologically, the esophageal wall consists of four distinct layers including the mucosa, submucosa, muscularis propria, and adventitia. In contrast to other segments of the luminal digestive tract, the esophagus does not have a serosal layer. The earliest pathologic (p) T stage of an esophageal cancer is classified as either pTis (ie, carcinoma in situ, for a squamous cell carcinoma) or high-grade dysplasia (for an adenocarcinoma). A pTis or high-grade dysplasia lesion is limited to the

Table 2–1. TUMOR-NODE-METASTASIS STAGING SYSTEM FOR ESOPHAGEAL CANCER*
Primary tumor (T)
TX Primary tumor cannot be assessed
T0 No evidence of primary tumor
Tis Carcinoma in situ
T1 Tumor invades lamina propria or submucosa
T2 Tumor invades muscularis propria
T3 Tumor invades adventitia
T4 Tumor invades adjacent structures
Regional lymph nodes (N)
NX Regional lymph nodes cannot be assessed
N0 No regional lymph node metastasis
N1 Regional lymph node metastasis
Distant metastasis (M)
MX Distant metastasis cannot be assessed
M0 No distant metastasis
M1 Distant metastasis
Tumors of the lower thoracic esophagus
M1a Metastasis in celiac lymph nodes
M1b Other distant metastasis
Tumors of the midthoracic esophagus
M1a Not applicable
M1b Nonregional lymph nodes and/or other distant metastasis
Tumors of the upper thoracic esophagus
M1a Metastasis in cervical lymph nodes
M1b Other distant metastasis

*American Joint Committee on Cancer (AJCC) classification.
Reprinted with permission from Fleming ID, Cooper JS, Henson DE, et al. editors. AJCC cancer staging manual. 5th ed. Philadelphia: Lippincott-Raven; 1997.

epithelial layer of the mucosa and represents noninvasive disease. A pT1 tumor represents the earliest stage of invasive disease and is a tumor that penetrates into the lamina propria (as can be seen in glandular epithelium associated with adenocarcinoma) or submucosa. A pT2 tumor invades deeper into the muscularis propria layer. A pT3 tumor penetrates through all esophageal wall layers and out into the adventitia. A locally advanced pT4 tumor invades adjacent mediastinal structures, such as the tracheobronchial tree, the pericardium, or the aorta. Nodal staging for esophageal cancer is based on the presence or absence of lymph node metastases. Documentation of metastatic disease is based on spread to distant metastatic foci and (in certain cases) may be dependent on the primary tumor location within the esophagus.

The AJCC divides the esophagus into four regions to assist localization and staging. Localization affects tumor classification, lymphatic drainage, and appropriate management options. The very superior portion of the esophagus, the cervical esophagus, extends from the lower edge of the cricoid cartilage to the thoracic inlet, located approximately 18 cm from the incisor teeth. The remainder of the esophagus is divided into upper, middle, and lower thoracic portions. The upper thoracic esophagus extends from the thoracic inlet to the level of the tracheal bifurcation, approximately 24 cm from the incisors. The middle thoracic esophagus extends from the tracheal bifurcation to the level of the distal esophagus, approximately 32 cm from the incisors. The lower thoracic esophagus is the approximate 8 cm of distal esophagus and includes the intra-abdominal portion and the esophagogastric junction, approximately 40 cm from the incisors.

As preoperative staging has evolved over the past two decades, the system has been modified to represent the clinical (cTNM) and pathologic (pTNM) staging of tumors separately because histopathologic confirmation of stage may not always be available when treatment decisions are being made. According to the AJCC, the determination of the pathologic nodal staging for an esophageal tumor is generally based on the evaluation of six or more lymph nodes removed from the mediastinal lymphadenectomy specimen. Nearby lymph node

groups are classified by the AJCC as either regional or distant nodes, depending on their relationship to the location of the primary esophageal tumor (Table 2–2). Lymph node involvement beyond the regional lymph nodes constitutes distant metastases. For example, when staging a tumor of the intrathoracic esophagus, involvement of the lymph nodes of the cervical or celiac axis would be considered to be metastatic (M1) disease.

The determination of M1 disease for an esophageal tumor may be based on the documentation of metastatic spread either to distant lymph nodes or to other solid organs. The most common sites for metastatic spread of esophageal cancer include the liver, lungs, bones, and the peritoneal cavity. Clearly, early determination of metastatic disease prior to the initiation of therapy is very important for determining operability, planning appropriate treatment, and determining potential eligibility for investigational treatment protocols.

The disease stage is determined according to the actual information for each of these T, N, and M factors (Table 2–3). For example, a tumor limited to the esophageal mucosa or submucosa and without lymph node or distant metastases (T1 N0 M0) represents stage I (early) disease whereas a tumor penetrating through the esophageal wall, invading an adjacent neighboring organ, and having regional

Table 2–2. CLASSIFICATION OF REGIONAL LYMPH NODES, BASED ON ESOPHAGEAL TUMOR LOCATION*
Regional lymph nodes
Cervical esophagus
Scalene
Internal jugular
Upper cervical
Periesophageal
Supraclavicular
Cervical, NOS
Intrathoracic esophagus (upper, middle, and lower)
Tracheobronchial
Superior mediastinal
Peritracheal
Carinal
Hilar (pulmonary roots)
Periesophageal
Perigastric
Paracardial
Mediastinal, NOS

*American Joint Committee on Cancer (AJCC) classification.
Adapted from Fleming ID, Cooper JS, Henson DE, et al., editors. AJCC cancer staging manual. 5th ed. Philadelphia: Lippincott-Raven; 1997.

Table 2–3. CLASSIFICATION OF STAGE GROUPINGS FOR ESOPHAGEAL CANCER*

Stage	TNM Classifications		
0	Tis	N0	M0
I	T1	N0	M0
IIA	T2	N0	M0
	T3	N0	M0
IIB	T1	N1	M0
	T2	N1	M0
III	T3	N1	M0
	T4	Any N	M0
IV	Any T	Any N	M1
IVA	Any T	Any N	M1a
IVB	Any T	Any N	M1b

TNM = tumor-node-metastasis.
*American Joint Committee on Cancer (AJCC) classification.
Adapted from Fleming ID, Cooper JS, Henson DE, et al., editors. AJCC cancer staging manual. 5th ed. Philadelphia: Lippincott-Raven; 1997.

lymph node involvement and distant metastases (T4 N1 M1) reflects stage IV (advanced) disease.

Staging of Cancer of the Esophagogastric Junction

The recent increase in the incidence of esophageal cancer has been associated with a rapid increase in the rate of adenocarcinomas of the distal esophagus and esophagogastric junction. However, physicians at different institutions (and even at the same institution) may not classify and approach tumors located in this region in the same way. Some physicians consider and treat these lesions as esophageal tumors whereas other physicians consider them to be proximal gastric cancers or even separate and distinct entities. To help to clarify this confusion, a recent consensus conference of the International Gastric Cancer Association (IGCA) and the International Society for Diseases of the Esophagus (ISDE) agreed that these tumors should be more clearly defined and classified so as to develop a more consistent approach to managing them.[4] These groups have defined adenocarcinomas of the esophagogastric junction as tumors that "have their center within 5 centimeters proximal and distal of the anatomical cardia."[4,5] Furthermore, they have developed a classification system for three distinct types of tumors of the esophagogastric junction, based on the tumor's apparent point of origin (Table 2–4).

The classification of adenocarcinomas located within the region of the esophagogastric junction

into more distinct tumor types may significantly help in the ongoing study and understanding of this potentially heterogenous group of tumors. Whereas type I adenocarcinomas are believed to arise predominantly from specialized intestinal Barrett's epithelium in the distal esophagus, there appears to be a low prevalence of intestinal metaplasia at or below the level of the gastric cardia in type II and III tumors (32% and 9%, respectively).[4] In addition, the development of dysplastic changes in segments of intestinal metaplasia at or below the gastric cardia appears to be much less frequent an occurrence as compared to such changes seen in distal esophageal intestinal metaplasia.[6] Furthermore, the differing behaviors of tumors of the esophagogastric junction may also be somewhat accounted for by different patterns of lymphatic spread. For tumors of the distal esophagus, main lymphatic pathways extend both cephalically into the mediastinum and caudally toward the region of the celiac axis, whereas tumors at or below the gastric cardia spread predominantly toward the regions of the celiac axis, the splenic hilum, and the para-aortic lymph nodes.[7,8]

The more precise classification and staging of distal esophageal tumors at or close to the esophagogastric junction may help physicians gain a better understanding of these tumors' natural history, patterns of spread, and expected response to therapy. This knowledge will be invaluable for the design of future clinical research protocols and treatment plans for managing patients with these tumors.

Table 2–4. CLASSIFICATION* OF CANCERS ARISING IN THE REGION OF THE ESOPHAGOGASTRIC JUNCTION

Type I tumor
 Adenocarcinoma of the distal esophagus, which usually arises from an area with specialized intestinal metaplasia of the esophagus (ie, Barrett's esophagus); may infiltrate the esophagogastric junction from above
Type II tumor
 True carcinoma of the cardia; arises from the cardiac epithelium or short segments with intestinal metaplasia at the esophagogastric junction; often referred to as a "junctional carcinoma"
Type III tumor
 Subcardial gastric carcinoma that infiltrates the esophagogastric junction and distal esophagus from below

*International Gastric Cancer Association and the International Society for Diseases of the Esophagus classification.
Adapted from Siewert JR, Stein HJ. Classification of adenocarcinoma of the oesophagogastric junction. Br J Surg 1998;85:1457–9.

METHODS FOR STAGING ESOPHAGEAL CANCER

Barium Radiography and Upper-Gastrointestinal Endoscopy

In a patient presenting with signs and symptoms suggestive of a possible esophageal malignancy, the diagnostic evaluation typically begins with either a single- or double-contrast barium swallow or an upper-gas- trointestinal (UGI) endoscopy. Both modalities provide a good structural assessment of the esophageal lumen and the overlying mucosa. On barium study, abnormal radiographic findings that suggest possible esophageal malignancy include an intraluminal mass–like filling defect, asymmetric stricturing, and mucosal irregularities (Figure 2–1). On occasion, however, an esophageal cancer may even present radiographically as an apparent smooth circumferential stricture.

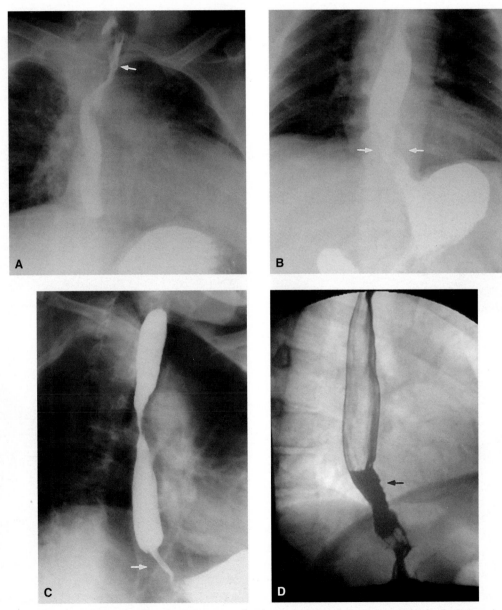

Figure 2–1.   *A,* Barium swallow demonstrates an "apple core" filling defect with associated luminal narrowing (*arrow*) resulting from a proximal esophageal cancer. *B,* Barium swallow demonstrates a distal esophageal tumor above a hiatal hernia (*arrows*). *C,* Barium swallow demonstrates circumferential narrowing (*arrow*) due to a distal esophageal tumor extending to the level of the esophagogastric junction. *D,* Barium swallow demonstrates distal esophageal wall infiltration (*arrow*) with minimal proximal dilatation caused by an esophageal carcinoma.

In one study of barium radiography in esophageal disease, four radiologists, blinded to the clinical history, reviewed the barium esophagrams from 35 patients (6 normal, 16 with benign esophageal disease, and 13 with small malignant tumors < 3.5 cm in diameter) and accurately diagnosed the small cancers in 73 percent of tumor cases.[9] Of the false-negative evaluations, 21 percent were interpreted as cases of benign esophageal disease and 6 percent as normal. Thus, although barium radiography may be a relatively good initial study in the assessment of symptomatic patients, small malignancies may be missed. In addition, all patients with abnormal barium studies need further investigation by UGI endoscopy (with biopsies and cytologic brushings) to rule out a potential malignancy (Figure 2–2).

In the United States, UGI endoscopy is currently the procedure of choice for the initial diagnostic evaluation of symptomatic patients. When combined with endoscopic biopsy, UGI endoscopy serves as the primary screening tool for patients with the pre-

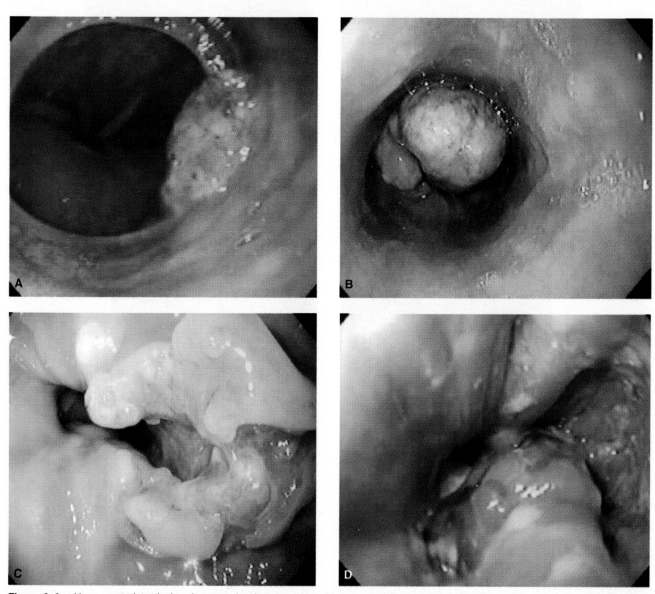

Figure 2–2. Upper gastrointestinal endoscopy, showing masses and tumors at various sites. *A,* Small esophageal cancer at the squamocolumnar junction. *B,* Bulky polypoid mass in the distal esophagus. *C,* Ulcerated mass in the distal esophagus. *D,* Infiltrative mass in the distal esophagus. *E,* Gastric cardia component of an infiltrative mass of the esophagogastric junction (same patient as in Figure 2–2D), seen during retroflexion in the proximal stomach (*arrow* indicates tumor). *F,* Submucosal infiltration of the gastric cardia, seen during retroflexion in the proximal stomach. *G,* Esophageal tumor undergoing biopsy. *H,* Esophageal tumor undergoing cytologic brushing.

malignant condition of Barrett's esophagus. Endoscopy not only permits the careful inspection and precise localization of any esophageal lesion but (most important) also allows targeted biopsies of abnormal areas, for a prompt and definitive histologic diagnosis.

Although barium radiography is a very good technique for diagnosing esophageal strictures in patients with dysphagia and although UGI endoscopy with biopsy and cytologic brushing is highly accurate in providing both a gross morphologic description and a histologic confirmation of malignancy, neither of these modalities alone is adequate to provide a complete preoperative staging assessment for esophageal malignancies. Although both techniques do provide an excellent structural examination of the esophageal lumen, neither modality can assess extraluminal disease. Thus, additional staging procedures are necessary (1) to provide accurate information regarding the depth of tumor invasion and the status of locoregional lymph nodes and (2) to assess for potential distant metastases.

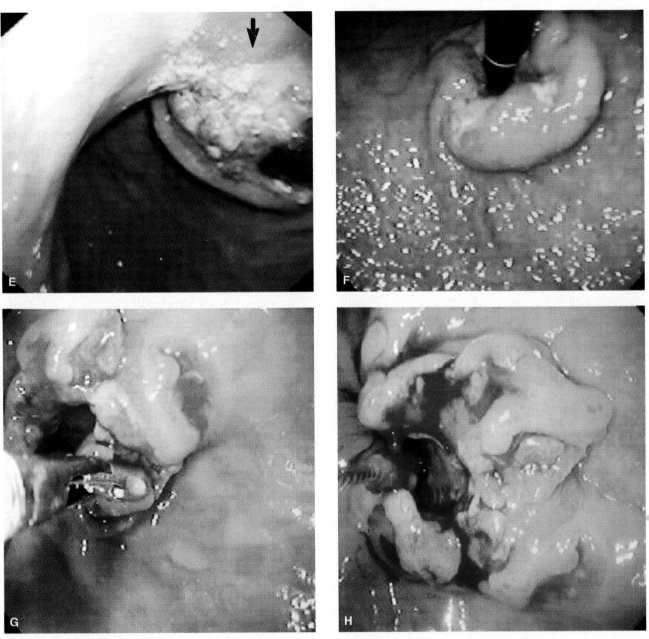

Figure 2–2.   *Continued*

Computed Tomography

Over recent years, computed tomography (CT) has become the method most used in the initial staging of newly diagnosed esophageal malignancies. Once an esophageal cancer has been confirmed by UGI endoscopy and biopsy, the patient's extent of disease evaluation often begins with a CT of the chest and abdomen. Current high-resolution helical CT is helpful in identifying metastatic disease to such sites as the liver, lungs, mediastinal and retroperitoneal lymph node areas, and intraperitoneal areas.

Imaging with CT can usually identify medium to large esophageal masses by the evident thickening of the esophageal wall and by the proximal luminal dilation caused by the obstruction (Figure 2–3, A to D). However, CT cannot accurately determine the depth of tumor invasion within the esophageal wall because of its inability to define individual layers of wall tissue and often cannot even identify the presence of small T1 and T2 masses. The resolution of current CT can only help to confirm the presence of an esophageal mass and the suspicion of invasion of adjacent mediastinal organs (T4), but it does not permit the accurate classification of T stage.

Lymph node metastases are identified on CT scans by the finding of enlarged and rounded hypodense structures in the mediastinum, adjacent to the stomach, and in the retroperitoneum or porta hepatis (see Figure 2–3, E to G). Mediastinal lymph nodes > 1.0 cm in maximum short-axis diameter in the transverse plane are considered to represent nodal metastases[10] and can sometimes be seen by CT.

On a CT scan, distant metastatic disease to the liver or lung usually appears as one or more hypodense round areas within the liver or lung parenchyma that enhance after the administration of intravenous contrast material (see Figure 2–3, H and I). Peritoneal disease can be strongly suggested by the finding of a thickening of the omentum or peritoneal surfaces, irregular contours on the bowel surface, or the presence of ascites.

When reviewing the many studies in the literature that report on the sensitivity, specificity, and accuracy of CT in the preoperative staging of esophageal cancer, one must take into account that many of these studies were not prospective, used early-generation CT technology, were limited by small sample sizes, and may have used varying definitions of metastatic disease (ie, celiac lymph node involvement) in their assessments.

One study from Duke University evaluated CT in the staging of 76 esophageal cancer and esophagogastric cancer patients.[11] The study compared the findings in these patients with the findings in 26 control patients without esophageal cancer and who had a normal mediastinum at surgery. A group of four radiologists were blinded to the patients' underlying diagnoses; they identified the CT scans of all 26 controls as normal. In the 61 cancer patients who were explored, there was an 88 percent accuracy rate for the detection of both local mediastinal invasion (depth of tumor penetration) and distant abdominal metastases. In a separate cohort of 12 patients, CT was less accurate in staging tumors of the esophagogastric junction and yielded accuracy rates of 50 percent for the prediction of both mediastinal invasion and distant metastases. In this study, CT correctly staged 94 percent of patients with esophageal cancer and 42 percent of those with cancers of the esophagogastric junction. Some of the difficulty with CT in assessing the T stage of distal tumors in the region of the esophagogastric junction may be related to poor gastric distention and/or the presence of a hiatal hernia in this region.

In a study from Vanderbilt University, CT findings in 18 esophageal cancer patients were compared with their operative findings and surgical pathology.[12] The accuracy of CT for localized tumor involvement was 77 percent whereas its accuracy was 94 percent for detecting direct aortic invasion and 88 percent for detecting tracheobronchial invasion. Computed tomography demonstrated a 72 percent accuracy for local lymph node involvement in mediastinal nodes; however, it was inaccurate for assessing distant lymph node metastases to intra-abdominal nodes in 11 of 18 patients. In 9 of these 11 cases (6 middle-thoracic and 3 lower-thoracic cases), positive celiac or left gastric nodes were found that were not detected by CT (false-negatives). In the other 2 cases, CT predicted abdominal lymph node involvement due to radiographically enlarged nodes (these were confirmed as being increased in size at surgery, but pathology failed to

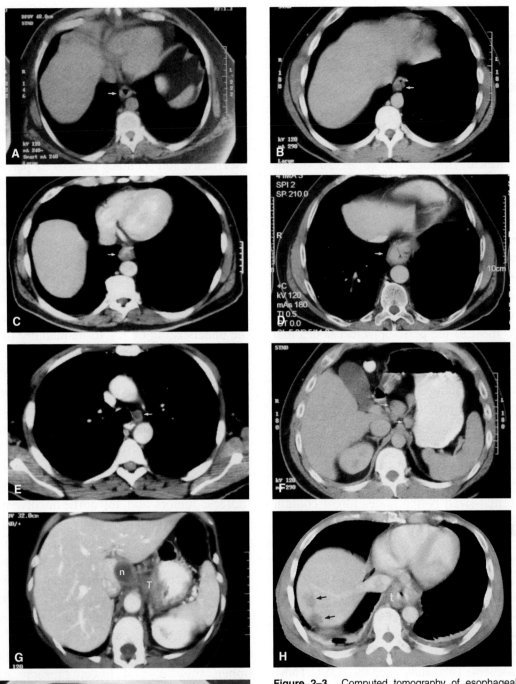

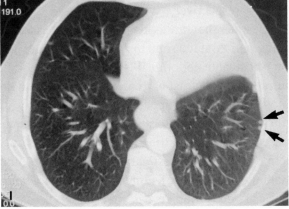

Figure 2–3. Computed tomography of esophageal masses and metastatic spread. *A,* An early-stage cancer of the esophagogastric junction (same patient as in Figure 2–2A) (*arrow* indicates tumor). *B,* A small distal esophageal tumor (*arrow*). *C,* An obstructing tumor (*arrow*) of the distal esophagus. *D,* A polypoid mass (*arrow*) filling the esophageal lumen. *E,* Metastatic spread of esophageal cancer to a subcarinal lymph node (*arrow*). This was confirmed by endoscopic ultrasonography (EUS)–guided fine-needle aspiration (FNA). *F,* Metastatic spread of esophageal cancer to perigastric and celiac lymph nodes (*arrow* indicates lymph node). This was confirmed by EUS-guided FNA. *G,* A suspicious-appearing necrotic celiac lymph node (*n*) in a patient with an esophagogastric-junction cancer (*T*). *H,* A distal esophageal tumor (*t*) and two hypodense liver metastases (*arrows*) *I,* Two small peripheral left lung metastases (*arrows*) in a patient with an esophageal cancer (confirmed by thoracoscopy).

demonstrate metastatic disease [false-positives]). Finally, accuracy for distant metastatic disease (not including the celiac or left gastric nodes) was 94 percent. Overall, surgical findings altered the TNM staging in 8 (73%) of 11 patients.

Another study of CT from Washington University (St. Louis, MO) reviewed CT findings in 30 esophageal cancer patients and correlated those findings with surgical findings, in 28 of 30 of the patients, or autopsy findings.[13] They reported findings similar to that of the Vanderbilt study, in that CT was demonstrated to be accurate for assessing tumor size, local invasion of the tracheobronchial tree, and metastatic disease to distant intra-abdominal lymph nodes (celiac and left gastric nodes) and solid organs (liver and adrenals), but to be inaccurate for assessing spread to regional periesophageal lymph nodes. Interestingly, most of the periesophageal nodes that were positive for metastatic tumor were not enlarged whereas the positive distant intra-abdominal nodes (M1 disease) were enlarged.

An important limitation of CT in staging esophageal tumors is its lack of sensitivity for accurately determining lymph node metastases (N stage). Also, an important factor, illustrated by both the Vanderbilt and Washington University studies, is that even normal-sized lymph nodes might contain microscopic foci of metastatic disease that is beyond the level of detection offered by CT.

In another retrospective study that assessed the accuracy of preoperative staging by CT in 33 patients with esophageal cancer, a comparison was made with surgical and pathologic findings.[14] Of note, this cohort of patients was preselected for having no evidence of liver metastases, based on preoperative staging assessment. This study used the AJCC TNM classification for tumor staging. Enlarged lymph nodes seen by CT were defined as being > 1 cm in diameter. The study reported excellent rates for sensitivity (100%), specificity (97%), and accuracy (97%) for the detection of tracheobronchial invasion but found that CT was not as accurate for determining aortic involvement (with rates of 100% for sensitivity, 52% for specificity, and 55% for accuracy). Once again, CT fared poorly in determining regional lymph node metastases (celiac nodes were defined as regional nodes for distal esophageal tumors whereas

they were defined as distant nodes for proximal and midesophageal tumors), demonstrating rates of only 61 percent for sensitivity, 60 percent for specificity, and 61 percent for accuracy. The authors perceived this to be related to the difficulty of CT in distinguishing periesophageal nodes from adjacent tumor. Computed tomography did somewhat better with distant lymph node involvement, showing sensitivity, specificity, and accuracy rates of 67 percent, 87 percent, and 85 percent, respectively. The sensitivity of CT for the detection of distant liver metastases could not be assessed in this study because the patients were preselected for not having liver metastases, but excellent specificity and accuracy rates (100% for both) were demonstrated for this modality. Overall, however, CT was able to correctly stage only 39 percent (13) of the 33 patients. The authors attributed the understaging by CT to its inability to accurately define depth of tumor invasion and to determine direct periesophageal mediastinal invasion.

An additional study that compared preoperative CT with surgical and pathologic findings in a cohort of 50 patients with esophageal cancer (University of Bern, Bern, Switzerland) found a very high accuracy rate for the detection of direct tumor invasion into the tracheobronchial tree (100%) for proximal thoracic tumors and for aortic involvement (95 to 100%) for proximal, middle, and distal tumors.[15] However, CT assessment of intra-abdominal lymph node metastases demonstrated sensitivity, specificity, and accuracy rates of 57 percent, 100 percent, and 80 percent, respectively. The low sensitivity for the detection of distal intra-abdominal nodes thus limited the overall accuracy rates for CT staging to only 80 percent, 68 percent, and 65 percent for upper, middle, and lower thoracic esophageal tumors, respectively.

Despite the limitations of CT for assessing T stage and N stage, our institution continues to rely on chest and abdominal spiral CT with oral and intravenous contrast early in the evaluation to detect those patients with apparent metastatic disease. The identification of metastatic disease at presentation permits immediate triage of these patients to systemic therapy or investigational treatment protocols, with the avoidance of surgery. Patients in whom initial CT does not reveal metastatic disease then undergo more advanced staging evaluations and are more appropriately offered curative surgical treatment or multimodality treatment protocols with curative intent.

Endoscopic Ultrasonography

Endoscopic ultrasonography (EUS) is a new and powerful imaging modality that has been developed over the past 15 years. It provides detailed imaging of the esophageal wall, nearby lymph nodes, and other adjacent structures. This modality makes use of the ability to introduce an ultrasound transducer directly into the gastrointestinal tract, thus bringing it into close proximity to the tumor. This eliminates the artifacts, created by intraluminal air and food, found in standard transcutaneous ultrasonography and CT.

Coupled with the development of new high-frequency ultrasound transducers, EUS permits the detailed evaluation of most areas of the gastrointestinal tract that are within the reach of standard endoscopes (Figure 2–4). While it does require sedation for most evaluations of the upper-gastrointestinal tract, EUS examinations are performed with the ease and comfort of most routine upper-gastrointestinal endoscopies. There is minimal risk, and EUS has proved to be well tolerated by most patients.

Many studies have shown that the resolution power of currently available EUS instruments provides superior assessment of almost all neoplasms of the esophagus, in addition to those involving the stomach, pancreas, and rectum. The 5-, 7.5-, and 12-MHz probes fitted on these scopes permit the assessment of microscopic tissue planes in the gastrointestinal tract, including the distinction of the normal multilayered histologic architecture of the mucosa, submucosa, muscularis propria, and serosa.[16–18] The first wall layer is bright and corresponds to a border echo and the superficial mucosa; the second is dark and corresponds to the deep mucosa (including the muscularis mucosae); the third is bright and corresponds to the submucosa and the acoustical interface between the submucosa and muscularis propria; the fourth is dark and corresponds to the muscularis propria; and the fifth is bright and corresponds to the adventitial interface (Figure 2–5). In contrast to CT, the ability of EUS to distinguish wall layers allows it to provide a more accurate determination of depth of invasion by tumors; EUS thus has the potential to identify early-stage intramural disease.

On EUS, normal esophageal wall thickness is about 0.3 cm.[19] On EUS, an esophageal malignancy appears as a hypoechoic abnormality within the wall, disrupting the normal wall echolayers. The lower-frequency transducers permit the evaluation of extramural disease (including local and regional lymphadenopathy and disease in adjacent organs such as the liver, spleen, and pancreas), in addition to the identification of ascites. Thus, EUS provides accurate assessment of depth of tumor invasion into and through the wall of the esophagus (Figure 2–6, A to C), detection of direct invasion into adjacent structures (see Figure 2–6, D and E), and identification of local lymph node metastases (see Figure 2–6, F and G), making it an ideal modality for determining clinical tumor stage according to the TNM method of cancer staging.

Computed tomography characterizes lymph nodes that are abnormally large (> 1 cm in diameter) as sus-

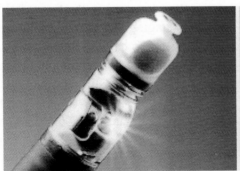 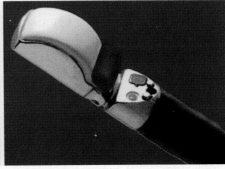

Figure 2–4.   Olympus mechanical radial (*left*) and Pentax linear (*right*) array endoscopic ultrasound scopes.

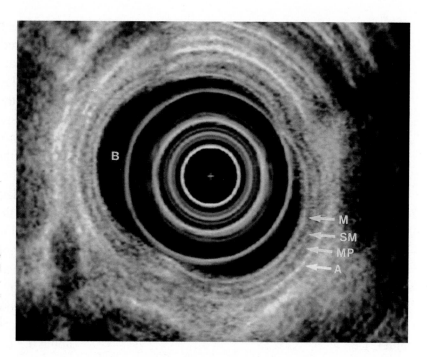

Figure 2–5. Endoscopic ultrasonography image of the normal echoarchitecture of the esophageal wall. The central concentric rings are artifacts created by the ultrasound scope. (M = mucosa; SM = submucosa; MP = muscularis propria; A = adventitia; B = water-filled balloon filling the esophageal lumen.)

picious for tumor involvement. In addition to size, EUS also uses additional criteria (such as rounded shape, homogeneous hypoechoic pattern, and sharply demarcated borders) to assess for metastatic lymph nodes.[20,21] Nodes that appear to be benign on EUS may be > 1 cm in diameter but are typically elongated in shape, demonstrate a hyperechoic pattern with distinct cortical and medullary areas, and have less sharply demarcated borders.[22]

In locoregional staging for esophageal cancer, EUS is superior to CT.[23] This is due to its more precise imaging of distinct esophageal wall layers and its better ability to assess malignant nodal disease.

In numerous studies of preoperative endosonographic assessment of esophageal cancer by EUS as compared with surgical pathology in resected specimens, the accuracy of EUS for determining depth of tumor invasion (T stage) has been reported to range from 75 to 90 percent.[24–34] In studies comparing EUS to CT for preoperative T staging, the accuracy of EUS ranges from 76 to 89 percent, and that of CT ranges from 49 to 59 percent.[21,26,27] At our institution, a prospective comparative study of preoperative EUS versus dynamic CT for esophageal cancer in 50 patients demonstrated an accuracy of 92 percent for T staging with EUS and 60 percent for T staging with CT ($p < .0003$).[19] A reasonable estimation of the overall accuracy of EUS for T staging,

based on the now extensive published literature, is approximately 85 percent.[23]

Although EUS is highly accurate for determining T stage, it may have some difficulty distinguishing between T1 (mucosal invasion) and T2 (submucosal invasion) tumors.[35] Since T2 tumors are associated with a high risk (30 to 70%) of lymph node metastases, this differentiation between early-stage T1 and T2 disease is extremely important if one is to consider the option of minimally invasive endoscopic resection to treat T1 lesions.[23] The accuracy of EUS for T staging superficial esophageal tumors has been reported to be 72 percent.[34] The use of small catheters (which can be passed through the instrument channel of a standard endoscope) containing higher-frequency 20-MHz transducers that offer higher resolution of esophageal wall layers may help overcome this issue in the future[36] (Figure 2–7).

For staging regional lymph node metastases (N stage), EUS has also been found to be more accurate than CT. The distinction between benign and malignant nodes is still a problem. Unlike CT, however, EUS not only can assess lymph node size but can also evaluate for additional criteria, such as well-circumscribed, rounded, and hypoechoic nodal characteristics, to predict metastatic nodal involvement. With CT, normal-sized lymph nodes containing occult microscopic metastases lead to understag-

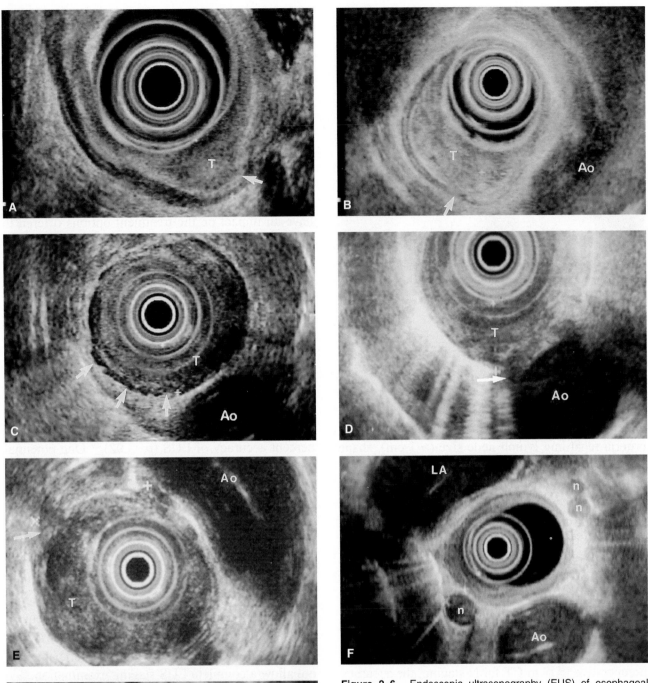

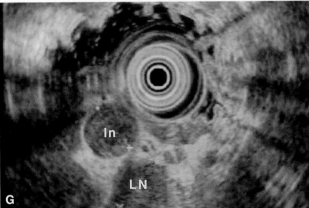

Figure 2–6. Endoscopic ultrasonography (EUS) of esophageal tumors and lymph node metastases. *A,* A T1 esophageal tumor (*T*) extending into the submucosa. (at *arrow*) in the same patient shown in Figure 2–2A. *B,* A T2 esophageal tumor extending into the muscularis propria (at *arrow*) (T = tumor, Ao = aorta.) *C,* A T3 esophageal tumor infiltrating through all wall layers and out into the adventitia (at *arrows*) (T = tumor, Ao = aorta.) *D,* A T4 esophageal tumor (*T*) invading the aorta (*Ao*) *arrow* indicates point of invasion. *E,* A T4 esophageal tumor (*T*) invading the trachea (*Tr*). Arrow indicates point of invasion. (Ao = aorta.) *F,* Locoregional lymph node metastases in a patient with an esophageal tumor. (n = periesophageal lymph node; Ao = aorta; LA = left atrium.) *G,* Lymph node metastases involving the perigastric (*In*) and celiac-axis (*LN*) lymph nodes in a patient with an esophageal tumor (confirmed by EUS-guided fine-needle aspiration).

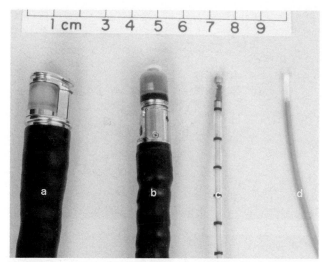

Figure 2–7. Size comparison of four different endoscopic ultrasonography (EUS) instruments. (a = Olympus EUS colonoscope; b = Olympus EUS gastroscope; c = Olympus prototype miniprobe; d = Boston Scientific EUS miniprobe.)

ing whereas benign enlarged inflammatory nodes lead to overstaging.

In a study from the Cleveland Clinic, EUS features of lymph node metastases were assessed in 100 patients with esophageal cancer.[37] When stringent criteria regarding lymph node size (> 1 cm), shape (round), border demarcation (sharp), and central echo pattern (homogeneous and hypoechoic) were applied, the sensitivity and specificity of EUS in detecting lymph node metastases were 89.1 percent and 91.7 percent, respectively; when all four features were present, accuracy of predicting lymph node metastases was 100 percent.

Multiple reports of preoperative EUS assessment of regional lymph node metastases in esophageal cancer since 1992 demonstrate accuracy rates ranging from 70 to 90 percent.[24,25,27–31,34,38] In comparing preoperative EUS to CT for N staging, the accuracy rates for EUS range from 72 to 80 percent whereas accuracy rates for CT range from 46 to 58 percent.[21,27,30] In the study from our institution that directly compared EUS and CT in this setting, we reported accuracy rates of 88 percent with EUS and 74 percent with CT.[19] Overall, the extensive published data suggest an EUS accuracy rate of approximately 75 percent for regional N staging.[23] As with CT, the reduced accuracy of EUS for N staging is related to the issue of distinguishing benign from malignant lymph nodes.

For the detection of advanced (T4) disease, EUS has been demonstrated to be more accurate than CT in determining vascular invasion of the aorta or pericardium.[39] In another series (a recent multicenter retrospective cohort study of 79 patients with stage T4 esophageal cancer as determined by preoperative EUS staging), EUS was more accurate than CT in determining T4 tumor invasion, with rates of 87.5 percent and 43.8 percent, respectively ($p = .0002$).[40] The accurate preoperative determination of locally advanced T4 disease would clearly have an impact on the treatment options offered to the patients as the patients would no longer be initial surgical candidates but would perhaps (in some centers) be eligible for investigational protocols evaluating the usefulness of preoperative neoadjuvant chemoradiotherapy.

In esophageal cancer patients, EUS is not as accurate as CT in the detection of distant metastatic disease to such common sites as the liver, lungs, and peritoneal cavity. In the series from our institution, CT demonstrated an accuracy of 90 percent in the staging of distant metastases, as compared to the 70 percent accuracy of EUS ($p < .02$).[19] One potential advantage of EUS, as compared to CT, may be in the more accurate detection of M1 disease related to celiac node involvement.

Another limitation of EUS in the preoperative assessment of esophageal cancer is its inability to completely evaluate severely strictured esophageal tumors. As it is common for patients to present with advanced disease, there have been reports of high-grade malignant strictures in 20 to 44 percent of patients at initial presentation.[41] These strictures may prevent passage of the echoendoscope and thus not allow a complete EUS staging examination.

An increased risk of perforation has been reported in patients with high-grade malignant strictures who undergo esophageal dilatation followed by EUS staging. In a study of 79 patients with esophageal cancer from the Cleveland Clinic, 26.6 percent presented with a high-grade malignant stricture; of these 21 patients, 24 percent developed an esophageal perforation as a result of the wire-guided dilatation or as a direct result of the EUS procedure.[42] However, some other ultrasonographers have reported that such high-grade malignant strictures can be safely dilated to allow passage of the echoendoscope just prior to the EUS staging procedure.[33]

As a result of the experience of several esophageal perforations at our institution, we do not typically dilate high-grade malignant esophageal strictures during EUS staging. Instead, our approach in these cases is to perform a limited ultrasonographic staging examination at the upper extent of the tumor or to use the new wire-guided thin-caliber EUS scope (MH 908, Olympus), which easily passes even obstructing tumors to permit full staging without the increased risk.

Endoscopic Ultrasonography–Guided Fine-Needle Aspiration

Although both CT and EUS can detect enlarged and suspicious-appearing lymph nodes, both techniques are limited to morphologic characterization. The presence of enlarged and inflammatory lymph nodes in esophageal cancer can reduce the specificity of both imaging modalities for detecting lymph node metastases. An important recent advance in the field of endoscopic ultrasonography was the use of EUS-guided fine-needle aspiration (FNA) to sample submucosal lesions, nearby lymph nodes, and other adjacent structures throughout the gastrointestinal tract.

The linear-array ultrasonographic endoscope provides scanning that is oriented parallel to the long axis of the endoscope and is capable of tracking the passage of a biopsy needle (Figure 2–8). Ultrasonography-guided tissue sampling can thus be obtained by the passage of a cytology needle through the instrument channel of the scope and directly into the plane of the ultrasonographic image (Figure 2–9), permitting very precise positioning of the needle in lesions and nodes as small as 1 cm and as far as 5 cm from the wall of the gastrointestinal tract.

In a series from the University of California at Irvine, EUS-guided FNA was used to assess submucosal gastrointestinal tract lesions and extraluminal lymph nodes and masses in 38 patients.[43] Of the 46 lesions that were sampled, 34 were extraluminal (8 periesophageal nodes, 1 mediastinal mass, 6 celiac nodes, 12 pancreatic masses, 1 perigastric mass, 1 liver mass, 1 periduodenal node, 2 pericolonic masses, 1 perirectal mass, and 1 perirectal node) and 12 were submucosal (8 gastric, 3 duodenal, and 1 esophageal). The overall diagnostic accuracy of FNA was 87 percent. In patients with known malignant lesions, the sensitivity and specificity of FNA was 91 percent and 100 percent, respectively. Celiac nodes were successfully sampled and diagnostic in 5 (83%) of 6 patients. In this study, EUS-guided FNA provided an initial tissue diagnosis of malignancy in 66 percent of cancer patients without a previous diagnosis, and the preoperative stage was changed for 44 percent of cancer patients. No complications were reported in this series.

Another group, from Indiana University, recently reported their experience with EUS-guided FNA in 288 patients with suspected gastrointestinal or mediastinal masses.[44] They reported an 87 percent overall diagnostic accuracy, an 89 percent sensitivity, and a 100 percent specificity. Within their cohort, subgroup analysis demonstrated that FNA had an accuracy of 95 percent for the diagnosis of mediastinal lymph nodes (n = 43) and an accuracy of 85 percent for intra-abdominal lymph nodes (n = 13). Their immediate complication rate was 2 percent, all

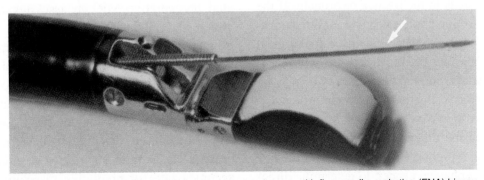

Figure 2–8.   Pentax linear array endoscopic ultrasound scope with fine-needle aspiration (FNA) biopsy needle (*arrow*).

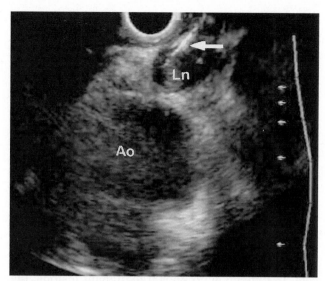

Figure 2–9. Endoscopic ultrasonography–guided fine-needle aspiration of a malignant mediastinal lymph node in a patient with esophageal cancer. *Arrow* indicates biopsy needle. (Ln = lymph node; Ao = aorta.)

related to FNA of pancreatic lesions (2 with bleeding and 2 with pancreatitis).

Endoscopic ultrasonography–guided FNA is rapidly becoming an important tool in the staging of patients with gastrointestinal cancers and other malignancies (including primary lung cancer) and has both diagnostic and therapeutic implications.

Bronchoscopy

Bronchoscopy has been performed by some physicians as part of the initial preoperative staging assessment in patients presenting with esophageal tumors involving the cervical and upper thoracic esophagus to assess for direct tracheobronchial invasion indicative of locally advanced stage T4 disease. Bronchoscopy allows direct visualization and biopsy of any suspicious areas in the trachea or bronchi. If the bronchoscopic examination is positive for direct invasion, the patient is no longer a candidate for surgical resection and may be offered treatment with combined chemotherapy and radiation therapy or may be offered available investigational treatment protocols.

A recent prospective study from Munich, Germany, evaluated the diagnostic usefulness of bronchoscopy in the preoperative assessment of 116 patients with esophageal cancer, to determine direct airway invasion and resectability.[45] The investigators compared the findings of 150 bronchoscopy examinations in this cohort with their intraoperative findings and surgical pathology. The overall accuracy of bronchoscopy (with brush cytology and biopsy) for determining direct tracheobronchial invasion in patients who were otherwise surgical candidates was 95.8 percent. In addition, the results of bronchoscopy and CT were discordant in 40 percent of the patients, with higher specificity and positive predictive value for bronchoscopy than for CT.

To date, we are not familiar with any comparative studies between bronchoscopy and EUS. At our institution, bronchoscopy is selectively used to assist in the staging of patients with cervical and upper thoracic esophageal malignancies.

Magnetic Resonance Imaging

The role of magnetic resonance imaging (MRI) in the preoperative staging of esophageal cancer is currently under investigation; however, results to date do not appear to demonstrate that MRI adds anything to CT imaging in this group of patients.

In a recent prospective study from Osaka, Japan, MRI and CT results were compared with surgical or autopsy findings in 31 patients with esophageal cancer.[46] The accuracy rates of MRI and CT for detecting regional lymph nodes were 68 percent and 65 percent, respectively; for distant nodes, it was 77 percent for both modalities. As with CT, MRI has a decreased accuracy for detecting regional lymph node metastases because it misses normal-size lymph nodes with metastases. Overall, the accuracy rates for predicting resectability were similar, being 87 percent for MRI and 84 percent for CT.

In a study from Milan, Italy, investigators evaluated preoperative MRI in assessing direct locoregional and mediastinal lymph node spread in 32 esophageal cancer patients and compared the results with surgical pathology.[47] They reported accuracy rates of 84 percent for the detection of mediastinal invasion, 87 percent for detecting tracheobronchial invasion, 91 percent for detecting aortic invasion, and 72 percent for detecting mediastinal lymph node metastases. Despite such good results, the overall accuracy rate for predicting resectability was only 75 percent for MRI in this study.

In an earlier study from the University of Michigan of the use of MRI for staging esophageal cancers, MRI and CT findings in 10 esophageal cancer patients were compared with their operative findings and surgical pathology, and with the MRI and CT assessments of 20 control patients with normal esophagi.[48] Both MRI and CT had low overall accuracy in staging (40% and 70%, respectively). The investigators attributed this poor accuracy primarily to the inability of MRI and CT to detect precise depth of tumor invasion (T stage).

Minimally Invasive Surgical Staging: Laparoscopy, Laparoscopic Ultrasonography, and Thoracoscopy

Over the past decade, improvements in anesthesia and laparoscopic techniques and instrumentation have fueled the development of minimally invasive surgery for the management of benign diseases as well as the diagnosis, staging, and treatment of many types of cancers. Adding to successful experiences with laparoscopic cholecystectomy, surgeons have worked to develop minimally invasive surgery for cancer management.

Initial studies of laparoscopy in the staging of upper-gastrointestinal malignancies indicate that laparoscopy is highly sensitive for detecting metastatic disease, particularly the identification of small tumor implants on the peritoneal surfaces and liver that are not detected by conventional imaging modalities (Figure 2–10, A to C). Laparoscopy also permits the evaluation of lymph nodes for metastatic disease (see Figure 2–10, D). In a study from our institution, laparoscopic exploration in 110 patients with gastric cancer accurately staged 94 percent of patients for metastatic disease, with a sensitivity of 84 percent and a specificity of 100 percent.[49] The prevalence rate of metastatic disease is 37 percent in all patients who had been preselected by an abnormal CT scan.

A large study of laparoscopic staging in 280 patients with cancer of the esophagus and 89 patients with gastric cardia cancer demonstrated metastatic disease to the liver, peritoneum, omentum, stomach, and lymph nodes in 52 patients (14%) and to the gastric wall or regional lymph nodes in 36

patients (9.7%).[50] The rate of false-negative findings by laparoscopy in this series was 4.4 percent (2.8% for liver metastases, 1.2% for peritoneal seeding, and 0.4% for omental implants).

A recent advance in minimally invasive surgical staging is the addition of laparoscopic ultrasonography (LUS) in the evaluation of patients with upper-gastrointestinal malignancies (Figure 2–11). One study from Denmark evaluated EUS, laparoscopy, LUS, CT, and transcutaneous ultrasonography in patients with upper-gastrointestinal malignancies.[51] Forty-four patients with esophageal, gastric, and pancreatic cancer were studied preoperatively, and the results of these examinations (which were used to determine the resectability and curability of the tumors, based on TNM staging) were compared to findings at laparotomy. The reported accuracy for predicting resectability and curability was 91 percent for EUS, 64 percent for CT and ultrasonography combined, 68 percent for laparoscopy alone, 95 percent for LUS alone, and 95 percent for EUS and LUS combined.

In a study from the University of Amsterdam, the Netherlands, laparoscopy and LUS was performed in 233 patients with upper-gastrointestinal tumors (tumors of the esophagus, gastric cardia, liver, bile duct, and pancreas) believed to be surgically resectable after conventional preoperative staging.[52] Of the 64 patients with esophageal or gastric cardia cancers (preoperative evaluation included EUS), findings at laparoscopy prevented laparotomy in 4 patients (6%) because of the detection of unsuspected metastatic disease.

The application of laparoscopic techniques and instruments in the chest has resulted in advances in video-assisted thoracoscopy and in the application of thoracoscopy to the surgical staging of esophageal cancer. Thoracoscopy allows the direct visualization of the entire thoracic esophagus, the accurate assessment of tumor invasion into the adventitia and adjacent mediastinal structures, and the evaluation and sampling of regional lymph nodes for histology.[53] It can also detect occult pleural and pulmonary metastases. However, to assess for intra-abdominal disease (including liver metastases and peritoneal implants) and to sample perigastric and celiac lymph nodes, thoracoscopy must be combined with diagnostic laparoscopy. Furthermore, tumors of the esophagogastric junction also require a combined laparoscopic approach to completely evaluate the inferior aspect of the primary tumor and to assess for intraabdominal disease.

A study from the University of Pittsburgh compared the accuracy of EUS with thoracoscopic and laparoscopic staging in evaluating lymph node metastases in 26 patients with surgically resectable esophageal cancer (24 patients with adenocarcinoma of the esophagogastric junction and 2 with squamous cell carcinoma of the midthoracic esophagus).[54] In 5 patients (19%), complete assessment by EUS was not possible due to high-grade malignant stricture that did not allow passage of the scope; in 3 of these 5 patients, laparoscopy and thoracoscopy revealed N1 disease. Endoscopic ultrasonography detected N1 disease in 13 patients, and laparoscopy and thoracoscopy confirmed N1 disease in 12 (92%) of these 13 patients. The sensitivity and specificity of EUS for nodal evaluation were 65 percent and 66 percent, respectively. The sensitivity of EUS decreased to 44 percent when EUS was used for detecting occult metastatic disease in lymph nodes less than 1 cm in diameter. No disease staged as T3 by EUS was up-

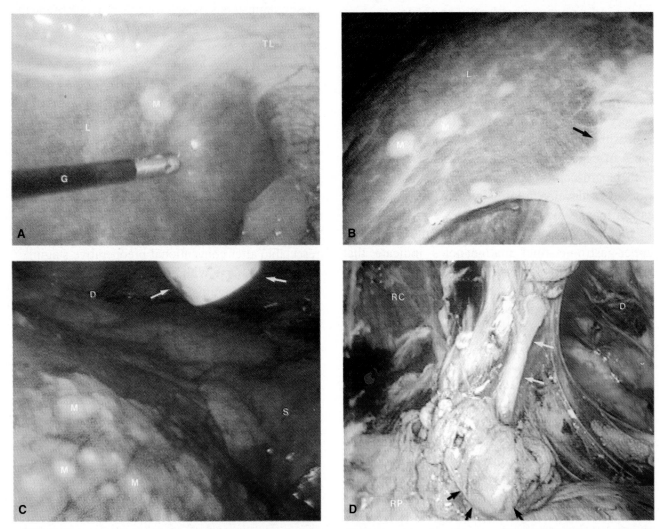

Figure 2–10.   *A,* Solitary liver metastasis, shown at laparoscopy. (M = liver metastasis; L = liver; G = grasper [instrument diameter = 0.3 cm]; D = diaphragm, TL = triangular ligament.) (×15 original magnification.) (Courtesy of Dr. Tracey Weigel.) *B,* Multiple small metastases involving the right lobe of the liver, shown at laparoscopy. *Arrow* indicates falciform ligament. (M = liver metastasis; L = liver.) (×15 original magnification.) (Courtesy of Dr. Tracey Weigel.) *C,* Multiple small (< 0.1cm in diameter) metastatic nodules studding the peritoneal surface in the region of the gastrohepatic ligament, shown at laparoscopy. *Arrows* indicate instrument port (port diameter = 0.5 cm). (M = metastatic peritoneal nodule; S = stomach; D = diaphragm.) (×15 original magnification.) (Courtesy of Dr. Tracey Weigel.) *D,* Metastatic disease to a left gastric artery lymph node, shown at laparoscopy. *Black arrows* indicate lymph node, *white arrows* indicate left gastric artery. (RP = retroperitoneum; RC = right crus of diaphragm; D = diaphragm.) (×15 original magnification.) (Courtesy of Dr. Tracey Weigel.)

staged to T4 by laparoscopy or thoracoscopy. However, whereas EUS did not detect distant metastases in any patient, laparoscopy identified M1 disease due to liver metastases in 4 (15%) of 26 patients.

In a more recent study from the Pittsburgh group, staging with laparoscopy and thoracoscopy was compared to conventional staging with CT and EUS in 53 patients with esophageal cancer.[55] In this cohort, after CT and EUS staging (1 case as carcinoma in situ, 1 case as stage I, 23 as stage II, 20 as stage III, and 8 as stage IV disease), laparoscopy and thoracoscopy changed the stage in 17 patients (32%), down-staging disease in 10 patients and up-staging disease in 7 patients.

In a study from the University of Rotterdam 'Dijkigt' in the Netherlands, conventional preoperative imaging (including EUS) was compared with laparoscopy and LUS in staging 40 patients with esophageal cancer and 20 patients with gastric cardia cancer.[56] In 1 (2.5%) of 40 patients with esophageal cancer, laparoscopy detected M1 disease due to a liver metastasis. Of the 20 patients with gastric cardia cancer, laparoscopy detected 4 (20%) with M1 disease (peritoneal seeding in 3 and omental metastases in 1) whereas LUS detected an additional 4 (20%) (liver metastasis in 2 and celiac lymph node metastasis in 2), demonstrating the detection of otherwise unsuspected M1 disease in 8 (40%) of the 20 patients by laparoscopy and LUS combined.

Minimally invasive surgical staging with thoracoscopy and laparoscopy for patients with cancers of the esophagus and the esophagogastric junction offers the ability to detect a small but significant number of patients with distant M1 disease that would not be detected by conventional preoperative imaging studies. In addition, direct tissue sampling of lymph node and peritoneal lesions increases the specificity for finding such abnormalities. The improved accuracy of preoperative staging offered by these procedures may improve the selection of patients for surgery and increase the curative resection rates at some hospitals while reducing the number of unnecessary laparotomies.

There are, however, limitations and risks related to thoracoscopy and laparoscopy staging procedures. Both procedures are invasive and are performed in an operating room under general anesthe-

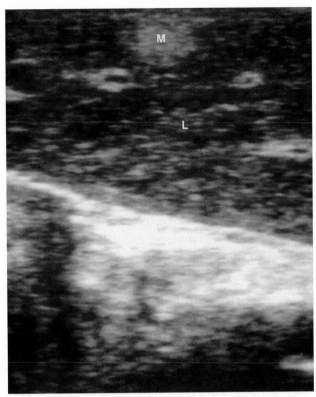

Figure 2–11. Laparoscopic ultrasonography (LUS) of a liver metastasis in a patient with an esophagogastric-junction tumor (M = metastasis; L = liver.) (Courtesy of Dr. Tracey Weigel.)

sia, which is associated with its own related costs and potential complications. In a small number of patients, laparoscopy may not be successful due to adhesions from prior abdominal surgery. There is a potential risk, albeit small, of tumor spillage and port site metastases related to these procedures. In addition, following thoracoscopy, a chest tube must be inserted, which requires the inconvenience and cost of a limited hospital stay for management and patient recovery.

The University of Pittsburgh group reported its procedure-related morbidities associated with thoracoscopic and laparoscopic staging.[54] In this study, 8 (30.8%) of the 26 patients developed "minor complications" (2 patients with prolonged ileus, 2 with atelectasis, 2 with urinary retention, and 2 with port site infections). One patient (3.8%) experienced a "major complication" (a small-bowel obstruction following laparoscopy). Thus, in this study, the overall rate of complications associated with thoracoscopy and laparoscopy for staging was 34.6 percent (9 of 26). Furthermore, the Pittsburgh group also reported its operating-room times and the length of hospital stays. The average operating-room time was 4.2 hours (a range of 1 to 6 hours), and the average length of hospital stay was 3.4 days (a range of 1 to 11 days). The authors did note, however, that both of these times decreased during the course of their study; for the last 10 patients, the average operating-room time was 3.6 hours and the average hospital stay was 1.8 days.

A potential role for minimally invasive preoperative staging is to complement the use of EUS or CT for properly stratifying (on the basis of optimal staging) those patients who are candidates for therapy in the context of a clinical trial.

Positron Emission Tomography

Positron emission tomography (PET) is a relatively new imaging modality that makes use of the ability to visualize tumors by virtue of differences in metabolic activity between tumor and normal tissue. Tumor tissues are generally more metabolically active than normal non-neoplastic tissues and have increased glycolytic activity. The administration of $[^{18}F]$-fluoro-2-deoxy-D-glucose (FDG) to an individual with cancer therefore results in a greater uptake of FDG by the tumor tissue than by most normal tissues. Once FDG enters cancer cells, it is phosphorylated and trapped within the cells, thereby rendering the cells radioactive. This enables cancerous tumors to be detected by the radioactivity emitted from the trapped radiolabeled FDG. Tumors of sufficient size and with a sufficient uptake of FDG are therefore readily detected by using a gamma camera. Through the technique of tomographic imaging, whole-body PET can provide detailed images that can be superimposed on conventional CT scans, correlating the areas of increased radioisotope activity with anatomic sites of disease (Figure 2–12).

Imaging by PET is currently under investigation to determine its potential role in preoperative staging for esophageal cancer. In a study from the University of Pittsburgh, PET was performed in 35 patients with esophageal cancer, and results were compared with surgical findings and pathology.[57] For the detection of locoregional lymph node metastases, PET demonstrated a sensitivity of 45 percent,

a specificity of 100 percent, and an overall accuracy of 48 percent. There were 11 false-negative PET study results for small (mean diameter of 0.52 cm), intracapsular locoregional nodal metastases. For detecting distant metastases, PET showed a sensitivity of 88 percent, a specificity of 93 percent, and an accuracy of 91 percent. It detected nine sites of distant metastases not identified by conventional scanning. One false-negative PET study result occurred in a patient with a small (0.2 cm) liver lesion. The investigators concluded that current PET technology was not accurate enough to detect small locoregional nodes. Its potential benefit in staging patients with esophageal cancer may be its ability to identify unsuspected distant metastases, which it accomplished in up to 20 percent of study patients who were found to be falsely negative for M1 disease by conventional preoperative staging modalities.

In a prospective study from Amsterdam, PET was evaluated in 26 patients with esophageal and esophagogastric cancers and was compared with CT and surgical findings, primarily to determine its ability to stage metastatic disease.[58] The rate of visualization of the primary tumor was 81 percent with CT and 96 percent with PET. Neither CT nor PET was good at determining the depth of wall penetration (T stage). For N staging, the sensitivity of CT was 38 percent, its specificity was 100 percent, and its overall accuracy was 62 percent whereas PET showed a sensitivity of 92 percent, a specificity of 88 percent, and an accuracy of 90 percent. In regard to determining M stage, CT detected distant metastases in 5 patients, with one false-positive liver hemangioma, and PET detected distant metastases in 8 patients, with one false-positive in the supraclavicular area (that was not confirmed on subsequent cytology assessment). The overall diagnostic accuracy for determining resectability was 65 percent for CT and 88 percent for PET.

In a more recent report, the investigators at the University of Pittsburgh updated their data to describe their prospective experience with 100 PET scans in 91 patients with esophageal cancer.[59] They compared PET with CT, bone scan, and surgical findings. In this study, a total of 70 distant metastases were confirmed in 39 patients by minimally invasive surgical staging or clinical correlation.

Positron emission tomography identified 51 metastases in 27 of the 39 cases, demonstrating a sensitivity of 69 percent, a specificity of 93.4 percent, and an accuracy of 84 percent, whereas CT detected only 26 metastases in 18 of the 39 cases, indicating a sensitivity of 46.1 percent, a specificity of 73.8 percent, and an accuracy of 63 percent ($p < .01$).

Another recent prospective comparison of PET with conventional staging modalities for preoperative assessment of esophageal cancer was reported from Leuven, Belgium.[60] The authors evaluated 43 patients with esophageal cancer and 31 with esophagogastric cancer and compared their findings with CT and EUS findings. Positron emission tomography detected the primary tumors in 70 (95%) of 74 patients and gave false-negative results in 4 patients with early-stage T1 lesions. In the 34 patients (46%) with advanced (stage IV) disease, PET demonstrated a higher accuracy rate (82%) for diagnosing stage IV disease than did the combination of both CT and EUS, which had an accuracy of 64 percent ($p = .004$). Positron emission tomography also demonstrated additional benefit in 16 patients (22%) by up-staging 11 patients (15%) and by down-staging 5 patients

(7%). In the 39 patients (53%) who underwent a 2- or 3-field lymphadenectomy, lymph node metastases were detected in 21 local and 35 regional or distant nodes. For the detection of local lymph node metastases, PET demonstrated a lower sensitivity (33% as compared to EUS at 81% [$p = .027$]) but a higher, although not statistically significant, specificity (89%, compared to 67% for EUS). For the detection of regional and distant nodal metastases, PET demonstrated a sensitivity of 46 percent, similar to that of the combination of CT and EUS (43%) ($p =$ not significant); however, its specificity was 98 percent, compared to 90 percent for the combination of CT and EUS ($p = .025$).

Positron emission tomography for staging these cancers remains investigational, but further study may prove it to be a useful adjunct as a preoperative staging tool.

Computed Tomography of the Head and Radionucleotide Bone Scan

Some clinicians routinely perform CT of the head and radionucleotide bone scan imaging in patients

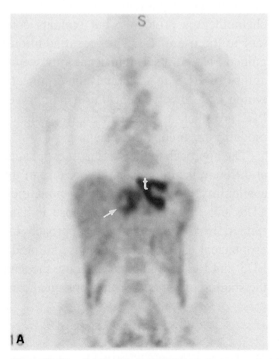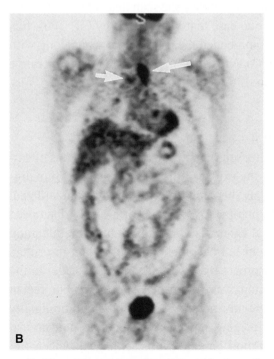

Figure 2–12. Positron emission tomography scans *A,* A tumor (*t*) of the gastroesophageal junction and fundus, with metastatic spread to celiac lymph nodes (confirmed by endoscopic ultrasonography–guided fine-needle aspiration) in same patient shown in Figure 2–6G) (*arrow* indicates celiac lymph node). *B,* A proximal esophageal tumor (*long arrow*) with metastatic spread to a right paraesophageal lymph node (*short arrow*).

with newly diagnosed esophageal carcinoma, on the rationale that it is crucial to rule out distant metastases (M1 disease) in these patients.

In a study from the University of Michigan, the records of 838 patients with esophageal cancer were retrospectively reviewed to assess the frequency and location of metastatic disease at initial presentation.[61] In this cohort, 147 patients (18%) had M1 disease. In 110 (75%) of these 147 patients, distant metastatic disease was detected preoperatively by conventional imaging or clinical examination; in 102 (69%) of the 147 patients, this was detected by CT of the chest or abdomen. The most common site of detected distant metastases was in the intra-abdominal lymph nodes (45%), followed by the liver (35%), lungs (20%), cervical/supraclavicular nodes (18%), bone (9%), adrenals (5%), peritoneum (2%), and brain (2%), and by the stomach, pancreas, pleura, skin/body wall, pericardium, and spleen (each 1%). In this study, neither bone scan nor CT of the head detected unsuspected metastatic disease in any case staged as M0 by chest and abdominal CT.

In a prospective study that compared several different imaging modalities for the preoperative staging assessment of 33 patients with esophageal cancer,[62] radionucleotide bone scan detected a metastatic lesion in one case that was missed by CT. Thus, this study recommended the use of bone scan, along with CT and bronchoscopy, in the standard preoperative evaluation of these patients.

SUMMARY

To provide a reproducible and practical means of categorizing the extent of disease, the staging of malignancies has become internationally standardized. Accurate preoperative staging of a newly diagnosed esophageal cancer is very important in the planning of treatment but becomes most important in centers where treatment may vary according to stage. In the past, staging was performed surgically, but recent technologic advances in radiographic and minimally invasive imaging now permit accurate nonsurgical staging in most patients with esophageal cancer.

Following a tissue confirmation of malignant disease (most commonly performed by UGI endoscopy with biopsy), we recommend that the initial staging evaluation be performed by CT of the chest and abdomen, primarily to rule out distant metastatic disease. In the absence of radiographic evidence of metastatic disease found by CT, EUS should be performed to determine the depth of tumor invasion into the esophageal wall and to identify any locoregional lymph node metastases. Although still investigational, PET seems to add important information about distant metastatic disease undetected by CT and EUS, and this modality may someday replace CT in the staging of gross distant metastases. Bronchoscopy remains important in the evaluation of upper and midthoracic esophageal tumors, to rule out locally advanced stage T4 disease due to direct tracheobronchial invasion, but this could be obviated by the use of EUS. The role of laparoscopy in staging tumors of the esophagogastric junction is currently being investigated, but its role in the assessment of cervical, upper thoracic, and middle thoracic esophageal cancer is minimal. Currently, there does not seem to be a role for bone scan, CT of the head, or MRI.

At this time, we feel that EUS provides accurate locoregional T and N staging in esophageal and esophagogastric-junction tumors, plays a vital role in the triage of patients to surgery or neoadjuvant chemotherapy protocols, but remains complementary to the use of CT. The recent addition of EUS-guided FNA offers a significant improvement in the ability of EUS to accurately determine metastatic lymph node involvement. Further improvements in PET are likely to result in greater reliance on this modality for preoperative staging.

The approach to the staging of esophageal cancer at different institutions varies because of the limited availability of different imaging modalities such as EUS and PET. However, as more individuals are trained in EUS, and as the approach to treating esophageal cancer becomes more tailored to stage, EUS and PET are likely to become the standards in the staging of patients with esophageal cancer.

REFERENCES

1. Pera M, Cameron AJ, Trastek VF, et al. Increasing incidence of adenocarcinoma of the esophagus and esophagogastric junction. Gastroenterology 1993;104:510–3.
2. Blot WJ, Devesa SS, Kneller RW, Fraumeni JF. Rising inci-

dence of adenocarcinoma of the esophagus and gastric cardia. JAMA 1991;265:1287–9.

3. Fleming ID, Cooper JS, Henson DE, et al., editors. AJCC cancer staging manual. 5th ed. American Joint Committee on Cancer. Philadelphia: Lippincott-Raven; 1997.

4. Siewert JR, Stein HJ. Classification of adenocarcinoma of the oesophagogastric junction. Br J Surg 1998;85:1457–9.

5. Siewert JR, Stein HJ. Adenocarcinoma of the gastroesophageal junction. Classification, pathology and extent of resection. Dis Esophagus 1996;9:173–82.

6. Weston AP, Krmpotich PT, Cherian R, et al. Prospective evaluation of intestinal metaplasia and dysplasia within the cardia of patients with Barrett's esophagus. Dig Dis Sci 1997;42:597–602.

7. Aikou T, Shimazu H. Difference in main lymphatic pathways from the lower esophagus and gastric cardia. Jpn J Surg 1989;19:290–5.

8. Tachimori Y, Kato H, Watanabe H, et al. Difference between carcinoma of the lower esophagus and the cardia. World J Surg 1996;20:507–10.

9. Moss AA, Koehler RE, Margulis AR. Initial accuracy of esophagograms in detection of small esophageal carcinoma. AJR Am J Roentgenol 1976;127:909–13.

10. Glazer GM, Gross BH, Quint LE, et al. Normal mediastinal lymph nodes: number and size according to American Thoracic Society mapping. AJR Am J Roentgenol 1985;144:261–5.

11. Thompson WM, Halvorsen RA, Foster WL Jr, et al. Computed tomography for staging esophageal and gastroesophageal cancer: reevaluation. AJR Am J Roentgenol 1983;141:951–8.

12. Lea JW 4th, Prager RL, Bender HW Jr. The questionable role of computed tomography in preoperative staging of esophageal cancer. Ann Thorac Surg 1984;38:479–81.

13. Picus D, Balfe DM, Koehler RE, et al. Computed tomography in the staging of esophageal carcinoma. Radiology 1983;146:433–8.

14. Quint LE, Glazer GM, Orringer MB, Gross BH. Esophageal carcinoma: CT findings. Radiology 1985;155:171–5.

15. Becker CD, Barbier P, Porcellini B. CT evaluation of patients undergoing transhiatal esophagectomy for cancer. J Comput Tomogr 1986;10:607–11.

16. Aibe T, Fuji T, Okita K, Takemoto T. A fundamental study of normal layer structure of the gastrointestinal wall visualized by endoscopic ultrasonography. Scand J Gastroenterol 1986;21 Suppl 123:6–15.

17. Tio TL, Tytgat GNJ. Endoscopic ultrasonography of normal and pathologic upper gastrointestinal wall structure: comparison of studies in vivo and in vitro with histology. Scand J Gastroenterol 1986;21 Suppl 123:27–33.

18. Kimmey MB, Martin RW, Haggitt RC, et al. Histologic correlates of gastrointestinal ultrasound images. Gastroenterology 1989;96:433–41.

19. Botet JF, Lightdale CJ, Zauber AF, et al. Preoperative staging of esophageal cancer: comparison of endoscopic US and dynamic CT. Radiology 1991;181:419–25.

20. Aibe T, Ito T, Yoshida T. Endoscopic ultrasonography of lymph nodes surrounding the upper GI tract. Scand J Gastroenterol 1986;21 Suppl 123:164–9.

21. Tio TL, Cohen P, Coene PP, et al. Endosonography and computed tomography of esophageal carcinoma: preoperative classification compared to the new (1987) TNM system. Gastroenterology 1989;96:1478–86.

22. Lightdale CJ. Practice guidelines: esophageal cancer. Am J Gastroenterol 1999;94:20–9.

23. Rösch T. Endosonographic staging of esophageal cancer: a review of literature results. Gastrointest Endosc Clin N Am 1995;5:537–47.

24. Dittler HJ, Siewert JR. Role of endoscopic ultrasonography in esophageal carcinoma. Endoscopy 1993;25:156–61.

25. Grimm H, Binmoeller K, Hamper K, et al. Endosonography for preoperative locoregional staging of esophageal and gastric cancer. Endoscopy 1993;25:224–30.

26. Hordijk ML, Zander H, van Blankenstein M, Tilanus HW. Influence of tumor stenosis on the accuracy of endosonography in preoperative T staging of esophageal cancer. Endoscopy 1993;25:171–5.

27. Kalantzis N, Kallimanis G, Laoudi F, et al. Endoscopic ultrasonography and computed tomography in preoperative (TNM) classification of oesophageal carcinoma [abstract]. Endoscopy 1992;24:653.

28. Nobre-Leito C, Santos AA, Mides Correia J, Costra Mira F. Esophageal carcinoma: preoperative staging with endosonography [abstract]. Endoscopy 1992;24 Suppl 1:379.

29. Rösch T, Lorenz R, Zenker K, et al. Local staging and assessment of resectability in carcinoma of esophagus, stomach and duodenum by endoscopic ultrasonography. Gastrointest Endosc 1992;38:460–7.

30. Souquet JC, Napoléon B, Pujol B, et al. Endosonography-guided treatment of eosphageal carcinoma. Endoscopy 1992;24 Suppl 1:324–8.

31. Grimm H. Binmoeller KF, Hamper K, Soehendra N. Accuracy of endoscopic ultrasound (EUS) in preoperative staging of esophageal carcinoma [abstract]. Endoscopy 1992;24:652.

32. Fok M, Cheng SWK, Wong J. Endosonography in patient selection for surgical treatment of esophageal carcinoma. World J Surg 1992;16:1098–103.

33. Kallimanis GE, Gupta PK, Al-Kawas FH, et al. Endoscopic ultrasound for staging cancer, with or without dilation, is clinically important and sage. Gastrointest Endosc 1995; 41:540–6.

34. Yoshikane H, Tsukamoto Y, Niwa Y, et al. Superficial esophageal carcinoma: evaluation by endoscopic ultrasonography. Am J Gastroenterol 1994;89:702–7.

35. Souquet JC, Napoléon B, Pujol B, et al. Endoscopic ultrasonography in the preoperative staging of esophageal cancer. Endoscopy 1994;26:764–6.

36. McLoughlin RF, Cooperberg PL, Mathieson JR, et al. High resolution endoluminal ultrasonography in the staging of esophageal carcinoma. J Ultrasound Med 1995;14:725–30.

37. Catalano MF, Sivak MV Jr, Rice T, et al. Endosonographic features predictive of lymph node metastasis. Gastrointest Endosc 1994;409:442–6.

38. Dittler HJ, Fink U, Siewert JR. Response to chemotherapy in esophageal cancer. Endoscopy 1994;26:769–71.

39. Ginsberg GG, Al-Kawas FH, Nguyen CC, et al. Endoscopic ultrasound evaluation of vascular involvement in esophageal cancer: a comparison with computed tomography [abstract]. Gastrointest Endosc 1993;39:276.

40. Chak A, Canto M, Gerdes H, et al. Prognosis of esophageal cancers preoperatively staged to be locally invasive (T4) by endoscopic ultrasound (EUS): a multicenter retrospective cohort study. Gastrointest Endosc 1995;42:501–6.

41. Van Dam J. Endoscopic evaluation of the patient with esophageal carcinoma. In: Wanebo HJ, editor. Surgery for gastrointestinal cancer: a multidisciplinary approach. Philadelphia: Lippincott-Raven Publishers; 1997.

42. Van Dam J, Rice TW, Catalano MF, et al. High-grade malignant stricture is predictive of esophageal tumor stage: risks of endosonographic evaluation. Cancer 1993;71: 2910–7.

43. Chang KJ, Datz KD, Durbin TE, et al. Endoscopic ultrasound-guided fine-needle aspiration. Gastrointest Endosc 1994;40:694–9.

44. Gress FG, Hawes RH, Savides TJ, et al. Endoscopic ultrasound-guided fine-needle aspiration biopsy using linear array and radial scanning endosonography. Gastrointest Endosc 1997;45:243–50.

45. Riedel M, Hauck RW, Stein HJ, et al. Preoperative bronchoscopic assessment of airway invasion by esophageal cancer: a prospective study. Chest 1998;113:687–95.

46. Takashima S, Takeuchi N, Shiozaki H, et al. Carcinoma of the esophagus: CT vs. MR imaging in determining resectability. AJR Am J Roentgenol 1991;156:297–302.

47. Petrillo R, Balzarini L, Bidoli P, et al. Esophageal squamous cell carcinoma: MRI evaluation of mediastinum. Gastrointest Radiol 1990;15:275–8.

48. Quint LE, Glazer GM, Orringer MB. Esophageal imaging by MR and CT: study of normal anatomy and neoplasms. Radiology 1985;156:727–31.

49. Burke EC, Karpeh MS, Conlon KC, Brennan MF. Laparoscopy in the management of gastric adenocarcinoma. Ann Surg 1997;225:262–7.

50. Dagnini G, Caldironi MW, Marin G, et al. Laparoscopy in abdominal staging of esophageal carcinoma: report of 369 cases. Gastrointest Endosc 1986;32:400–2.

51. Mortensen MB, Scheel-Hincke JD, Madsen MR, et al. Combined endoscopic ultrasonography and laparoscopic ultrasonography in the pretherapeutic assessment of resectability in patients with upper gastrointestinal malignancies. Scand J Gastroenterol 1996;31:1115–9.

52. van Dijkum EJMN, de Wit LT, van Delden OM, et al. The efficacy of laparoscopic staging in patients with upper gastrointestinal tumors. Cancer 1997;79:1315–9.

53. Sugarbaker DJ, Jaklitsch MT, Liptay MJ. Thoracoscopic staging and surgical therapy for esophageal cancer. Chest 1995;107:218S–23S.

54. Luketich JD, Schauer P, Landreneau R, et al. Minimally invasive surgical staging is superior to endoscopic ultrasound in detecting lymph node metastases in esophageal cancer. J Thorac Cardiovasc Surg 1997;114:817–23.

55. Luketich JD, Meehan M, Nguyen NT, et al. Minimally invasive surgical staging for esophageal cancer. Surg Endosc 2000;14:700–2.

56. Romijn MG, van Overhagen H, Spillenaar Bilgen EJ, et al. Laparoscopy and laparoscopic ultrasonography in staging of oesophageal and cardial carcinoma. Br J Surg 1998; 85:1010–2.

57. Luketich JD, Schauer PR, Meltzer CC, et al. Role of positron emission tomography in staging esophageal cancer. Ann Thorac Surg 1997;64:765–9.

58. Kole AC, Plukker JT, Nieweg OE, Vaalburg W. Positron emission tomography for staging of oesophageal and gastroesophageal malignancy. Br J Cancer 1998;78:521–7.

59. Luketich JD, Friedman DM, Weigel TL, et al. Evaluation of distant metastases in esophageal cancer: 100 consecutive positron emission tomography scans. Ann Thorac Surg 1999;68:1133–6.

60. Flamen P, Lerut A, Van Cutsem E, et al. Utility of positron emission tomography for the staging of patients with potentially operable esophageal carcinoma. J Clin Oncol 2000;18:3202–10.

61. Quint LE, Hepburn LM, Francis IR, et al. Incidence and distribution of distant metastases from newly diagnosed esophageal carcinoma. Cancer 1995;76:1120–5.

62. Inculet RI, Keller SM, Dwyer A, Roth JA. Evaluation of noninvasive tests for the preoperative staging of carcinoma of the esophagus: a prospective study. Ann Thorac Surg 1985;40:561–5.

3

Molecular Biology of Esophageal Cancer

EZRA E.W. COHEN, MD

CHARLES M. RUDIN, MD, PhD

Cancer of the esophagus remains a leading cause of cancer mortality worldwide. Over 300,000 new cases are reported each year, and the 5-year survival rate is less than 10 percent. Incidence rates vary widely: The majority of cases are recorded in Asia, and localized areas of high incidence are reported in South Africa, France, and Brazil. In the United States, there are an estimated 12,300 new cases per year, with a male-female ratio of 3:1.[1] The majority of cases fall into two distinct histologic types: squamous cell carcinoma (SCC) and adenocarcinoma (ADC). There has been an unexplained dramatic rise in the incidence of ADC in the last two decades throughout the Occident, resulting in an approximately equal number of cases of each type in the United States.

Certain risk factors have been linked to esophageal cancer. Squamous cell carcinoma has been associated with smoking and alcohol use. In the developing world, diet and human papillomavirus may also play a role.[2] In contrast, ADC is not as closely related to tobacco and alcohol use but has been linked with obesity, higher socioeconomic status, and white race.[3] Barrett's esophagus (BE), conversion of the normal squamous epithelium to metaplastic columnar morphology, has been recognized as a predisposing condition to ADC.[4] It is estimated that 10 percent of individuals with BE will develop ADC, with BE conferring a 30- to 125-fold increased risk.[3–6] Despite allelic heterogeneity within tumors and between tumors and adjacent epithelia,[7] there is strong evidence suggesting that BE represents a direct precursor of ADC through clonal proliferation.[8] To illustrate the link between BE and ADC and the predisposing nature of the former lesion, several investigators have examined tumors and adjacent dysplastic tissue and have found identical allelic loss and microsatellite alterations in premalignant and malignant lesions.[3,9]

Intensive work by many groups over the past decade is generating a rapidly expanding body of knowledge of the molecular alterations associated with esophageal cancer. These disparate observations have begun to coalesce into an improved understanding of the basis of this disease, with implications for chemoprevention, early intervention, improved prognostication, and perhaps most importantly, a host of new therapeutic targets for this frustrating disease. This chapter will outline progress in defining molecular pathways implicated in esophageal carcinogenesis. The two principal histologic types, SCC and ADC, will be discussed separately.

ESOPHAGEAL CANCER AND THE G_1 CHECKPOINT

Many of the genetic alterations that contribute to esophageal carcinogenesis involve factors known to mediate critical cell-cycle control mechanisms in the G_1 phase of the cell cycle (Figure 3–1). Although a detailed molecular description of the regulatory mechanisms controlling cell-cycle progression is beyond the scope of this chapter, a brief overview of the critical G_1 regulators may provide a context for the observed alterations described in detail in later sections.

Cell-cycle progression is dependent on an ordered sequence of events required to allow a cell to complete division.[10] Commitment to cell replication is made during the G_1 phase of the cell cycle, following passage through what has been referred to as the "restriction point." The G_1 phase is characterized by high mitogenic responsiveness, cell growth, and protein synthesis as the cell prepares for entry into the S phase (genomic replication).[11]

Cell-cycle progression has been found to be dependent on the activity of a series of kinases called cyclin-dependent kinases (CDKs), which are active only in specific phases of the cell cycle. The predominant G_1 CDKs—CDK4 and CDK6—become active in late G_1 phase upon complexing with their regulatory partner, cyclin D. There are three cyclin D genes: cyclin D1, D2, and D3. Of these, cyclin D1 has been most clearly related to aberrant growth in malignancy.[12] Activity of the G_1 CDKs is highly dependent on stimulation from various mitogenic signaling pathways. Among the critical substrates for cyclin D:CDK4 is the Rb protein. Phosphorylation of Rb by cyclin D:CDK4 is a key determinant of passage through the restriction point and S phase entry (see Figure 3–1B).

Tight control of the activity of the G_1 CDKs to prevent inappropriate or unregulated clonal proliferation is a critical anticancer mechanism. The G_1 CDKs are suppressed by the action of two families of inhibitors: the p21 family (p21, p27, p57) and the p16 or INK4 family (p15, p16, p18, p19) (see Figure 3–1B).[12] In turn, these inhibitors are themselves subject to complex regulation. For example, the p21 gene is transcriptionally induced by the critical tumor-suppressor p53, leading to cell-cycle arrest upon p53 expression. Expression of p21 is used as a measure of intact p53 functional activity following p53-inducing stimuli such as deoxyribonucleic acid (DNA) damage; p21 can also be induced by p53-independent mechanisms that are less well characterized to date.

Activity of cyclin D:CDK4 in the G_1 phase of the cell cycle therefore serves as an integrator of multiple signals determining whether a cell is to undergo replication, remain quiescent, or undergo cell death. These signals include cell surface–mediated growth factor signaling cascades, sensors of cellular metabolic reserve, and monitors of genomic integrity. The cancer cell can evade these regulatory mechanisms in many ways. Loss of p53 function leads to loss of appropriate responses to DNA damage (including loss of critical cell death responses) as well as to loss of G_1 arrest mediated through p21 (see Figure 3–1B). Inactivation of p16 or other related inhibitors leads to deregulated cyclin:CDK activity and cell proliferation. Mutations in growth factor receptor signaling pathways lead to the perceived constitutive activity of these signals and inappropriate cell-cycle entry. Finally, activating muta-

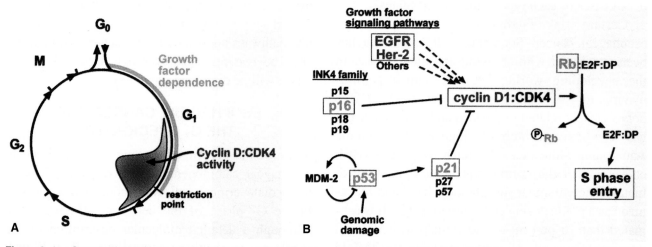

Figure 3–1. Genetic alterations in esophageal cancer affect G_1 cell-cycle progression. *A,* Diagrammatic representation of the phases of the cell cycle. The highly growth factor–dependent period of the G_1 phase prior to passage through the restriction point is indicated in orange. Activity of the critical cyclin D1:CDK4 complex is highly cell-cycle dependent and is schematically indicated in green. *B,* Regulatory factors controlling late G_1 phase cell-cycle progression. Oncogenes found to be frequently up-regulated in esophageal malignancy are indicated in green; tumor-suppressor genes frequently inactivated are indicated in red. This figure does not distinguish squamous cell carcinoma from adenocarcinoma. Details regarding specific genetic alterations may be found in the text. (CDK4 = cyclin-dependent kinase 4; EGFR = epidermal growth factor receptor.)

tions of cyclin D or loss of the suppressive function of Rb can directly lead to loss of G_1 cell-cycle control and unregulated proliferation. Mutations in genes contributing to the multiple branches of this web of interactions are discussed later.

CYTOGENETICS

Cytogenetic analyses represent the largest body of work to date on the molecular alterations associated with esophageal carcinogenesis. Identification of common sites of gross chromosomal alteration in premalignant and malignant tissue provides insight both into the locations of genes that are critical to malignant growth and into the order in which these genetic alterations occur in the process of carcinogenesis. Sites of consistent genetic amplification are likely to contain oncogenes with deregulated activity in can-

cers. In contrast, sites of consistent loss of heterozygosity (LOH) may contain tumor-suppressor genes that are inactivated in cancers. Patterns of chromosomal alteration also provide information on whether the genetic alterations associated with a particular cancer derive primarily from chromosomal instability or defects in fidelity of replication (microsatellite instability). The chromosomal alterations and the genes located therein associated with esophageal cancer are listed in Table 3–1.

Flow cytometry studies have consistently revealed high degrees of aneuploidy in esophageal SCC. Robaszkiewicz and colleagues demonstrated aneuploidy in up to 90 percent of tumor cells in poorly differentiated cancers while 91 percent of their samples contained some degree of DNA content derangement.[13] The link between alterations in gross DNA content and either tumor behavior or carcinogenic pro-

Table 3–1. LOCALIZATION, FUNCTION, AND PATHOGENESIS OF GENETIC ALTERATIONS IN ESOPHAGEAL CANCER

Chromosome	Gene*	Alternative Names	Function†	Alteration
2p21	MSH2	hMSH-2	DNA repair	LOH
3p21	β-Catenin	CTNNB1	Cellular adhesion, gene transcription	—
3p21	MLH1	hMLH-1	DNA repair	LOH
5q21	APC	FAP gene	Tumor suppressor	LOH
6p12	VEGF	—	Endothelial cell growth factor	—
6p21	p21	WAF1, CIP1	Tumor suppressor	—
7p12-13	EGFR	c-erb B1, Her-1	Growth factor receptor	Gene amplification, up-regulation
7p22	PDGFa	—	Growth factor	—
8q24	Myc	—	Regulates transcription of cell growth genes	Gene amplification
9p21	p16	INK4a, CDKN2, CDKN2A, CDK4I, MTS1	Tumor suppressor	LOH, mutation, hypermethylation
9p21	p15	CDKN2b, INK4b, MTS2	Tumor suppressor	LOH
11q13	Cyclin D1	PRAD1, EXP2, CCND1	Promotes transition from G_1 to S phase	Gene amplification
11q13	FGF	hst-1, bFGF	Growth factor	—
11q13	HBGF	int-2	Growth factor	—
12p13	p27	KIP1	Tumor suppressor	—
13q14	Rb	Retinoblastoma	Inhibits entry into S phase	LOH, mutation
16q22	E-cadherin	CDH1	Cellular adhesion	—
17p13	p53	—	Tumor suppressor	LOH, mutation
17q21	Her-2	EGFR2, c-erb B2	Growth factor receptor	Gene amplification
18q21	DPC4	—	TGF-β pathway	LOH
18q21	Bcl-2	—	Antiapoptotic	—
18q21	DCC	—	Cellular adhesion	LOH
19q13	Bax	Bcl-2 associated X	Proapoptotic	—
22q13	PDGFb	c-sis	Growth factor	—
—	Bcl-x$_L$	—	Antiapoptotic	—

APC = adenomatous polyposis coli; DCC = deleted-in-colon-cancer; DNA = deoxyribonucleic acid; DPCH = deleted-in-pancreatic-cancer-locus-4; EGFR = epidermal growth factor receptor; FGF = fibroblast growth factor; HBGF = heparin-binding growth factor; LOH = loss of heterozygosity; PDGF = platelet-derived growth factor; TGF-β = transforming growth factor-β; VEGF = vascular endothelial growth factor.

*Name as referred to in text.
†See text for details.

gression has remained somewhat controversial.[2,14]

Several series have examined the frequency of LOH in SCC in an attempt to delineate candidate genes involved in carcinogenesis.[15] Loss of heterozygosity has been reported to occur most frequently at 5q, 13q, 17p, and 18q.[16–18] Of these, 17p loss appears most commonly (50 to 62% of cases) and is thought to correspond with p53 gene deletion.

Aneuploidy has also been reported to occur at high rates in ADC,[4,5] reflecting the accumulation of genetic alterations in the progression from dysplasia to carcinoma. Aneuploidy appears as an early event in the progression to ADC and is found more frequently as a lesion advances.[7,19,20] In a retrospective review of 80 patients with ADC, Nakamura and colleagues found a rate of aneuploidy of 86 percent and correlated this with lymph node metastasis.[21] Reid and colleagues found that more advanced lesions were more likely to be aneuploid[22] and that patients who had aneuploid BE lesions were far more likely to develop high-grade dysplasia or ADC (69% vs 0%).[23,24] Moreover, there appeared to be multiple aneuploid clones in each tumor, reflecting the association between aneuploidy and global genomic instability.

Several authors examined the loss or gain of specific chromosomes or alleles. Two independent studies demonstrated gains at 8q and 20q.[7,19] The c-*myc* oncogene is located within the amplified region on 8q. Losses are frequently observed at 17p, 5q, 9p,

13q, 18q, and 3p.[3,7,25–27] These sites represent putative tumor-suppressor genes, and their significance is discussed below. Once again, loss of 17p is the most frequently reported, with a prevalence of up to 100 percent.

There are several areas of LOH that are emerging as novel potential loci of undefined tumor-suppressor genes. One of these regions is located on 17q.[26–28] Swift and colleagues observed LOH in 56 percent of their patients at 17q whereas Dolan and colleagues and Petty and colleagues demonstrated loss of a distal locus on this arm. Of interest, tylosis, a disorder of palmoplantar keratoderma associated with SCC of the esophagus, has been linked to distal 17q loss. The implication of this finding in ADC has yet to be clarified.

CELL-CYCLE REGULATORS

Specific genes altered during carcinogenesis fall into one of two categories: proto-oncogenes that are overexpressed or tumor-suppressor genes that are inactivated (Figure 3–2). Oncogene overexpression has been shown to derive from gene amplification, increased gene transcription, or the inhibition of degradative pathways. Loss of tumor-suppressor gene activity may occur through gene deletion, mutation, or promoter hypermethylation. This section will review the modifications of specific oncogenes and

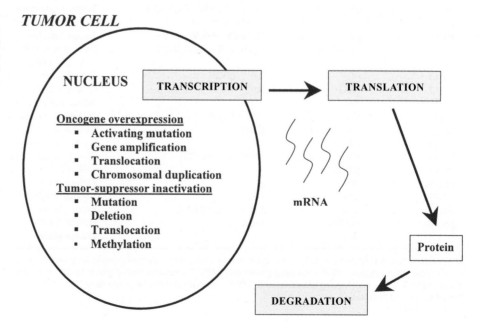

Figure 3–2. Altered protein expression in cancer cells. Expression of factors regulating oncogenesis can be altered by changes in the level of gene transcription, messenger ribonucleic acid (mRNA) translation, protein degradation, or protein structure.

tumor-suppressors directly associated with the regulation of cell-cycle entry in esophageal cancer.

Mutation of p53

Mutation of p53 is one of the most frequently observed mutations in human cancer,[29] and this gene has been extensively investigated in esophageal cancer. The LOH studies discussed above suggest that loss of p53 (located on 17p) is a significant event in both SCC and ADC.

The incidence of p53 mutation in SCC has been reported to be as high as 93 percent[30] but is likely closer to 50 percent overall.[2,15] The mutation rate seems to increase in dysplastic mucosa, with the risk of subsequent malignant transformation reported at rates as high as 80 percent.[15,30–33] Mutations most commonly occur in the DNA-binding region of the protein encoded by exons 5 through 8.[2,32] A variety of less frequent mutations outside this core domain have also been reported. Approximately 31 to 41 percent of mutations have been reported to occur at A: (adenine: thymine) base pairs[15,31] and are changes similar to those induced by acetaldehyde, a cellular metabolite of ethanol. An additional 15 percent of cases display mutations characteristic of other tobacco-related malignancies. In contrast, C (cytosine) to T (thymine) transitions, the predominant type of mutation in the more distal gastrointestinal malignancies, are found in only 10 to 18 percent of esophageal SCCs.[15,34] A direct correlation between the incidence of p53 mutation and tobacco exposure has been noted.

Several studies have attempted to address the timing of p53 mutation in the process of carcinogenesis. Analogous to other mucosal tumors, squamous carcinogenesis in the esophagus is thought to progress through distinct histologic stages of hyperplasia, dysplasia, and carcinoma in situ (Figure 3–3). Shi and colleagues examined the prevalence of p53 mutation in tumor tissue and adjacent mucosa from 43 patients after resection of SCC.[32] An increased incidence of p53 mutation was noted as the histology changed from hyperplasia to dysplasia and from dysplasia to carcinoma. Additionally, all the mutations found in early lesions were present in the corresponding SCC. Shi and colleagues concluded that dysplasia is indeed a precancerous lesion and that p53 mutation

is frequently an early event in tumorigenesis. Individual pre-invasive lesions can contain heterogeneous p53 mutations, reflecting the strong selective pressure for loss of the critical tumor-suppressor gene and the genetic instability of these lesions.[35]

Consistent with the results of p53 sequencing, immunohistochemically detectable abnormality of p53 expression also demonstrates progressive increase from normal epithelium to hyperplasia to dysplasia. No clear correlation between p53 immunostaining and the expression of other factors involved in the G_1 checkpoint (p21, p16, Rb) has been evident.[33] Some authors have noted an overexpression of p53 (considered evidence of mutant p53), particularly at the periphery of tumor nests, in a pattern distinct from p21 staining.[2,33] Mutation of p53 appears to precede Rb loss: Rb LOH is frequent in tumors with p53 mutation and is rarely seen in the context of wild-type p53.[36]

The prognostic value of p53 alteration remains controversial. Some authors have noted a worse prognosis when p53 is overexpressed.[37–40] However, in only two of these studies did p53 retain its prognostic significance after multivariate analysis. Others have noted a shorter survival when p53 is not expressed.[41] Still other studies have failed to show a survival correlation with p53.[42–45] It is notable that when several markers are examined simultaneously (as in the latter studies), p53 expression begins to lose prognostic value. As with other tumor types, the disparity in reported results of p53 analysis may be partly explained by differences in technique or interpretation, as well as by difficulty in correlating various assays with p53 functional status.

The incidence of p53 deletion in ADC is, as mentioned, quite high. Mutation rates at this locus range in the literature from 45 to 75 percent.[20,46] Kubba and colleagues reviewed publications from 1988 to 1998.[47] Of the 364 ADC samples analyzed, 63.4 percent displayed evidence of p53 mutation. The vast majority of these mutations were found within the DNA-binding site of the protein, exons 5 to 8.[15,48] A remarkable 80 percent of these mutations involved base transitions at CpG dinucleotides, a higher frequency than reported even for other adenocarcinomas.[15,49]

As it became increasingly evident that BE was a precursor lesion of ADC, researchers have attempted to place the p53 mutation in the metaplasia-dysplasia-carcinoma sequence (see Figure 3–3B) and to order its occurrence relative to other genetic alterations. Mutation of the p53 gene can occur early in this histologic progression, and it becomes more prevalent as lesions advance. Ramel and colleagues found a 5 percent mutation rate in Barrett's metaplasia, a 15 percent rate in low-grade dysplasia, a 45 percent rate in high-grade dysplasia, and a 53 percent rate in ADC; several other groups subsequently reported similar frequencies.[46,50–52] Identical mutations have been reported in dysplastic and malignant epithelium from the same individuals,[52] highlighting the clonal relationship between invasive tumors and the surrounding dysplastic lesion, which can expand to involve large areas of epithelium.[48]

Mutation of the p53 locus typically appears to precede the development of aneuploidy. Alteration of p53 can be detected in diploid cell populations within dysplastic mucosa. These cells demonstrate an increased propensity to arrest at the G_2 phase (thought to be indicative of aberrant replicative cycles), with subsequent development of aneuploidy and progression to carcinoma.[24,52,53]

Distinct aspects of G_1 cell-cycle progression are regulated by p53 and p16. Repression of p16 or deletion of its chromosomal arm (9p) is another frequent finding (discussed below). Alterations of these two genes are often found in concert although the mechanisms of their inactivation are likely different.[54,55] It is difficult to ascertain which genetic aberration occurs first, but one study was able to detect 9p LOH preceding 17p LOH in their samples.[55] Recent evidence suggests that 9p LOH (corresponding to p16 inactivation) most often precedes 17p LOH (corresponding to p53 inactivation). Both lesions have been reported to precede 5q, 13q, and 18q LOH,[54,56–58] and clones without p53 or p16 abnormalities fail to progress.

The prognostic value of p53 determination has also been analyzed in the context of ADC. Casson

Figure 3–3. Esophageal carcinogenesis progresses through defined morphologic stages. *A,* Squamous cell carcinogenesis typically develops in the upper portion of the esophagus through stages of progressive squamous dysplasia. The surrounding dysplastic lesion and even the histologically normal mucosa may share some of the characteristic clonal alterations of the fully transformed malignancy. *B,* Adenocarcinoma frequently arises in regions of gastric or intestinal metaplasia (Barrett's esophagus) in the lower portion of the esophagus. Barrett's metaplasia is thought to progress through stages demonstrating no dysplasia, low-grade dysplasia, and high-grade dysplasia, ultimately progressing to invasive adenocarcinoma.

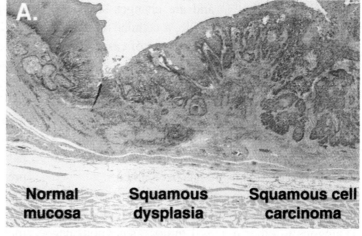

Normal mucosa   Squamous dysplasia   Squamous cell carcinoma

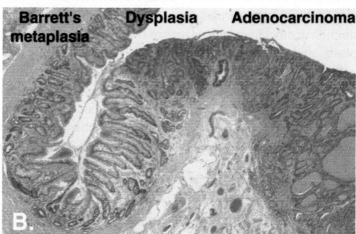

Barrett's metaplasia   Dysplasia   Adenocarcinoma

and colleagues studied 52 patients prospectively and found p53 mutation to be a poor prognostic indicator, even by multivariate analysis.[59] This has been upheld by others,[60] but the finding is not universal.[15,47]

Taken together, these findings support the hypothesis that p53 alteration occurs frequently as an early event in the tumor progression of both SCC and ADC. Field cancerization—the concept that the entire mucosal field subject to carcinogenic exposure contains many independent lesions in different stages of malignant progression—is supported by the presence of heterogeneous p53 mutations at distant sites within histologically normal epithelium.

Expression of p21

The p21 gene functions as a tumor-suppressor gene transcriptionally regulated by both p53-dependent and p53-independent mechanisms.[61] As discussed above, p21 functions as a CDK inhibitor, causing arrest predominantly in the G_1 phase of the cell cycle.[62,63] Inactivation of the p21 gene may partly mimic the loss of p53. The role of this gene has been more extensively studied in SCC than in ADC.

Expression of p21 is retained in approximately 50 percent of SCC tumors.[44,64–66] Whereas p21 is expressed predominantly in the basal cell layer in normal esophageal mucosa, its expression in neoplastic tissue has been reported to be limited to the upper epithelial layers.[64,67] The significance of this finding has yet to be determined. In cells with evidence of p53 mutation, p21 continues to be expressed, implying p53-independent regulation.[64]

Sequence analysis of p21 in esophageal cancers in a population in India found that 84 percent of the patients exhibited variation at codon 149, significantly higher than 16 percent of 50 normal individuals.[68] The polymorphism at this codon occurred almost exclusively when p53 was not mutated, suggesting that this alteration may play a significant role in the p53-dependent p21 regulatory pathway.

As discussed above, the correlation between p53 expression and survival is difficult to demonstrate. Therefore, a number of investigators have examined its downstream effector for its prognostic value and have found that p21 expression does appear to have a stronger predictive value than p53 in multivariate analyses.[41,44,65,69,70] Five-year survival rates were 68 percent and 31 percent in high and low p21 expressers, respectively.[70] Furthermore, p21 also predicted survival after adjuvant chemotherapy: 5-year survival rates for p21-positive and p21-negative tumors were 50 percent and 13 percent, respectively.[41] An outlying study of 172 surgically treated patients, however, found high p21 expression to be surprisingly correlated with poor survival.[67]

Relatively little is known about p21 expression in ADC. It appears that p21 levels are high in dysplasia and increase progressively in ADC. Once again, there is evidence of a p53-independent phenomenon that may not be effective at halting tumor proliferation because of other molecular derangements or other critical p53-dependent pathways.[71] Paradoxically, p21-negative tumors have been associated with improved survival in at least one study.[72]

Alteration of p27

The p21 family member p27 appears to be an important tumor-suppressor gene in a number of solid tumors.[73] Decreased levels of p27 have been reported in about 40 percent of SCCs;[43,74,75] few reports exist on p27 alteration in ADC. Loss of p27 is rarely a feature of metaplasia but has been found in intermediate-stage lesions.[43] Conflicting studies have correlated p27 loss with worsened survival,[74] no effect on survival,[75] and improved survival.[76] These disparate results illustrate the relatively few data available on p27 and (in all likelihood) the minor role it plays in esophageal carcinogenesis.

Alteration of p16 and p15

Like p21 and p27, these INK4 family members inhibit the cyclin D CDK4/6 complex and promote G_1 cell-cycle arrest.[77] In addition to loss of function through LOH or mutation, hypermethylation of the p16 promoter region seems to play an important role in silencing its transcription in many cancers.[78,79] This gene has been extensively studied in both SCC and ADC. Alteration of p15 has not been well defined but is discussed here because of the similarity in these two proteins' function and their location at 9p21.

Loss of heterozygosity of the 9p chromosome occurs in 30 to 50 percent of SCCs.[80] Reduction of p16 expression has a reported incidence of approximately 50 to 86 percent.[33,43,74,81–83] The greater extent of functional inactivation than LOH appears to be due primarily to promoter hypermethylation.[2] In a Chinese population, Xing and colleagues documented hypermethylation in 50 percent of their cases while rarely finding p16 mutation. Others have reported similar findings.[84,85] The relatively rare mutations discovered in p16 have usually been in the coding regions of exons 1 and 2.[15,86,87]

Whether p16 expression is predictive of survival is controversial. It has most often been studied in this respect with other cell-cycle control proteins, and for the most part, it has not proved to be prognostic in multivariate analysis.[74] Nevertheless, some authors have correlated its decreased expression with poorer survival[2,83] but note that further studies need to be done.

Much less is known about p15, other than that deletion seems to be the major mechanism of aberrant expression.[80,84] Of interest, hypermethylation of p15 has also been observed (17% incidence), but only in the company of p16 hypermethylation.[80]

Loss of p16 expression has been studied at all stages of premalignant progression. The fact that p16 and p15 are located in proximity to each other on 9p21 makes it difficult to discern which protein derangement plays a more significant role in carcinogenesis. However, it is believed that underexpression of p16 is a significant event in the progression to ADC.[55] Loss of heterozygosity of 9p is found in 50 to 90 percent of ADC samples.[3,26,54,55,88,89] One contrasting study, on a Japanese population, found only 1 of its 34 ADC samples lacking in p16 expression,[81] but this is inconsistent with the majority of reports.

The rate of 9p loss increases significantly as lesions progress from BE to ADC,[54] with rates of 9p LOH as high as 59 percent found in BE.[55] In BE, 9p LOH can be found before 17p LOH,[55] and it appears to typically precede aneuploidy in the evolution of cancer.[56,88] The significance of 9p LOH was further illustrated when specimens from sequential biopsies of neoplastic lesions were examined; 9p LOH and p16 mutation or hypermethylation appear to be early events in carcinogenesis, preceding LOH at 5q and 13q.[56] As noted previously, clones that did not have alterations in either p53 or p16 did not progress to cancer. Other authors have also demonstrated the importance of p16 loss in the promotion of widespread genomic instability.[26,89]

Inactivation of p16 in ADC, as in SCC, is accomplished by hypermethylation[90] and (to a lesser extent) by mutation.[88] In contrast to SCC, however, mutation of p16 in ADC is not a rare event, being present in approximately 25 percent of samples.

Cyclin D1

The cyclin D1 gene, located on chromosome 11q13, encodes a protein that complexes with a cyclin-dependent protein kinase (CDK) to phosphorylate Rb and promote a cell's advancement from the G_1 phase to the S phase (see Figure 3–1B).[15] Overexpression of cyclin D1 is thought to override the G_1 checkpoint, driving tumor cell proliferation. Its significance in SCC has been extensively studied, but its role in ADC is less clear.

Cyclin D1 overexpression in esophageal SCC has been reported in 23 to 73 percent of tumor samples, with the larger series finding a prevalence of approximately 40 percent.[39,65,82,83,85,91–95] The level of expression appears to be relatively constant between dysplastic lesions and carcinomas, with aberrant expression preceding the alteration of several other oncogenes.[43] Expression of cyclin D1 correlates with markers of proliferation, suggesting that this protein may be vital for tumor progression.[82]

Cyclin D1 overexpression frequently appears to result from gene amplification. Two studies from Italy and Japan demonstrated cyclin D1 gene amplification rates of 31 percent in 55 and 45 patients, respectively.[85,96] Cyclin D1 gene amplification correlates well with messenger ribonucleic acid (mRNA) and protein overexpression.[96,97]

Several authors have analyzed cyclin D1 expression as a prognostic tool, examining rates of local recurrence, lymph node metastasis, distant spread, and survival. Shimada and colleagues[98] examined the expression of 11 different molecular markers in 116 patients who underwent curative esophagectomy. Despite its retrospective nature and a single method of tissue analysis (immunohistochemistry), their research supported cyclin D1, E-cadherin, and cell regrowth capability as independent prognostic factors. Others correlated cyclin D1 overexpression with recurrence in distant organs and shortened survival.[83,95,96] Three series examined the relationship of cyclin D1 with survival after therapy including surgery, chemotherapy, radiotherapy, or a combination of these.[42,91,99] All three series found a lower survival rate when cyclin D1 was overexpressed. When patients are pooled irrespectively of stage or treatment, cyclin D1 positivity still confers a worse prognosis.[75,92,93] In fact, only two studies failed to show a correlation between cyclin D1 and survival.[39,65] Despite the retrospective nature of the data, the various analytic techniques employed, and the fact that each study was single institutional, the bulk of the evidence strongly supports cyclin D1 overexpression as a negative prognostic factor for SCC.

Cyclin D1 overexpression in ADC has been observed,[3,100] with rates as high as 92 percent. The mechanism of overexpression appears distinct as gene amplification seems to play an insignificant role.[85] Information on the predictive or prognostic value of cyclin D1 in ADC is lacking.

Retinoblastoma Protein

Retinoblastoma (Rb) protein is a critical negative regulator of cell entry into the S phase. Induction of Rb by phosphorylation (in normal cells) or mutation/deletion (in cancer cells) releases a constraint on transcription and allows the cell cycle to proceed. Altered expression of Rb is a feature of many malignancies and has been studied in both major subtypes of esophageal cancer.

From 30 to 50 percent of esophageal SCC cases exhibit reduced expression of Rb.[2] Loss of heterozygosity is an important mechanism underlying this process and is more frequent in the presence of other genetic alterations, including p53 mutation, cyclin D1 overexpression, and p16 underexpression.[36,43] In fact, Rb alteration appears to be a relatively late phenomenon in SCC.

Examination of outcomes in relation to Rb expression has yielded conflicting results. Some authors have noted poorer survival in patients with Rb-negative tumors[85,101] although this finding does not hold in multivariate analysis. Furthermore, other authors have reported no correlation between Rb and survival.[40,93] Overall, the findings suggest that Rb alteration is a late event in SCC tumorigenesis and may result from widespread genetic instability in many cases.

Loss of heterozygosity in Rb can be demonstrated in 35 to 50 percent of ADC cases.[5,102] Although Rb loss occurs in early lesions and although the rate of loss increases in dysplasia and carcinoma,[103] the significance of this event in ADC progression or aggressiveness in not known.

GROWTH FACTOR RECEPTORS

In addition to factors that directly regulate cell-cycle progression, a second major class of oncogenic factors is comprised of cell surface–bound growth factor receptors and their soluble ligands. Several of the critical growth factor receptors fall into a class known as receptor tyrosine kinases due to their related signaling mechanisms.[104] There has been tremendous progress recently in the understanding of the role of the receptor tyrosine kinase family of growth factor receptors in cancer. Over 50 receptor tyrosine kinases have been identified in mammalian cells, and many of these receptors and their cognate growth factor ligands have been implicated in carcinogenesis. Many tumors express both a receptor and its ligand, leading to an autocrine growth stimulus; tumors have also been found to induce surrounding stromal cells to secrete growth factors (Figure 3–4). The two receptor tyrosine kinases that have been most extensively studied are the closely related epidermal growth factor receptor (EGFR, also known as c-erb B1) and epidermal growth facor receptor 2 (EGFR2, also known as Her-2 or c-erb B2).

Epidermal Growth Factor Receptor

The EGFR ligands epidermal growth factor (EGF) and transforming growth factor-α (TGF-α) stimulate the growth of SCC.[2] Although there is little evidence to suggest that growth factors themselves are overexpressed in SCC, several authors have documented the amplification and up-regulation of EGFR. Recent data suggest that EGFR is highly expressed in 40 to 70 percent of SCC cases.[45,105–107] Itakura and colleagues demonstrated overexpression

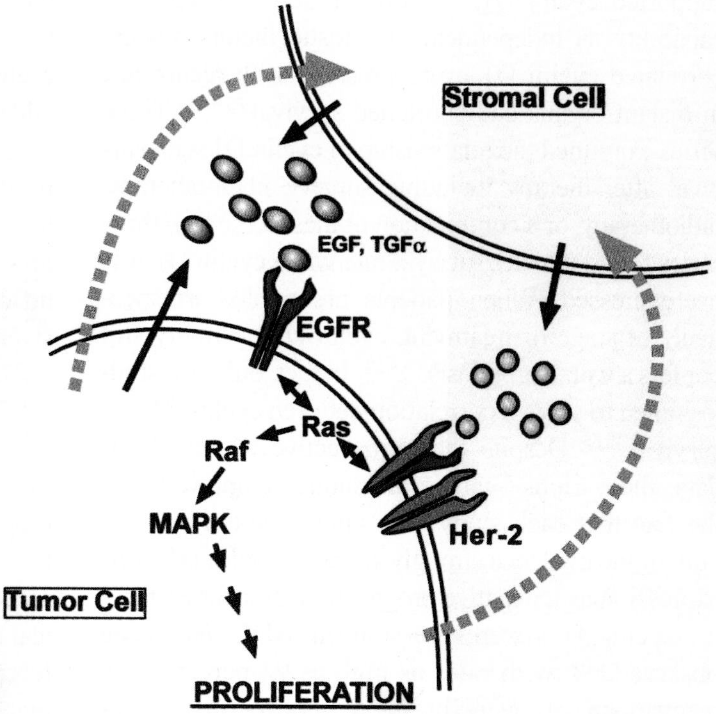

Figure 3–4. Secretion of growth factors by tumor and stromal cells. *Black arrows* represent the secretion of growth factors by tumor or stromal cells. *Gray arrows* represent the secretion of chemokines by tumor cells to induce stromal cells to secrete growth factors. Stimulation of growth factor receptors leads to the activation of tyrosine kinases that in turn activate internal pathways (ras, raf, and mitogen-activated protein [MAP] kinase) to promote cell proliferation. Both epidermal growth factor (EGF) and transforming growth factor-α (TGF-α) can stimulate the epidermal growth factor receptor (EGFR). Although the Her-2 receptor can homodimerize, no known ligand for the homodimeric receptor has been defined. Her-2 can heterodimerize to signal with EGFR (as shown) or with other EGFR family members (not shown). (MAPK = MAP kinase.)

of EGFR in 71 percent of primary tumors and 88 percent of lymph node metastases analyzed. They noted gene amplification in 21 percent of the tumors, which universally corresponded with overexpression.[105] When comparing malignant mucosa with normal mucosa, Friess and colleagues revealed a fourfold increase in EGFR mRNA levels, again corresponding to receptor overexpression.[106]

The impact of overexpression of EGFR on survival is controversial, but most studies show a negative correlation. Two retrospective postresection studies found 5-year survival rates of 38 percent and 14 percent in EGFR-positive patients as opposed to 68 percent and 69 percent survival rates in EGFR-negative patients.[45,72] In fact, the study by Inada and colleagues found a 5-year survival rate of 91.7 percent when the primary tumor was EGFR negative and E-cadherin positive (discussed below). There is also a tendency for EGFR-expressing tumors to have higher degrees of local invasion,[45] hematogenous recurrence,[98] and lymph node metastasis.[105] Other investigators, however, have failed to show an influence of EGFR on survival.[106,107]

There is evidence of involvement of the EGFR signaling pathway in ADC although the number of studies available is less than for SCC. Both TGF-α and EGFR are overexpressed in BE, with increasing prevalence in dysplasia and ADC.[5,108–110] This is partly accomplished through gene amplification[109] rather than by re-arrangement.[15] Although alteration of EGFR signaling has been correlated with lymph node metastasis, it does not appear to have independent value as a prognostic marker in cases of ADC.[5,106,109,110]

Epidermal growth factor receptor 2 (or Her-2) has received attention for its role in ADC of the breast. Research into its expression and significance has extended to other malignancies (especially ADCs). It is now also the target of a monoclonal antibody, trastuzumab, which has shown efficacy in breast cancer trials. Thus, it is not surprising that Her-2 has been more extensively studied and plays a more significant role in ADC than in SCC. A ligand for the homodimeric Her-2 receptor has not been identified; Her-2 has been shown to heterodimerize with at least three other EGFR family members and is believed to signal predominantly through these heterodimeric receptor complexes.

Approximately 10 to 20 percent of esophageal cancers overexpress Her-2, with SCC being at the lower end of that range and ADC at the upper. In SCC, Her-2 positivity does not appear to predict behavior, correlate with histologic or molecular abnormalities, or alter prognosis.[111,112]

Conversely, in ADC, Her-2 expression correlates with aneuploidy[20,21] and has been used to prospectively predict which lesions will progress to cancer.[113] Gene amplification has been found to be the principal mechanism underlying overexpression.[109,114] In three separate multivariate analyses, Her-2 status remained independently prognostic.[21,114,115]

Other Growth Factors and Growth Factor Receptors

Epidermal growth factor receptor and Her-2 have been the most intensely investigated molecules in this area, but researchers are beginning to appreciate the role of other related signaling pathways, including those activated by vascular endothelial growth factor (VEGF), fibroblast growth factor (FGF), platelet-derived growth factor (PDGF), and heparin-binding growth factor (HBGF). Vascular endothelial growth factor is up-regulated in both SCC and ADC. Koide and colleagues found that VEGF was overexpressed in 58 percent of 52 patients with SCC and that this correlated with venous invasion, lymph node metastasis, and survival.[116] In ADC, increased VEGF expression appears in metaplastic lesions and more frequently in invasive tumors.[117]

Fibroblast growth factor and HBGF have also been linked to metastatic disease and are often coamplified as a result of their proximity to each other on 11q13.[15,117] Another study examining PDGF found its expression to correlate with microvessel count, VEGF levels, venous invasion, and survival in SCC patients.[118] At this point, the data on these growth factors and their receptors are sparse and preliminary. More information will need to be gathered before firm conclusions can be made regarding the role of these molecules in esophageal cancer.

ADHESION MOLECULES

The two protein families in this category that have been best studied in esophageal cancer are the cadherins and the catenins. The cadherin family of transmembrane glycoproteins is involved in maintaining cell-cell adhesion. In this regard, E-cadherin appears to be particularly important in mucosal tissues.[119] E-cadherin is anchored to the cytoskeleton by cytoplasmic proteins, including the α-, β-, and γ-catenins (Figure 3–5). Down-regulation of cellular adhesion molecules may facilitate cell migration and has been implicated in cancer metastasis.[120]

β-Catenin has been shown to have critical functions other than cell adhesion.[121,122] Accumulation of cytoplasmic β-catenin leads to translocation of the protein to the nucleus, where it complexes with DNA-binding transcription factors (see Figure 3–5). The activation of these transcription factors by β-catenin appears to both inhibit apoptosis and promote cellular proliferation.[123] The tumor-suppressor function of the adenomatous polyposis coli (APC) gene appears to depend on its ability to bind cytoplasmic β-catenin, promoting its degradation. Inactivation of the APC gene, therefore, may lead to the accumulation and nuclear transposition of β-catenin. It has been recognized that it may be important not only to measure

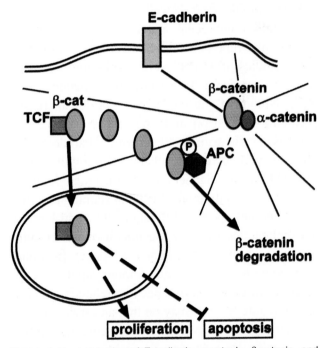

Figure 3–5. Interaction of E-cadherin, α-catenin, β-catenin, and adenomatous polyposis coli (APC). E-cadherin normally interacts with α-catenin and β-catenin to attach to the cellular cytoskeleton. When E-cadherin is intact, β-catenin is phosphorylated and forms a complex with APC for degradation. Free β-catenin otherwise accumulates in the cytoplasm and becomes associated with TCF. This complex can be transported to the nucleus where it can inhibit apoptosis and promote deoxyribonucleic acid (DNA) transcription.

levels of these proteins in malignant cells but also to ascertain their distribution within the cell.[119]

E-cadherin expression is lost or reduced in 45 to 80 percent of SCC, with lower levels correlating with the extent of metastasis.[45,98,124–126] Some observers have noted that as cells become less differentiated, E-cadherin localization shifts to the cytoplasm, especially at the invading edge of the tumor.[119] The mechanism underlying these alterations has not been elucidated.

E-cadherin expression has been linked to prognosis in several studies. A multivariate analysis of 11 molecular markers found E-cadherin to be prognostic of survival.[98] Tamura and colleagues examined E-cadherin expression in 62 patients and found that those who had low levels of expression were more likely to have histologic evidence of blood vessel invasion, had higher rates of hematogenous metastasis, and had higher rates of mortality. Others have reported similar findings, with 5-year survival rates of 87 percent versus 19 percent in E-cadherin–positive and E-cadherin–negative patients, respectively.[45] These results have been observed in low-risk geographic areas as well.[127]

In light of the recent appreciation of the multiple intracellular functions of β-catenin, many of the previous studies of its pattern of expression may need to be reconsidered. In a study of 22 patients with SCC, Ninomiya and colleagues reported increased β-catenin expression in 14 percent of patients and decreased expression in 40 percent.[128] Paradoxically, all cases with lowered levels also had a mutation of the APC gene. Sanders and colleagues found a decrease in membranous β-catenin staining as carcinomas became poorly differentiated,[119] and Kimura and colleagues found a fourfold increase in cytoplasmic staining in carcinomas.[129] As yet, β-catenin mutations have not been demonstrated, and β-catenin expression has not been correlated with clinical outcome.[126,129] It may be that as carcinogenesis proceeds, β-catenin shifts from being membrane associated at E-cadherin adhesion sites to accumulating in the cytoplasm, with subsequent nuclear translocation.

Several authors have demonstrated lower E-cadherin expression in the progression of BE to ADC.[130–132] Loss of heterozygosity at the E-cadherin

locus has been observed in 65 percent of ADC cases, but mutations in this gene appear to be rare.[133] As with SCC, a change in β-catenin expression from the membrane to the cytoplasm has also been observed.[131] Only one study has been able to correlate cadherin and catenin expression with survival[134] whereas other series have not shown a prognostic value to these markers.[132,135,136] Given the complex interaction and function of these proteins, it will be necessary to learn more about their role in ADC before any conclusions can be made regarding their significance.

APOPTOTIC REGULATORS

Programmed cell death, or apoptosis, is the physiologic process by which an organism deletes specified cells. Many factors influence whether a cell undergoes apoptosis, and some proteins favor its initiation whereas others favor its inhibition (Table 3–2). Several lines of evidence demonstrate that the inhibition of normal apoptotic pathways plays a critical role in carcinogenesis. Thorough discussion of the pathways involved is beyond the scope of this chapter. One important family of apoptotic regulators that has been examined in esophageal cancer is related to the Bcl-2 protein. The Bcl-2 family includes both inhibitors of cell death (eg, Bcl-2 and Bcl-x_L) and promoters of cell death (eg, Bax), and the relative ratio of pro- and antiapoptotic proteins in a given cell is thought to determine the apoptotic threshold.

Overexpression of Bcl-2 has been documented in 30 to 70 percent of SCC cases in studies.[2] Many of these studies did not examine interacting proteins or measure any index of apoptosis. It appears that the number of cells undergoing apoptosis actually increases as lesions advance from hyperplasia to carcinoma, correlating with proliferation.[137] Con-

Table 3–2. PROTEINS MOST OFTEN IMPLICATED IN PROMOTION OR INHIBITION OF APOPTOSIS IN HUMAN CANCER	
Proapoptotic	Antiapoptotic
Bad	Bcl-2
Bid	Bcl-x_L
Bax	MCL-1
Bak	Bwc-w
Bcl-x_s	

versely, poorly differentiated carcinomas reveal lower degrees of apoptosis, compared with well-differentiated cancers.[138] An apparently paradoxical decrease in expression of the Bcl-2–related factor Bcl-x_L in SCC has been reported.[139] Some reports have suggested that antiapoptotic proteins are overexpressed early in carcinogenesis but may be progressively lost as carcinomas evolve.[140]

Attempting to use apoptotic proteins as markers for survival has been difficult, and most studies show no correlation.[139,141] One study, however, did demonstrate poorer survival in multivariate analysis when Bcl-x_L was weakly expressed.[69]

In ADC, the evidence seems to point to similar derangements. Expression of Bcl-2 has been reported to be increased in early neoplastic lesions and decreased in carcinomas.[142] Apoptotic indices are elevated in high-grade dysplasia and carcinoma.[143,144] Soslow and colleagues examined the ratio of Bcl-2 to Bax and found that this correlated with histologic severity and proliferative index,[145] emphasizing the need to examine several apoptotic proteins to begin to understand the alterations taking place. The data thus far do not allow definitive conclusions regarding the roles of specific apoptotic regulators in esophageal cancer.

OTHER POTENTIAL ONCOGENES

Several other genes have been implicated in different cancers, and their expression in cases of esophageal carcinoma has been studied.

Adenomatous Polyposis Coli

Germline mutation in one allele of the APC gene is found in patients with APC, who are at extremely high risk for colon cancer. Mutations of the APC gene have also been found in a large fraction of spontaneous colon cancers. The product of the APC gene regulates β-catenin degradation and may have other anticancer activities as well (see Figure 3–5).[146] Its alteration in other malignancies has led to its study in esophageal cancer.

Loss of heterozyosity at 5q occurs in approximately 30 percent of SCCs, but mutation of the remaining APC allele is reported to be an uncommon event.[16,147] Similarly, in ADC, 5q LOH has been reported in the range of 20 to 55 percent of cases.[54,57,102,148] Identical APC gene mutations have been found in dysplastic lesions and adjacent carcinomas, but the frequency of these mutations is consistently under 10 percent.[6,147] When examined in conjunction with other genetic alterations, APC loss appears to occur later and does not have any evident prognostic value.[54,57,58] Patients with APC do not have high rates of esophageal cancers. These observations all suggest that APC is of minor importance in esophageal cancer.

Deleted-in-Colon-Cancer and Deleted-in-Pancreatic-Cancer Locus-4 Genes

These two tumor-suppressor genes are located on 18q. The deleted-in-colon-cancer (DCC) gene, a participant in cellular adhesion, has been implicated in colon cancer development whereas the deleted-in-pancreatic-cancer locus-4 (DPC4) gene, functioning in the transforming growth factor-β (TGF-β) signaling pathway, plays a role in pancreatic carcinogenesis.[149] Their modification in esophageal cancer has been explored in LOH analyses. Chromosome 18q is deleted in 25 to 45 percent of SCC cases[15,18] and in 25 to 70 percent of ADC cases.[15,57,102,148,150] Miyake and colleagues, examining 51 cases of lymph node metastatic SCC, found only 2 cases with mutation of DCC and 10 cases (23%) with deletions of DCC. These alterations were more common the farther away the lymph nodes were from the primary lesion.[151] However, other authors studying 18q LOH have found that the DCC locus remains intact.[15,18]

Loss of heterozygosity of 18q is found in the premalignant tissue of ADC and portended a marginally worse prognosis (a hazard ratio of 1.7) in one study.[57,148] Barrett and colleagues analyzed DPC4 deletion in ADC and found a 46 percent rate of 18q LOH, but the DPC4 locus remained unaltered.[150]

The evidence therefore suggests that while 18q deletion is common in esophageal cancer, the putative genes involved have yet to be elucidated. Despite their roles in other ADCs, DCC and DPC4 do not appear to be significant contributors to esophageal carcinogenesis.

Cyclooxygenase-2 and the *myc* Oncogene

Cyclooxygenase-2 (COX-2) is a membrane-bound glycoprotein involved in the synthesis of prostaglandins from arachidonic acid. Its expression is restricted to certain tissues and is stimulated by inflammatory insults. Increased levels of COX-2 have been implicated in the pathogenesis of colo-rectal and gastric carcinomas.[152] Furthermore, inhibitors of prostaglandin synthesis have been linked with reduced rates of colonic adenoma formation.[153] Clinical trials evaluating the use of COX-2 inhibitors as chemopreventive agents are under way. In esophageal cancers, this enzyme is of interest because of its implication in carcinogenesis and as a target for therapy. Research on COX-2 has been almost exclusively in regard to ADC, but studies on its involvement in SCC are being initiated as well.

Levels of COX-2 are increased in BE, with a progressive rise in expression in dysplasia and carcinoma.[152,154,155] It is unclear, however, whether this is a result of deregulation of COX-2 expression in neoplastic tissues or a response to acid and bile exposure. The role of increased COX-2 levels in carcinogenesis, its effects on tumor behavior, and the benefits of inhibiting this enzyme are not known.

The *myc* oncogene regulates cell-cycle progression and cell death. Its amplification has been demonstrated in both SCC and ADC but is relatively infrequent.[2,5,15,20] It does not appear to play a major role in esophageal cancer.

IMMUNE ESCAPE

It has been suggested that both SCC and ADC may evade immune destruction by altering cell surface markers and inducing apoptosis of tumor-infiltrating lymphocytes (TILs).[140] Normal and metaplastic esophageal mucosa express cell surface Fas (CD95), a "death receptor" that initiates an apoptotic response when engaged. Both SCC and ADC have been reported to lose surface expression of Fas.[103,156,157] The down-regulation of Fas has been found in conjunction with overexpression of the membrane-bound ligand for Fas, Fas-L.[156,158,159] Expression of Fas-L can induce apoptosis in adjacent cells expressing Fas, including antitumor lym-

phocytes. Expression of Fas-L is often localized to the periphery of tumor nests, is associated with higher rates of lymph node invasion, and has been shown to result in a mean fourfold decrease in the number of TILs. Some cases of esophageal cancers also exhibit down-regulation of human leukocyte antigen (HLA) class I antigens and the T-cell co-stimulatory molecules B7 and intercellular adhesion molecule 1 (ICAM-1).[160] All of these mechanisms may contribute to the evasion of immunologic responses to esophageal carcinomas.

MICROSATELLITE INSTABILITY

Microsatellite instability (MSI) has been recognized as a marker of defects in DNA repair genes and has been linked with gastric and colo-rectal carcinomas.[161] The two best studied of these genes are MSH2 and MLH1, located on chromosomes 2p and 3p, respectively. These genes essentially function as tumor suppressors, with inactivation resulting in ineffective DNA mismatch repair and a dramatic increase in the genomic replicative error rate. Microsatellite insability in esophageal cancer has been found more frequently in ADC cases than in SCC cases.[3,5,15,162] Even in ADC, however, MSI is demonstrated in only 10 to 20 percent of tumors.[17,163,164] Thus, MSI appears to have at most a minor role in the pathogenesis of esophageal cancer.

CONCLUSION

The past two decades have been notable for remarkable progress in the understanding of the molecular basis of esophageal cancer. A clearer appreciation of the mechanisms of action of various oncogenic factors has sometimes called into question the results of earlier studies that used limited analytic techniques or that combined distinct carcinoma subtypes. Nevertheless, a number of conclusions can be drawn.

Detailed chromosomal and molecular analyses coupled with careful histologic observation have begun to permit an ordering of the many genetic alterations associated with esophageal carcinogenesis and have clearly separated, at a molecular and etiologic level, the two principal histologic subtypes of esophageal cancer (Figure 3–6). Loss of p53 func-

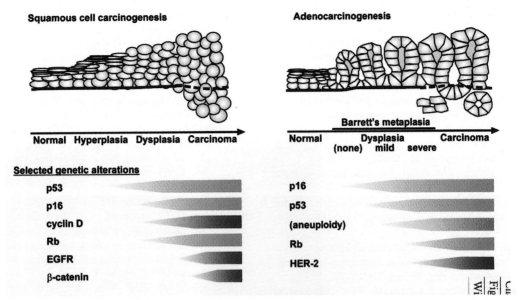

Figure 3–6. Molecular models of esophageal carcinogenesis. Stages of carcinogenic progression for the two predominant types of esophageal carcinoma are presented schematically above. Selected characteristic genetic alterations for each tumor type, with approximate time of onset in carcinogenesis, are indicated below. Green indicates oncogenes up-regulated in carcinogenesis; red indicates tumor-suppressor genes inactivated in carcinogenesis. (EGFR = epidermal growth factor receptor.)

tion typically occurs early in SCC and likely contributes to subsequent genomic instability. Derangements of other critical G_1 checkpoint regulators such as p16 and cyclin D1 fuel this process. The acquisition of autocrine growth stimulus through up-regulation of EGFR, the loss of contact inhibition through down-regulation of E-cadherin, and a variety of other alterations may ultimately lead to full transformation of the malignant clone.

The development of ADC presents a somewhat different spectrum of molecular alterations. Loss of p16 through hypermethylation appears to be a frequent and important early alteration. Inactivation of p53, through a spectrum of mutational alterations distinct than that found in SCC, is a somewhat later event. Similar to other ADCs that have been analyzed, up-regulation of Her-2 appears to be a particularly important growth factor receptor derangement in ADC of the esophagus.

Challenges for the future include filling in the many gaps in the current understanding of esophageal carcinogenesis and, most important, converting this improved understanding into novel preventative and therapeutic strategies for this disease. Despite advances in the understanding of its molecular basis, esophageal carcinoma remains a

typically fatal diagnosis with a relatively short median survival. A number of approaches derived from these molecular analyses (including chemopreventative studies involving COX-2 inhibitors, as well as therapeutic trials focused on interrupting growth factor signaling pathways) are currently under investigation in patients with esophageal cancer. The groundwork of molecular understanding may support the development of more effective treatments of this vexing malignancy.

REFERENCES

1. Greenlee RT, Murray T, Bolden S, Wingo PA. Cancer statistics, 2000. CA Cancer J Clin 2000;50:7–33.
2. Lam AK. Molecular biology of esophageal squamous cell carcinoma. Crit Rev Oncol Hematol 2000;33:71–90.
3. Jankowski JA, Wright NA, Meltzer SJ, et al. Molecular evolution of the metaplasia-dysplasia-adenocarcinoma sequence in the esophagus. Am J Pathol 1999;154:965–73.
4. Ortiz-Hidalgo C, De La Vega G, Aguirre-Garcia J. The histopathology and biologic prognostic factors of Barrett's esophagus: a review. J Clin Gastroenterol 1998;26:324–33.
5. Fitzgerald RC, Triadafilopoulos G. Recent developments in the molecular characterization of Barrett's esophagus. Dig Dis 1998;16:63–80.
6. Aldulaimi D, Jankowski J. Barrett's esophagus: an overview of the molecular biology. Dis Esophagus 1999;12:177–80.
7. Walch AK, Zitzelsberger HF, Bruch J, et al. Chromosomal imbalances in Barrett's adenocarcinoma and the metaplasia-

dysplasia-carcinoma sequence. Am J Pathol 2000;156:555–66.

8. Raskind WH, Norwood T, Levine DS, et al. Persistent clonal areas and clonal expansion in Barrett's esophagus. Cancer Res 1992;52:2946–50.

9. Gleeson CM, Sloan JM, McGuigan JA, et al. Barrett's oesophagus: microsatellite analysis provides evidence to support the proposed metaplasia-dysplasia-carcinoma sequence. Genes Chromosomes Cancer 1998;21:49–60.

10. Ford HL, Pardee AB. Cancer and the cell cycle. J Cell Biochem 1999;Suppl 32–33:166–72.

11. Donjerkovic D, Scott DW. Regulation of the G_1 phase of the mammalian cell cycle. Cell Res 2000;10:1–16.

12. Sherr CJ, Roberts JM. CDK inhibitors: positive and negative regulators of G_1-phase progression. Genes Dev 1999;13:1501–12.

13. Robaszkiewicz M, Reid BJ, Volant A, et al. Flow-cytometric DNA content analysis of esophageal squamous cell carcinomas. Gastroenterology 1991;101:1588–93.

14. Chanvitan A, Puttawibul P, Casson AG. Flow cytometry in squamous cell esophageal cancer and precancerous lesions. Dis Esophagus 1997;10:206–10.

15. Montesano R, Hollstein M, Hainaut P. Genetic alterations in esophageal cancer and their relevance to etiology and pathogenesis: a review. Int J Cancer 1996;69:225–35.

16. Aoki T, Mori T, Du X, et al. Allelotype study of esophageal carcinoma. Genes Chromosomes Cancer 1994;10:177–82.

17. Ikeguchi M, Unate H, Maeta M, Kaibara N. Detection of loss of heterozygosity at microsatellite loci in esophageal squamous-cell carcinoma. Oncology 1999;56:164–8.

18. Shibagaki I, Shimada Y, Wagata T, et al. Allelotype analysis of esophageal squamous cell carcinoma. Cancer Res 1994;54:2996–3000.

19. Barnas C, Henn T, Stark M, et al. Detection of genetic alterations in cancers of the esophagus and esophagogastric junction by comparative genomic hybridization: frequent involvement of chromosome 4q. Proc Am Assoc Cancer Res 1999;40:539.

20. Persons DL, Croughan WS, Borelli KA, Cherian R. Interphase cytogenetics of esophageal adenocarcinoma and precursor lesions. Cancer Genet Cytogenet 1998;106:11–7.

21. Nakamura T, Nekarda H, Hoelscher AH, et al. Prognostic value of DNA ploidy and c-erbB-2 oncoprotein overexpression in adenocarcinoma of Barrett's esophagus [published erratum appears in Cancer 1994 Oct 15;74(8):2396]. Cancer 1994;73:1785–94.

22. Reid BJ, Sanchez CA, Blount PL, Levine DS. Barrett's esophagus: cell cycle abnormalities in advancing stages of neoplastic progression. Gastroenterology 1993;105:119–29.

23. Reid BJ, Blount PL, Rubin CE, et al. Flow-cytometric and histological progression to malignancy in Barrett's esophagus: prospective endoscopic surveillance of a cohort. Gastroenterology 1992;102:1212–9.

24. Galipeau PC, Cowan DS, Sanchez CA, et al. 17p (p53) allelic losses, 4N (G2/tetraploid) populations, and progression to aneuploidy in Barrett's esophagus. Proc Natl Acad Sci U S A 1996;93:7081–4.

25. Barrett MT, Galipeau PC, Sanchez CA, et al. Determination of the frequency of loss of heterozygosity in esophageal adenocarcinoma by cell sorting, whole genome amplifi-

cation and microsatellite polymorphisms. Oncogene 1996;12:1873–8.

26. Dolan K, Garde J, Gosney J, et al. Allelotype analysis of oesophageal adenocarcinoma: loss of heterozygosity occurs at multiple sites. Br J Cancer 1998;78:950–7.

27. Swift A, Risk JM, Kingsnorth AN, et al. Frequent loss of heterozygosity on chromosome 17 at 17q11.2-q12 in Barrett's adenocarcinoma. Br J Cancer 1995;71:995–8.

28. Petty EM, Kalikin LM, Orringer MB, Beer DG. Distal chromosome 17q loss in Barrett's esophageal and gastric cardia adenocarcinomas: implications for tumorigenesis. Mol Carcinog 1998;22:222–8.

29. Levine AJ. p53, the cellular gatekeeper for growth and division. Cell 1997;88:323–31.

30. Wang LD, Zhou Q, Hong JY, et al. p53 protein accumulation and gene mutations in multifocal esophageal precancerous lesions from symptom free subjects in a high incidence area for esophageal carcinoma in Henan, China. Cancer 1996;77:1244–9.

31. Robert V, Michel P, Flaman JM, et al. High frequency in esophageal cancers of p53 alterations inactivating the regulation of genes involved in cell cycle and apoptosis. Carcinogenesis 2000;21:563–5.

32. Shi ST, Yang GY, Wang LD, et al. Role of p53 gene mutations in human esophageal carcinogenesis: results from immunohistochemical and mutation analyses of carcinomas and nearby non-cancerous lesions. Carcinogenesis 1999;20:591–7.

33. Yang G, Zhang Z, Liao J, et al. Immunohistochemical studies on Waf1p21, p16, pRb and p53 in human esophageal carcinomas and neighboring epithelia from a high-risk area in northern China. Int J Cancer 1997;72:746–51.

34. Hollstein M, Sidransky D, Vogelstein B, Harris CC. p53 mutations in human cancers. Science 1991;253:49–53.

35. Bennett WP, Hollstein MC, Metcalf RA, et al. p53 mutation and protein accumulation during multistage human esophageal carcinogenesis. Cancer Res 1992;52:6092–7.

36. Xing EP, Yang GY, Wang LD, et al. Loss of heterozygosity of the Rb gene correlates with pRb protein expression and associates with p53 alteration in human esophageal cancer. Clin Cancer Res 1999;5:1231–40.

37. Wang DY, Xiang YY, Tanaka M, et al. High prevalence of p53 protein overexpression in patients with esophageal cancer in Linxian, China and its relationship to progression and prognosis [published erratum appears in Cancer 1995 Mar 15;75(6):1404]. Cancer 1994;74:3089–96.

38. Lam KY, Tsao SW, Zhang D, et al. Prevalence and predictive value of p53 mutation in patients with oesophageal squamous cell carcinomas: a prospective clinico-pathological study and survival analysis of 70 patients. Int J Cancer 1997;74:212–9.

39. Ikeda G, Isaji S, Chandra B, et al. Prognostic significance of biologic factors in squamous cell carcinoma of the esophagus. Cancer 1999;86:1396–405.

40. Hashimoto N, Tachibana M, Dhar DK, et al. Expression of p53 and RB proteins in squamous cell carcinoma of the esophagus: their relationship with clinicopathologic characteristics. Ann Surg Oncol 1999;6:489–94.

41. Kuwahara M, Hirai T, Yoshida K, et al. p53, p21(Waf1/Cip1) and cyclin D1 protein expression and prognosis in esophageal cancer. Dis Esophagus 1999;12:116–9.

42. Shimada Y, Imamura M, Shibagaki I, et al. Genetic alterations in patients with esophageal cancer with short- and long-term survival rates after curative esophagectomy. Ann Surg 1997;226:162–8.

43. Shamma A, Doki Y, Shiozaki H, et al. Cyclin D1 overexpression in esophageal dysplasia: a possible biomarker for carcinogenesis of esophageal squamous cell carcinoma. Int J Oncol 2000;16:261–6.

44. Natsugoe S, Nakashima S, Matsumoto M, et al. Expression of p21WAF1/Cip1 in the p53-dependent pathway is related to prognosis in patients with advanced esophageal carcinoma. Clin Cancer Res 1999;5:2445–9.

45. Inada S, Koto T, Futami K, et al. Evaluation of malignancy and the prognosis of esophageal cancer based on an immunohistochemical study (p53, E-cadherin, epidermal growth factor receptor). Surg Today 1999;29:493–503.

46. Moskaluk CA, Heitmiller R, Zahurak M, et al. p53 and p21(WAF1/CIP1/SDI1) gene products in Barrett esophagus and adenocarcinoma of the esophagus and esophagogastric junction. Hum Pathol 1996;27:1211–20.

47. Kubba AK, Poole NA, Watson A. Role of p53 assessment in management of Barrett's esophagus. Dig Dis Sci 1999;44:659–67.

48. Prevo LJ, Sanchez CA, Galipeau PC, Reid BJ. p53-mutant clones and field effects in Barrett's esophagus. Cancer Res 1999;59:4784–7.

49. Gleeson CM, Sloan JM, McGuigan JA, et al. Base transitions at CpG dinucleotides in the p53 gene are common in esophageal adenocarcinoma. Cancer Res 1995;55:3406–11.

50. Ramel S, Reid BJ, Sanchez CA, et al. Evaluation of p53 protein expression in Barrett's esophagus by two-parameter flow cytometry. Gastroenterology 1992;102:1220–8.

51. Casson AG, Manolopoulos B, Troster M, et al. Clinical implications of p53 gene mutation in the progression of Barrett's epithelium to invasive esophageal cancer. Am J Surg 1994;167:52–7.

52. Neshat K, Sanchez CA, Galipeau PC, et al. p53 mutations in Barrett's adenocarcinoma and high-grade dysplasia. Gastroenterology 1994;106:1589–95.

53. Blount PL, Galipeau PC, Sanchez CA, et al. 17p allelic losses in diploid cells of patients with Barrett's esophagus who develop aneuploidy. Cancer Res 1994;54:2292–5.

54. Gonzalez MV, Artimez ML, Rodrigo L, et al. Mutation analysis of the p53, APC, and p16 genes in the Barrett's oesophagus, dysplasia, and adenocarcinoma. J Clin Pathol 1997;50:212–7.

55. Galipeau PC, Prevo LJ, Sanchez CA, et al. Clonal expansion and loss of heterozygosity at chromosomes 9p and 17p in premalignant esophageal (Barrett's) tissue. J Natl Cancer Inst 1999;91:2087–95.

56. Barrett MT, Sanchez CA, Prevo LJ, et al. Evolution of neoplastic cell lineages in Barrett oesophagus. Nat Genet 1999;22:106–9.

57. Wu TT, Watanabe T, Heitmiller R, et al. Genetic alterations in Barrett esophagus and adenocarcinomas of the esophagus and esophagogastric junction region. Am J Pathol 1998;153:287–94.

58. Blount PL, Meltzer SJ, Yin J, et al. Clonal ordering of 17p and 5q allelic losses in Barrett dysplasia and adenocarcinoma. Proc Natl Acad Sci U S A 1993;90:3221–5.

59. Casson AG, Kerkvliet N, O'Malley F. Prognostic value of p53 protein in esophageal adenocarcinoma. J Surg Oncol 1995;60:5–11.

60. Schneider PM, Stoeltzing O, Roth JA, et al. p53 mutational status improves estimation of prognosis in patients with curatively resected adenocarcinoma in Barrett's esophogus. Clin Cancer Res 2000;6:3147–52.

61. Michieli P, Chedid M, Lin D, et al. Induction of WAF1/CIP1 by a p53-independent pathway. Cancer Res 1994;54:3391–5.

62. Harper JW, Adami GR, Wei N, et al. The p21 Cdk-interacting protein Cip1 is a potent inhibitor of G_1 cyclin-dependent kinases. Cell 1993;75:805–16.

63. el-Deiry WS, Tokino T, Velculescu VE, et al. WAF1, a potential mediator of p53 tumor suppression. Cell 1993;75:817–25.

64. Shirakawa Y, Naomoto Y, Kimura M, et al. Topological analysis of p21WAF1/CIP1 expression in esophageal squamous dysplasia. Clin Cancer Res 2000;6:541–50.

65. Hirai T, Kuwahara M, Yoshida K, et al. The prognostic significance of p53, p21 (Waf1/Cip1), and cyclin D1 protein expression in esophageal cancer patients. Anticancer Res 1999;19:4587–91.

66. Ohashi K, Nemoto T, Eishi Y, et al. Expression of the cyclin dependent kinase inhibitor p21WAF1/CIP1 in oesophageal squamous cell carcinomas. Virchows Arch 1997;430:389–95.

67. Sarbia M, Stahl M, zur Hausen A, et al. Expression of p21WAF1 predicts outcome of esophageal cancer patients treated by surgery alone or by combined therapy modalities. Clin Cancer Res 1998;4:2615–23.

68. Bahl R, Arora S, Nath N, et al. Novel polymorphism in p21(waf1/cip1) cyclin dependent kinase inhibitor gene: association with human esophageal cancer. Oncogene 2000;19:323–8.

69. Sarbia M, Gabbert HE. Modern pathology: prognostic parameters in squamous cell carcinoma of the esophagus. Recent Results Cancer Res 2000;155:15–27.

70. Nita ME, Nagawa H, Tominaga O, et al. p21Waf1/Cip1 expression is a prognostic marker in curatively resected esophageal squamous cell carcinoma, but not p27Kip1, p53, or Rb. Ann Surg Oncol 1999;6:481–8.

71. Hanas JS, Lerner MR, Lightfoot SA, et al. Expression of the cyclin-dependent kinase inhibitor p21(WAF1/CIP1) and p53 tumor suppressor in dysplastic progression and adenocarcinoma in Barrett esophagus. Cancer 1999;86:756–63.

72. Hirai T, Kuwahara M, Yoshida K, et al. Clinical results of transhiatal esophagectomy for carcinoma of the lower thoracic esophagus according to biological markers. Dis Esophagus 1998;11:221–5.

73. Slingerland J, Pagano M. Regulation of the cdk inhibitor p27 and its deregulation in cancer. J Cell Physiol 2000;183:10–7.

74. Shamma A, Doki Y, Tsujinaka T, et al. Loss of p27(KIP1) expression predicts poor prognosis in patients with esophageal squamous cell carcinoma. Oncology 2000;58:152–8.

75. Itami A, Shimada Y, Watanabe G, Imamura M. Prognostic value of p27(Kip1) and cyclin D1 expression in esophageal cancer. Oncology 1999;57:311–7.

76. Anayama T, Furihata M, Ishikawa T, et al. Positive correlation between p27Kip1 expression and progression of human esophageal squamous cell carcinoma. Int J Cancer 1998;79:439–43.

77. Morgan DO. Principles of CDK regulation. Nature 1995; 374:131–4.

78. Herman JG, Merlo A, Mao L, et al. Inactivation of the CDKN2/p16/MTS1 gene is frequently associated with aberrant DNA methylation in all common human cancers. Cancer Res 1995;55:4525–30.

79. Merlo A, Herman JG, Mao L, et al. 5' CpG island methylation is associated with transcriptional silencing of the tumour suppressor p16/CDKN2/MTS1 in human cancers. Nat Med 1995;1:686–92.

80. Xing EP, Nie Y, Wang LD, et al. Aberrant methylation of p16INK4a and deletion of p15INK4b are frequent events in human esophageal cancer in Linxian, China. Carcinogenesis 1999;20:77–84.

81. Hayashi K, Metzger R, Salonga D, et al. High frequency of simultaneous loss of p16 and p16beta gene expression in squamous cell carcinoma of the esophagus but not in adenocarcinoma of the esophagus or stomach. Oncogene 1997;15:1481–8.

82. Shamma A, Doki Y, Shiozaki H, et al. Effect of cyclin D1 and associated proteins on proliferation of esophageal squamous cell carcinoma. Int J Oncol 1998;13:455–60.

83. Takeuchi H, Ozawa S, Ando N, et al. Altered p16/MTS1/CDKN2 and cyclin D1/PRAD-1 gene expression is associated with the prognosis of squamous cell carcinoma of the esophagus. Clin Cancer Res 1997;3:2229–36.

84. Xing EP, Nie Y, Song Y, et al. Mechanisms of inactivation of p14ARF, p15INK4b, and p16INK4a genes in human esophageal squamous cell carcinoma. Clin Cancer Res 1999;5:2704–13.

85. Roncalli M, Bosari S, Marchetti A, et al. Cell cycle-related gene abnormalities and product expression in esophageal carcinoma. Lab Invest 1998;78:1049–57.

86. Gamieldien W, Victor TC, Mugwanya D, et al. p53 and p16/CDKN2 gene mutations in esophageal tumors from a high-incidence area in South Africa. Int J Cancer 1998; 78:544–9.

87. Busatto G, Shiao YH, Parenti AR, et al. p16/CDKN2 alterations and pRb expression in oesophageal squamous carcinoma. Mol Pathol 1998;51:80–4.

88. Barrett MT, Sanchez CA, Galipeau PC, et al. Allelic loss of 9p21 and mutation of the CDKN2/p16 gene develop as early lesions during neoplastic progression in Barrett's esophagus. Oncogene 1996;13:1867–73.

89. Morgan RJ, Newcomb PV, Bailey M, et al. Loss of heterozygosity at microsatellite marker sites for tumour suppressor genes in oesophageal adenocarcinoma. Eur J Surg Oncol 1998;24:34–7.

90. Wong DJ, Barrett MT, Stoger R, et al. p16INK4a promoter is hypermethylated at a high frequency in esophageal adenocarcinomas. Cancer Res 1997;57:2619–22.

91. Sarbia M, Stahl M, Fink U, et al. Prognostic significance of cyclin D1 in esophageal squamous cell carcinoma patients treated with surgery alone or combined therapy modalities. Int J Cancer 1999;84:86–91.

92. Matsumoto M, Furihata M, Ishikawa T, et al. Comparison of deregulated expression of cyclin D1 and cyclin E with that of cyclin-dependent kinase 4 (CDK4) and CDK2 in human oesophageal squamous cell carcinoma. Br J Cancer 1999;80:256–61.

93. Ishikawa T, Furihata M, Ohtsuki Y, et al. Cyclin D1 overexpression related to retinoblastoma protein expression as a prognostic marker in human oesophageal squamous cell carcinoma. Br J Cancer 1998;77:92–7.

94. Chetty R, Chetty S. Cyclin D1 and retinoblastoma protein expression in oesophageal squamous cell carcinoma. Mol Pathol 1997;50:257–60.

95. Shinozaki H, Ozawa S, Ando N, et al. Cyclin D1 amplification as a new predictive classification for squamous cell carcinoma of the esophagus, adding gene information. Clin Cancer Res 1996;2:1155–61.

96. Inomata M, Uchino S, Tanimura H, et al. Amplification and overexpression of cyclin D1 in aggressive human esophageal cancer. Oncol Rep 1998;5:171–6.

97. Morgan RJ, Newcomb PV, Hardwick RH, Alderson D. Amplification of cyclin D1 and MDM-2 in oesophageal carcinoma. Eur J Surg Oncol 1999;25:364–7.

98. Shimada Y, Imamura M, Watanabe G, et al. Prognostic factors of oesophageal squamous cell carcinoma from the perspective of molecular biology. Br J Cancer 1999;80:1281–8.

99. Samejima R, Kitajima Y, Yunotani S, Miyazaki K. Cyclin D1 is a possible predictor of sensitivity to chemoradiotherapy for esophageal squamous cell carcinoma. Anticancer Res 1999;19:5515–21.

100. Wild CP, Bani-Hani K, Hardie LJ, et al. A prospective study of cyclin D1 overexpression in Barrett's esophagus patients: association with an increased risk of progression to adenocarcinoma. Proc Am Assoc Cancer Res 1999;40:203.

101. Ikeguchi M, Oka S, Gomyo Y. Clinical significance of retinoblastoma protein (pRb) expression in esophageal squamous cell carcinoma. J Surg Oncol 2000;73:104–8.

102. Reid BJ, Barrett MT, Galipeau PC, et al. Barrett's esophagus: ordering the events that lead to cancer. Eur J Cancer Prev 1996;5 Suppl 2:57–65.

103. Coppola D, Schreiber RH, Mora L, et al. Significance of Fas and retinoblastoma protein expression during the progression of Barrett's metaplasia to adenocarcinoma. Ann Surg Oncol 1999;6:298–304.

104. Porter AC, Vaillancourt RR. Tyrosine kinase receptor-activated signal transduction pathways which lead to oncogenesis. Oncogene 1998;17:1343–52.

105. Itakura Y, Sasano H, Shiga C, et al. Epidermal growth factor receptor overexpression in esophageal carcinoma. An immunohistochemical study correlated with clinicopathologic findings and DNA amplification. Cancer 1994;74: 795–804.

106. Friess H, Fukuda A, Tang WH, et al. Concomitant analysis of the epidermal growth factor receptor family in esophageal cancer: overexpression of epidermal growth factor receptor mRNA but not of c-erbB-2 and c-erbB-3. World J Surg 1999;23:1010–8.

107. Torzewski M, Sarbia M, Verreet P, et al. The prognostic significance of epidermal growth factor receptor expression in squamous cell carcinomas of the oesophagus. Anticancer Res 1997;17:3915–9.

108. Brito MJ, Filipe MI, Linehan J, Jankowski J. Association of transforming growth factor alpha (TGFA) and its precursors with malignant change in Barrett's epithelium: biological and clinical variables. Int J Cancer 1995;60:27–32.

109. Moy JR, Orringer MB, Beer DG. Gene amplification in esophageal Barrett's adenocarcinoma. AACR 1998;39:132.

110. Yacoub L, Goldman H, Odze RD. Transforming growth factor-alpha, epidermal growth factor receptor, and MiB-1 expression in Barrett's-associated neoplasia: correlation with prognosis. Mod Pathol 1997;10:105–12.

111. Hardwick RH, Barham CP, Ozua P, et al. Immunohistochemical detection of p53 and c-erbB-2 in oesophageal carcinoma; no correlation with prognosis. Eur J Surg Oncol 1997;23:30–5.

112. Lam KY, Tin L, Ma L. C-erbB-2 protein expression in oesophageal squamous epithelium from oesophageal squamous cell carcinomas, with special reference to histological grade of carcinoma and pre-invasive lesions. Eur J Surg Oncol 1998;24:431–5.

113. Kim R, Clarke MR, Melhem MF, et al. Expression of p53, PCNA, and C-erbB-2 in Barrett's metaplasia and adenocarcinoma. Dig Dis Sci 1997;42:2453–62.

114. Brien TP, Odze RD, Sheehan CE, et al. HER-2/neu gene amplification by FISH predicts poor survival in Barrett's esophagus-associated adenocarcinoma. Hum Pathol 2000;31:35–9.

115. Flejou JF, Paraf F, Muzeau F, et al. Expression of c-erbB-2 oncogene product in Barrett's adenocarcinoma: pathological and prognostic correlations. J Clin Pathol 1994;47:23–6.

116. Koide N, Nishio A, Kono T, et al. Histochemical study of vascular endothelial growth factor in squamous cell carcinoma of the esophagus. Hepatogastroenterology 1999;46:952–8.

117. Park JM, Danenberg K, Lord RV, et al. Induction of vascular endothelial growth factor and basic fibroblast growth factor in Barrett's esophagus and Barrett's associated adenocarcinomas. Proc Am Assoc Cancer Res 1999;40:229.

118. Koide N, Watanabe H, Yazawa K, et al. Immunohistochemical expression of thymidine phosphorylase/platelet-derived endothelial cell growth factor in squamous cell carcinoma of the esophagus. Hepatogastroenterology 1999;46:944–51.

119. Sanders DS, Bruton R, Darnton SJ, et al. Sequential changes in cadherin-catenin expression associated with the progression and heterogeneity of primary oesophageal squamous carcinoma [published erratum appears in Int J Cancer 1999 Jun 21;84(3):336]. Int J Cancer 1998;79:573–9.

120. Jankowski JA, Bruton R, Shepherd N, Sanders DS. Cadherin and catenin biology represent a global mechanism for epithelial cancer progression. Mol Pathol 1997;50:289–90.

121. Bullions LC, Levine AJ. The role of beta-catenin in cell adhesion, signal transduction, and cancer. Curr Opin Oncol 1998;10:81–7.

122. Resnik E. beta-Catenin—one player, two games. Nat Genet 1997;16:9–11.

123. Korinek V, Barker N, Morin PJ, et al. Constitutive transcriptional activation by a beta-catenin-Tcf complex in APC-/-colon carcinoma. Science 1997;275:1784–7.

124. Sato F, Shimada Y, Watanabe G, et al. Expression of vascular endothelial growth factor, matrix metalloproteinase-9 and E-cadherin in the process of lymph node metastasis in oesophageal cancer. Br J Cancer 1999;80:1366–72.

125. Tamura S, Shiozaki H, Miyata M, et al. Decreased E-cadherin expression is associated with haematogenous recurrence and poor prognosis in patients with squamous cell carcinoma of the oesophagus. Br J Surg 1996;83:1608–14.

126. Nakanishi Y, Ochiai A, Akimoto S, et al. Expression of E-cadherin, alpha-catenin, beta-catenin and plakoglobin in esophageal carcinomas and its prognostic significance: immunohistochemical analysis of 96 lesions. Oncology 1997;54:158–65.

127. Jian WG, Darnton SJ, Jenner K, et al. Expression of E-cadherin in oesophageal carcinomas from the UK and China: disparities in prognostic significance. J Clin Pathol 1997;50:640–4.

128. Ninomiya I, Endo Y, Fushida S. Alteration of beta-catenin in esophageal squamous-cell carcinoma. Int J Cancer 2000;85:757–61.

129. Kimura Y, Shiozaki H, Doki Y, et al. Cytoplasmic beta-catenin in esophageal cancers. Int J Cancer 1999;84:174–8.

130. Swami S, Kumble S, Triadafilopoulos G. E-cadherin expression in gastroesophageal reflux disease, Barrett's esophagus, and esophageal adenocarcinoma: an immunohistochemical and immunoblot study. Am J Gastroenterol 1995;90:1808–13.

131. Bailey T, Biddlestone L, Shepherd N. Altered cadherin and catenin complexes in the Barrett's esophagus-dysplasia-adenocarcinoma sequence: correlation with disease progression and dedifferentiation. Am J Pathol 1998;152:135–44.

132. Washington K, Chiappori A, Hamilton K, et al. Expression of beta-catenin, alpha-catenin, and E-cadherin in Barrett's esophagus and esophageal adenocarcinomas. Mod Pathol 1998;11:805–13.

133. Wijnhoven BP, de Both NJ, van Dekken H, et al. E-cadherin gene mutations are rare in adenocarcinomas of the oesophagus. Br J Cancer 1999;80:1652–7.

134. Krishnadath KK, Tilanus HW, van Blankenstein M, et al. Reduced expression of the cadherin-catenin complex in oesophageal adenocarcinoma correlates with poor prognosis. J Pathol 1997;182:331–8.

135. Pomp J, Blom J, van Krimpen C, et al. E-cadherin expression in oesophageal carcinoma treated with high-dose radiotherapy; correlation with pretreatment parameters and treatment outcome. J Cancer Res Clin Oncol 1999;125:641–5.

136. Turner JR, Torres CM, Wang HH, et al. Preoperative chemoradiotherapy alters the expression and prognostic significance of adhesion molecules in Barrett's-associated adenocarcinoma. Hum Pathol 2000;31:347–53.

137. Wang LD, Zhou Q, Yang WC, Yang CS. Apoptosis and cell proliferation in esophageal precancerous and cancerous lesions: study of a high-risk population in northern China. Anticancer Res 1999;19:369–74.

138. Ohashi K, Nemoto T, Eishi Y, et al. Proliferative activity and p53 protein accumulation correlate with early invasive trend, and apoptosis correlates with differentiation grade in oesophageal squamous cell carcinomas. Virchows Arch 1997;430:107–15.

139. Torzewski M, Sarbia M, Heep H, et al. Expression of Bcl-X(L), an antiapoptotic member of the Bcl-2 family, in esophageal squamous cell carcinoma. Clin Cancer Res 1998;4:577–83.

140. O'Connell J, Bennett MW, O'Sullivan GC, et al. Resistance to Fas (APO-1/CD95)-mediated apoptosis and expression of Fas ligand in esophageal cancer: the Fas counterattack. Dis Esophagus 1999;12:83–9.

141. Sarbia M, Stahl M, Fink U, et al. Expression of apoptosis-regulating proteins and outcome of esophageal cancer

patients treated by combined therapy modalities. Clin Cancer Res 1998;4:2991–7.

142. Katada N, Hinder RA, Smyrk TC, et al. Apoptosis is inhibited early in the dysplasia-carcinoma sequence of Barrett esophagus. Arch Surg 1997;132:728–33.

143. Goldblum JR, Rice TW. Bcl-2 protein expression in the Barrett's metaplasia-dysplasia-carcinoma sequence. Mod Pathol 1995;8:866–9.

144. Lauwers GY, Kandemir O, Kubilis PS, Scott GV. Cellular kinetics in Barrett's epithelium carcinogenic sequence: roles of apoptosis, bcl-2 protein, and cellular proliferation. Mod Pathol 1997;10:1201–8.

145. Soslow RA, Remotti H, Baergen RN, Altorki NK. Suppression of apoptosis does not foster neoplastic growth in Barrett's esophagus. Mod Pathol 1999;12:239–50.

146. Sparks AB, Morin PJ, Vogelstein B, Kinzler KW. Mutational analysis of the APC/beta-catenin/Tcf pathway in colorectal cancer. Cancer Res 1998;58:1130–4.

147. Powell SM, Papadopoulos N, Kinzler KW, et al. APC gene mutations in the mutation cluster region are rare in esophageal cancers. Gastroenterology 1994;107:1759–63.

148. Dolan K, Garde J, Walker SJ, et al. LOH at the sites of the DCC, APC, and TP53 tumor suppressor genes occurs in Barrett's metaplasia and dysplasia adjacent to adenocarcinoma of the esophagus. Hum Pathol 1999;30:1508–14.

149. DeVita Jr. VT, Hellmans S, Rosenberg SA. Cancer: principles and practice of oncology. Philadelphia: Lippincott, 1997.

150. Barrett MT, Schutte M, Kern SE, Reid BJ. Allelic loss and mutational analysis of the DPC4 gene in esophageal adenocarcinoma. Cancer Res 1996;56:4351–3.

151. Miyake S, Nagai K, Yoshino K, et al. Point mutations and allelic deletion of tumor suppressor gene DCC in human esophageal squamous cell carcinomas and their relation to metastasis. Cancer Res 1994;54:3007–10.

152. Shirvani VN, Ouatu-Lascar R, Kaur BS, et al. Cyclooxygenase 2 expression in Barrett's esophagus and adenocarcinoma: ex vivo induction by bile salts and acid exposure. Gastroenterology 2000;118:487–96.

153. Baron JA, Sandler RS. Nonsteroidal anti-inflammatory drugs and cancer prevention. Annu Rev Med 2000;51:511–23.

154. Lord RV, Danenberg K, Peters JH, DeMeester TR. Increased COX-2 and iNOS expression and decreased COX-1 expression in Barrett's esophagus and Barrett's associated adenocarcinomas. Proc Am Assoc Cancer Res 1999;40:318.

155. Wilson KT, Fu S, Ramanujam KS, Meltzer SJ. Increased expression of inducible nitric oxide synthase and cyclooxygenase-2 in Barrett's esophagus and associated adenocarcinomas. Cancer Res 1998;58:2929–34.

156. Gratas C, Tohma Y, Barnas C, et al. Up-regulation of Fas (APO-1/CD95) ligand and down-regulation of Fas expression in human esophageal cancer. Cancer Res 1998;58:2057–62.

157. Hughes SJ, Nambu Y, Soldes OS, et al. Fas/APO-1 (CD95) is not translocated to the cell membrane in esophageal adenocarcinoma. Cancer Res 1997;57:5571–8.

158. Bennett MW, O'Connell J, O'Sullivan GC, et al. The Fas counterattack in vivo: apoptotic depletion of tumor-infiltrating lymphocytes associated with Fas ligand expression by human esophageal carcinoma. J Immunol 1998;160:5669–75.

159. Younes M, Schwartz MR, Ertan A, et al. Fas ligand expression in esophageal carcinomas and their lymph node metastases. Cancer 2000;88:524–8.

160. Hosch SB, Izbicki JR, Pichlmeier U, et al. Expression and prognostic significance of immunoregulatory molecules in esophageal cancer. Int J Cancer 1997;74:582–7.

161. Naidoo R, Chetty R. DNA repair gene status in oesophageal cancer. Mol Pathol 1999;52:125–30.

162. Meltzer SJ, Yin J, Manin B, et al. Microsatellite instability occurs frequently and in both diploid and aneuploid cell populations of Barrett's-associated esophageal adenocarcinomas. Cancer Res 1994;54:3379–82.

163. Gleeson CM, Sloan JM, McGuigan JA, et al. Ubiquitous somatic alterations at microsatellite alleles occur infrequently in Barrett's-associated esophageal adenocarcinoma. Cancer Res 1996;56:259–63.

164. Muzeau F, Flejou JF, Belghiti J, et al. Infrequent microsatellite instability in oesophageal cancers. Br J Cancer 1997;75:1336–9.

4

Barrett's Esophagus with High-Grade Dysplasia and/or Esophageal Adenocarcinoma

JOHN HART, MD

Esophageal adenocarcinoma arising in the setting of Barrett's esophagus is an important cause of morbidity and mortality in the United States. Epidemiologic studies have documented a striking rise in the incidence of this tumor, which surpassed squamous cell carcinoma as the most common esophageal tumor, beginning about 1990. According to data collected by the Centers for Disease Control in the National Health Interview Survey, there were an estimated 808,000 prevalent cases of Barrett's esophagus in the United States in 1998. Based on this estimate, a study conducted by the American Gastroenterological Association calculated a total direct cost of $350 million in 1998 for the diagnosis and treatment of Barrett's esophagus and its complications.

HISTOLOGIC DIAGNOSIS OF DYSPLASIA IN BARRETT'S ESOPHAGUS

The light-microscopic assessment of biopsy specimens of Barrett's mucosa for dysplasia remains the cornerstone of surveillance programs implemented to decrease the mortality from esophageal adenocarcinoma. Unfortunately, the histologic diagnosis of dysplasia has never been highly reproducible, even among surgical pathologists who see many cases of Barrett's esophagus. Many factors are responsible for the poor performance by pathologists, and several methods have been proposed to aid in making a more "objective" diagnosis of dysplasia; of course, these techniques add to the cost, labor, and time needed to arrive at a diagnosis.

Dysplasia is defined as an unequivocal neoplastic change in an epithelium confined by a basement membrane that is recognized microscopically by certain cytologic and architectural features. The fact that dysplasia is considered to represent a neoplastic state implies at least the potential for malignant degeneration. Most pathologists rely on the five-tiered classification scheme for dysplasia originally proposed in 1988 by a panel of expert gastrointestinal pathologists.[1] The criteria established in this system are summarized below (the reader is referred to the original article[1] for a full description), as follows:

1. Negative for dysplasia: The mucosal architecture is normal. There may be focal nuclear stratification and small numbers of "dystrophic" goblet cells, but the nuclear-to-cytoplasmic (N:C) ratio is normal, and nuclear pleomorphism is minimal. Nucleoli are not markedly enlarged, and mitotic figures are variable in number. A greater degree of nuclear alterations is expected in the presence of inflammation, erosion, or ulceration (Figures 4–1 and 4–2).

2. Indefinite for dysplasia: Cytologic and architectural changes that are worrisome but insufficient for the diagnosis of dysplasia (Figure 4–3).

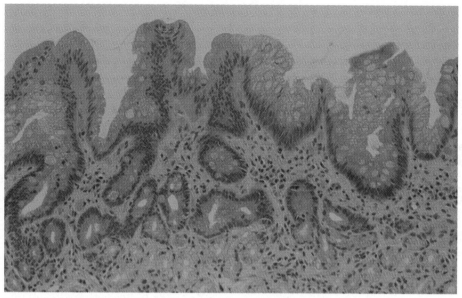

Figure 4–1. Barrett's mucosa without dysplasia. The biopsy specimen consists of specialized columnar mucosa (hematoxylin and eosin; ×100 original magnification).

3. Positive for low-grade (Figures 4–4 and 4–5) and high-grade (Figures 4–6 and 4–7) dysplasia: The diagnosis of dysplasia is based on the presence of significant cytologic or architectural abnormalities, and high-grade dysplasia can be diagnosed if *either* is sufficiently severe. The cytologic features include nuclear pleomorphism, hyperchromatism, increased N:C ratio, markedly enlarged nucleoli, cytoplasmic basophilia, excessive nuclear stratifi-cation, and increased number of abnormal mitotic figures. The architectural features include irregularly shaped, crowded, or budded glands; papillary extensions into gland lumina; and a villiform configuration of the surface.

4. Intramucosal carcinoma: "…defined as carcinoma which has penetrated through the basement membrane of the glands into the lamina propria but that has not invaded through the muscularis

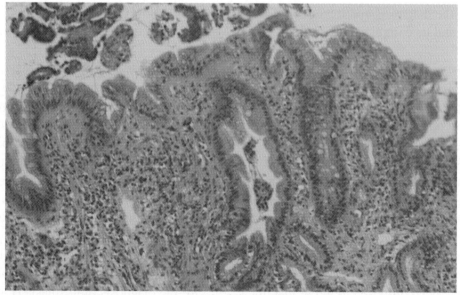

Figure 4–2. Barrett's mucosa without dysplasia. In this biopsy specimen, there is minimal cytologic atypia that is considered reactive in origin (hematoxylin and eosin; ×200 original magnification).

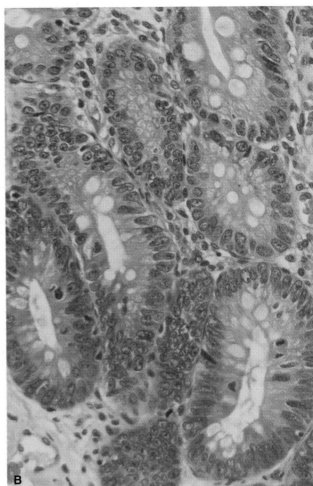

Figure 4–3. Barrett's mucosa, with focus indefinite for dysplasia. *A,* This low-power view demonstrates mild cytologic atypia in the deep portions of the glands but good maturation toward the surface (hematoxylin and eosin; ×100 original magnification). *B,* A view at higher power, to highlight the mild nuclear enlargement and crowding. Note the absence of significant acute inflammation (hematoxylin and eosin; ×400 original magnification).

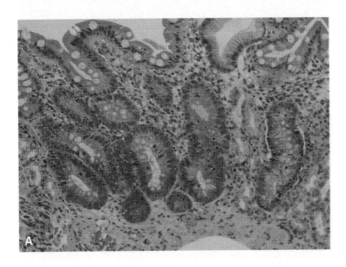

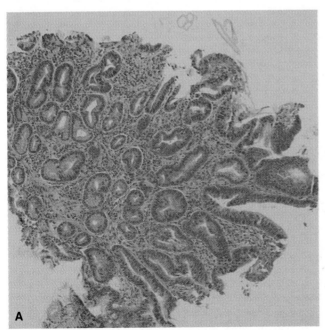

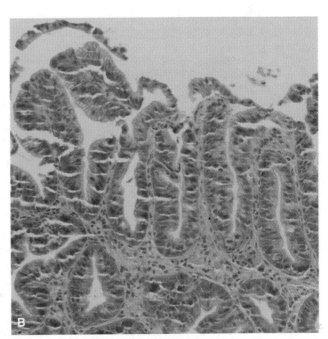

Figure 4–4. Barrett's mucosa with low-grade dysplasia. *A,* No nondysplastic mucosa is present at low power (hematoxylin and eosin; ×40 original magnification). *B,* The cytologic features are very similar to those of a colonic adenomatous polyp (hematoxylin and eosin; ×100 original magnification).

Figure 4–5. Barrett's mucosa with low-grade dysplasia. *A,* A low-power view reveals a distinct focus that exhibits cytologic atypia (hematoxylin and eosin; ×40 original magnification). *B,* A view of this focus at higher power reveals the lack of cytologic maturation toward the luminal surface(hematoxylin and eosin; ×100 original magnification).

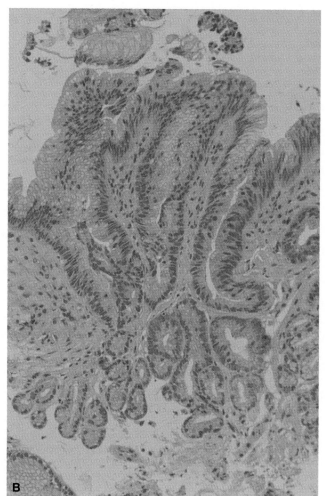

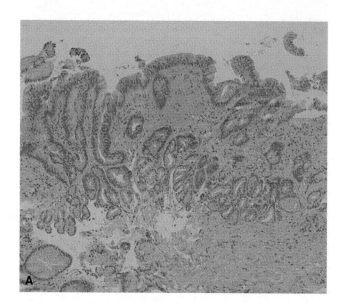

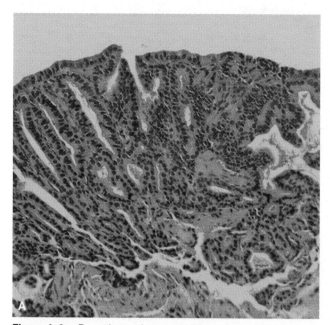

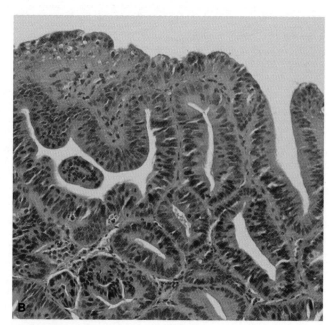

Figure 4–6. Barrett's esophagus with high-grade dysplasia. *A,* Note the glandular crowding and complexity, features not seen in low-grade dysplasia (hematoxylin and eosin; ×400 original magnification). *B,* Marked cytologic atypia is evident in this view at a higher power (hematoxylin and eosin; ×100 original magnification).

mucosae…"[1] (Figure 4–8). In contrast, invasive tumor is diagnosed when tumor cells have infiltrated into the submucosa (Figures 4–9 and 4–10).

REPRODUCIBILITY OF THE DIAGNOSIS OF DYSPLASIA

Clearly, the histologic criteria described above are entirely subjective. In current daily practice, unfortunately, there is no objective molecular marker that can ensure the accuracy of the pathologic diagnosis. The experience of the surgical pathologist is

undoubtedly a factor in proper diagnosis, which has led to the recommendation that the diagnosis of dysplasia be confirmed by a second expert consultant before surgical or ablative therapy is considered.[2] This point was well illustrated in a study of the risk of progression following a diagnosis of low-grade dysplasia. When the biopsy specimens showing low-grade dysplasia were re-reviewed by a group of pathologists, there was considerable disagreement regarding the diagnoses. However, among those cases in which there was agreement on the diagnosis of low-grade dysplasia, there was a significant risk

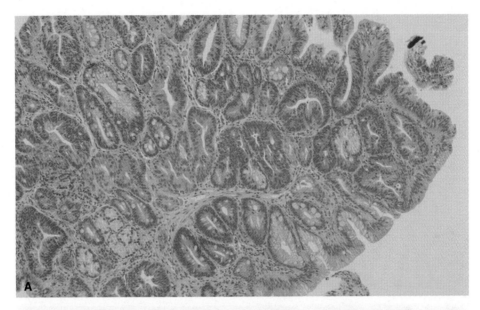

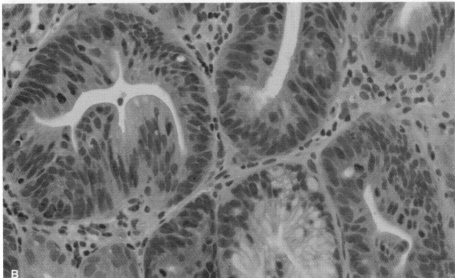

Figure 4–7. Barrett's esophagus with high grade-dysplasia. *A,* Marked glandular crowding is evident at low power (hematoxylin and eosin; ×40 original magnification). *B,* Cribriforming of the glands is focally evident (hematoxylin and eosin; ×400 original magnification).

of progression to high-grade dysplasia or cancer whereas among those cases in which there was no agreement on the diagnosis of low-grade dysplasia, no patient progressed.[3]

The reproducibility of the five diagnostic tiers among the authors of the original classification was considerable when the clinically most relevant stratification of high-grade dysplasia and intramucosal carcinoma versus all other diagnoses was considered. The reproducibility declined progressively, however, as each additional diagnostic tier was included in the analysis. The separation of low-grade dysplasia from indefinite-for-dysplasia and indefinite-for-dysplasia from negative-for-dysplasia was most problematic. Recently, a reproducibility study that included a larger number of biopsies, a more rigorous experimental design, and a more sophisticated statistical analysis of the result was reported by 12 experienced gastrointestinal pathologists.[4] Once again, however, while the interobserver reproducibility of the diagnoses of negative-for-dysplasia, high-grade dysplasia, and invasive carcinoma was satisfactory (kappa values of 0.44, 0.40, and 0.67, respectively), the reproducibility of the diagnoses of low-grade dyspla-

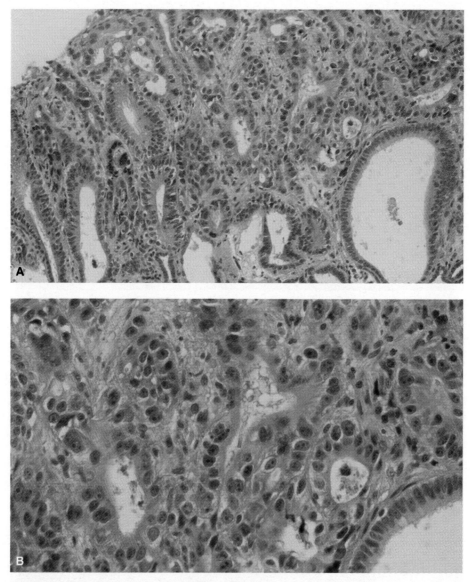

Figure 4–8.   Barrett's mucosa with intramucosal carcinoma. *A,* Marked cytologic atypia is evident even in this low-power view (hematoxylin and eosin; ×100 original magnification). *B,* At high power, the presence of single cell invasion into the lamina propria is obvious (hematoxylin and eosin; ×400 original magnification).

sia and of indefinite-for-dysplasia was poor (kappa values of 0.23 and 0.14). The poor reproducibility for the indefinite and low-grade dysplasia categories (both intra- and interobserver) has led to the recommendation that they be lumped together for daily practice in terms of patient follow-up.

A major factor contributing to interobserver disagreement by pathologists is suboptimal biopsy histology. Poor biopsy technique and poor fixation, sectioning, or staining of biopsy specimens make accurate histologic interpretation much more difficult. Another important cause of diagnostic confusion is the presence of acute inflammation, particularly due to erosion or ulceration. Acute inflammation can result in marked inflammatory epithelial atypia, which is sometimes difficult to distinguish from true dysplasia.[2] Unfortunately, while ulceration can occur simply as a result of severe reflux, it is also a worrisome feature because it often occurs in areas of carcinoma.

Another factor that contributes to poor diagnostic reproducibility revolves around the lack of criteria regarding the minimum area of cytologic or architectural atypia necessary to make a diagnosis of

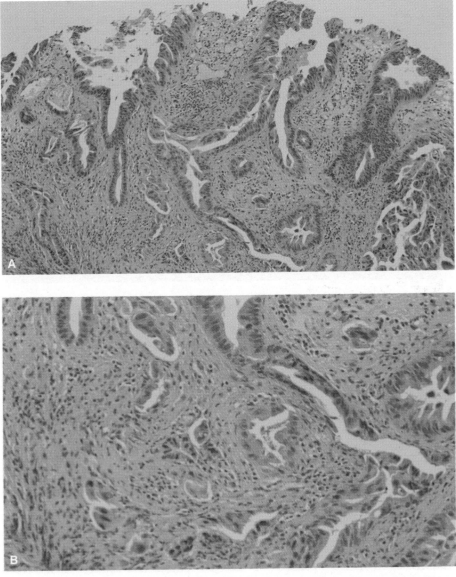

Figure 4–9. Barrett's mucosa with invasive adenocarcinoma. *A,* The invasive glands have irregular and angulated contours (hematoxylin and eosin; ×40 original magnification). *B,* A desmoplastic stroma surrounding the tumor is indicative of submucosal invasion (hematoxylin and eosin; ×200 original magnification).

dysplasia. Disparity between the degree of cytologic and architectural abnormality can also lead to variation in diagnoses among pathologists in some cases.

CLINICAL SIGNIFICANCE OF DYSPLASIA

Very few studies have reported the long-term follow-up of patients diagnosed with low-grade dysplasia on biopsy. In a study from 1989 that included 6 patients with low-grade dysplasia, 2 patients continued to exhibit low-grade dysplasia after 3.5 and 8 years of follow-up, 1 patient developed high-grade dysplasia after 4 years, and 3 patients progressed to cancer

after 1.5, 3.5, and 4.0 years. It should be noted, however, that the rate of progression to cancer in this study is the highest reported in the English literature.[5] In a more recent and larger study, which reported a follow-up of a median of 26 months and a mean of 40 months, 4 of 25 patients who were originally diagnosed with low-grade dysplasia developed adenocarcinoma, and a 5th patient developed high-grade dysplasia.[6] In the study involving consensus diagnoses by 12 gastrointestinal pathologists, invasive cancer developed in 4 of 25 patients with low-grade dysplasia diagnosed by biopsy, with a median follow-up of 60 months. Interestingly, progression to

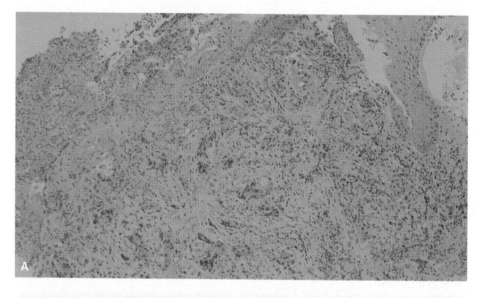

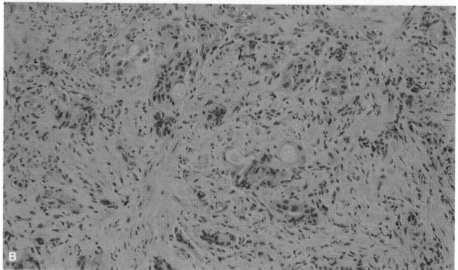

Figure 4–10.   Invasive moderately differentiated esophageal adenocarcinoma. *A,* This biopsy specimen reveals no evidence of pre-existing Barrett's mucosa (hematoxylin and eosin; ×40 original magnification). *B,* A view at higher power highlights the presence of small malignant glands that are haphazardly invading fibrous stroma (hematoxylin and eosin; ×200 original magnification).

invasive adenocarcinoma also occurred in 4 of 22 patients with a consensus diagnosis of indefinite-for-dysplasia on the initial biopsy, which suggested that this group of patients should receive the same clinical follow-up as patients with low-grade dysplasia.[4]

Of course, sampling error can be a significant obstacle in evaluating all such studies (eg, areas of high-grade dysplasia might have been missed in the initial evaluation). In addition, it seems reasonable to assume that the interval from the diagnosis of low-grade dysplasia to the development of high-grade dysplasia or cancer might be shorter for a patient who was discovered to have low-grade dysplasia upon initial screening ("prevalent dysplasia") than for a patient who developed low-grade dysplasia while already enrolled in a surveillance program and whose prior endoscopies revealed no dysplasia ("incident dysplasia").

A diagnosis of high-grade dysplasia consistently appears to confer a significantly greater risk for the development of adenocarcinoma. In the consensus study, for example, invasive adenocarcinoma developed in 20 of 33 patients whose biopsy specimens showed high-grade dysplasia, at a mean interval of only 8 months.[7] In a meta-analysis of surgical series reporting patients who underwent immediate esophagectomy following a diagnosis of high-grade dysplasia by biopsy, adenocarcinoma was discovered in 56 of 119 patients.[8] Although 41 tumors were found to be stage I, stage II tumors were diagnosed in 12 patients, and stage III tumors were diagnosed in 3 patients. In one of the studies included in the review,[9] however, no invasive tumors were evident in any of seven patients (although high-grade dysplasia was confirmed in the esophagectomy of each of them). This report emphasized that it was possible to differentiate high-grade dysplasia from early adenocarcinoma by (1) the use of a very aggressive biopsy protocol (four-quadrant jumbo biopsies for every 2 cm of Barrett's mucosa, plus multiple biopsies from any endoscopically visible lesions), (2) the examination of well-oriented serial sections of these biopsy specimens by an expert gastrointestinal pathologist, and (3) the performance of an immediate repeat endoscopy and biopsy in any patient with suspicious biopsy findings. Unfortunately, this high standard of care is not available in most centers. In a prospective study reported by the same group,[10] progression from high-grade dysplasia to cancer in five patients occurred at a mean of 14 months (range, 5 to 21 months). Moreover, in the most recent report by this group, there was a 59% incidence of cancer developing among 76 patients with high-grade dysplasia over a cumulative 5-year period.[11]

In a smaller study (15 patients), there was a 27% rate of progression from unifocal high-grade dysplasia to cancer over a 3-year follow-up period.[12] The significance of the anatomic extent of high-grade dysplasia was rigorously addressed in another report, involving 100 patients. In this study, the extent of high-grade dysplasia was defined as focal if five or fewer crypts in one biopsy specimen showed high-grade dysplasia and diffuse if it involved more than five crypts or was evident in more than one biopsy specimen. The incidence of cancer at 3 years was 14% for the focal high-grade dysplasia group and 56% for the diffuse group.[13] The data from these studies indicate that a diagnosis of high-grade dysplasia, particularly when more than a single microscopic focus is involved, is an ominous finding that requires very close clinical follow-up, with serious consideration of immediate esophagectomy in patients who are reasonable surgical candidates.

However, it should be noted that there is one center that has consistently reported a significantly lower cancer risk in patients with high-grade dysplasia. Indeed, in their most recent study, which included 79 patients with high-grade dysplasia, only 12 patients (16%) developed cancer during a mean follow-up period of 7.3 years.[14] However, the possibility of an "overdiagnosis" of high-grade dysplasia by the single pathologist for this study has been raised,[15] emphasizing again the importance of consensus diagnoses in research studies.

PROGNOSTIC MARKERS: p53 IMMUNOHISTOCHEMISTRY

The poor reproducibility of the light-microscopic diagnosis of dysplasia has led to attempts to define more "objective" markers of risk for the development of adenocarcinoma. Although studies have suggested that both a decrease in sialomucin[16] and an increase in sulfomucin[17] may increase the risk of developing cancer, neither of these retrospective studies provided convincing data or long-term follow-ups. A larger prospective study[18] revealed that the presence of sulfomucin did not predict the development of dysplasia or cancer. More recently, study of the expression of individual mucin genes by immunohistochemistry and in situ hybridization has replaced the cruder histochemical assessment of mucin subtypes (Figures 4–11 and 4–12). There is evidence to suggest that the pattern of mucin gene expression does vary during the progression from metaplasia to dysplasia to frank carcinoma.[19] Cyclin D1 overexpression, as assessed by immunohistochemical staining, has also been proposed as a prognostic marker for the future development of invasive adenocarcinoma.[20] This finding has been considered potentially significant because, unlike most reports promoting prognostic markers, this study was prospective, was well controlled, and involved a sizable cohort (307 patients followed for an average of 3.5 years). The analyses showed that there was a significantly increased risk of developing adenocarcinoma (odds ratio = 6.85; 95% confidence interval [CI], 1.57 to 29.91) among patients with initial-biopsy specimens that overexpressed cyclin D1.[20] Of course, these results would have to be independently verified before this marker could be used in clinical practice.[21] Flow cytometry has also provided predictive information regarding the develop-

ment of cancer,[22] but this technology is unlikely to become routinely available.

Immunohistologic demonstration of the nuclear accumulation of p53 protein, on the other hand, can be easily performed in most centers, and a vast amount of literature on its value in predicting the progression to cancer has been amassed. In almost every published study, the incidence of p53 positivity by immunohistochemistry progressively increases as the degree of dysplasia in Barrett's mucosa increases from no dysplasia to low-grade dysplasia to high-grade dysplasia[23] (Figure 4–13). The percentages vary somewhat from study to study as one would expect, given the variety of antibodies and technical conditions used. In two large studies[24,25] in which microwave antigen retrieval was not used, none of the biopsy specimens (a total of 87) without dysplasia exhibited nuclear staining for p53 protein.[23,24] In these studies, a combined 6 (12%) of 51 biopsy specimens graded as indefinite or low-grade dysplasia were p53 positive, compared to a combined 7 (47%) of 15 biopsy specimens graded as high-grade dysplasia. In contrast, in two studies[26,27] that did use microwave antigen retrieval, p53 staining was evident in 11% of biopsies without dysplasia (a total of 61 biopsies), 42% of biopsies with low-grade dysplasia (53 biopsies), and 86% of biopsies with high-grade dysplasia (22 biopsies). The authors of one of

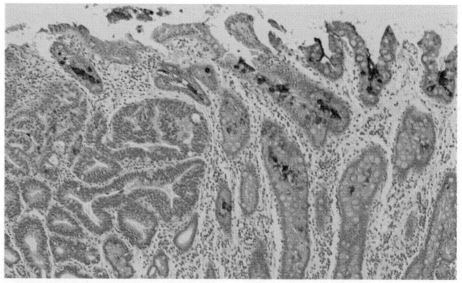

Figure 4–11.   Immunohistochemical stain for Muc5AC mucin gene protein (×200 original magnification). Note the decreased staining (*brown*) in the area of dysplasia (courtesy of Dr. S.F. Kuan, University of Chicago).

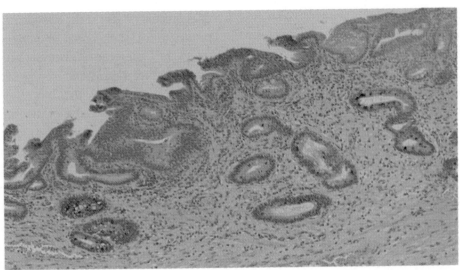

Figure 4–12. Immunohistochemical stain for Muc2 mucin gene protein (×100 original magnification). Note the absence of staining (*brown*) in the area of dysplasia (courtesy of Dr. S.F. Kuan, University of Chicago).

these studies emphasized the extreme sensitivity of this method, noting that gastric mucosa and especially the basal cell layer of squamous mucosa contained in the biopsy specimens sometimes exhibited nuclear p53 staining.

Unfortunately, p53 immunohistochemistry has not consistently been shown to add prognostic information as to the likelihood of progression to adenocarcinoma.[23] In the one study in which p53 positivity did appear to be of prognostic value, biopsy specimens from 9 of 25 patients with low-grade dysplasia were p53 positive, and 5 patients later developed high-grade dysplasia or adenocarcinoma.

In contrast, none of the other 16 patients with low-grade dysplasia that was p53 negative developed high-grade dysplasia or adenocarcinoma.[6] Although the sensitivity of p53 positivity for the development of malignancy was 100% and the specificity was 93%, the predictive value of a positive test was only 0.56 (compared to a 100% sensitivity, a 64% specificity, and a 0.20 predictive value for the light-microscopic diagnosis of low-grade dysplasia). This result needs to be confirmed by additional investigators before any recommendation can be made regarding the use of p53 immunohistochemistry for patient management.

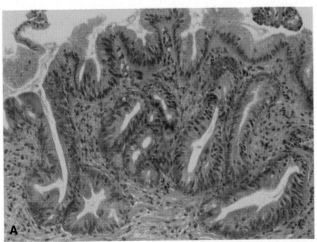
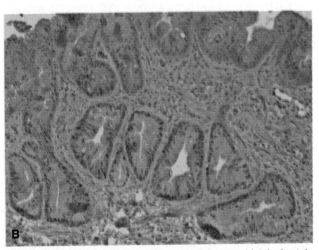

Figure 4–13. *A*, Barrett's mucosa with low-grade dysplasia (hematoxylin and eosin; ×100 original magnification). *B*, Immunohistologic stain with a p53 monoclonal antibody, revealing nuclear reactivity (*in brown*) within the dysplastic glands (×100 original magnification).

The incidence of p53 positivity in invasive adenocarcinomas (in both biopsy and esophagectomy specimens) is generally in the range of 65% in most large studies.[23] To date, no study has demonstrated a survival difference for p53-positive versus p53-negative (by immunohistochemical analysis) esophageal adenocarcinoma.[23]

It is important to keep in mind that p53 immunohistochemistry does not correlate precisely with the actual presence of a mutation in the p53 gene. The antibodies that are used for p53 immunohistochemistry recognize both mutant and wild-type p53 proteins. Normal tissues generally do not exhibit nuclear p53 positivity because the wild-type protein is quickly degraded and does not accumulate to a significant degree. Most of the mutant p53 proteins, however, are resistant to degradation and therefore accumulate in the nucleus to the point at which they can be detected immunohistochemically. In a published review of a large number of studies comparing p53 immunohistochemistry with direct mutational analysis in a wide range of tumor types, the sensitivity of immunohistochemistry for predicting a p53 mutation was 75%, with a positive predictive value of 63%.[28] Obviously, the degree of correlation will depend on the tumor type, the specific antibody, and the methods used for immunohistochemistry. In the two published direct comparisons, correlation of immunohistologic results with deoxyribonucleic acid (DNA) analysis in esophageal adenocarcinomas was good although the number of cases was small.[23]

CLINICAL MANAGEMENT OF DYSPLASIA

The studies published to date do not allow for rigid protocols regarding the proper surveillance strategy for management of patients with Barrett's esophagus who exhibit dysplasia on biopsy. A substantial proportion of patients whose biopsy specimens show high-grade dysplasia will have adenocarcinoma found by esophagectomy, and resection in patients with a low likelihood of operative morbidity and mortality seems defensible. On the other hand, many such patients will not be found to have an invasive tumor. The literature appears to support the contention that the presence of an endoscopically obvious lesion or mass increases the likelihood that cancer is present,[2,8] and at the very least, multiple biopsy specimens of such areas should be obtained. The American College of Gastroenterology has recommended either repeat endoscopy every 3 months or resection in patients with a biopsy diagnosis of high-grade dysplasia.[29] Because of the importance of accuracy in the diagnosis of high-grade dysplasia, it was also recommended that confirmation by an experienced gastrointestinal pathologist be obtained.[29] Endoscopic esophageal ultrasonography can be helpful in identifying early invasive tumors. The recent development of photodynamic laser ablation of high-grade dysplasia and early cancers with the use of mucosal-specific photosensitizer chemicals makes it particularly important that no more than superficially invasive tumor is present as this technique may not be effective for more advanced tumors.[30]

The proper management of patients whose biopsy specimens show low-grade dysplasia is even more uncertain. In most centers, early repeat endoscopy (with numerous additional biopsies) is performed, similar to the recommended management of dysplasia in ulcerative colitis. The recommendation of the American College of Gastroenterology is repeat endoscopy at 6 and 12 months, followed by yearly examinations.[29] The proper management strategy is complicated by the possibility of regression of at least low-grade dysplasia following intensive medical management with proton pump inhibitors. Partial and even near-total regression of Barrett's mucosa has been documented to occur with omeprazole therapy, but the true incidence of regression of dysplasia is unknown because of the problem of sampling error (Figures 4–14 and 4–15). In addition, it is well documented that squamous mucosa can regrow over persistent foci of columnar mucosa, making future endoscopic assessment difficult.[31] A similar problem has been identified after ablative therapies for high-grade dysplasia.[30]

Some have questioned the usefulness of endoscopic surveillance programs in patients with Barrett's esophagus, on a cost-benefit basis.[32,33] Most commentators, however, have concluded that screening is justifiable although they admit that certain recommendations (eg, the optimal interval between examinations and the number of biopsy specimens that should be obtained) have not been well defined.[34,35] Obviously, the appropriateness of surveillance is critically dependent on an accurate assessment of the incidence of adenocarcinoma in patients with Barrett's esophagus. Estimates based on prospective data (with 3 to 5 years of follow-up) have ranged from as high as 1 per 52 to as low as 1 per 98 patient-years of follow-up. Two more recent studies, with larger numbers of patients and longer follow-ups, reported rates of 1 cancer per 208 to 1 cancer per 285 patient-years of follow-up.[36,37]

ENDOSCOPIC AND GROSS APPEARANCE OF BARRETT'S DYSPLASIA

Dysplasia can occur anywhere in the segment of Barrett's mucosa; it most often has no distinctive appearance that allows macroscopic recognition (Figures 4–16 and 4–17). In fact, the presence of a grossly evident lesion or mass is a worrisome feature that is most often indicative of an underlying invasive adenocarcinoma. One exception, reported rarely, is the presence of a distinct polypoid lesion, grossly similar to a colonic adenomatous polyp (Figure 4–18). These so-called Barrett's adenomas may consist merely of dysplastic epithelium or may contain a focus of invasive adenocarcinoma.[38] Dysplasia may be multifocal, but it occurs most often as a patch with irregular borders. There may be small foci of high-grade dysplasia randomly located in a larger field of low-grade dysplasia.[39]

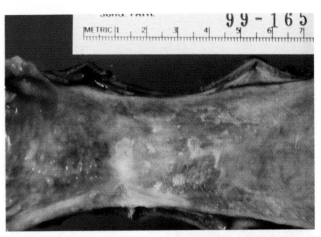

Figure 4–15. Esophagectomy specimen demonstrating regression of Barrett's mucosa. Note the presence of pearly white islands of squamous mucosa.

ENDOSCOPIC AND GROSS APPEARANCE OF BARRETT'S ADENOCARCINOMA

The risk of development of adenocarcinoma does not differ significantly in patients with short-segment Barrett's esophagus (defined as a segment less than 3 cm long) when compared to those with longer segments.[40] The gross configuration of the tumor is similar to that seen with squamous cell carcinomas, except that polypoid adenocarcinomas are slightly less common. Most often, the tumor is an ulcerative and infiltrative mass or has a plaque-like appearance (Figures 4–19 and 4–20). Exten-

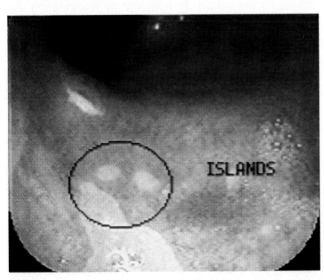

Figure 4–14. Endoscopic photograph illustrating regression due to medical therapy. Note the regrowth of squamous mucosa in the form of isolated islands in a background of salmon-colored Barrett's mucosa.

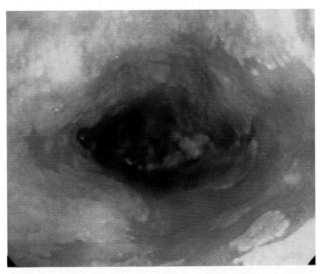

Figure 4–16. Endoscopic photograph of Barrett's esophagus. Random biopsy specimens revealed high-grade dysplasia that was not endoscopically apparent.

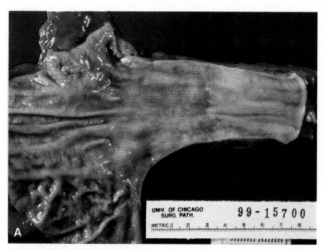
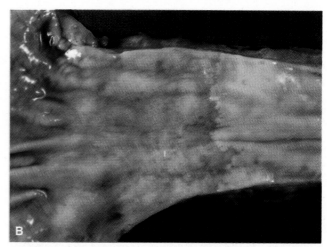

Figure 4–17. Esophagectomy specimen with Barrett's mucosa. Histologic sections revealed multifocal high-grade dysplasia and focal intramucosal adenocarcinoma. There was no definitive gross evidence of the tumor.

sive sampling will usually reveal dysplastic epithelium adjacent to invasive cancers, but in some cases (particularly of very large cancers), it may be difficult even to simply document the presence of any Barrett's mucosa. This is a particular problem when the invasive tumor is centered close to the esophagogastric junction (Figure 4–21), making it difficult to distinguish between gastric and esophageal origin.[41]

MICROSCOPIC FEATURES OF BARRETT'S ADENOCARCINOMAS

Barrett's adenocarcinomas are usually deeply invasive at the time of resection, which explains the low 5-year survival rates associated with these tumors.

The histologic features of these tumors closely resemble those of gastric adenocarcinomas although signet-ring cell differentiation is much less common in the Barrett's tumors (Figure 4–22). Grading depends on the degree of glandular differentiation and on the severity of cytologic atypia (Figures 4–23 to 4–25). The lymphatic drainage of the esophagus is oriented parallel to the long axis of the organ, which means that the tumor can spread along the lymphatic channels for some distance beneath intact squamous mucosa. Since much of the esophagus is not bounded by a serosa, there is no anatomic barrier against invasion into adjacent tissues or organs. These two anatomic features are important factors that contribute to the relatively low rate of resectability for cure in cases of Barrett's adenocarcinoma.

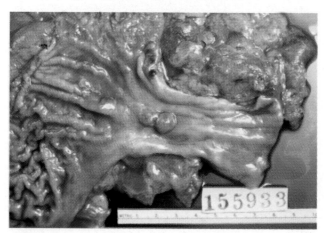

Figure 4–18. Esophagectomy specimen demonstrating Barrett's adenoma.

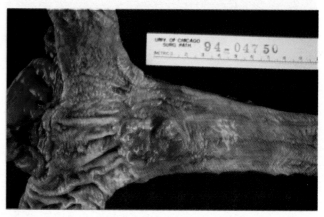

Figure 4–19. A specimen from an esophagectomy for early plaquelike adenocarcinoma arising at the gastroesophageal junction in short-segment Barrett's mucosa.

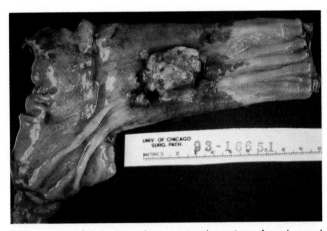

Figure 4–20. A specimen from an esophagectomy for advanced polypoid adenocarcinoma arising in a long segment of Barrett's mucosa.

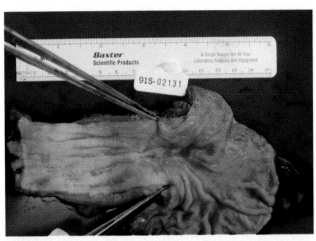

Figure 4–21. Adenocarcinoma at the gastroesophageal junction. Histologic sections revealed no evidence of Barrett's mucosa.

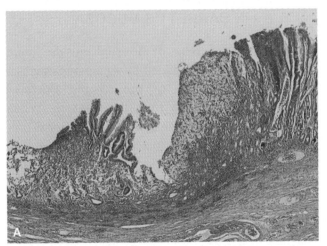

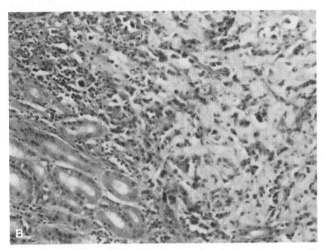

Figure 4–22. Barrett's adenocarcinoma with signet-ring cell differentiation. *A,* Note the Barrett's mucosa adjacent to the invasive tumor. *B,* Signet-ring cell differentiation can be seen at the far right of the photograph.

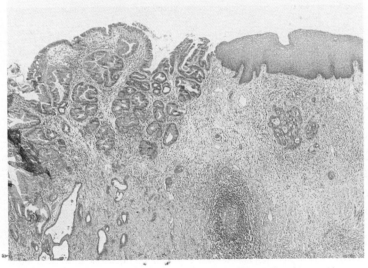

Figure 4–23. Small superficial well-differentiated Barrett's adenocarcinoma.

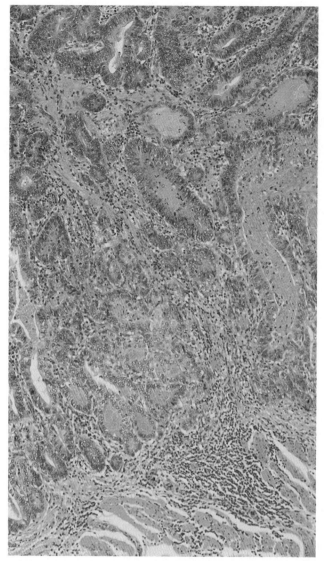

Figure 4–24.   Moderately differentiated Barrett's adenocarcinoma.

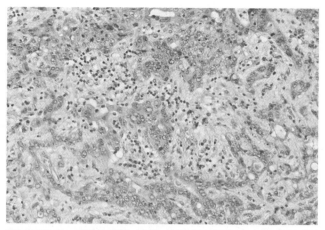

Figure 4–25.   Poorly differentiated Barrett's adenocarcinoma.

TUMORS WITH GLANDULAR DIFFERENTIATION NOT ARISING IN BARRETT'S MUCOSA

Rarely, adenocarcinomas of the esophagus are found to be completely surrounded by squamous mucosa, without any evidence of pre-existing Barrett's esophagus or extension from the stomach. When located in the upper esophagus, such a tumor is presumed to arise from a patch of ectopic gastric epithelium, termed a "gastric inlet patch."[42] Glandular tumors arising in the middle or lower third of the esophagus are thought to arise from submucosal glands or their ducts. Very rarely, tumors originating from these glands exhibit histologic features that closely resemble salivary gland tumors of the upper aerodigestive tract (Figures 4–26 and 4–27).

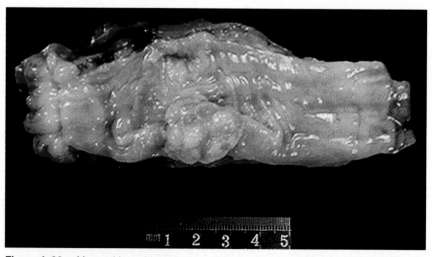

Figure 4–26.   Mucoepidermoid carcinoma arising in the midesophagus. Note the absence of Barrett's mucosa.

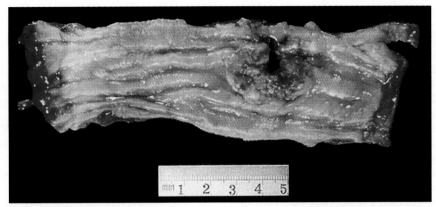

Figure 4–27. Adenoid cystic carcinoma arising in the midesophagus. Note the absence of Barrett's mucosa.

Mucoepidermoid and adenoid cystic carcinomas have been most commonly reported.[43,44]

REFERENCES

1. Reid BJ, Haggitt RC, Rubin CE, et al. Observer variation in the diagnosis of dysplasia in Barrett's esophagus. Hum Pathol 1988;19:166–78.

2. Haggitt RC. Barrett's esophagus, dysplasia, and adenocarcinoma. Hum Pathol 1994;25:982–93.

3. Skacel M, Petras RE, Gramlich TL, et al. The diagnosis of low-grade in Barrett's esophagus and its implications for disease progression. Am J Gastroenterol 2000;95:3383–7.

4. Montgomery E, Bronner MP, Goldblum JR, et al. Reproducibility of the diagnosis of dysplasia in Barrett esophagus. Hum Pathol 2001;32:368–78.

5. Hameeteman W, Tytgat GNJ, Houthoff HJ, et al. Barrett's esophagus: development of dysplasia and adenocarcinoma. Gastroenterology 1989;96:1249–56.

6. Younes M, Ertan A, Lechago LV, et al. p53 accumulation is a specific marker of malignant potential in Barrett's metaplasia. Dig Dis Sci 1997;42:697–701.

7. Montgomery E, Goldblum JR, Greenson JK, et al. Dysplasia as a predictive marker for invasive carcinoma in Barrett esophagus: a follow-up study based on 138 cases from a diagnostic variability study. Hum Pathol 2001;32:379–8.

8. Ferguson MK, Naunheim KS. Resection for Barrett's esophagus with high grade dysplasia: implications for photodynamic therapy. J Thorac Cardiovasc Surg 1997;114:824–9.

9. Levine DS, Haggitt RC, Blount PL, et al. An endoscopic biopsy protocol can differentiate high-grade dysplasia from early adenocarcinoma in Barrett's esophagus. Gastroenterology 1993;105:40–50.

10. Reid BJ, Blount PL, Rubin CE, et al. Predictors of progression to malignancy in Barrett's esophagus: endoscopic, histologic and flow cytometric follow-up of a cohort. Gastroenterology 1992;102:1212–9.

11. Reid BJ, Levine DS, Longton G, et al. Predictors of progression to cancer in Barrett's esophagus: baseline histology and flow cytometry identify low- and high-risk patient subsets. Am J Gastroenterol 2000;95:1669–76.

12. Weston AP, Sharma P, Topalovski M, et al. Long-term follow-up of Barrett's high-grade dysplasia. Am J Gastroenterol 95:1888–93.

13. Buttar NS, Wang KK, Sebo TJ, et al. Extent of high-grade dysplasia in Barrett's esophagus correlates with risk of adenocarcinoma. Gastroenterology 2001;120:1630–9.

14. Schnell TG, Sontag SJ, Chejfec G, et al. Long-term nonsurgical management of Barrett's esophagus with high-grade dysplasia. Gastroenterology 2001;120:1607–19.

15. Spechler SJ. Disputing dysplasia [editorial]. Gastroenterology 2001;120:1864–7.

16. Peuchmaur M, Potet F, Goldfain D. Mucin histochemistry of the columnar epithelium of the oesophagus (Barrett's oesophagus): a prospective biopsy study. J Clin Pathol 1984;37:607–10.

17. Jass JR. Mucin histochemistry of the columnar epithelium of the oesophagus: a retrospective study. J Clin Pathol 1984;34:866–70.

18. Lapertosa G, Baracchini P, Fulcheri E, et al. Mucin histochemical analysis in the interpretation of Barrett's esophagus. Results of a multicenter study. Am J Clin Pathol 1992;98:61–6.

19. Arul GS, Moorghen M, Myerscough N, et al. Mucin gene expression in Barrett's oesophagus: an in situ hybridization and immunohistochemical study. Gut 2001;47:753–61.

20. Bani-Hani K, Martin IG, Hardie LJ, et al. Prospective study of cyclin D1 overexpression in Barrett's esophagus: association with increased risk of adenocarcinoma. J Natl Cancer Inst 2000;92:1316–21.

21. Weissfeld JL. Cyclin D1 and esophageal adenocarcinoma risk: how good does a marker have to be [editorial]. J Natl Cancer Inst 2000;92:1282–3.

22. Haggitt RC, Reid BJ, Rubin CE, et al. Barrett's esophagus: correlation between mucin histochemistry, flow cytometry and histologic diagnosis for predicting increased cancer risk. Am J Pathol 1988;131:53–61.

23. Ireland AP, Clark GWB, DeMeester TR. Barrett's esophagus. The significance of p53 in clinical practice. Ann Surg 1997;225:17–30.

24. Younes M, Lebovitz RM, Lechago LV, et al. p53 protein accumulation in Barrett's metaplasia, dysplasia and carcinoma: a follow-up study. Gastroenterology 1993;105:1637–42.

25. Symmans PJ, Linehan JM, Brito MJ, et al. p53 expression in Barrett's oesophagus, dysplasia, and adenocarcinoma using antibody DO-7. J Pathol 1994;173:221–6.

26. Krishnadath KK, Tilanus HW, van Blankenstein M, et al. Accumulation of p53 protein in normal, dysplastic, and neoplastic Barrett's oesophagus. J Pathol 1995;175:175–80.

27. Kim R, Clarke MR, Melmmem MF, et al. Expression of p53, PCNA, and C-erb-2 in Barrett's metaplasia and adenocarcinoma. Dig Dis Sci 1997;42:2453–62.

28. Greenblatt MS, Bennett WP, Hollstein MC, et al. Mutations in the p53 tumor supressor gene: clues to cancer etiology and molecular pathogenesis. Cancer Res 1994;54:4855–78.

29. Sampliner RE. Practice guidelines on the diagnosis, surveillance, and therapy of Barrett's esophagus. Am J Gastroenterol 1998;93:1028–31.

30. Gossner L, Stolte M, Sroka R, et al. Photodynamic ablation in high-grade dysplasia and early cancer in Barrett's esophagus by means of 5-aminolevulinic acid. Gastroenterology 1998;114:448–55.

31. Sharma P, Morales TG, Bhattacharyya A, et al. Squamous islands in Barrett's esophagus: what lies underneath? Am J Gastroenterol 1998;93:332–5.

32. Achkar E, Carey W. The cost of surveillance for adenocarcinoma complicating Barrett's esophagus. Am J Gastroenterol 1988;83:291–4.

33. van der Burgh A, Dees J, Hop WCJ, et al. Oesophageal cancer is an uncommon cause of death in patients with Barrett's esophagus. Gut 1996;39:5–8.

34. Spechler SJ. Endoscopic surveillance for patients with Barrett's esophagus: Does the cancer risk justify the practice [editorial]. Ann Intern Med 1987;106:902–4.

35. Grimm I, Shaheen N, Bozymski EM. Surveillance for Barrett's esophagus: are we saving lives [selected summary]? Gastroenterology 1997;112:661–2.

36. Drewitz DJ, Sampliner RE, Garewal HS. The incidence of adenocarcinoma in Barrett's esophagus: a prospective study of 170 patients followed 4.8 years. Am J Gastroenterol 1997;92:212–5.

37. O'Connor JB, Falk GW, Richer JE. The incidence of adenocarcinoma and dysplasia in Barrett's esophagus. Am J Gastroenterol 1999;94:2037–42.

38. Lee RG. Adenomas arising in Barrett's esophagus. Am J Clin Pathol 1986;83:629–32.

39. McArdle JE, Lewin KJ, Randell G, Weinstein W. Distribution of dysplasia and early invasive carcinoma in Barrett's esophagus. Hum Pathol 1992;23:479–82.

40. Rudolph RE, Vaughan TL, Storer BE, et al. Effect of segment length on risk for neoplastic progression in patients with Barrett esophagus. Ann Intern Med 2000;132:612–20.

41. Cameron AJ, Lomboy CT, Pera M, et al. Adenocarcinoma of the esophagogastric junction and Barrett's esophagus. Gastroenterology 1995;1541–6.

42. Christensen W, Sternberg SS. Adenocarcinoma of the upper esophagus arising in ectopic gastric mucosa. Am J Surg Pathol 1987;11:397–402.

43. Epstein JI, Sears DL, Tucker RS, Eagan JW. Carcinoma of the esophagus with adenoid cystic differentiation. Cancer 1984;53:1131–6.

44. Osamura RY, Sato S, Mira M, et al. Mucoepidermoid carcinoma of the esophagus. Report of an unoperated autopsy case and a review of the literature. Am J Gastroenterol 1978;69:467–70.

5

Adenocarcinoma of the Esophagus and Gastroesophageal Junction

NORA T. JASKOWIAK, MD

MITCHELL C. POSNER, MD

The incidence of adenocarcinoma of the esophagus and gastroesophageal (GE) junction has risen dramatically in the United States and other Western countries over the last decades of the twentieth century.[1–3] At midcentury, esophageal adenocarcinoma was a rare entity compared to squamous cell cancer of the esophagus, but adenocarcinomas now outnumber squamous cell carcinomas in many series. This increase has been particularly impressive in white men, in whom the incidence of adenocarcinoma of the esophagus has risen by more than 350 percent since the mid-1970s.[3] The causes of this startling increase and its pattern are poorly understood although intense work on risk factors and etiology has yielded some insights.

The transitional nature of the anatomic GE junction has added further confusion to the understanding of this disease. Adenocarcinomas of the distal esophagus, GE junction, and gastric cardia have all increased in incidence, and many studies have grouped tumors at these locations together. Although there is a rationale for this grouping (increasing incidence rates in all locations, anatomic continuity, and similar pathologies), differences among these tumors exist as well (differing rates of increased incidence, proportion of cases involving Barrett's metaplasia, possible differing patterns of nodal spread). Recently proposed classification schemes aim to further define the anatomic regions.[4]

The specialized intestinal metaplasia that defines Barrett's esophagus[5] is recognized as a precursor lesion in most cases of esophageal adenocarcinoma and in many cases of adenocarcinoma at the GE junction. Barrett's esophagus is a result of chronic gastroesophageal reflux disease (GERD), but only about 10 percent of patients with chronic GERD will develop Barrett's changes.[6] Predisposing factors to development of Barrett's esophagus have yet to be defined, despite intense research. Molecular factors are beginning to be recognized.[7] Asymptomatic Barrett's esophagus occurs as well, complicating attempts at screening.

This chapter reviews the facts and controversies surrounding adenocarcinomas of the esophagus and GE junction, with particular attention to etiology, staging, and surgical therapy.

CLASSIFICATION

The classification of tumors, particularly at the GE junction, has been a problematic issue that has complicated the reporting of results. A consensus conference of the International Gastric Cancer Association (IGCA) and the International Society for Diseases of the Esophagus (ISDE) in 1998 defined and described adenocarcinomas of the GE junction as tumors that have their center within 5 cm proximally and distally of the anatomic cardia.[4] Within this area, tumors are differentiated into the following three distinct entities (Figure 5–1):

Type I: Adenocarcinoma of the distal esophagus, usually arising from an area with specialized intestinal metaplasia of the esophagus (ie, Barrett's esophagus); it may infiltrate the esophagogastric junction from above.

Type II: True carcinoma of the cardia, arising from the cardiac epithelium or short segments of intestinal metaplasia at the gastroesophageal junction; this entity is often referred to as "junctional carcinoma."

Type III: Subcardial gastric carcinoma that infiltrates the esophagogastric junction and distal esophagus from below.[4]

This chapter focuses on adenocarcinomas of the distal esophagus and on type I and II tumors of the GE junction. For the purposes of this chapter, type III tumors are categorized as gastric tumors.

INCIDENCE AND EPIDEMIOLOGY

It was estimated that there would be 13,200 new cases of esophageal carcinoma diagnosed in the United States and 12,500 deaths due to esophageal cancer in the year 2001.[8] These numbers represent all cancers of the esophagus (both squamous cell cancer and adenocarcinoma). Although squamous cell carcinoma was the predominant histology for most of the twentieth century, the incidence of adenocarcinoma has increased over the past several decades. In surgical series from the mid–twentieth century, adenocarcinomas represented a distinct minority, ranging from 1.3 to 10.0 percent of cases.[9–11] Recent major surgical series have reported rates of adenocarcinoma incidence of between 59 and 70 percent.[12–15] A single-institution study from the Johns Hopkins Tumor Registry reported sharp increases in cases of adenocarcinoma of the esophagus, beginning in 1978 and continuing to rise through 1994[16] (Figure 5–2). In 1994, the number of adenocarcinoma cases surpassed the number of squamous cell cancer cases for the first time since cases began to be recorded (in 1959).[16]

This rise has been confirmed by data from the National Cancer Institute's Surveillance, Epidemiology, and End Results (SEER) program showing adenocarcinoma cases exceeding squamous cell cancer cases in white males in 1990.[3] Blot and colleagues, using SEER data, reported in 1991 that the occurrence of adenocarcinoma of the esophagus was increasing at a rate of 4 to 10 percent per year in the United States, faster than the rate of increase in any other cancer.[1] During the period in question, squamous cell carcinoma trends were stable and the rates of adenocarcinoma of the distal stomach were decreasing.[1] A report from the National Cancer Data Base (NCDB) looked at rates of esophageal cancer in 1988 and 1993.[17] During this period, the rate of adenocarcinoma of the esophagus rose from 33.2 to 43.1 percent of all cases of esophageal cancer while the rate of squamous cell carcinoma fell from 66.2 to 56.0 percent of all cases.[17] Similar trends have been observed in Denmark, Switzerland, Sweden, Norway, and the United Kingdom. [6]

Rates of adenocarcinoma of the GE junction and gastric cardia have also risen in a similar (though less steep) fashion. Data from the SEER program reveal that in white males, annual rates of adenocarcinoma of the gastric cardia rose from 2.1 cases per year per 100,000 population in 1974 to 1976 to 3.3 cases per year per 100,000 in 1992 to 1994.[3] Rates rose in African American males also, from 1.0 cases per 100,000 in 1974 to 1976 to 1.9 per 100,000 in 1992 to 1994.[3] A study of rates of gastric cardia cancer in Connecticut revealed even greater rates of increase in

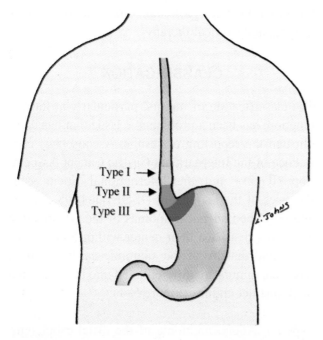

Figure 5–1. Classification of gastroesophageal junction tumors. (Adapted from Siewert JR, Stein HJ. Classification of adenocarcinoma of the oesophagogastric junction. Br J Surg 1998;85:1457–9.)

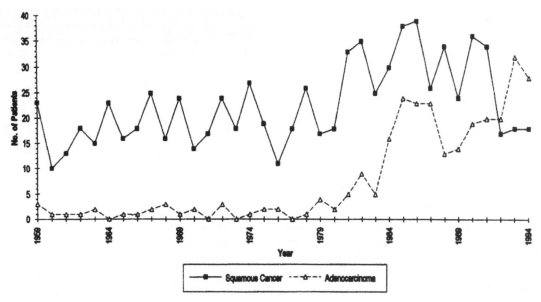

Figure 5–2. Trends in esophageal squamous cell carcinoma and adenocarcinoma by year at the Johns Hopkins Hospital, 1959 to 1994. (Reproduced with permission from Heitmiller RF, Sharma RR. Comparison of prevalence and resection rates in patients with esophageal squamous cell carcinoma and adenocarcinoma. J Thorac Cardiovasc Surg 1996;112:130–6.)

males, from 0.6 cases per 100,000 in 1955 to 1959 to 3.0 per 100,000 in 1985 to 1989, a fivefold increase.[18] Similar rates of increase occurred in females, although with lower absolute numbers (from 0.1 cases per 100,000 in 1965 to 1969 to 0.6 per 100,000 in 1985 to 1989).[18]

Pera and colleagues observed similar rates of increase in a population-based study in Olmsted County, Minnesota.[19] Adenocarcinoma of the esophagus rose from 0.13 cases per 100,000 person-years in 1935 to 1971 to 0.74 cases per 100,000 person-years in 1974 to 1984 while adenocarcinoma of the GE junction rose from 0.25 cases per 100,000 person-years in 1935 to 1971 to 1.34 cases per 100,000 person-years in 1974 to 1984.[19]

Overall rates of increase vary according to age, gender, and race, although increases are seen among all groups. Blot and colleagues showed a very high male-to-female ratio (~7.6:1) among white persons.[1] In SEER data, the rising incidence of esophageal adenocarcinoma tended to affect all age groups[1,2] whereas NCDB data showed the greatest rate of rise in older men.[17] Multiple studies have revealed the greatest rate of rise to be among white males, with smaller but increasing rates in African Americans (males and females) and white females[3,17–19] (Figure 5–3).

ETIOLOGY

The exact cause of this increased incidence is unclear. Table 5–1 lists factors identified in numerous reports to be associated with an increased or decreased risk of adenocarcinoma of the esophagus.

Barrett's esophagus is the single most important factor for the development of adenocarcinoma of the esophagus and GE junction. Myriad studies have been conducted, and these studies place patients with Barrett's esophagus at a 30 to 125 times increased risk of developing esophageal adenocarcinoma.[20] The definition of Barrett's esophagus has evolved over the last several decades, with wide variations over time and between investigators. For the purposes of this chapter, Barrett's esophagus is defined as an acquired disorder of the distal esophagus, in which (due to chronic GE reflux and resultant reflux esophagitis) squamous epithelium is eroded and replaced by columnar epithelium, either by metaplasia or by the extension of columnar epithelium from the stomach.[21]

The controversies surrounding Barrett's esophagus go back to Norman Barrett himself. Barrett, an influential British surgeon, wrote in 1950 that the "peptic" ulcers seen below the squamocolumnar junction were in a "pouch of stomach" drawn up into the chest by scar.[22] In 1953, Allison and Johnstone demonstrated that these ulcers actually occurred in a portion of the tubular foregut that had normal esophageal musculature, esophageal-type glands, and no peritoneal covering.[23] In 1957, Barrett conceded that in some cases, columnar epithelium extended up into the esophagus, calling this "columnar-lined lower esophagus," which has since been referred to as "Barrett's esophagus."[24] Barrett, Allison, and others thought that the condition was congenital, but in 1959, Moersch recognized it as acquired.[25] The association between columnar-lined esophagus and GERD was first shown in the landmark paper of Bremner in 1970, in an experimental

Table 5–1. FACTORS ASSOCIATED WITH RISK OF ESOPHAGEAL ADENOCARCINOMA

Association Factor	Odds Ratio
Positive	
Barrett's esophagus	NA
GERD	7.7
Tobacco	2.0–2.4
Obesity	2.5–16.2
Liquor consumption	—
Colon cancer (men only)	—
Breast cancer (radiation only)	—
LES-relaxing drugs	—
Negative	
Helicobacter pylori (cagA+ strains)	0.4
Wine consumption	0.6
High income	—
High education level	—

GERD = gastroesophageal reflux disease; LES = lower esophageal sphincter; NA = not available.

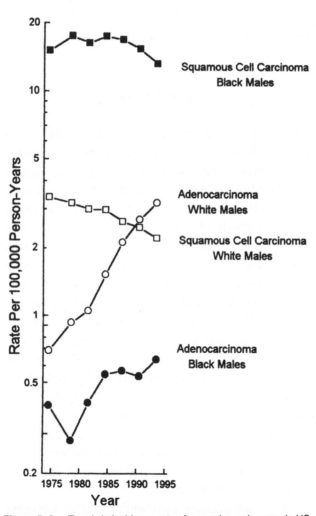

Figure 5–3. Trends in incidence rates for esophageal cancer in US males by race and cell type, from the years 1974 to 1976 to the years 1992 to 1994. (Reproduced with permission from Devesa SS, Blot WJ, Fraumeni JF Jr. Changing patterns in the incidence of esophageal and gastric carcinoma in the United States. Cancer 1998;83:2049–53.)

model in dogs.[26] The association between Barrett's esophagus and adenocarcinoma of the esophagus has been recognized since the 1970s.[21]

Other controversies of definition have existed as well, related to anatomy, cell pattern, extent, and etiology. Three types of columnar mucosa have been identified in the distal esophagus: the gastric-fundic type, which contains chief cells and parietal cells; the junctional type, which contains mucous cells without parietal cells; and the specialized type, which has intestinal characteristics.[21,27,28] The specialized type, which is referred to as specialized intestinal metaplasia (SIM), is characterized by goblet cells, which stain with Alcian blue at a pH of 2.5.[27] Of the three types of columnar mucosa, only SIM is known to be preneoplastic, with adenocarcinomas frequently being surrounded by SIM.[21,27,28]

Anatomically, the exact GE junction is defined variously by anatomists, radiologists, endoscopists, and physiologists. There is no "gold standard" for precise localization of the GE junction, which makes characterizing the extent of columnar mucosa imprecise.[21] Because of this, Barrett's esophagus has been defined by some authors as a minimal length of columnar mucosa (most commonly 3 cm, with a range of from 2 to 5 cm), largely to avoid false-positives when studying the entity. At present, Barrett's esophagus is referred to as "long-segment" Barrett's esophagus (LSBE) when its length is ≥ 3 cm of columnar mucosa and as "short-segment" Barrett's esophagus (SSBE) when it is < 3 cm in length.[29,30] Dysplasia and cancer have been found to arise from both LSBE and SSBE.[31,32] As well, there has been confusion between the cardiac region of the stomach, which is located distal to the GE junction and has oxyntic mucosa, and the cardia, which is located at and proximal to the GE junction in the distal esophagus and which may be lined with squamous mucosa or with junctional (cardiac) mucosa (only columnar cells and mucous cells).[28] Specialized intestinal metaplasia has been documented in biopsy specimens of the cardia,[28,30] and some investigators believe that it is the precursor for adenocarcinomas of the cardia.[21,31,33]

Estimates of the frequency of Barrett's esophagus depend on whether length (ie, ≥ 3 cm) or histologic characteristics (ie, the presence of SIM) or a combination of the two is the defining characteristic. Commonly presented numbers indicate that Barrett's esophagus is present in 0.45 to 2.2 percent of all patients undergoing upper endoscopy and in up to 10 to 12 percent of patients undergoing upper endoscopy for symptoms of reflux.[28,30,34] In one study, SIM was found on biopsy of the GE junction in 18 percent of patients who underwent endoscopy in a general endoscopy unit.[35] It has been hypothesized that many patients suffer reflux without typical symptoms and that columnar epithelium may be more acid resistant than normal squamous epithelim, and therefore less symptomatic, leading to a large number of patients with asymptomatic Barrett's esophagus.[34]

It is widely believed (and there is much evidence to support the concept) that Barrett's esophagus is the result of prolonged GE reflux.[26,28,34] Studies have documented a correlation between the degree of dysfunction of the lower esophageal sphincter, the amount of time that esophageal pH is < 4, and the poor esophageal clearance of acid with the extent of Barrett's changes in the distal esophagus.[34,36-38] Whereas previously it was thought that acid alone was the major injurious agent, there has been mounting evidence in the last decade that the presence of duodenal juice (principally bile) in the refluxate may lead to worsening of the injury, higher rates of Barrett's esophagus, and complications of Barrett's esophagus (ulcers, strictures, dysplasia, cancer).[27,34,37-40] Patients with higher bilirubin exposure (determined by use of a Bilitec probe) have a greater prevalence of Barrett's esophagus and its complications than patients without bilirubin in the refluxate.[37,39,40] Fein and colleagues demonstrated that patients with dysplasia and Barrett's esophagus had greater exposure to duodenal juice than did those with uncomplicated Barrett's esophagus ($p = .04$), with the same overall acid exposure time.[40] Stein and colleagues showed that there was an exponential increase in mean esophageal bile exposure time in those with erosive esophagitis and Barrett's esophagus when compared to those with GERD without esophagitis ($p < .01$) and that pathologic bile exposure occurred in 54 percent of patients with Barrett's esophagus and 78 percent of those with early adenocarcinomas in Barrett's esophagus.[37] The cause of SIM of the cardia is controversial; some investigators believe it to be reflux[28,41] whereas others believe it is related to *Helicobacter pylori* infection and intestinal metaplasia of the stomach.[42] These and similar data have led many to conclude that the combination of gastric and duodenal reflux may lead to the most severe esophageal mucosal damage and to Barrett's esophagus and its complications. A possible sequence that has been proposed is shown in Figure 5–4.[27,28]

The frequency with which Barrett's esophagus degenerates into dysplasia and adenocarcinoma and

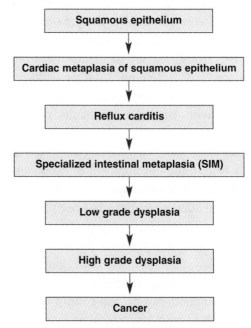

Figure 5–4. Sequence in the development of esophageal adenocarcinoma.

the frequency with which adenocarcinomas are found with surrounding Barrett's esophagus have been examined in multiple series. In a study examining the prevalence of SIM in all patients undergoing upper endoscopy, Hirota and colleagues found that the overall prevalence of SIM was 13.2 percent (1.6% for LSBE, 6.0% for SSBE, and 5.6% for GE-junction SIM).[43] Dysplasia or cancer was found in 31 percent of LSBE cases, 10 percent of SSBE cases, and 6.4 percent of GE-junction SIM cases ($p \leq .043$).[43] Examining the question from the opposite angle (ie, what is the prevalence of Barrett's esophagus in patients with adenocarcinomas of the distal esophagus and GE junction?), Clark and colleagues found that SIM was identified in histologic sections of resected specimens in 79 percent of esophageal adenocarcinomas, 42 percent of cardiac/GE-junction adenocarcinomas, and only 5 percent of subcardiac adenocarcinomas.[41] Cameron and colleagues found Barrett's esophagus in 100 percent of esophageal adenocarcinomas, 42 percent of GE-junction adenocarcinomas, and 0 percent of esophageal squamous cell cancers.[20] Of note, both Clark and Cameron commented that in GE-junction adenocarcinomas, segments of Barrett's esophagus/SIM tended to be short and had been missed on endoscopy in many cases.[20,41] The incidence of adenocarcinoma in patients with known Barrett's esophagus was examined by Drewitz and colleagues in 177 patients with Barrett's esophagus observed for a mean of 4.8 years. Four adenocarcinomas developed during the study, for an incidence of 1 per 208 patient-years of follow-up.[44] Other authors have stated that the annual incidence of adenocarcinoma in patients with Barrett's esophagus ranges from 0.23 to 0.8 percent.[21,36,45]

Factors other than Barrett's esophagus are thought to play a role in the development of esophageal and GE-junction adenocarcinomas. The role of smoking in esophageal adenocarcinoma has been identified in several studies, although its impact in adenocarcinoma is less than in squamous cell carcinoma. In a landmark study, Gammon and colleagues examined risk factors for esophageal adenocarcinoma.[46] A multicenter population-based case-control design was used. The risk of both esophageal and gastric adenocarcinomas was increased in current smokers, with

an odds ratio (OR) of 2.4.[46] A dose-response relation was demonstrated. Furthermore, no reduction in risk was observed until 30 years after smoking cessation. These results led to the conclusion that smoking is a major risk factor for esophageal and gastric cardiac adenocarcinomas and raised the possibility that the impact is at an early stage of carcinogenesis as no reduction was seen for many years after cessation. This may partly explain the rising incidence of these cancers, as rates of smoking increased steadily through the first two-thirds of the twentieth century.[46]

These findings of a more than doubly increased risk are consistent with the results of six other case-control studies, which showed a statistically significant association between cigarette smoking and adenocarcinoma of the esophagus and gastric cardia.[47] Zhang and colleagues reported that the odds ratio for risk of adenocarcinoma of the esophagus and gastric cardia was 2.36 if a patient's smoking history was one of > 60 pack-years of smoking (contrasted with an odds ratio of 5.9 for esophageal squamous cell cancer in a patient with a history of > 40 pack-years).[48] Although not as dominating a factor as in esophageal squamous cell cancer, tobacco use remains a reproducible, significant, and preventable risk factor for adenocarcinoma of the esophagus and gastric cardia.

Past data concerning the impact of body weight on esophageal adenocarcinoma have been weak and inconsistent. Several recent studies identified excess weight as a strong risk factor. In a multicenter population-based case-control study, Chow and colleagues showed that the OR for esophageal adenocarcinoma increased with increasing adult body mass index (BMI).[49] The magnitude was greatest in the youngest patients. Increased BMI posed a less impressive but still greater risk for GE-junction adenocarcinoma. No association was seen between increased BMI and esophageal squamous cell carcinoma or noncardiac gastric cancer.[49] On the basis of these findings, the authors concluded that the increasing prevalence of obesity in the United States might contribute to the upward trend in esophageal and esophagogastric adenocarcinomas. An even stronger and dose-dependent association emerged from a Swedish study by Lagergren and colleagues.[50] In a population-based case-control study, they demonstrated that among obese patients (BMI > 30 kg/m^2), the OR for esophageal adenocarcinoma was 16.2 (compared to the leanest group [BMI < 22 kg/m^2]) and that the OR was 4.3 for gastric cardia adenocarcinoma.[50] No association was seen between BMI and esophageal squamous cell carcinoma. The mechanism of this increased risk is unclear. It has been proposed that increased BMI may lead to increased GERD and hiatal hernia, but one study found no association between GERD symptoms and BMI.[51] In a case-control study, Zhang and colleagues found that a high intake of calories and fat was associated with an increased risk of adenocarcinoma of the esophagus, more suggestive of a dietary than a mechanical effect.[52]

Special attention has been paid in recent years to the role of *Helicobacter pylori* in gastrointestinal-tract cancers. Whereas there is a positive association of atrophic gastritis and gastric cancers with cagA+ strains of *H. pylori*, there is a negative association for esophageal, GE-junction, and gastric cardia tumors. In a multicenter case-control study, Chow and colleagues demonstrated an inverse relation between *H. pylori* infection and esophageal cancer in the United States. The OR for cagA+ strains of *H. pylori* and esophageal adenocarcinoma was 0.4.[53] In another study, the presence of cagA+ *H. pylori* appeared to be protective against the development of esophageal adenocarcinoma.[54] The exact mechanism of the protective effect is unclear, but one theory states that there is decreased acid production in the presence of cagA+ *H. pylori* and therefore less acid reflux. Others have stated the opposite—that *H. pylori* infection is responsible for SIM of the cardia.[42] Work is ongoing, but serious questions exist about the effects of widespread eradication of *H. pylori* on the rates of esophageal and GE-junction adenocarcinomas.

The role of alcohol consumption in the occurrence of esophageal and GE-junction adenocarcinomas is likely minimal, in direct contrast to the known impact of ethanol on the risk of squamous cell cancers of the esophagus. In the study of Gammon and colleagues, there was no association seen between consumption of beer or liquor and rates of esophageal and GE-junction adenocarcinoma (ORs of 0.8 for beer and 1.1 for liquor).[46] Wine drinking was associated with a reduced risk of these cancers (OR = 0.6). Levi and colleagues demonstrated an OR of 1.8 for esophageal and GE-junction adenocarcinomas if more than 21 drinks per week were consumed (contrasted with an OR of 9.5 for esophageal squamous cell carcinoma, with the same level of intake).[55]

The impact of various medications on the rate of esophageal and GE-junction adenocarcinomas has been examined as well. Two major categories of concern have been H$_2$ blockers and drugs that relax the lower esophageal sphincter (LES). Data from a case-control study conducted through the National Cancer Institute revealed no increased risk of adenocarcinoma of the esophagus and GE junction in users of H$_2$ blockers.[56] Data on LES-relaxing drugs are conflicting at present. Theoretically, cancer risk would increase if LES pressure was reduced by drugs such as nitroglycerine, anticholinergics, β-adrenergic agonists, aminophyllines, benzodiazepines, and calcium channel blockers, secondary to increased reflux and development of Barrett's changes. A study in the United States by Vaughn and colleagues found no increased risk with the use of calcium channel blockers (OR = 1.0) but found a positive increased risk with the long-term use of certain asthma medications. The OR was 2.5 for theophylline use and 1.7 for β adrenergic agonists.[57] In a large Swedish case-control study, Lagergren and colleagues found an increased risk of adenocarcinoma of the esophagus in long-term (> 5 years) users of LES-relaxing drugs.[58] (Calcium channel blockers were not examined in that study.) No consistent association was seen with these drugs and the incidence of adenocarcinoma of the gastric cardia or squamous cell cancer of the esophagus. The authors concluded that ~10 percent of esophageal adenocarcinomas in Sweden might be caused by the long-term use of drugs that promote LES relaxation.[58]

In addition, interest has focused on whether the use of acetylsalicylic acid (ASA) and nonsteroidal anti-inflammatory drugs (NSAIDs) might reduce the risk of some gastrointestinal-tract malignancies as it has reduced the risk of colon cancers. A population-based case-control study demonstrated a decreased risk of esophageal adenocarcinoma, noncardia gastric tumors, and squamous cell carcinoma of the esophagus with the use of ASA and NSAIDs.[59] An OR of 0.37 was found for esophageal adenocarcinoma in current users of ASA. Further investigation is needed to confirm these results.

The role of GERD, independent of Barrett's esophagus, has been examined. Reflux is thought to increase cancer risk by promoting cellular proliferation and by exposing esophageal epithelium to potentially genotoxic gastric and intestinal contents.[57] Lagergren and colleagues demonstrated a dose-dependent relationship between the symptoms of GERD and the development of adenocarcinoma of the esophagus and GE junction.[60] Patients with recurrent symptomatic reflux had an OR of 7.7 for esophageal adenocarcinoma and 2.0 for gastric cardia adenocarcinoma. More frequent, more severe, and longer-lasting symptoms were associated with an even higher risk. In another population-based case-control study, the risk of esophageal adenocarcinoma increased with the increasing frequency of GERD symptoms, with an OR of 5.5 among patients with daily symptoms.[61] No further increased risk was seen with the use of H_2 blockers.

DIAGNOSIS AND STAGING

Most patients with esophageal cancer present with advanced-stage disease. Symptoms at presentation include dysphagia, weight loss, and bleeding. Precise histologic diagnosis and accurate tumor staging are prerequisites for the selection of the most suitable treatment, especially if the patient is being considered for clinical trials.[62]

Clinical staging is determined by the extent of disease, which is established by a variety of diagnostic tests and imaging studies. Pathologic staging is determined by evaluating a surgical specimen after resection. The most recent American Joint Committee on Cancer (AJCC) staging system, based on the primary tumor (T)–nodal involvement (N)–distant metastasis (M) system, is shown in Table 5–2. The current staging system has been criticized, and revisions have been suggested. Because this staging system is largely based on retrospective data from Japan, it is most applicable to patients with squamous cell tumors of the upper and middle thirds of the esophagus. In particular, the classification of involved celiac lymph nodes as M1 disease has been questioned. A recent study evaluating sur-

Table 5–2. AMERICAN JOINT COMMITTEE ON CANCER STAGING FOR ESOPHAGEAL CANCER

Tumor-Node-Metastasis Staging
  Primary tumor (T)
    TX: Primary tumor cannot be assessed
    T0: No evidence of primary tumor
    Tis: Carcinoma in situ
    T1: Tumor invades lamina propria or submucosa
    T2: Tumor invades muscularis propria
    T3: Tumor invades adventitia
    T4: Tumor invades adjacent structures
  Regional lymph nodes (N)
    NX: Regional lymph nodes cannot be assessed
    N0: No regional lymph node metastasis
    N1: Regional lymph node metastasis
  Distant metastasis (M)
    General
      MX: Distant metastasis cannot be assessed
      M0: No distant metastasis
      M1: Distant metastasis
    Tumors of the lower thoracic esophagus
      M1a: Metastasis in celiac lymph nodes
      M1b: Other distant metastasis
    Tumors of the midthoracic esophagus
      M1a: Not applicable
      M1b: Nonregional lymph nodes and/or other distant metastasis
    Tumors of the upper thoracic esophagus
      M1a: Metastasis in cervical lymph nodes
      M1b: Other distant metastasis
Stage groupings
  0: Tis, N0, M0
  I: T1, N0, M0
  IIA: T2, N0, M0
      T3, N0, M0
  IIB: T1, N1, M0
      T2, N1, M0
  III: T3, N1, M0
      T4, any N, M0
  IV: any T, any N, M1
  IVA: any T, any N, M1a
  IVB: any T, any N, M1b

Adapted from American Joint Committee on Cancer. Esophagus. In: AJCC cancer staging manual. Lippincott-Raven Publishers; 1997. p. 65–9.

vival with respect to lymph node involvement demonstrated that both lymph node location and number significantly influenced survival.[12] A proposed staging system that reserves M1 status for visceral metastases and reclassifies extensive lymph node metastases as N2 reflects prognosis more accurately than the current AJCC system.[12]

A general schema for the work-up of esophageal and GE-junction adenocarcinomas is shown in Figure 5–5. The diagnosis of esophageal cancer and the assessment of a tumor's longitudinal extent are usually accomplished by endoscopy with biopsy, with emphasis on both orthograde and retroflexed views of the GE junction.[63] Barium studies (Figure 5–6) are useful in evaluating the morphology of the tumor and have a high sensitivity (~98%) for demonstrating esophageal tumors.[64] A barium swallow provides essential information concerning gastric anatomy, the location and extent of the lesion, and whether there is pathology proximal or distal to the primary lesion.[65] Though rarely the case with adenocarcinomas, bronchoscopy is recommended to rule out tracheal invasion when tumors lie at or above the carina.

Once the histologic diagnosis of esophageal cancer is established, staging of the extent of disease is done. Computed tomography (CT) of the chest and abdomen is considered the initial imaging study of choice for evaluating lymph node metastases, distant metastases, and extraesophageal tumor infiltration into mediastinal organs[62] (Figure 5–7). Abdominal

ultrasonography and magnetic resonance imaging (MRI) are occasionally useful in evaluating liver metastases. The use of positron emission tomography (PET) for staging patients with esophageal adenocarcinoma has recently been reported.[66–68] In an early experience, Flamen and colleagues found that PET significantly improves the detection of stage IV disease, compared to the combination of CT and endoscopic ultrasonography (EUS).[67] Patients in whom distant metastases are found are candidates for palliative treatment.

Much investigation has been done in the past decade into the role of EUS in the locoregional staging of esophageal cancer. It is the most accurate diagnostic modality for locoregional staging, providing detailed images of the mass and its relationship with the layers of the esophageal wall.[69] Most studies of EUS have included both adenocarcinomas

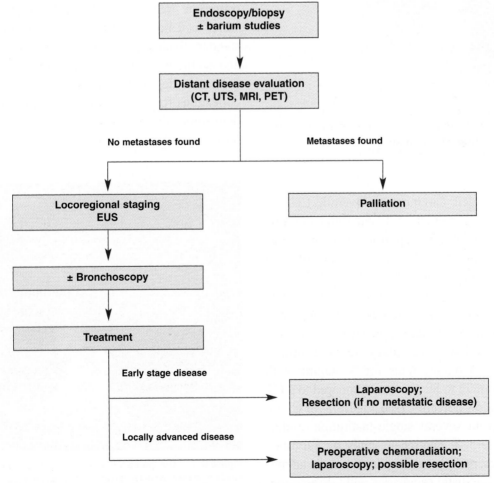

Figure 5–5. Algorithm for the work-up of esophageal adenocarcinoma patients. (CT = computed tomography; MRI = magnetic resonance imaging; PET = positron emission tomography; UTS = ultrasonography.)

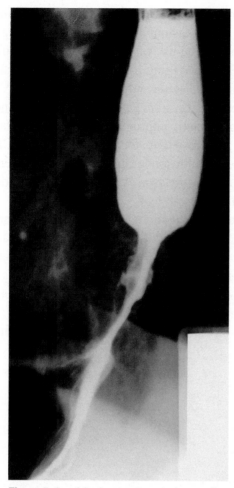

Figure 5–6.   A barium swallow study, revealing irregular narrowing of the distal esophageal lumen, with proximal dilation and air-contrast level. (Courtesy of A. Dachman, MD.)

conclusion of many of these studies is that although EUS has distinct advantages in staging tumors and planning therapy, it has limitations as well, and that caution must be exercised when deciding resectability on the basis of EUS as it tends to err in the direction of up-staging tumors.[72] A more direct approach to evaluating regional lymph node involvement is with EUS-guided fine-needle aspiration (FNA). Reports show that this technique of tissue sampling is safe and effective[70] (Figure 5–9). Reed and colleagues recently reported an 88 percent confirmation of node positivity with EUS-guided FNA when EUS identified suspicious celiac lymph nodes.[73] This improvement in staging may help guide treatment in patients with locally advanced esophageal adenocarcinomas.

Some of the limitations of EUS (eg, the inability of the probe to pass through near-obstructing tumors, and an inability to differentiate between intramucosal and intramural tumors) are now being overcome with microprobe EUS. These probes, which can be passed through the working ports of standard endoscopes, have been shown to be safe and accurate, with a particularly improved ability to determine depth of invasion. A study by Murata and colleagues focused on the ability of microprobes to determine the depth of invasion of superficial tumors and found an overall accuracy of 75 percent

and squamous cell carcinomas. Overall, EUS is highly accurate in predicting T stage and multiple studies have found it to be superior to CT for T stage evaluation[70] (Figure 5–8, A and B). The accuracy of EUS for T staging ranges from 76 to 89 percent whereas the accuracy of CT for T staging is between 43 and 59 percent.[70,71] Endoscopic ultrasonography tends to overestimate T stage, particularly in T1 and T2 lesions (perhaps secondary to peritumoral inflammation). Accuracy rates for N staging with EUS range from 72 to 80 percent, compared to a CT range of 46 to 58 percent[70] (see Figure 5–8, C and D). Results from several single-institution studies appear in Table 5–3. The recent study by Salminen and colleagues includes only patients with adenocarcinoma of the distal esophagus and GE junction; its results were similar to those of prior studies. The

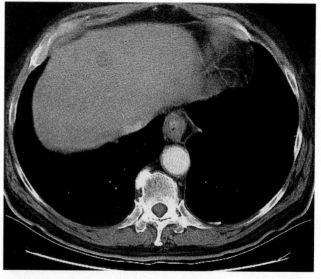

Figure 5–7.   Computed tomography scan of the gastroesophageal junction shows wall-thickening at the gastroesophageal junction, consistent with tumor. Note the sharply marginated liver mass, consistent with metastasis.

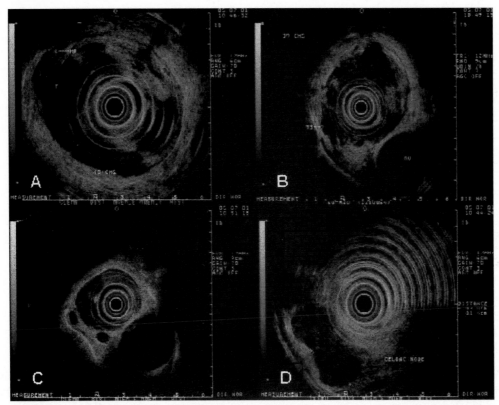

Figure 5–8. Endoscopic ultrasonographic images of the esophagus and periesophageal lymph nodes. *A*, Tumor to muscularis propria. *B*, Tumor through esophageal wall (T3). *C*, Peritumoral lymph nodes. *D*, Celiac node, 2 cm. (Courtesy of I. Waxman, MD.)

and an 84 percent accuracy for predicting tumor containment by the lamina propria.[74] A more recent comparative study looked at 53 stenosing tumors, 58 percent of which were adenocarcinomas, and examined the tumors with both conventional EUS and microprobe EUS microprobe sonography (MPS). Accuracy for both T and N staging markedly improved with the MPS device (T stage, 87% vs 62%; N stage, 83% vs 70%).[75]

There have been several recent reports looking at the role of laparoscopy and thoracoscopy in staging esophageal cancer patients. Both modalities are used to determine suitability for surgical resection. In one study of laparoscopy, contraindications to resection included evidence of hepatic metastases, peritoneal involvement, extensive lymph node involvement, direct invasion of the liver or colon, and poor tolerance of laparoscopy.[76] Using these criteria, 42 percent of 244 patients were found to have contraindications to resection (38% had contraindications secondary to advanced local or metastatic disease and 4% had contraindications secondary to poor tolerance of laparoscopy). Laparoscopy was highly effective in detecting hepatic metastases and had sensitivity, specificity, and overall accuracy of 96 percent, 100 percent, and 98 percent, respectively.[76] In a study from Stein and colleagues, diagnostic laparoscopy with laparoscopic ultrasonography and

Table 5–3. ACCURACY OF ENDOSCOPIC ULTRASONOGRAPHY FOR ESOPHAGEAL CANCER STAGING					
Study, Year	Ref. No.	n	% Not Traversable with Probe	T Stage Accuracy (%)	N Stage Accuracy (%)
Rice, 1991	210	28	21	59	70
Dittler, 1993	211	167	NA	86	73
Peters, 1994	71	42	19	76	82
Salminen, 1999	72	32	19	66	72

NA = not available; n = sample size.

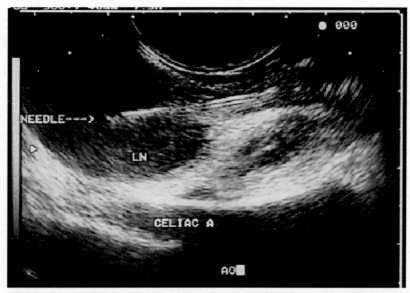

Figure 5–9. Endoscopic ultrasonography-guided fine-needle aspiration of a celiac lymph node. (Courtesy of I. Waxman, MD.)

peritoneal lavage was found to be safe and to frequently provide therapeutically relevant new information in patients with locally advanced adenocarcinoma of the distal esophagus or cardia.[77] Studies of thoracoscopy have shown it to be effective in intrathoracic tumor-node-metastasis (TNM) staging, allowing evaluation of direct mediastinal invasion and mediastinal nodal status.[78] The overall accuracy of thoracoscopy and laparoscopy for detecting lymph node involvement was 94 percent.[78]

PROGNOSIS, NATURAL HISTORY, AND PATTERN OF TUMOR SPREAD

The prognosis of esophageal adenocarcinoma is highly dependent on stage and is quite poor overall since most tumors are advanced at presentation. As reported by the AJCC,[79] the 5-year survival rates for both esophageal adenocarcinoma and squamous cell cancer are 68 percent for stage I, 35 percent for stage II, 18 percent for stage III, and 5 percent for stage IV. Overall 10-year survival for all patients with esophageal cancer was 12.3 percent.[80] For adenocarcinoma of the GE junction, Steup and colleagues reported an overall 5-year actuarial survival rate of 33 percent in surgically treated patients. The 5-year survivals were 100 percent for stage I, 68 percent for stage II, 37 percent for stage III, and 10 percent for stage IV.[81] A recent report on radical surgery for

esophageal and GE-junction adenocarcinoma demonstrated an overall 5-year survival of 35.3 percent in surgically treated patients.[82] Obviously, these figures do not reflect those patients who were ineligible for surgery.

A variety of factors have proved to have prognostic significance in esophageal and GE-junction adenocarcinoma. These are summarized in Table 5–4 and include T stage, N stage, M stage, positive esophageal margin at resection, R0 (no residual disease at surgery) versus R1 (microscopic residual disease)/R2 (macroscopic residual disease) resection, and occurrence of postoperative complications.[81,83–86] The number of diseased lymph nodes and the ratio of involved to removed lymph nodes have shown prognostic significance in some studies.[33,83,85]

Table 5–4. FACTORS INFLUENCING PROGNOSIS OF ADENOCARCINOMA OF THE ESOPHAGUS AND GASTROESOPHAGEAL JUNCTION	
By Univariate Analysis	**By Multivariate Analysis**
T stage	T stage
N stage	N stage
M stage	M stage
Number of disease nodes	R0 resection
Positive esophageal margin	Ratio of positive to removed nodes
Occurrence of postoperative complications	

Adapted from Siewert et al,[63] Steup et al,[81] Thomas et al,[83] Nigro et al.[85]

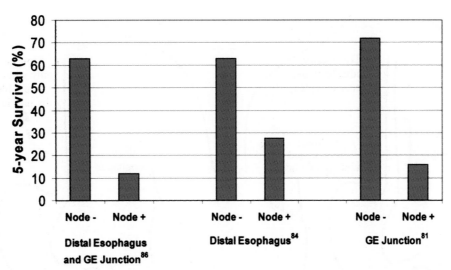

Figure 5–10. The impact of lymph node status on 5-year survival rates. (GE = gastroesophageal.) (Data from Lerut,[86] Holscher et al,[84] Steup et al.[81])

Lymph node status appears to be the single most important factor for prognosis in esophageal adenocarcinoma. Figure 5–10 summarizes a number of these studies. In a report from Lerut, node-negative patients had a 5-year survival of 63 percent, compared with 12 percent for node-positive patients.[86] Holscher and colleagues reported that in patients undergoing R0 resection for distal esophageal tumors, pN0 patients had a 63 percent 5-year survival compared to a 27.5 percent 5-year survival for pN1 patients ($p < .02$).[84] Steup and colleagues, in a study of adenocarcinoma at the GE junction, found that the 5-year survival rate for node-negative patients was 72 percent, versus 16 percent for node-positive patients ($p < .005$).[81] A study looking at the absolute number of positive lymph nodes in patients with GE-junction adenocarcinomas showed that patients with four or fewer involved lymph nodes had a statistically significant survival advantage compared to patients with more than four metastatic nodes ($p < .05$).[33] In patients with transmural distal esophageal adenocarcinomas, Nigro and colleagues demonstrated that patients with more than four involved nodes had a worse prognosis than those with no positive nodes or one to four positive nodes.[85]

Patterns of lymph node spread from the esophagus and esophageal cancer have been studied extensively. Siewert states that the embryologic development of the distal esophagus from the primitive intestinal loop dictates that lymph flow is primarily directed toward the large lymphatic collection area around the celiac axis.[87] Tanabe used an injection of radiolabeled colloid into the esophageal wall to examine patterns of lymph flow[88] (Figure 5–11). Injection into the midesophagus resulted in flow both up into the superior mediastinum and cervical nodes and down into the abdomen. Injection into the wall of the lower esophagus showed that the main direction of flow was down, into the abdomen.[88] Reports of surgery for esophageal adenocarcinoma have documented the pattern of positive nodes in various nodal basins[33,84–87] (Figure 5–12). A summary of these results is presented in Table 5–5. The percentage of positive nodes varies across these studies largely because of the different percentages of T stages included. A general pattern can be identified, with the highest rate of involved nodes being in the lower paraesophageal, paracardial (cardia of the GE junction), and parahiatal level and with lower rates of involvement of the splenic, hepatoduodenal, superior mediastinal, and cervical nodes.

The depth of invasion of the primary tumor is prognostically significant and correlates with nodal positivity. In the study by Holscher and colleagues, patients with pT1 tumors had a significantly better 5-year survival rate (83%) compared with those with pT2 tumors (36.8%) ($p = .001$), and the 5-year survival rate of the pT4 cases (7%) was significantly less than that for pT3 cases (27.5%) ($p < .05$).[84] In that study, pT1 tumors had a low rate of nodal positivity

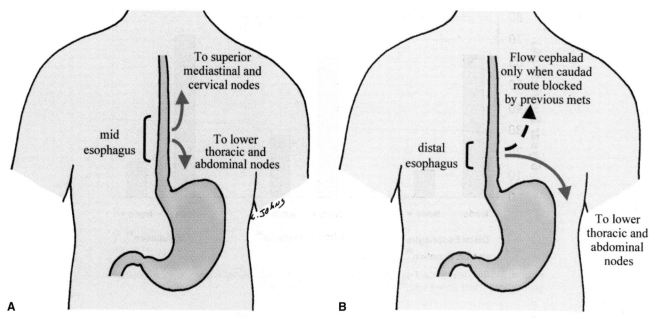

Figure 5–11. Pattern of lymph flow from the esophagus. *A*, Flow from the midesophagus is both cephalad and caudad. *B*, Flow from the distal esophagus is principally caudad. (Adapted from Tanabe G, Baba M, Kuroshima K, et al. [Clinical evaluation of the esophageal lymph flow system based on RI uptake of dissected regional lymph nodes following lymphoscintigraphy]. Nippon Geka Gakkai Zasshi 1986;87:315–23.)

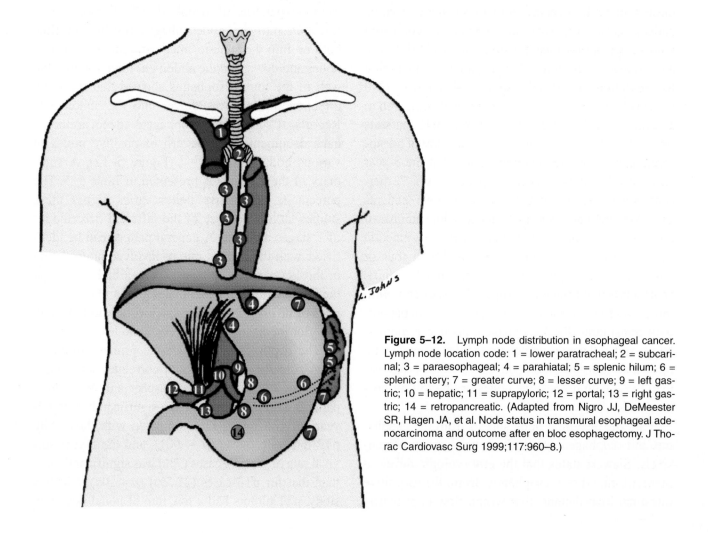

Figure 5–12. Lymph node distribution in esophageal cancer. Lymph node location code: 1 = lower paratracheal; 2 = subcarinal; 3 = paraesophageal; 4 = parahiatal; 5 = splenic hilum; 6 = splenic artery; 7 = greater curve; 8 = lesser curve; 9 = left gastric; 10 = hepatic; 11 = suprapyloric; 12 = portal; 13 = right gastric; 14 = retropancreatic. (Adapted from Nigro JJ, DeMeester SR, Hagen JA, et al. Node status in transmural esophageal adenocarcinoma and outcome after en bloc esophagectomy. J Thorac Cardiovasc Surg 1999;117:960–8.)

(13.2%), significantly different from pT2 tumors (77%), pT3 tumors (83%), and pT4 tumors (96%) ($p < .001$).[84] In a study from the University of Southern California (USC) by Clark and colleagues using the wall node metastasis (WNM) system, positive nodes occurred in 33 percent (2 of 6) of intramucosal tumors, 67 percent (6 of 9) of intramural tumors, and 89 percent (25 of 28) of transmural tumors ($p < .01$).[33]

Three-field lymph node dissection (abdominal, mediastinal, and cervical) has been proposed by some surgeons who favor radical en bloc resections.[89,90] When patients with esophageal adenocarcinoma have undergone three-field dissections, positive cervical nodes have been identified. In a study of three-field lymphadenectomies in 30 patients, half of whom had adenocarcinoma, Altorki found that 27 percent of the adenocarcinoma patients had occult cervical node metastases, irrespective of T status.[90] In no patient with adenocarcinoma were the cervical nodes the only involved nodal basin. It has been suggested by Siewert that drainage of lymph into the cervical nodes occurs only when the aboral route is blocked by previous nodal metastases.[87]

MOLECULAR-BIOLOGIC ASPECTS

In recent years, a variety of molecular studies have been carried out to increase understanding of the metaplasia-dysplasia-carcinoma sequence and to attempt to identify early markers of malignant transformation. The molecular and genetic abnormalities identified include deoxyribonucleic acid (DNA) content, growth factors, oncogenes, tumor-suppressor genes, adhesion molecules, microsatellite instability, and specific genetic anomolies. Of interest, several molecular factors that have been found to be important in some cancers (such as the *ras* oncogene, the retinoblastoma (Rb) gene, and bcl-2) have been found to play no definitive role in esophageal adenocarcinoma as yet.[91]

Phenotypic Abnormalities

On the phenotypic level, increased expression or changes in patterns of expression in a number of molecular factors have been identified. Many studies have used immunohistochemical staining of spe-

Table 5–5. ANATOMIC DISTRIBUTION OF LYMPH NODE METASTASES

Study	n	Position of Tumor	T Levels Included	Cervical/High Paratracheal	Subcarinal	Lower Paraesophageal	Paracardial/ Hiatal	Lesser Curvature	Celiac Axis	Splenic Artery/Hilum	Greater Curvature	Hepatoduodenal Ligament
Nigro, 1999	8	Distal esophagus	"Transmural"	ND	13	50	25	25	25	13	0	0
Lerut, 1998	11	Distal esophagus	T3 N+	36	20	↑ 50	↓	NI	10	14	NI	0
Holscher, 1995	134	Distal esophagus	All T levels	ND	2	38	55	10	↑	24	↓	12
Clark, 1994	43	Low esophagus + cardia	All T levels (²/₃ transmural)	2	9	28	35	42	21	7	9	5
Nigro, 1999	36	GEJ	"Transmural"	ND	8	33	56	22	53	22	6	3
Lerut, 1998	16	GEJ	T3 N+	17	22	↑ 8.3	↓	NI	38	61	NI	0
Siewert, 2000	186	Type II GEJ	All T levels	NI	NI	16	62	68	↑ 27	↓	16	5

ND = not done; NI = no information; GEJ = gastroesophageal junction.
Adapted from Clark et al,[33] Siewert et al,[63] Holscher et al,[84] Nigro et al,[85] Lerut.[86]

cific antigens. A nuclear antigen that is expressed in proliferating cells (G_1, S, G_2, and M phases) but not in resting cells (G_0 phase) is Ki-67. Hong and colleagues examined Ki-67 patterns in various degrees of dysplasia and adenocarcinoma. The pattern of Ki-67 nuclear staining correlated with the histologic findings, with increased size of the proliferative zone and spread of proliferation through the entire thickness of the epithelium in high-grade dysplasia and cancer ($p < .001$).[92] Other studies have confirmed these results.[93] It has been suggested that the Ki-67 staining pattern may represent an additional parameter for differentiating patients with dysplasia from those without dysplasia.

The overexpression of certain growth factors has been noted. Studies of epidermal growth factor receptor (EGFR) and transforming growth factor-α (TGF-α) show a steady increase from nonmetaplastic through adenocarcinoma tissues. One hundred percent of Barrett's adenocarcinomas were positive for TGF-α, and 64 percent were positive for EGFR; EGFR expression correlated with poorer survival on univariate analysis.[93] Data on the overexpression of c-erb B2 in Barrett's dysplasia and adenocarcinoma are conflicting. While several studies have shown no change or a decreased expression of c-erb B2 in esophageal adenocarcinomas,[94,95] other studies have demonstrated overexpression of c-erb B2. Hardwick and colleagues reported no immunostaining for nondysplastic columnar-lined esophagus whereas 26 percent (8 of 31) of adenocarcinomas stained positive for c-erb B2.[96] They concluded that overexpression of c-erb B2 is a relatively late event in some Barrett's adenocarcinomas. Flejou and colleagues found that 11 percent (7 of 66) of Barrett's adenocarcinomas overexpressed c-erb B2 and that this correlated with a poorer prognosis.[97]

Abnormally decreased expression of adhesion molecules has been documented in cases of esophageal adenocarcinoma. This altered expression is thought to lead to decreased cell-cell interaction, possibly increasing the propensity for metastases. Washington and colleagues studied specimens of Barrett's esophagus (with and without dysplasia) and esophageal adenocarcinomas and found that abnormally decreased expression of β-catenin, α-catenin, and E-cadherin was significantly associated with higher degrees of dysplasia.[98] Fourteen of 16 cases (87.5%) of high-grade dysplasia and 7 of 7 cases (100%) of intramucosal carcinoma showed abnormal expression of β-catenin, compared with 3 of 6 cases (50%) that were indefinite for dysplasia and 11 of 17 cases (65%) with low-grade dysplasia ($p = .022$).[98] This alteration in adhesion molecules appears to occur relatively early in the dysplasia-carcinoma sequence.

Abnormalities in Deoxyribonucleic Acid Content

In Barrett's epithelium, a sequence of DNA content changes has been identified along the metaplasia-dysplasia-carcinoma sequence, with an increased S phase in metaplasia, an increased tetraploid ($4N$) fraction in low-grade dysplasia, and aneuploidy in high-grade dysplasia and carcinoma. In a prospective cohort study, Reid and colleagues observed 62 patients with Barrett's esophagus. Of 13 patients with aneuploidy or increased tetraploidy ($4N$) on initial flow cytometry, 9 developed high-grade dysplasia or cancer during follow-up (mean = 34 months). None of the 49 patients without these abnormalities progressed ($p < .0001$).[99] This suggests that neoplastic progression in Barrett's esophagus may occur in patients who have an acquired genomic instability that generates abnormal clones of cells. It has been suggested that flow cytometry for aneuploidy may help identify those patients who warrant more frequent endoscopic surveillance. In addition to aneuploidy, other cytogenetic abnormalities principally related to chromosome loss have been noted. Frequent losses of chromosomes 4, 18, 21, and Y have been noted.[100] Few data exist, however, as to the sequence or timing of these losses.

Specific Genetic Abnormalities

Several specific gene alterations in Barrett's esophagus and adenocarcinoma have been identified by single-strand confirmation polymorphism (SSCP), sequence analysis, immunohistochemistry, and other techniques. Of these, abnormalities in p53 at the gene and protein level have been most extensively studied.

The gene for p53 resides on the short arm of chromosome 17 (17p). Mutations in the p53 gene are the most common mutations found in human cancers to date; approximately one-half of all human cancers contain a p53 mutation. The normal p53 protein has important regulatory functions related to the cell cycle and acts as a tumor suppressor. It has been referred to as the "guardian of the genome" because of its role in G_1-S checkpoint regulation, DNA repair, and induction of apoptosis when repair is not possible. Loss of normal p53, therefore, leads to cell-cycle abnormalities, lack of DNA repair, and avoidance of apoptosis. Loss of normal p53 also results in increased angiogenesis, possibly due to a lack of thrombospondins.[7]

Data concerning p53 in the metaplasia-dysplasia-carcinoma sequence are many, although questions have arisen as to the reliability of some methods of detecting abnormal p53. Immunohistochemical detection of abnormal p53 is possible because mutated p53 accumulates in the cell nucleus; this has been the technique most commonly used. However, it is not specific because (1) normal p53 can be detected at times in the nucleus and (2) not all p53 mutations lead to an excess accumulation of protein. The most sensitive method is sequencing of DNA.[7]

Studies show that a loss of p53 function plays a role in the transition of Barrett's metaplasia to dysplasia and cancer. This conclusion was first published in 1991 by Casson and colleagues, who identified p53 gene mutations in specific codons in both Barrett's epithelium and adenocarcinomas.[101] Since then, many investigators have confirmed abnormal p53, by immunohistochemical techniques and by SSCP/sequencing. The frequency of p53 mutation in high-grade dysplasia and adenocarcinoma ranges from 45 to 88 percent in various studies.[7,102–105] The question of exactly when the p53 mutation occurs in the metaplasia-dysplasia-carcinoma sequence has been investigated. Data indicate that mutation of p53 is found only occasionally in metaplastic and low-grade dysplastic tissues. It has been hypothesized that mutation of p53 is an event in the progression to carcinoma in Barrett's metaplasia, possibly following increased S phase and 4*N* fractions but preceding aneuploidy, thereby acting as a switch from low-grade to high-grade dysplasia[106] (Figure 5–13). Gimenez and colleagues demonstrated a statistically significant increase in positive staining for p53 and abnormal cytometric data (increasing aneuploidy) throughout the metaplasia-dysplasia-carcinoma sequence, with a marked increase in p53 mutation in tissues with low- and high-grade dysplasia and with increased aneuploidy in high-grade dysplasia and adenocarcinoma.[107] Mutations are generally found in exons 5 to 8, and the majority are CpG transitions.[108,109] It has been suggested that p53 (along with other antibodies) could be helpful in the distinction between low-grade and high-grade dysplasia.[110] Ribeiro and colleagues showed a positive correlation between p53 point mutations and pTNM stage ($p = .03$) as well as between p53 mutations and residual disease in the resected specimen, following neoadjuvant chemoradiotherapy ($p = .01$).[105] Further, both overall survival ($p = .0038$) and disease-free survival ($p = .0004$) were significantly lower for patients with p53 mutations than for those without mutations[105] (Figure 5–14). Other studies also have suggested an association between p53 overexpression and reduced overall survival.[111,112]

Other tumor-suppressor genes have been investigated, and these may play a role in the development of esophageal adenocarcinoma. These include p16 (chromosome 9q), APC (5q), and DCC/DPC (18q).[100,113–117] Many of the studies of these genes have used the microsatellite analysis technique to identify sites of allelic loss or loss of heterozygosity (LOH). Studies of APC have shown that loss of APC occurs as a late event, after loss of p53, as opposed to its early loss in the colon cancer sequence.[114] Data

	Barrett's alone	LGD	HGD	Adenoca
Abnormal p53 By IHC	5.3%	20%	65.6%	64.7%

Figure 5–13. Protein p53 in Barrett's esophagus. (Adenoca = adenocarcinoma; IHC = immunohistochemistry; HGD = high-grade dysplasia; LGD = low-grade dysplasia.) (Data from Ireland AP, Clark GW, DeMeester TR. Barrett's esophagus. The significance of p53 in clinical practice. Ann Surg 1997;225:17–30.)

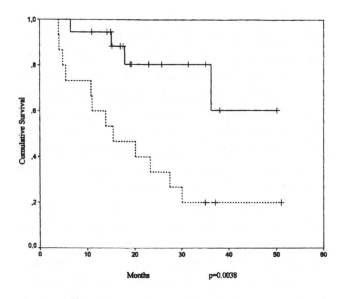

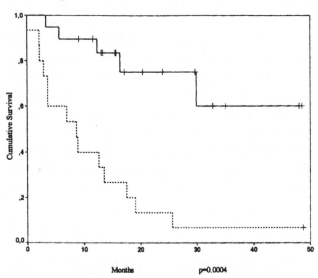

Figure 5–14. The influence of p53 status on survival in esophageal cancer patients. Overall (*A*) and disease-free (*B*) survival curves for patients with (*broken line*) and without (*solid line*) p53 mutations. (Reproduced with permission from Ribeiro U Jr, Finkelstein SD, Safatle-Ribeiro AV, et al. p53 sequence analysis predicts treatment response and outcome of patients with esophageal carcinoma. Cancer 1998;83:7–18.)

concerning LOH at 18q and 9q are variable; some investigators identify an early loss of chromosomal material, even in diploid cell populations[115,116] whereas others find these abnormalities only as a late event.[113,117] Attempts to further define the order of specific gene loss in the metaplasia-dysplasia-carcinoma sequence are ongoing. Figure 5–15 summarizes some of the proposed molecular and genetic changes in the malignant progression to esophageal adenocarcinoma.

TREATMENT

Barrett's Esophagus without Dysplasia or with Low-grade Dysplasia

There are several components in the "treatment" of Barrett's esophagus without dysplasia or with low-grade dysplasia. These include attempts to (1) treat its symptoms, (2) cause its regression, (3) prevent its progression, and (4) detect progression if it occurs. The components of a possible treatment plan for Barrett's include a surveillance program, medical therapy, and surgical therapy. While all of these play a part in the successful management of Barrett's esophagus, the exact role of each continues to evolve.

Many studies have shown that relief of symptomatic reflux can be achieved with both medical and surgical therapy although the significance of symptomatic relief has been questioned. Barrett's esophagus is often asymptomatic or minimally symptomatic, and reflux of gastric and duodenal contents can persist even in the face of improved symptoms. The possibility that the columnar-lined esophagus may have decreased pain sensitivity has been raised as well.[118] Treatment with proton pump inhibitors and H_2 blockers can lead to the complete eradication of symptoms, while esophageal pH remains abnormal. For this reason, some have recommended 24-hour pH monitoring to titrate drug doses.[119] Also, proton pump and H_2 blocker therapy has no effect on bile reflux and may place esophageal pH into a range in which bile is more damaging to the mucosa.[28] Prokinetic agents may assist in decreasing the bile reflux.

Both laparoscopic and open anti-reflux procedures are very effective in resolving symptoms, and abolishing both bile and acid reflux into the esophagus.[37,120] Patti and colleagues showed that laparoscopic Nissen fundoplication led to resolution of heartburn in 95 percent of patients, of regurgitation in 93 percent of patients, and of cough in 100 percent of patients.[120] A randomized study by the Department of Veterans Affairs assigned patients to either medical or surgical therapy for "complicated" GERD; both were effective for relief of symptoms and improved endoscopic signs of GERD, but in the initial report, surgical therapy was statistically significantly more effective ($p < .003$).[121] However, a recently published follow-up report stated

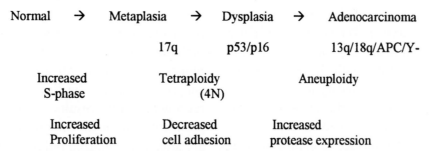

Figure 5–15. Summary of molecular and histopathologic changes in the malignant progression of Barrett's esophagus. (Adapted from Mueller J, Werner M, Siewert JR. Malignant progression in Barrett's esophagus: pathology and molecular biology. Recent Results Cancer Res 2000;155:29–41.)

that at a median follow-up of ~ 7 years, the majority of patients in both groups were taking anti-reflux medications regularly and that there was no difference in the frequency of treatment for esophageal stricture between the two groups.[45] Furthermore, there was no significant difference between groups in the incidence of esophageal cancer (~0.4% per year in patients with Barrett's esophagus at baseline, ~0.07% per year in those without Barrett's esophagus).[45] Finally, survival at 140 months was significantly lower in the surgical group in comparison with the medical group. These findings at follow-up call into question the role of anti-reflux surgery in the era of proton pump inhibitor therapy, as well as the role of routine surveillance, given the extremely low incidence of adenocarcinoma in this high-risk population.[45]

The next issue is the effect medical or surgical therapy has on the regression of Barrett's esophagus or on the prevention of progression. Data suggest that neither acid-suppression therapy nor anti-reflux surgery results in the predictable disappearance or regression of Barrett's esophagus. Malesci and colleagues found that 60 mg/d of omeprazole consistently improved gastric pH and decreased the amount of time that esophageal pH was < 4.0 over a 1-year period and that this resulted in a partial but significant regression in the length of Barrett's epithelium.[122] However, investigators at the University of Arizona in Tucson found that both H_2 blocker therapy and proton pump inhibitor therapy led to an improvement in symptoms but to no consistent reduction in the extent of Barrett's epithelium.[123,124] Of 64 patients who underwent anti-reflux procedures at USC, 35 patients were

unchanged, 12 had complete regressions (all had SSBE initially), 12 had partial length regressions, and 5 had progressions in length or degree of dysplasia.[27] In a randomized study of medical versus surgical therapy for Barrett's esophagus, Ortiz and colleagues found that the length of Barrett's esophagus decreased more often after surgical therapy (25% vs 7%) and increased more commonly with medical therapy (40% vs 9%).[125] Progression to low-grade dysplasia occurred in several patients on medical therapy and progression to high-grade dysplasia occurred in one patient on medical therapy and in one surgical patient after failed fundoplication.[125] In a prospective study of treatment of Barrett's esophagus in the United Kingdom, Attwood and colleagues found that surgical therapy was statistically significantly superior to medical therapy for both the control of symptoms and the prevention of complications of Barrett's esophagus.[126] However, progression to adenocarcinoma has been documented in the setting of both medical and surgical therapy.[118,127] Therefore, surveillance is required regardless of the type of therapy undertaken.

The rationale for surveillance in Barrett's esophagus is clear: there is a documented 30 to 125 times increased risk of adenocarcinoma in people with Barrett's esophagus compared to the general population, and the disease is often fatal if discovered at an advanced stage. If a patient with Barrett's esophagus has a reasonable life expectancy and is a candidate for therapy, surveillance is mandatory since neither medical nor surgical therapy reliably protects against malignant degeneration.[27] Though there are no controlled trials, surveillance has been shown in several reports to increase survival. Peters and colleagues demonstrated that endoscopically surveyed patients had better outcomes postoperatively than nonsurveyed patients, principally secondary to earlier-stage tumors.[128] Similarly, Streitz and colleagues found that endoscopically surveyed patients had tumors detected at an earlier stage and that this led to improved long-term survival,[129] as was also the case in the report of Thomas and colleagues.[83] Current published recommendations for surveillance are for "traditional" (ie, > 3 cm in length) Barrett's esophagus since adequate data on SSBE do not yet exist. The surveillance intervals suggested are based on the time to progression from metaplasia to dysplasia and cancer in a number of reports and are by no means absolute. Surveillance endoscopy should be accompanied by systematic biopsy (ie, four-quadrant biopsies done along at least every 2 cm of Barrett's mucosa, with additional specific biopsies of any abnormal [eroded, ulcerated, nodular, strictured] mucosa). The current surveillance guidelines are summarized in Table 5–6.[5] As discussed earlier, many different markers (DNA content, specific gene abnormalities, proliferative indices, etc.) have been investigated to assist in the discrimination of surveillance biopsy specimens, but none (besides histopathologic confirmation of dysplasia) have been proven to conclusively predict progression to adenocarcinoma.

A relatively recent development in terms of treatment for Barrett's metaplasia is endoscopic mucosal ablation. The concept is to ablate the abnormal epithelium and allow squamous mucosa to re-epithelialize the area, thus obviating the cancer risk. This has been proposed for Barrett's metaplasia and low-grade dysplasia as well as for high-grade dysplasia and intramucosal adenocarcinomas in high-risk patients. Various methods have been attempted, including chemical, thermal, and ultrasonic techniques. Common to all approaches is acid reflux suppression during healing, to optimize squamous regrowth. Early results with all modalities are promising although complications and recurrence are already recognized pitfalls.

Thermal ablation, by multipolar electrocoagulation or laser (argon, neodymium:yttrium-aluminum-garnet [Nd:YAG], neodymium:potassium titany/phosphate [KTP]), has been used with some success. In an early report from Berenson and colleagues, argon laser was used to ablate metaplastic tissue, with repeat endoscopy/ablation/biopsies every 2 to 5 weeks.[130] This resulted in the partial or complete disappearance of columnar tissue and the re-epithelialization with squamous mucosa in 38 of 40 locations treated in 10 patients.[130] Such results are complicated, however, by frequent relapse at 1 year (47%) despite proton pump inhibitor therapy and by the presence of residual Barrett's glands under new squamous epithelium.[130,131] In addition, the development of invasive adenocarcinoma under new squamous mucosa has been documented.[132]

Photodynamic therapy (PDT) uses a systemic photosensitizer (such as sodium porfimer [Photofrin] or 5-aminolevulinic acid [5-ALA]) and the intraesophageal application of light to chemically ablate abnormal mucosa.[133] Initially used to treat severe dysplasia, this technique has been applied to metaplastic and low-grade dysplastic mucosa as well. Early studies that used Photofrin reported a high incidence of stricture formation (40 to 58%).[27] Sensitivity to sunlight for several weeks after administration of Photofrin was a frequently reported side effect although this is avoided with newer agents such as 5-ALA. In a recent prospective randomized controlled trial, investigators in the United Kingdom randomized 18 patients to 5-ALA administration followed by laser endoscopy and 18 patients to placebo administration followed by laser endoscopy. A response was obtained in terms of decreased area (a median decrease in area of 30%) in 16 (89%) of 18 treated patients and the disappearance of low-grade dysplasia in 18 (100%) of 18 patients in the treated group. This compares favorably to a 10 percent decrease in area in 2 of 18 control patients (a

Table 5–6. RECOMMENDED SURVEILLANCE INTERVALS FOR BARRETT'S ESOPHAGUS	
Dysplasia	Follow-Up Endoscopy
None	After 2 negative, every 2–3 years
Low grade	Every 6 months × 2, then every year
High grade	Immediate re-endoscopy and biopsy; expert confirmation; resection for surgical candidates

Adapted with permission from Sampliner RE. Practice guidelines on the diagnosis, surveillance, and therapy of Barrett's esophagus. The Practice Parameters Committee of the American College of Gastroenterology. Am J Gastroenterol 1998;93:1028–32.

median decrease in area of 0%) and the disappearance of dysplasia in 33 percent of the control group ($p < .001$).[134] No side effects were seen, and the effects of treatment were maintained for up to 24 months.[134] The investigators concluded that 5-ALA–induced PDT can provide safe and effective ablation of low-grade dysplastic epithelium.[134]

The use of ultrasonic energy to ablate columnar mucosa has also been investigated. The Cavitron ultrasonic surgical aspirator can be used to ablate only the epithelium superficial to the muscularis mucosa.[135] An advantage of this method is that tissue can be aspirated for cytologic studies, not destroyed as in the above techniques. At present, the use of this method has been reported only in animal models; all cases demonstrated complete squamous re-epithelialization and no stricture formation.[135]

Barrett's Esophagus with High-Grade Dysplasia

The treatment of Barrett's esophagus with high-grade dysplasia is controversial for several reasons. First, the diagnosis itself is difficult. Interobserver variation between pathologists is high, and confirmation of high-grade dysplasia by an experienced pathologist is prerequisite for any definitive therapy. Second, although high-grade dysplasia is a recognized premalignant condition, the timetable for the development of invasive adenocarcinoma is highly variable, and the natural history is less than completely understood. Sampliner and colleagues reported that 21 of 61 patients with high-grade dysplasia developed invasive adenocarcinoma over 0.2 to 4.5 years.[5] In a prospective study by Hameeteman and colleagues, adenocarcinoma following low-grade and high-grade dysplasia developed in 1.5 to 4 years.[136] Others have observed patients with high-grade dysplasia for up to 44 months without seeing the development of cancer.[137] This has prompted a call for less aggressive intervention until invasive cancer is documented.[137] Third, when invasive adenocarcinoma occurs, it can be fatal, prompting others to call for early aggressive therapy. The current options for treating high-grade dysplasia include esophagectomy, surveillance endoscopy with biopsy, and endoscopic mucosal ablation techniques.

The standard therapy for high-grade dysplasia in patients with acceptable operative risk is esophagectomy. Proponents of this approach base their argument on the fact that occult adenocarcinomas are found in 36 to 55 percent of esophagectomies for preoperatively diagnosed high-grade dysplasia.[120,128,138–140] These are often (but not always) early-stage tumors, with an improved survival rate as compared to more advanced disease.[128,138] In a report from Heitmiller and colleagues, 30 patients underwent esophagectomy for high-grade dysplasia, and 13 (43%) of these patients had invasive adenocarcinoma (8 patients with AJCC stage I, 2 patients with stage II, and 3 patients with stage III)[138] (Figure 5–16). In a

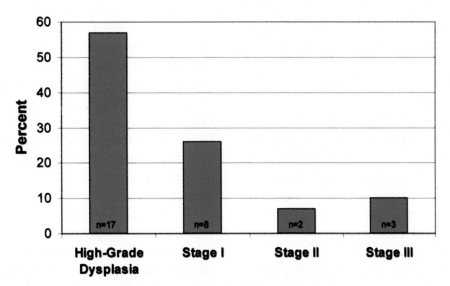

Figure 5–16. Pathologic findings at surgery for high-grade dysplasia.

meta-analysis of the published results of 119 patients undergoing esophagectomy for high-grade dysplasia, Ferguson and Naunheim reported an operative mortality rate of 2.6 percent, a 47 percent incidence of invasive adenocarcinoma, and an 82 percent 5-year survival rate for patients with invasive carcinoma.[139] Based on these results, many believe that esophagectomy for high-grade dysplasia is safe, effective, and necessary.

The surgical approach to esophagectomy may vary. Most surgeons accept a transhiatal esophagectomy with a gastric pull-up; others have done more radical resections, believing that the removal of lymph nodes has an impact on survival; still others have advocated vagal-sparing esophagectomy, with colon interposition for improved quality of life.[28] No randomized studies exist to compare the outcomes of these various approaches.

Some argue that a procedure with the morbidity and mortality of esophagectomy should be done only for histologically proven invasive cancer. These investigators advocate surveillance endoscopy with systematic biopsy (following a specific protocol with four-quadrant biopsy specimens taken every 2 cm of metaplasia) as proper treatment for high-grade dysplasia.[137,141] Levine and colleagues found that analysis of endoscopic biopsy specimens was accurate in detecting high-grade dysplasia and differentiating it from early adenocarcinoma in 50 patients studied, 28 of whom underwent surgery and 22 of whom had continued surveillance and biopsy. Furthermore, operative mortality was 14 percent (1 in 7) in patients with high-grade dysplasia only on final pathology whereas no patient in the observation group died from missed esophageal adenocarcinoma.[141] A recent report from this group at the University of Washington revealed that a four-quadrant 1-cm biopsy protocol most consistently detects early cancers arising in high-grade dysplasia.[142] (Intervals between endoscopies are individualized.) Critics of this approach claim that cancer will be missed during surveillance and will be advanced beyond the curable stage, leading to higher mortality,[143] and that such intensive surveillance protocols are untenable in the nonuniversity setting.[144]

Studies of endoscopic ablation for high-grade dysplasia have proliferated in recent years. Photodynamic therapy is the principal approach that has been used. Several studies have documented the eradication of high-grade dysplasia in the majority of patients treated, with squamous regeneration in the setting of acid suppression with a proton pump inhibitor.[145–147] Some of these studies have been troubled by the occurrence of subsquamous islands of nondysplastic Barrett's epithelium[145,147] and, in one case, a subsquamous adenocarcinoma.[147] In the PDT study by Overholt and colleagues, esophageal stricture occurred at a rate of 34 percent with Photofrin, but this has not been reported with 5-ALA.[147] Endoscopic mucosal resection has been used and is addressed below. At present, the results of PDT are promising, but examination of the results of long-term follow-up is necessary before PDT can replace surgery as the standard therapy for high-grade dysplasia.

TREATMENT OF ADENOCARCINOMA OF THE ESOPHAGUS AND GASTROESOPHAGEAL JUNCTION

Esophageal Resection

Resection of the esophagus for treatment of esophageal cancer was first successfully performed in the early part of the twentieth century and became standard practice in the decades that followed. Torek used a transthoracic approach in 1913,[148] and Denk described the concept of a transhiatal esophagectomy the same year.[149] In 1933, Turner refined this "blunt" transhiatal technique.[150] The first series of esophagectomy with immediate esophagogastrostomy was published by Ohsawa[151] in 1933 and first reported in the United States by Adams and Phemister in 1938.[152] Significant milestones in esophageal surgery since then include the description by Ivor Lewis of a combined right thoracotomy and laparotomy for esophagectomy in 1946[153] and Orringer's re-introduction of Turner's "esophagectomy without thoracotomy" in 1978.[154]

At present, esophagectomy represents the only known potentially curative treatment for esophageal cancer, and it is the best palliative method as well. Surgery remains the primary treatment modality in the absence of known metastatic disease or medical

Table 5–7. APPROACHES TO ESOPHAGECTOMY FOR CANCER

Transhiatal esophagectomy
Ivor Lewis (right thoracotomy and laparotomy)
Left thoracotomy
Left thoracoabdominal
Radical esophagectomy/extended en bloc esophagectomy
Esophagectomy with three-field lymph node dissection
Distal esophagectomy with total gastrectomy
Laparoscopic esophagectomy
Endoscopic mucosectomy

contraindications to surgery. The primary goal of treatment is a prolonged disease-free state, with relief of dysphagia. Outcomes vary with stage, and esophageal wall penetration and lymph node involvement rank as the major prognostic factors in almost all studies. Although survival rates vary between different studies, an approximate 20 percent overall 5-year survival rate is reported in the majority of series.

The choice of operation for adenocarcinoma of the esophagus and GE junction depends on several factors, which were summarized in a 1988 report by Mathisen. These include surgeon preference, tumor location, body habitus, prior operations, overall medical condition of the patient, choice of esophageal substitute, and history of prior radiation therapy.[15] Much has been written and much controversy generated about the choice of surgical approach for esophageal cancer. The various approaches are listed in Table 5–7. Each of the major approaches, with their principal strengths and weaknesses, are summarized below, in Table 5–8, and in Figure 5–17, followed by what comparative data exist to assess the various techniques.

Transhiatal Esophagectomy

Originally described by Denk in 1913 and Turner in 1933, "esophagectomy without thoracotomy" was re-introduced and popularized by Orringer, beginning with his 1978 publication.[154] Orringer described undertaking the procedure in 22 patients with esophageal cancer but not with a curative intent.[154] Since that time, the procedure and its results have been reported by Orringer [155–157] and others[84,158–162] as a choice in the armamentarium of potentially curative procedures for esophageal cancer. The purported advantages are as follows:

1. Cervical anastomotic leak is less devastating as it is rarely associated with mediastinitis.
2. Thoracotomy is avoided, leading to less pulmonary morbidity.
3. The procedure can be curative, with a reported survival equivalent to transthoracic or en bloc radical resection.

Opponents of this technique argue that complete lymphadenectomy is compromised with transhiatal esophagectomy and is a necessary component for resection of esophageal carcinoma, primarily for staging and possibly for cure.

Results of transhiatal esophagectomy have been reported widely although most extensively by Orringer. Mortality rates range from 4 to 7 percent,[157,163,164] with a trend toward decreased mortality in the past decade. Common complications include pulmonary compromise (atelectasis, pneumonia, etc.) and anastomotic leak, with complications such as delayed gastric emptying, bleeding, gastric tube necrosis, recurrent laryngeal nerve paralysis, chy-

Table 5–8. SURGICAL APPROACHES TO ESOPHAGECTOMY: SUMMARY

Approach	Location of Tumor	Location of Anastomosis	Advantages	Disadvantages
Transhiatal	Entire esophagus; cardia	Cervical	Low-morbidity anastomosis; avoids thoracotomy	Lack of exposure of midesophagus
Ivor Lewis	Middle third	Thoracic or cervical	Direct exposure of midesophagus	Intrathoracic anastomosis; requires thoracotomy
Left thoracotomy/ thoracoabdominal	Lower third or cardia	Thoracic	Excellent exposure of lower esophagus	Requires thoracotomy; intrathoracic anastomosis; postoperative reflux
Radical en bloc	Entire esophagus; cardia	Cervical or thoracic	More extensive lymph node dissection	Increased operative risk with no proven benefit
Laparoscopic	Entire esophagus; cardia	Cervical or thoracic	Lower morbidity; better tolerated	Technically demanding

lothorax, tracheal laceration, and pneumothorax occurring less frequently.[157,165] Late complications include dumping syndrome, regurgitation, and dysphagia, often secondary to anastomotic stricture.[157,165]

Anastomotic strictures occur often in the setting of a prior cervical anastomotic leak and can be a major long-term problem. That pattern of complications led Orringer to explore techniques that would minimize

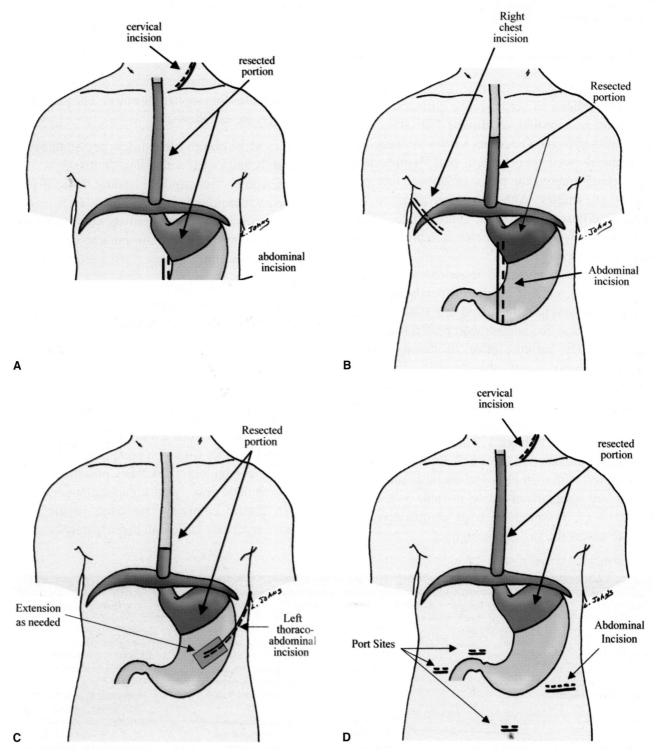

Figure 5–17. Surgical approaches to esophagectomy. *A*, Transhiatal esophagectomy. *B*, Ivor Lewis esophagectomy. *C*, Left thoracotomy/thoracoabdominal approach. *D*, Laparoscopy assisted transhiatal esophagectomy.

the chances of anastomotic leak.[166] Using the side-to-side stapled technique, Orringer was able to decrease the leak rate from the 10 to 15 percent range, as seen in over 1,000 hand-sewn anastomoses, to 2.7 percent.[166] The survival rate for patients after transhiatal esophagectomy has been reported as in the range of 23 to 40 percent at 5 years.[87,157]

Ivor Lewis Esophagectomy

The combined right thoractomy and laparotomy for resection of esophageal cancer was first presented in 1946 by Ivor Lewis in the Hunterian Lecture to the Royal College of Surgeons.[153] Originally described as a two-stage procedure, the one-stage variation has been used routinely since that time and is described by many as the procedure of choice for lesions of the middle third of the esophagus.[167,168] The anastomosis can also be done in the neck, using a three-incision technique initially described in 1985 by McKeown, who used a right cervical incision.[169] Advantages of the combined abdominal and thoracic approach include direct visualization of the midportion of the esophagus and exposure for complete regional (thoracic) lymph node dissection, including the periesophageal, subcarinal, and upper mediastinal nodes. Disadvantages include the physiologic insult of combined chest and abdominal incisions and the risk of mediastinal anastomotic leaks, which historically have a high fatality rate.

Many series of esophagectomies via the Ivor Lewis approach have been reported; these were recently summarized (in comparison to transhiatal esophagectomy) by Rindani and colleagues. Mortality rates range from < 2.0[168] to 9.5 percent.[164] Over the last decades, these rates have dropped significantly with improvements in intraoperative and postoperative care. Complications include anastomotic leak, atelectasis/pneumonia, cardiovascular complications, wound infections, and chylothorax. While anastomotic leak in the thorax previously had an associated mortality rate of nearly 50 to 60 percent, the rate has now decreased due to improved intensive care practices and the wide application of parenteral or enteral nutritional supplementation. Late complications include anastomotic stricture, dysphagia, dumping syndrome, and reflux. Five-year survival

rates for patients after Ivor Lewis esophagectomy for adenocarcinoma range from 8[15] to 26 percent.[164,170]

Left Thoracotomy or Left Thoracoabdominal Approach

The left transthoracic approach to the lower esophagus is performed via a left lateral thoracotomy or a left thoracoabdominal approach. Historically, this has been an approach to tumors in the lower third of the esophagus and in the gastric cardia. Advantages include excellent exposure to the lower third of the esophagus and the fact that the patient does not need to be repositioned intraoperatively.[171] The disadvantages are that (1) the heart and aorta limit the proximal extent of the esophageal dissection and make intrathoracic anastomosis difficult, (2) the gastric drainage procedure and the Kocher maneuver can be difficult to perform via a left thoracotomy, and (3) postoperative reflux esophagitis occurs in many patients.

Radical En Bloc Esophagectomy

First proposed by Logan in 1963[172] in an attempt to apply accepted oncologic resection techniques to carcinoma of the esophagus and cardia, the radical en bloc esophagectomy has been championed by Skinner and associates[173,174] as well as by DeMeester[175] and Akiyama.[176] The objective of this approach is a more extensive removal of tissues adjacent to the esophagus in order to resect all nodal metastases. This approach adheres to Halsted's view that cancer progresses in an orderly fashion to the lymph nodes prior to becoming a systemic disease. Originally stated to be indicated for patients with limited (stage I to IIB) disease (by preoperative assessment), a recent paper from Altorki and Skinner supports it as the procedure of choice in stage III disease as well.[174] Supporters claim (1) that a more complete cancer resection decreases the likelihood of local recurrence and improves long-term survival without substantial morbidity or mortality, (2) that the technique allows better and more accurate staging, and (3) that prolonged survival and even cure may occasionally be possible after extended lymphadenectomy with positive nodes. Detractors state that "radical" esophagectomy has no clear survival advantage over any other approach and that considerable postoperative complications are associated with this approach. To date, no randomized trials exist comparing this radical approach to any other surgical approach.

The overall principles of the approach include proximal and distal margins of at least 10 cm whenever possible, with total excision of adjacent tissues with the arterial and venous supply and lymphatic drainage. For tumors of the lower third of the esophagus or at the GE junction, the spleen, a large portion of stomach, and a rim of diaphragm are routinely removed. In the chest, the azygous vein, thoracic duct, and a portion of pericardium and pleura are taken en bloc. Either the remaining stomach or a colon interposition can be used to restore gastrointestinal continuity. A cervical anastomosis and possibly a cervical lymph node dissection may be included in the procedure. An extensive mediastinal and abdominal lymph node dissection is an important aspect of the radical resection.

Mortality rates for the radical operation range from 2.4 to 11.0 percent in institutions that commonly perform the procedure.[176,177] Complications occur in ~50 percent of cases and include respiratory and cardiac problems, anastomotic leak, chylothorax, and ischemia or necrosis of the esophageal substitute.

Three-Field Lymphadenectomy

The three-field lymphadenectomy approach, which stresses the dissection of lymph nodes in the abdomen, mediastinum, and cervical region, is a variation of the radical esophagectomy. This technique was pioneered at several Japanese centers after recurrence was noted in cervical lymph nodes in 30 to 40 percent of patients in which abdominal and mediastinal lymph nodes had been dissected.[89] Interesting data as to the pattern of lymph node spread have been generated, including the fact that metastases to the cervical nodes occurred in 20 percent of tumors of the lower third of the esophagus.[90] Those who support this technique state that survival is improved after three-field resection, compared to survival after two-field resection.[89] Detractors point out that all of the survival data are derived from noncontrolled retrospective series; that the worth of

lymphadenectomy, especially distant lymph node excision, has never been proven; and that greater morbidity (particularly secondary to paralysis of the recurrent laryngeal nerve) is common with this more extensive procedure.

Total Gastrectomy for Tumors at the Gastroesophageal Junction

Recently, Siewert and colleagues reported on surgery in 1,002 patients with GE-junction tumors.[63] For type II and type III tumors, an extended total gastrectomy was recommended, with transhiatal resection for distal esophageal tumors only. The extended total gastrectomy is done via a midline laparotomy only, and an extensive lymph node dissection similar to that suggested for gastric cancer is performed. An esophagojejunostomy is done to restore gastrointestinal continuity.[63]

Choice of Esophageal Substitute

With resection of the esophagus, a substitute must be fashioned to traverse the mediastinum. In the early part of the twentieth century, this was sometimes accomplished with rubber tubing (either externally or subcutaneously). At present, there are typically two choices for esophageal substitute: the stomach or the colon. Both have advantages and disadvantages.

The stomach is now considered the preferred substitute following esophageal resection. The stomach has the advantage that gastrointestinal continuity is restored with a single anastomosis. Given the potential morbidity and mortality of an anastomotic leak, this is a serious consideration. Further, the gastric mobilization is technically easier than the colonic mobilization, and the blood supply of the gastric remnant is more consistent and reliable than that of the colon. However, the stomach may not be available or appropriate in the setting of prior gastric surgery or severe ulcer disease. Additional disadvantages include the fact that reflux esophagitis and stricture formation occur with gastric substitutes, especially with an intrathoracic anastomosis.

The colon is an excellent esophageal substitute when needed. Either the right or left colon can be used although the left is better suited to the intrathoracic transposition. This can be done via either a substernal or posterior mediastinal route. The advantages include the colon's availability in cases in which the stomach cannot be used and the ability to place the substitute in an isoperistaltic orientation to minimize reflux. The disadvantages include the fact that the colon can become elongated and redundant, leading to obstructive symptoms, and that this procedure is more difficult technically and requires a total of three anastomoses (esophagocolic, cologastric, and colocolonic).

Laparoscopic Esophagectomy

As laparoscopic and thoracoscopic techniques and instrumentation have improved, the ability to do more complex procedures has increased. Laparoscopic and thoracoscopic approaches to esophagectomy for cancer and high-grade dysplasia have been reported. A variety of approaches have been used, including endoscopic Ivor Lewis esophagectomy,[178] combined laparoscopic and thoracoscopic techniques,[179,180] completely laparoscopic transhiatal

esophagectomy,[179,181,182] and hand-assisted laparoscopic transhiatal esophagectomy.[183] Overall, feasibility has been demonstrated. The potential advantages include lower morbidity and mortality and better patient tolerance of the procedure (shorter recovery times, etc.). Survival results are pending.

Endoscopic Techniques for Early Esophageal Adenocarcinoma

Endoscopic resection techniques have been attempted in patients with early-stage esophageal adenocarcinoma, as they have for patients with high-grade dysplasia. Indications include small (< 2 cm), superficial (intraepithelial or microinvasive, not into submucosa), and early (N0) tumors in high-surgical-risk patients and in those refusing surgery. Endoscopic ultrasonography staging is essential, with the high-frequency (20 MHz) probe preferred. Treatment options include resection or destruction of the tumor. Resection is done by endoscopic mucosal resection (EMR) (Figure 5–18), which provides tissue for

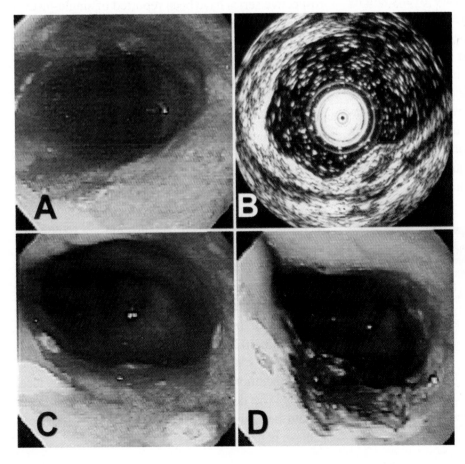

Figure 5–18. Endoscopic mucosal resection (EMR) of intramucosal adenocarcinoma. *A,* Patch of intramucuosal adenocarcinoma in Barrett's esophagus at 25 cm from incisors. *B,* HFUS (20 MHz), showing no invasive disease. *C,* Periphery of lesion is marked for resection with BICAP. *D,* Site after EMR with strip biopsy technique. At a 2-year follow-up, there was no recurrence at the site with Barrett's epithelium only. (Courtesy of I. Waxman, MD.)

pathologic evaluation; this is done by piecemeal excision, using a plastic overtube and snare electrocautery.[184] Early results from Japan demonstrated the effective removal of superficial cancers, with a 6.8 percent rate of major complications (hemorrhage, perforation, and stenosis), a 3 to 7 percent local recurrence rate, and a 5-year survival rate of 80 percent.[185]

Tumor destruction is accomplished by either Nd:YAG laser or PDT. These are easier to perform than EMR, but no pathologic specimen is obtained. The experience for both modalities in early cancer is limited, but reports demonstrate the effective ablation of cancer in 73 percent of cases with Nd:YAG laser[186] and in 87 percent of cases using PDT.[187] Overall, these procedures must be viewed as experimental, given the inaccuracies of preoperative staging modalities in differentiating mucosal from submucosal tumors.

Results of Surgery

Mortality rates following esophageal resection in recent series range from 2 to 10 percent; the acceptable 30-day mortality is approximately 5 percent.[13,15,157] Overall, this does not vary greatly among the surgical techniques used.[164] Frequently seen complications of esophageal resections (for all pathologies) with the transhiatal and Ivor Lewis approaches are summarized and compared in Table 5–9. Pulmonary complications are the most frequent. Anastomotic leak is also a commonly reported complication, with rates varying from 0[15] to 15 percent.[157] In the summary report of Rindani and colleagues, anastomotic leaks occurred more frequently in the transhiatal group (16%) than in the transthoracic group

(10%). Similarly, the rate of recurrent laryngeal nerve injury was slightly higher with the transhiatal approach (11.2%) than with the transthoracic approach (4.8%).[164] Postoperative mortality (ie, 30-day mortality) was higher in the transthoracic group (9.5%) than in the transhiatal group (6.3%).[164]

Survival after esophagectomy for adenocarcinoma of the esophagus and gastroesophageal junction is dependent on stage, as discussed above. Table 5–10 presents a summary of complications and survival in a number of series looking exclusively at adenocarcinoma of the esophagus and GE junction. Five-year survival rates range from 13 to 34 percent.[63,81,83,84,129,188,189]

The issue of whether one surgical approach is superior to another has been debated in the literature for decades. No randomized trials exist comparing one technique with another for adenocarcinoma of the esophagus and GE junction. Two prospective randomized trials in squamous cell carcinoma of the esophagus have shown no differences in morbidity, 30-day mortality, or long-term survival between transhiatal and transthoracic techniques.[158,159] Many retrospective series have been reported of single-institution experiences with transhiatal and transthoracic esophagectomy, usually for a mixture of histologies. These have shown no differences between the transhiatal and transthoracic approaches with respect to operative mortality or overall survival.[160–162] The summarized results of comparative trials published by Rindani and colleagues confirm the similarity in overall survival, with a 5-year survival of 24 percent for transhiatal esophagectomy and 26 percent for Ivor Lewis esophagectomy.[164] Reports of improved survival with radical extended en bloc resections have involved highly selected patients and are impossible to interpret. All the existing data point to the conclusion that one technique is not superior to another oncologically and that the surgical approach is to be individualized according to patient factors (location and extent of tumor, body habitus, prior surgery, medical condition) and surgeon factors (preference, experience). As stated by Pairolero of the Mayo Clinic, "[the] operation for cancer of the esophagus is local therapy. The debate about which operation is better should be laid to rest once and for all as we try to achieve better control of this malignancy."[15]

Table 5–9. MORBIDITY AND MORTALITY AFTER ESOPHAGECTOMY		
Mortality and Morbidity	Transhiatal (%)	Ivor Lewis (%)
30-day mortality	6.3	9.5
Respiratory complications	24.0	25.0
Cardiovascular complications	12.4	10.5
Wound infection	8.8	6.2
Chylothorax	2.1	3.4
Anastomotic leak	16.0	10.0
Anastomotic stricture	28.0	16.0
Recurrent laryngeal nerve injury	11.2	4.8

Adapted from Rindani R, Martin CJ, Cox MR. Transhiatal versus Ivor Lewis oesophagectomy: is there a difference? Aust N Z J Surg 1999;69:187–94.

Table 5–10. OUTCOMES OF SURGERY FOR ADENOCARCINOMA OF THE ESOPHAGUS AND GASTROESOPHAGEAL JUNCTION

Study Author	Year	n	Complication Rate (%)	Anastomotic Leak Rate (%)	Mortality (%)		5-yr Survival (%)		Ref. No.
					30-Day	90-Day/Inhosp	Total	RO	
Distal esophagus/GE									
Streitz et al	1991	61	21.3	3.3	3.3	—	23.7	—	212
Menke-Pluymers et al	1992	85	34.0	9.4	7.0	—	24.0	30.0	188
Moon et al	1992	88	43.0	21.5	10.3	18.2	13.0	—	189
Holsher et al	1995	165	43.0	20.5	6.1	12.7	34.0	41.4	84
Thomas et al	1997	164	41.0	11.0	6.0	—	17.0	—	83
Esophagogastric junction									
Steup et al	1996	95	46.0	9.7	—	6.2	33.0	—	81
Siewert et al	2000	1,002	—	—	3.8	—	32.3	38.7	63

inhosp = in-hospital; R0 = R0 resection (no residual tumor at surgery); n = sample size.

MULTIMODALITY THERAPIES FOR ADENOCARCINOMA OF ESOPHAGUS AND GASTROESOPHAGEAL JUNCTION

Given the overall poor prognosis obtained with surgery alone, especially for advanced-stage tumors, other strategies have been used to improve survival in patients with adenocarcinoma of the esophagus and GE junction. These strategies include neoadjuvant chemoradiotherapy, neoadjuvant chemotherapy, and chemoradiotherapy alone as primary treatment. Many of these studies combined patients with adenocarcinoma and squamous cell histologies; few examined adenocarcinoma exclusively. The rationales, results, and conclusions of these approaches will be reviewed briefly.

Neoadjuvant Chemoradiotherapy Followed by Surgery

The theoretical foundations of neoadjuvant chemoradiotherapy include the following:

1. Local control will be better than chemoradiotherapy alone because residual disease is removed.
2. Regional control will be better because the chemoradiotherapy will eradicate disease that might remain at the margins of resection.
3. Distant control will improve after early exposure to chemotherapy, eliminating occult micrometastatic disease.

Important components in planning for neoadjuvant chemoradiation include accurate staging, drug choice, and method of administration.

Neoadjuvant chemoradiation for esophageal cancer has been studied in numerous phase II trials and in several phase III trials. Upon examination of the phase II trials, several principles emerge. Responses were seen with many regimens, and pathologic complete responses occured in ~24 to 40 percent of cases.[190–193] These protocols used 5-fluorouracil (5-FU) and cisplatin, with and without additional agents that include vinblastine,[190] etoposide,[191] and interferon-α (IFN-α).[193] Radiation was given concurrently, with doses ranging from 40 to 45 Gy. Improvement in survival has been seen in comparison to historical controls.[190] Further, in patients with pathologic complete responses, survival was improved when compared to those with residual disease at surgery.[192] An exemplary phase II study was that carried out at Johns Hopkins Hospital by Forastiere and colleagues.[192] In a study of 50 patients, 33 had adenocarcinoma of the esophagus. All were staged by preoperative CT and contrast esophagography. Neoadjuvant treatment included cisplatin, 5-FU, and 44 Gy of radiation. Two deaths occurred preoperatively, and there was a 94 percent operability rate and a 90 percent resectability rate. No operative mortality occurred. The pathologic complete response rate was 40 percent. Median survival was 31 months, and the 2-year survival was 58 percent, which compared favorably with institutional controls. Survival analysis by histologic type showed no difference between squamous cancers and adenocarcinoma. Survival by pathologic response did show a significant difference: the 2-year survival with pathologic complete response (CR) was 78 percent (median survival, 58 months) compared with a 2-

year survival of 46 percent with positive pathology (median survival, 22.4 months).[192]

Two prospective randomized trials of neoadjuvant chemoradiotherapy have included patients with adenocarcinoma, and the results were conflicting. The often cited study by Walsh and colleagues included only patients with adenocarcinoma; these patients were randomized to surgery alone or to preoperative treatment with 5-FU, cisplatin, and 40 Gy of radiation.[194] The pathologic complete-response (pCR) rate was 25 percent. Median survival in the multimodality-treated group was 16 months as compared to 11 months in the surgery-alone group (p = .01) (Figure 5–19, A).[194] Three-year survival was 32 percent in the multimodality group and 6 percent in the surgery-alone group (p = .01). This study has been criticized for inadequate prerandomization staging methods, for including both esophageal and cardia adenocarcinoma, and for including patients with early-stage disease.[195] Also, the 6 percent 3-year survival rate with surgery alone is well below that of most historical controls.

A much anticipated study from a group at the University of Michigan was published recently. This study was based on the promising results of a phase II trial at that institution. In the pilot study, half (21) of the 43 patients had adenocarcinoma. The median survival of patients treated with intensive cisplatin, fluorouracil, and vinblastine concurrently administered with 45 Gy of radiation was 29 months, compared to a 12-month median survival in historical institutional controls.[190] Histologic complete responders had a 70-month median survival. Based on these results, a prospective randomized trial was designed comparing transhiatal esophagectomy to treatment with cisplatin, 5-FU, vinblastine, and radiation (45 Gy) followed by transhiatal esophagectomy. The study included 100 patients with esophageal cancer, 75 of whom had adenocarcinoma. The results showed no significant difference in survival between the two arms at a median follow-up of 8.2 years.[196] Median survival was 17.6 months in the surgery-alone arm and 16.9 months in the combined-therapy arm. Three-year survival was 16 percent with surgery alone and 30 percent for combination therapy, but this was not statistically significant (p = .15) (see Figure 5–19, B).[196] The study has been criticized for including patients with positive celiac nodes and for being inadequately powered to detect small yet potentially clinically significant differences in outcome.[197] At present, neoadjuvant chemoradiotherapy remains an experimental approach, to be pursued in the clinical trial setting. Large randomized trials will be necessary to show a benefit if one exists. New agents, including paclitaxel,[198] are under investigation in phase II studies but have yet to be tested widely.

Neoadjuvant Chemotherapy Followed by Surgery

Preoperative chemotherapy alone, without concurrent radiation, has been investigated extensively. Two advantages are that the intact primary can be used to determine sensitivity to a specific chemotherapy regimen and that chemotherapy is introduced early to act against microscopic distant disease. The combination of 5-FU and cisplatin produces an objective response rate (> 50% tumor shrinkage) in approximately 50 percent of patients in several phase II studies. However, complete responses occur in only ~5 percent.

Several small randomized trials have investigated these regimens versus surgery alone, primarily for squamous cell carcinoma of the esophagus.[199–201] Response rates of ~50 percent and no benefit for survival were findings common to all three trials. A larger intergroup trial was reported in 1998.[202] In this prospective trial, 440 patients with either squamous cell carcinoma or adenocarcinoma were randomized to surgery alone or to preoperative chemotherapy with cisplatin and 5-FU followed by surgery. No differences were found in median survival (14.9 months vs 16.1 months) or 2-year survival (35% vs 37%).[202] No differences were found between squamous cell carcinoma and adenocarcinoma responses, and there was no increase in operative morbidity in patients who received preoperative chemotherapy. In summary, neoadjuvant chemotherapy can lead to response rates of ~50 percent, but complete responses are rare, and no survival advantage has been identified to date.

Chemoradiotherapy without Surgery for Locally Advanced Disease

Interest in nonsurgical approaches to potentially resectable esophageal cancer developed in the 1980s

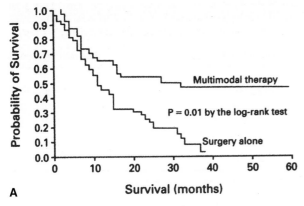

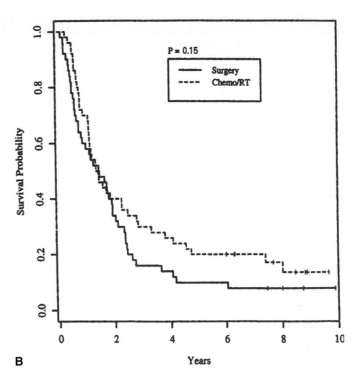

Figure 5–19. Results of prospective, randomized trials of surgery for esophageal cancer versus neoadjuvant treatment plus surgery for esophageal cancer. *A*, Results of study by Walsh and colleagues. (Reproduced with permission from Walsh TN, Noonan N, Hollywood D, et al. A comparison of multimodal therapy and surgery for esophageal adenocarcinoma. N Engl J Med 1996;335:462–7.) *B*, Results of study by Urba and colleagues. (Chemo/RT = chemoradiotherapy.) (Reproduced with permission from Urba SG, Orringer MB, Turrisi A, et al. Randomized trial of preoperative chemoradiation versus surgery alone in patients with locoregional esophageal carcinoma. J Clin Oncol 2001;19:305–13.)

in response to poor 5-year survival rates in some surgical series and high surgical mortality rates that sometimes exceeded the percentage of 5-year survivors. These studies generally combined external beam radiation with multiagent chemotherapy in order to target distant disease and to enhance radiation effects locoregionally. Higher doses of radiation were used than in the neoadjuvant setting. Several phase II trials (mostly involving patients with squamous cell cancer) supported feasibility and effect. This prompted a multicenter intergroup phase III study.[203] Initially restricted to patients with squamous cell cancer, patients with adenocarcinomas were added after the 1st year of the trial, and these ultimately made up 15 percent of the overall study population of 192 patients. This study, most recently reported by Cooper in 1999, included patients with locally advanced esophageal cancer (T1–3, N0–1, M0) who were treated with 50 Gy of radiation concurrent with cisplatin and 5-FU, with additional postradiation chemotherapy, versus patients treated with 64 Gy of radiation alone. An additional group of patients received combination therapy after the period of randomization; this group is reported separately in the final analysis. The results demonstrated a survival benefit of combined-modality treatment greater than that of radiation alone, with

5-year survivals of 26 percent and 0 percent and median survivals of 14.1 months and 9.3 months ($p < .001$), respectively.[203] No statistical difference was seen in relation to histologic type. Of note, local disease persisted in 26 percent of the combined-modality group, and locoregional failures alone occurred in an additional ~16 percent, accounting for the majority of treatment failures (Table 5–11). Results from trials examining the worth of preoperative chemoradiotherapy confirm that the vast majority of patients have residual disease following induction chemoradiotherapy. These data strongly suggest that definitive chemoradiotherapy should not be used to treat potentially resectable disease but should be reserved for patients with T4 disease or with medical risks that preclude surgery.[193,204]

Treatment for Metastatic Adenocarcinoma of the Esophagus and Gastroesophageal Junction

Many patients with adenocarcinoma of the esophagus and GE junction have inoperable disease at the time of diagnosis (70 to 80% in the Western Hemisphere), contributing to the grim prognosis for esophageal adenocarcinoma. Numerous options exist for palliative treatment of these patients,

Table 5–11. LOCATION OF DISEASE AT FIRST TREATMENT FAILURE

| First Failure | No. (%) Patients Alive after Radiation Therapy | No. (%) Patients Alive after Combined-Modality Therapy | |
	Randomized	Randomized	Nonrandomized
None	0 (0)	13 (21)	4 (6)
Persistent	23 (37)	15 (25)	19 (28)
Locoregional	10 (16)	8 (13)	14 (20)
Distant only	9 (15)	5 (8)	11 (16)
Locoregional and distant	9 (15)	5 (8)	7 (10)
Death	11 (18)	15 (24)	14 (20)

Adapted from Cooper JS, Guo MD, Herskovic A, et al. Chemoradiotherapy of locally advanced esophageal cancer: long-term follow-up of a prospective randomized trial (RTOG 85-01). Radiation Therapy Oncology Group. JAMA 1999;281:1623–7.

including chemotherapy, radiation, and local endoscopic therapies. Effective chemotherapy regimens exist for metastatic esophagogastric carcinoma. A recent study of therapy with the combination of epirubicin, cisplatin, and fluorouracil (ECF) reported overall response rates of 61 percent (11% CR) and acceptable toxicity.[205] A randomized trial comparing the ECF regimen with the standard combination of 5-FU, doxorubicin (Adriamycin), and methotrexate (FAMTX) for patients with advanced esophagogastric cancer showed improved response and survival for ECF, with additional benefits in quality of life and cost-effectiveness. Patients receiving ECF had an overall response rate of 45 percent, versus 21 percent for patients receiving FAMTX ($p = .0002$).[206] The median survival was 8.9 months with ECF and 5.7 months with FAMTX ($p = .0009$), and the 1-year survival was 36 percent with ECF, versus 21 percent with FAMTX.[206]

Local palliative options exist as well, with the goal of improving quality of life by improving swallowing ability. Options include palliative surgery, esophageal dilatation, esophageal stenting, PDT, Nd:YAG laser excision, endoesophageal BICAP cauterization, local injection therapies, and brachytherapy.[207] Radiochemotherapy has been attempted for metastatic disease, with some success.[208,209] Treatment decisions for patients with advanced disease should be individualized, with a clear understanding of the goals of therapy.

CONCLUSION

Exploring the biologic basis of adenocarcinoma of the esophagus and GE junction will be central to expanding and improving the therapeutic options necessary to alter the natural history of this disease. The urgency for defining effective treatment is more pronounced when it is apparent that the incidence of esophageal adenocarcinoma continues to increase at an alarming rate. Properly designed clinical trials will be crucial to confirm the promise of novel therapeutic agents and approaches developed in the laboratory. Focusing on active prevention and targeting known premalignant conditions will likely constitute a high-yield endeavor.

REFERENCES

1. Blot WJ, Devesa SS, Kneller RW, Fraumeni JF Jr. Rising incidence of adenocarcinoma of the esophagus and gastric cardia. JAMA 1991;265:1287–9.
2. Blot WJ, Devesa SS, Fraumeni JF Jr. Continuing climb in rates of esophageal adenocarcinoma: an update [letter]. JAMA 1993;270:1320.
3. Devesa SS, Blot WJ, Fraumeni JF Jr. Changing patterns in the incidence of esophageal and gastric carcinoma in the United States. Cancer 1998;83:2049–53.
4. Siewert JR, Stein HJ. Classification of adenocarcinoma of the oesophagogastric junction. Br J Surg 1998;85:1457–9.
5. Sampliner RE. Practice guidelines on the diagnosis, surveillance, and therapy of Barrett's esophagus. The Practice Parameters Committee of the American College of Gastroenterology. Am J Gastroenterol 1998;93:1028–32.
6. Pera M. Epidemiology of esophageal cancer, especially adenocarcinoma of the esophagus and esophagogastric junction. Recent Results Cancer Res 2000;155:1–14.
7. Ireland AP, Clark GW, DeMeester TR. Barrett's esophagus. The significance of p53 in clinical practice. Ann Surg 1997;225:17–30.
8. Greenlee RT, Hill-Harmon M, Murray T, Thur M. Cancer statistics. CA Cancer J Clin 2001;51:15–36.
9. Puestow CB, Gillesby WJ, Guynn VL. Cancer of the esophagus. Arch Surg 1955;70:662–8.
10. Raphael HA, Ellis FH, Dockerty MB. Primary adenocarcinoma of the esophagus. Ann Surg 1966;162:785.

11. Turnbull A, Goodner J. Primary adenocarcinoma of the esophagus. Cancer 1968;22:915–8.

12. Korst RJ, Rusch VW, Venkatraman E, et al. Proposed revision of the staging classification for esophageal cancer. J Thorac Cardiovasc Surg 1998;115:660–70.

13. Ellis FH Jr, Heatley GJ, Krasna MJ, et al. Esophagogastrectomy for carcinoma of the esophagus and cardia: a comparison of findings and results after standard resection in three consecutive eight-year intervals with improved staging criteria. J Thorac Cardiovasc Surg 1997;113:836–48.

14. Dalrymple-Hay MJ, Evans KB, Lea RE. Oesophagectomy for carcinoma of the oesophagus and oesophagogastric junction. Eur J Cardiothorac Surg 1999;15:626–30.

✗ 15. Mathisen DJ, Grillo HC, Wilkins EW Jr, et al. Transthoracic esophagectomy: a safe approach to carcinoma of the esophagus. Ann Thorac Surg 1988;45:137–43.

16. Heitmiller RF, Sharma RR. Comparison of prevalence and resection rates in patients with esophageal squamous cell carcinoma and adenocarcinoma. J Thorac Cardiovasc Surg 1996;112:130–6.

17. Daly JM, Karnell LH, Menck HR. National Cancer Data Base report on esophageal carcinoma. Cancer 1996;78:1820–8.

18. Zheng T, Mayne ST, Holford TR, et al. The time trend and age-period-cohort effects on incidence of adenocarcinoma of the stomach in Connecticut from 1955–1989. Cancer 1993;72:330–40.

19. Pera M, Cameron AJ, Trastek VF, et al. Increasing incidence of adenocarcinoma of the esophagus and esophagogastric junction. Gastroenterology 1993;104:510–3.

20. Cameron AJ, Lomboy CT, Pera M, Carpenter HA. Adenocarcinoma of the esophagogastric junction and Barrett's esophagus. Gastroenterology 1995;109:1541–6.

21. Spechler SJ, Goyal RK. The columnar-lined esophagus, intestinal metaplasia, and Norman Barrett. Gastroenterology 1996;110:614–21.

22. Barrett NR. Chronic peptic ulcer of the esophagus and "esophagitis." Br J Surg 1950;38:175–82.

23. Allison RR, Johnstone AS. The esophagus lined with gastric mucus membrane. Thorax 1953;8:87–101.

24. Barrett NR. The lower esophagus lined by columnar epithelium. Surgery 1957;41:881–94.

25. Moersch R, Ellis F, McDonald JR. Pathologic changes occurring in severe reflux esophagitis. Surg Gynecol Obstet 1959;108:476–84.

26. Bremner CG, Lynch VP, Ellis HF. Barrett's esophagus: congenital or acquired? An experimental study of esophageal mucosal regeneration in the dog. Surgery 1970;68:209–16.

27. Bremner CG, Demeester TR. Proceedings from an international conference on ablation therapy for Barrett's mucosa. Brittany, France, 31 August-2 September 1997. Dis Esophagus 1998;11:1–27.

28. DeMeester SR, DeMeester TR. Columnar mucosa and intestinal metaplasia of the esophagus: fifty years of controversy. Ann Surg 2000;231:303–21.

29. Clark GWB, Ireland AP, Peters JH, et al. Short-segment Barrett's esophagus: a prevalent complication of gastroesophageal reflux disease with malignant potential. J Gastrointest Surg 1997;1:113–22.

30. Sharma P, Morales TG, Sampliner RE. Short segment Barrett's esophagus—the need for standardization of the definition and of endoscopic criteria. Am J Gastroenterol 1998;93:1033–6.

31. Schnell TG, Sontag SJ, Chejfec G. Adenocarcinomas arising in tongues or short segments of Barrett's esophagus. Dig Dis Sci 1992;37:137–43.

32. Sharma P, Morales TG, Bhattacharyya A, et al. Dysplasia in short-segment Barrett's esophagus: a prospective 3-year follow-up. Am J Gastroenterol 1997;92:2012–6.

33. Clark GW, Peters JH, Ireland AP, et al. Nodal metastasis and sites of recurrence after en bloc esophagectomy for adenocarcinoma. Ann Thorac Surg 1994;58:646–54.

34. Attwood SE, DeMeester TR, Bremner CG, et al. Alkaline gastroesophageal reflux: implications in the development of complications in Barrett's columnar-lined lower esophagus. Surgery 1989;106:764–70.

35. Spechler SJ, Zeroogian JM, Antonioli DA, et al. Prevalence of metaplasia at the gastro-oesophageal junction. Lancet 1994;344:1533–6.

36. Ortiz-Hidalgo C, De La Vega G, Aguirre-Garcia J. The histopathology and biologic prognostic factors of Barrett's esophagus: a review. J Clin Gastroenterol 1998;26:324–33.

37. Stein HJ, Kauer WK, Feussner H, Siewert JR. Bile reflux in benign and malignant Barrett's esophagus: effect of medical acid suppression and Nissen fundoplication. J Gastrointest Surg 1998;2:333–41.

38. Oberg S, DeMeester TR, Peters JH, et al. The extent of Barrett's esophagus depends on the status of the lower esophageal sphincter and the degree of esophageal acid exposure. J Thorac Cardiovasc Surg 1999;117:572–80.

39. Kauer WK, Peters JH, DeMeester TR, et al. Mixed reflux of gastric and duodenal juices is more harmful to the esophagus than gastric juice alone. The need for surgical therapy re-emphasized. Ann Surg 1995;222:525–33.

40. Fein M, Ireland AP, Ritter MP, et al. Duodenogastric reflux potentiates the injurious effects of gastroesophageal reflux. J Gastrointest Surg 1997;1:27–33.

41. Clark GW, Smyrk TC, Burdiles P, et al. Is Barrett's metaplasia the source of adenocarcinomas of the cardia? Arch Surg 1994;129:609–14.

42. Goldblum JR, Vicari JJ, Falk GW, et al. Inflammation and intestinal metaplasia of the gastric cardia: the role of gastroesophageal reflux and *H. pylori* infection. Gastroenterology 1998;114:633–9.

43. Hirota WK, Loughney TM, Lazas DJ, et al. Specialized intestinal metaplasia, dysplasia, and cancer of the esophagus and esophagogastric junction: prevalence and clinical data. Gastroenterology 1999;116:277–85.

44. Drewitz DJ, Sampliner RE, Garewal HS. The incidence of adenocarcinoma in Barrett's esophagus: a prospective study of 170 patients followed 4.8 years. Am J Gastroenterol 1997;92:212–5.

45. Spechler SJ, Lee E, Ahnen D, et al. Long-term outcome of medical and surgical therapies for gastroesophageal reflux disease: follow-up of a randomized controlled trial. JAMA 2001;285:2331–8.

46. Gammon MD, Schoenberg JB, Ahsan H, et al. Tobacco, alcohol, and socioeconomic status and adenocarcinomas of the esophagus and gastric cardia. J Natl Cancer Inst 1997;89:1277–84.

47. Zhang ZF, Kurtz RC, Marshall JR. Cigarette smoking and

esophageal and gastric cardia adenocarcinoma [editorial; comment]. J Natl Cancer Inst 1997;89:1247–9.

48. Zhang ZF, Kurtz RC, Sun M, et al. Adenocarcinomas of the esophagus and gastric cardia: medical conditions, tobacco, alcohol, and socioeconomic factors. Cancer Epidemiol Biomarkers Prev 1996;5:761–8.

49. Chow WH, Blot WJ, Vaughan TL, et al. Body mass index and risk of adenocarcinomas of the esophagus and gastric cardia. J Natl Cancer Inst 1998;90:150–5.

50. Lagergren J, Bergstrom R, Nyren O. Association between body mass and adenocarcinoma of the esophagus and gastric cardia. Ann Intern Med 1999;130:883–90.

51. Lagergren J, Bergstrom R, Nyren O. No relation between body mass and gastro-oesophageal reflux symptoms in a Swedish population based study. Gut 2000;47:26–9.

52. Zhang ZF, Kurtz RC, Yu GP, et al. Adenocarcinoma of the esophagus and gastric cardia: the role of diet. Nutr Cancer 1997;27:298–309.

53. Chow WH, Blaser MJ, Blot WJ, et al. An inverse relation between cagA+ strains of *Helicobacter pylori* infection and risk of esophageal and gastric cardia adenocarcinoma. Cancer Res 1998;58:588–90.

54. Richter JE, Falk GW, Vaezi MF. *Helicobacter pylori* and gastroesophageal reflux disease: the bug may not be all bad. Am J Gastroenterol 1998;93:1800–2.

55. Levi F, Ollyo JB, La Vecchia C, et al. The consumption of tobacco, alcohol and the risk of adenocarcinoma in Barrett's oesophagus. Int J Cancer 1990;45:852–4.

56. Chow WH, Finkle WD, McLaughlin JK, et al. The relation of gastroesophageal reflux disease and its treatment to adenocarcinomas of the esophagus and gastric cardia. JAMA 1995;274:474–7.

57. Vaughan TL, Farrow DC, Hansten PD, et al. Risk of esophageal and gastric adenocarcinomas in relation to use of calcium channel blockers, asthma drugs, and other medications that promote gastroesophageal reflux. Cancer Epidemiol Biomarkers Prev 1998;7:749–56.

58. Lagergren J, Bergstrom R, Adami HO, Nyren O. Association between medications that relax the lower esophageal sphincter and risk for esophageal adenocarcinoma. Ann Intern Med 2000;133:165–75.

59. Farrow DC, Vaughan TL, Hansten PD, et al. Use of aspirin and other nonsteroidal anti-inflammatory drugs and risk of esophageal and gastric cancer. Cancer Epidemiol Biomarkers Prev 1998;7:97–102.

60. Lagergren J, Bergstrom R, Lindgren A, Nyren O. Symptomatic gastroesophageal reflux as a risk factor for esophageal adenocarcinoma. N Engl J Med 1999;340:825–31.

61. Farrow DC, Vaughan TL, Sweeney C, et al. Gastroesophageal reflux disease, use of H2 receptor antagonists, and risk of esophageal and gastric cancer. Cancer Causes Control 2000;11:231–8.

62. Meyenberger C, Fantin AC. Esophageal carcinoma: current staging strategies. Recent Results Cancer Res 2000;155:63–72.

63. Siewert JR, Feith M, Werner M, Stein HJ. Adenocarcinoma of the esophagogastric junction: results of surgical therapy based on anatomical/topographic classification in 1,002 consecutive patients. Ann Surg 2000;232:353–61.

64. Levine MS, Chu P, Furth EE, et al. Carcinoma of the esophagus and esophagogastric junction: sensitivity of radiographic diagnosis. AJR Am J Roentgenol 1997;168:1423–6.

65. Whyte RI, Orringer MB. Surgery for carcinoma of the esophagus: the case for transhiatal esophagectomy. Semin Radiat Oncol 1994;4:146–56.

66. Block MI, Patterson GA, Sundaresan RS, et al. Improvement in staging of esophageal cancer with the addition of positron emission tomography. Ann Thorac Surg 1997;64:770–7.

67. Flamen P, Lerut A, Van Cutsem E, et al. Utility of positron emission tomography for the staging of patients with potentially operable esophageal carcinoma. J Clin Oncol 2000;18:3202–10.

68. Luketich JD, Schauer PR, Meltzer CC, et al. Role of positron emission tomography in staging esophageal cancer. Ann Thorac Surg 1997;64:765–9.

69. Brugge WR, Lee MJ, Carey RW, Mathisen DJ. Endoscopic ultrasound staging criteria for esophageal cancer. Gastrointest Endosc 1997;45:147–52.

70. Van Dam J. Endosonographic evaluation of the patient with esophageal cancer. Chest 1997;112:184S–90S.

71. Peters JH, Hoeft SF, Heimbucher J, et al. Selection of patients for curative or palliative resection of esophageal cancer based on preoperative endoscopic ultrasonography. Arch Surg 1994;129:534–9.

72. Salminen JT, Farkkila MA, Ramo OJ, et al. Endoscopic ultrasonography in the preoperative staging of adenocarcinoma of the distal oesophagus and oesophagogastric junction. Scand J Gastroenterol 1999;34:1178–82.

73. Reed CE, Mishra G, Sahai AV, et al. Esophageal cancer staging: improved accuracy by endoscopic ultrasound of celiac lymph nodes. Ann Thorac Surg 1999;67:319–22.

74. Murata Y, Suzuki S, Ohta M, et al. Small ultrasonic probes for determination of the depth of superficial esophageal cancer. Gastrointest Endosc 1996;44:23–8.

75. Menzel J, Hoepffner N, Nottberg H, et al. Preoperative staging of esophageal carcinoma: miniprobe sonography versus conventional endoscopic ultrasound in a prospective histopathologically verified study. Endoscopy 1999;31:291–7.

76. Molloy RG, McCourtney JS, Anderson JR. Laparoscopy in the management of patients with cancer of the gastric cardia and oesophagus. Br J Surg 1995;82:352–4.

77. Stein HJ, Kraemer SJ, Feussner H, et al. Clinical value of diagnostic laparoscopy with laparoscopic ultrasound in patients with cancer of the esophagus or cardia. J Gastrointest Surg 1997;1:167–73.

78. Krasna MJ. Minimally invasive staging for esophageal cancer. Chest 1997;112:191S–4S.

79. American Joint Committee on Cancer. Esophagus. In: AJCC cancer staging manual. Lippincott-Raven Publishers, 1997. p. 65–9.

80. Iizuka T, Isono K, Kakegawa T, Watanabe H. Parameters linked to ten-year survival in Japan of resected esophageal carcinoma. Japanese Committee for Registration of Esophageal Carcinoma Cases. Chest 1989;96:1005–11.

81. Steup WH, De Leyn P, Deneffe G, et al. Tumors of the esophagogastric junction. Long-term survival in relation to the pattern of lymph node metastasis and a critical analysis of the accuracy or inaccuracy of pTNM classification. J Thorac Cardiovasc Surg 1996;111:85–95.

82. Collard JM. Exclusive radical surgery for esophageal adeno-carcinoma. Cancer 2001;91:1098–104.

83. Thomas P, Doddoli C, Lienne P, et al. Changing patterns and surgical results in adenocarcinoma of the oesophagus. Br J Surg 1997;84:119–25.

84. Holscher AH, Bollschweiler E, Bumm R, et al. Prognostic factors of resected adenocarcinoma of the esophagus. Surgery 1995;118:845–55.

85. Nigro JJ, DeMeester SR, Hagen JA, et al. Node status in transmural esophageal adenocarcinoma and outcome after en bloc esophagectomy. J Thorac Cardiovasc Surg 1999;117:960–8.

86. Lerut T. Esophageal surgery at the end of the millennium. J Thorac Cardiovasc Surg 1998;116:1–20.

87. Siewert JR, Stein HJ. Barrett's cancer: indications, extent, and results of surgical resection. Semin Surg Oncol 1997;13:245–52.

88. Tanabe G, Baba M, Kuroshima K, et al. [Clinical evaluation of the esophageal lymph flow system based on RI uptake of dissected regional lymph nodes following lymphoscintigraphy]. Nippon Geka Gakkai Zasshi 1986;87:315–23.

89. Isono K, Sato H, Nakayama K. Results of a nationwide study on the three-field lymph node dissection of esophageal cancer. Oncology 1991;48:411–20.

90. Altorki NK, Skinner DB. Occult cervical nodal metastasis in esophageal cancer: preliminary results of three-field lymphadenectomy. J Thorac Cardiovasc Surg 1997;113:540–4.

91. Fitzgerald RC, Triadafilopoulos G. Recent developments in the molecular characterization of Barrett's esophagus. Dig Dis 1998;16:63–80.

92. Hong MK, Laskin WB, Herman BE, et al. Expansion of the Ki-67 proliferative compartment correlates with degree of dysplasia in Barrett's esophagus. Cancer 1995;75:423–9.

93. Yacoub L, Goldman H, Odze RD. Transforming growth factor-alpha, epidermal growth factor receptor, and MiB-1 expression in Barrett's-associated neoplasia: correlation with prognosis. Mod Pathol 1997;10:105–12.

94. Sauter ER, Keller SM, Erner S, Goldberg M. HER-2/neu: a differentiation marker in adenocarcinoma of the esophagus. Cancer Lett 1993;75:41–4.

95. Houldsworth J, Cordon-Cardo C, Ladanyi M, et al. Gene amplification in gastric and esophageal adenocarcinomas. Cancer Res 1990;50:6417–22.

96. Hardwick RH, Shepherd NA, Moorghen M, et al. c-erbB-2 overexpression in the dysplasia/carcinoma sequence of Barrett's oesophagus. J Clin Pathol 1995;48:129–32.

97. Flejou JF, Paraf F, Muzeau F, et al. Expression of c-erbB-2 oncogene product in Barrett's adenocarcinoma: pathological and prognostic correlations. J Clin Pathol 1994;47:23–6.

98. Washington K, Chiappori A, Hamilton K, et al. Expression of beta-catenin, alpha-catenin, and E-cadherin in Barrett's esophagus and esophageal adenocarcinomas. Mod Pathol 1998;11:805–13.

99. Reid BJ, Blount PL, Rubin CE, et al. Flow-cytometric and histological progression to malignancy in Barrett's esophagus: prospective endoscopic surveillance of a cohort. Gastroenterology 1992;102:1212–9.

100. Mueller J, Werner M, Siewert JR. Malignant progression in Barrett's esophagus: pathology and molecular biology. Recent Results Cancer Res 2000;155:29–41.

101. Casson AG, Mukhopadhyay T, Cleary KR, et al. p53 gene mutations in Barrett's epithelium and esophageal cancer. Cancer Res 1991;51:4495–9.

102. Hamelin R, Flejou JF, Muzeau F, et al. TP53 gene mutations and p53 protein immunoreactivity in malignant and pre-malignant Barrett's esophagus. Gastroenterology 1994; 107:1012–8.

103. Neshat K, Sanchez CA, Galipeau PC, et al. p53 mutations in Barrett's adenocarcinoma and high-grade dysplasia. Gastroenterology 1994;106:1589–95.

104. Schneider PM, Casson AG, Levin B, et al. Mutations of p53 in Barrett's esophagus and Barrett's cancer: a prospective study of ninety-eight cases. J Thorac Cardiovasc Surg 1996;111:323–33.

105. Ribeiro U Jr, Finkelstein SD, Safatle-Ribeiro AV, et al. p53 sequence analysis predicts treatment response and outcome of patients with esophageal carcinoma. Cancer 1998;83:7–18.

106. Reid BJ, Barrett MT, Galipeau PC, et al. Barrett's esophagus: ordering the events that lead to cancer. Eur J Cancer Prev 1996;5 Suppl 2:57–65.

107. Gimenez A, Minguela A, Parrilla P, et al. Flow cytometric DNA analysis and p53 protein expression show a good correlation with histologic findings in patients with Barrett's esophagus. Cancer 1998;83:641–51.

108. Hollstein M, Shomer B, Greenblatt M, et al. Somatic point mutations in the p53 gene of human tumors and cell lines: updated compilation. Nucleic Acids Res 1996;24:141–6.

109. Jones PA, Buckley JD, Henderson BE, et al. From gene to carcinogen: a rapidly evolving field in molecular epidemiology. Cancer Res 1991;51:3617–20.

110. Polkowski W, Baak JP, van Lanschot JJ, et al. Clinical decision making in Barrett's oesophagus can be supported by computerized immunoquantitation and morphometry of features associated with proliferation and differentiation. J Pathol 1998;184:161–8.

111. Casson AG, Kerkvliet N, O'Malley F. Prognostic value of p53 protein in esophageal adenocarcinoma. J Surg Oncol 1995;60:5–11.

112. Harris CC, Hollstein M. Clinical implications of the p53 tumor-suppressor gene. N Engl J Med 1993;329:1318–27.

113. Wu TT, Watanabe T, Heitmiller R, et al. Genetic alterations in Barrett esophagus and adenocarcinomas of the esophagus and esophagogastric junction region. Am J Pathol 1998;153:287–94.

114. Blount PL, Meltzer SJ, Yin J, et al. Clonal ordering of 17p and 5q allelic losses in Barrett dysplasia and adenocarcinoma. Proc Natl Acad Sci U S A 1993;90:3221–5.

115. Barrett MT, Sanchez CA, Galipeau PC, et al. Allelic loss of 9p21 and mutation of the CDKN2/p16 gene develop as early lesions during neoplastic progression in Barrett's esophagus. Oncogene 1996;13:1867–73.

116. Barrett MT, Schutte M, Kern SE, Reid BJ. Allelic loss and mutational analysis of the DPC4 gene in esophageal adenocarcinoma. Cancer Res 1996;56:4351–3.

117. Gonzalez MV, Artimez ML, Rodrigo L, et al. Mutation analysis of the p53, APC, and p16 genes in the Barrett's oesophagus, dysplasia, and adenocarcinoma. J Clin Pathol 1997;50:212–7.

118. Stein HJ, Feith M, Siewert JR. Malignant degeneration of

Barrett's esophagus: clinical point of view. Recent Results Cancer Res 2000;155:42–53.

119. Ouatu-Lascar R, Triadafilopoulos G. Complete elimination of reflux symptoms does not guarantee normalization of intraesophageal acid reflux in patients with Barrett's esophagus. Am J Gastroenterol 1998;93:711–6.

120. Patti MG, Arcerito M, Feo CV, et al. Barrett's esophagus: a surgical disease. J Gastrointest Surg 1999;3:397–404.

121. Spechler SJ. Comparison of medical and surgical therapy for complicated gastroesophageal reflux disease in veterans. The Department of Veterans Affairs Gastroesophageal Reflux Disease Study Group. N Engl J Med 1992;326:786–92.

122. Malesci A, Savarino V, Zentilin P, et al. Partial regression of Barrett's esophagus by long-term therapy with high-dose omeprazole. Gastrointest Endosc 1996;44:700–5.

123. Sampliner RE, Garewal HS, Fennerty MB, Aickin M. Lack of impact of therapy on extent of Barrett's esophagus in 67 patients. Dig Dis Sci 1990;35:93–6.

124. Sharma P, Sampliner RE, Camargo E. Normalization of esophageal pH with high-dose proton pump inhibitor therapy does not result in regression of Barrett's esophagus. Am J Gastroenterol 1997;92:582–5.

125. Ortiz A, Martinez de Haro LF, Parrilla P, et al. Conservative treatment versus antireflux surgery in Barrett's oesophagus: long-term results of a prospective study. Br J Surg 1996;83:274–8.

126. Attwood SE, Barlow AP, Norris TL, Watson A. Barrett's oesophagus: effect of antireflux surgery on symptom control and development of complications. Br J Surg 1992;79:1050–3.

127. McDonald ML, Trastek VF, Allen MS, et al. Barretts's esophagus: does an antireflux procedure reduce the need for endoscopic surveillance? J Thorac Cardiovasc Surg 1996;111:1135–40.

128. Peters JH, Clark GW, Ireland AP, et al. Outcome of adenocarcinoma arising in Barrett's esophagus in endoscopically surveyed and nonsurveyed patients. J Thorac Cardiovasc Surg 1994;108:813–22.

129. Streitz JM, Andrews CW, Ellis FH. Endoscopic surveillance of Barrett's esophagus. Does it help? J Thorac Cardiovasc Surg 1993;105:383–8.

130. Berenson MM, Johnson TD, Markowitz NR, et al. Restoration of squamous mucosa after ablation of Barrett's esophageal epithelium. Gastroenterology 1993;104:1686–91.

131. Van Laethem JL, Cremer M, Peny MO, et al. Eradication of Barrett's mucosa with argon plasma coagulation and acid suppression: immediate and mid term results. Gut 1998;43:747–51.

132. Van Laethem JL, Peny MO, Salmon I, et al. Intramucosal adenocarcinoma arising under squamous re-epithelialisation of Barrett's oesophagus. Gut 2000;46:574–7.

133. Bremner CG, Bremner RM. Barrett's esophagus. Surg Clin North Am 1997;77:1115–37.

134. Ackroyd R, Brown NJ, Davis MF, et al. Photodynamic therapy for dysplastic Barrett's oesophagus: a prospective, double blind, randomised, placebo controlled trial. Gut 2000;47:612–7.

135. Bremner RM, Mason RJ, Bremner CG, et al. Ultrasonic epithelial ablation of the lower esophagus without stric-

ture formation. A new technique for Barrett's ablation. Surg Endosc 1998;12:342–7.

136. Hameeteman W, Tytgat GN, Houthoff HJ, van den Tweel JG. Barrett's esophagus: development of dysplasia and adenocarcinoma. Gastroenterology 1989;96:1249–56.

137. Reid BJ, Weinstein WM, Lewin KJ, et al. Endoscopic biopsy can detect high-grade dysplasia or early adenocarcinoma in Barrett's esophagus without grossly recognizable neoplastic lesions. Gastroenterology 1988;94:81–90.

138. Heitmiller RF, Redmond M, Hamilton SR. Barrett's esophagus with high-grade dysplasia. An indication for prophylactic esophagectomy. Ann Surg 1996;224:66–71.

139. Ferguson MK, Naunheim KS. Resection for Barrett's mucosa with high-grade dysplasia: implications for prophylactic photodynamic therapy. J Thorac Cardiovasc Surg 1997;114:824–9.

140. Pera M, Trastek VF, Carpenter HA, et al. Barrett's esophagus with high-grade dysplasia: an indication for esophagectomy? Ann Thorac Surg 1992;54:199–204.

141. Levine DS, Haggitt RC, Blount PL, et al. An endoscopic biopsy protocol can differentiate high-grade dysplasia from early adenocarcinoma in Barrett's esophagus. Gastroenterology 1993;105:40–50.

142. Reid BJ, Blount PL, Feng Z, Levine DS. Optimizing endoscopic biopsy detection of early cancers in Barrett's high-grade dysplasia. Am J Gastroenterol 2000;95:3089–96.

143. Spechler SJ, Goyal RK. Cancer surveillance in Barrett's esophagus: what is the end point? Gastroenterology 1994;106:275–7.

144. Clark GW, Ireland AP, DeMeester TR. Dysplastic Barrett's: is continued surveillance appropriate? Gastroenterology 1994;106:1128.

145. Barr H, Shepherd NA, Dix A, et al. Eradication of high-grade dysplasia in columnar-lined (Barrett's) oesophagus by photodynamic therapy with endogenously generated protoporphyrin IX. Lancet 1996;348:584–5.

146. Gossner L, Stolte M, Sroka R, et al. Photodynamic ablation of high-grade dysplasia and early cancer in Barrett's esophagus by means of 5-aminolevulinic acid. Gastroenterology 1998;114:448–55.

147. Overholt BF, Panjehpour M, Haydek JM. Photodynamic therapy for Barrett's esophagus: follow-up in 100 patients. Gastrointest Endosc 1999;49:1–7.

148. Torek F. The first successful case of resection of the thoracic portion of the oesophagus for carcinoma. Surg Gynecol Obstet 1913;16:614–7.

149. Denk W. Zur Radikaloperation des Oesophaguskarzinoms. Zentralbl Chir 1913;40:1065–8.

150. Turner G. Excision of the thoracic oesophagus for carcinomas with construction of a extrathoracic gullet. Lancet 1933;2:1315.

151. Ohsawa T. The surgery of the oesophagus. Jpn Chir 1933;10:604.

152. Adams W, Phemister D. Carcinoma of the lower thoracic esophagus: report of a successful resection and esophagogastrostomy. J Thorac Surg 1938;7:621–32.

153. Lewis I. The surgical treatment of carcinoma of the esophagus: with special reference to a new operation for growths of the middle third. Br J Surg 1946;34:18–31.

154. Orringer MB, Sloan H. Esophagectomy without thoracotomy. J Thorac Cardiovasc Surg 1978;76:643–54.

155. Orringer MB. Transhiatal esophagectomy without thoracotomy for carcinoma of the thoracic esophagus. Ann Surg 1984;200:282–8.

156. Orringer MB, Marshall B, Stirling MC. Transhiatal esophagectomy for benign and malignant disease. J Thorac Cardiovasc Surg 1993;105:265–77.

157. Orringer MB, Marshall B, Iannettoni MD. Transhiatal esophagectomy: clinical experience and refinements. Ann Surg 1999;230:392–403.

158. Chu KM, Law SY, Fok M, Wong J. A prospective randomized comparison of transhiatal and transthoracic resection for lower-third esophageal carcinoma. Am J Surg 1997;174:320–4.

159. Goldminc M, Maddern G, Le Prise E, et al. Oesophagectomy by a transhiatal approach or thoracotomy: a prospective randomized trial. Br J Surg 1993;80:367–70.

160. Boyle MJ, Franceschi D, Livingstone AS. Transhiatal versus transthoracic esophagectomy: complication and survival rates. Am Surg 1999;65:1137–42.

161. Gluch L, Smith RC, Bambach CP, Brown AR. Comparison of outcomes following transhiatal or Ivor Lewis esophagectomy for esophageal carcinoma. World J Surg 1999;23:271–6.

162. Pommier RF, Vetto JT, Ferris BL, Wilmarth TJ. Relationships between operative approaches and outcomes in esophageal cancer. Am J Surg 1998;175:422–5.

163. Katariya K, Harvey JC, Pina E, Beattie EJ. Complications of transhiatal esophagectomy. J Surg Oncol 1994;57:157–63.

164. Rindani R, Martin CJ, Cox MR. Transhiatal versus Ivor-Lewis oesophagectomy: is there a difference? Aust N Z J Surg 1999;69:187–94.

165. Horvath OP, Lukacs L, Cseke L. Complications following esophageal surgery. Recent Results Cancer Res 2000;155:161–73.

166. Orringer MB, Marshall B, Iannettoni MD. Eliminating the cervical esophagogastric anastomotic leak with a side-to-side stapled anastomosis. J Thorac Cardiovasc Surg 2000;119:277–88.

167. Mathisen DJ. Ivor Lewis procedure. In: Pearson FG, editor. Esophageal surgery. New York: Churchill Livingston; 1995. p. 669–76.

168. Lee RB, Miller JI. Esophagectomy for cancer. Surg Clin North Am 1997;77:1169–96.

169. McKeown KC. The surgical treatment of carcinoma of the oesophagus. J R Coll Surg Edinb 1985;30:1–14.

170. Karl RC, Schreiber R, Boulware D, et al. Factors affecting morbidity, mortality, and survival in patients undergoing Ivor Lewis esophagogastrectomy. Ann Surg 2000;231:635–43.

171. Akiyama H, Miyazono H, Tsurumaru H, et al. Thoracoabdominal approach for carcinoma of the cardia of the stomach. Am J Surg 1979;137:345–9.

172. Logan A. The surgical treatment of carcinoma of the esophagus and cardia. J Thorac Cardiovasc Surg 1963;46:150.

173. Skinner D. En bloc resection for neoplasms of the esophagus and cardia. J Thorac Cardiovasc Surg 1983;85:59–71.

174. Altorki NK, Girardi L, Skinner DB. En bloc esophagectomy improves survival for stage III esophageal cancer. J Thorac Cardiovasc Surg 1997;114:948–56.

175. DeMeester TR. Esophageal carcinoma: current controversies. Semin Surg Oncol 1997;13:217–33.

176. Akiyama H, Tsurumaru M, Udagawa H, Kajiyama Y. Radical lymph node dissection for cancer of the thoracic esophagus. Ann Surg 1994;220:364–73.

177. Skinner DB. En bloc resection for esophageal cancer. In: Pearson FG, editor. Esophageal surgery. New York: Churchill Livingston; 1995. p. 709–18.

178. Watson DI, Davies N, Jamieson GG. Totally endoscopic Ivor Lewis esophagectomy. Surg Endosc 1999;13:293–7.

179. Luketich JD, Nguyen NT, Weigel T, et al. Minimally invasive approach to esophagectomy. J Soc Laparoendosc Surg 1998;2:243–7.

180. Nguyen NT, Follette DM, Wolfe BM, et al. Comparison of minimally invasive esophagectomy with transthoracic and transhiatal esophagectomy. Arch Surg 2000;135:920–5.

181. DePaula AL, Hashiba K, Ferreira EA, et al. Laparoscopic transhiatal esophagectomy with esophagogastroplasty. Surg Laparosc Endosc 1995;5:1–5.

182. Swanstrom LL, Hansen P. Laparoscopic total esophagectomy. Arch Surg 1997;132:943–9.

183. Gerhart CD. Hand-assisted laparoscopic transhiatal esophagectomy using the dexterity pneumo sleeve. J Soc Laparoendosc Surg 1998;2:295–8.

184. Endo M. Endoscopic resection as local treatment of mucosal cancer of the esophagus. Endoscopy 1993;25:672–4.

185. Kodama M, Kakegawa T. Treatment of superficial cancer of the esophagus: a summary of responses to a questionnaire on superficial cancer of the esophagus in Japan. Surgery 1998;123:432–9.

186. Yang GR, Zhao LQ, Li SS, et al. Endoscopic Nd:YAG laser therapy in patients with early superficial carcinoma of the esophagus and the gastric cardia. Endoscopy 1994;26:681–5.

187. Sibille A, Lambert R, Souquet JC, et al. Long-term survival after photodynamic therapy for esophageal cancer. Gastroenterology 1995;108:337–44.

188. Menke-Pluymers MB, Schoute NW, Mulder AH, et al. Outcome of surgical treatment of adenocarcinoma in Barrett's oesophagus. Gut 1992;33:1454–8.

189. Moon MR, Schulte WJ, Haasler GB, Condon RE. Transhiatal and transthoracic esophagectomy for adenocarcinoma of the esophagus. Arch Surg 1992;127:951–5.

190. Forastiere AA, Orringer MB, Perez-Tamayo C, et al. Preoperative chemoradiation followed by transhiatal esophagectomy for carcinoma of the esophagus: final report. J Clin Oncol 1993;11:1118–23.

191. Stewart JR, Hoff SJ, Johnson DH, et al. Improved survival with neoadjuvant therapy and resection for adenocarcinoma of the esophagus. Ann Surg 1993;218:571–8.

192. Forastiere AA, Heitmiller RF, Lee DJ, et al. Intensive chemoradiation followed by esophagectomy for squamous cell and adenocarcinoma of the esophagus. Cancer J Sci Am 1997;3:144–52.

193. Posner MC, Gooding WE, Landreneau RJ, et al. Preoperative chemoradiotherapy for carcinoma of the esophagus and gastroesophageal junction. Cancer J Sci Am 1998;4:237–46.

194. Walsh TN, Noonan N, Hollywood D, et al. A comparison of multimodal therapy and surgery for esophageal adenocarcinoma. N Engl J Med 1996;335:462–7.

195. Wilke H, Fink U. Multimodal therapy for adenocarcinoma of the esophagus and esophagogastric junction. N Engl J Med 1996;335:509–10.

196. Urba SG, Orringer MB, Turrisi A, et al. Randomized trial of preoperative chemoradiation versus surgery alone in patients with locoregional esophageal carcinoma. J Clin Oncol 2001;19:305–13.

197. Kelsen D. Preoperative chemoradiotherapy for esophageal cancer. J Clin Oncol 2001;19:283–5.

198. Meluch AA, Hainsworth JD, Gray JR, et al. Preoperative combined modality therapy with paclitaxel, carboplatin, prolonged infusion 5-fluorouracil, and radiation therapy in localized esophageal cancer: preliminary results of a Minnie Pearl Cancer Research Network phase II trial. Cancer J Sci Am 1999;5:84–91.

199. Roth JA, Pass HI, Flanagan MM, et al. Randomized clinical trial of preoperative and postoperative adjuvant chemotherapy with cisplatin, vindesine, and bleomycin for carcinoma of the esophagus. J Thorac Cardiovasc Surg 1988;96:242–8.

200. Nygaard K, Hagen S, Hansen HS, et al. Pre-operative radiotherapy prolongs survival in operable esophageal carcinoma: a randomized, multicenter study of pre-operative radiotherapy and chemotherapy. The second Scandinavian trial in esophageal cancer. World J Surg 1992;16:1104–10.

201. Schlag PM. Randomized trial of preoperative chemotherapy for squamous cell cancer of the esophagus. The Chirurgische Arbeitsgemeinschaft fuer Onkologie der Deutschen Gesellschaft fuer Chirurgie Study Group. Arch Surg 1992;127:1446–50.

202. Kelsen DP, Ginsberg R, Pajak TF, et al. Chemotherapy followed by surgery compared with surgery alone for localized esophageal cancer. N Engl J Med 1998;339:1979–84.

203. Cooper JS, Guo MD, Herskovic A, et al. Chemoradiotherapy of locally advanced esophageal cancer: long-term follow-up of a prospective randomized trial (RTOG 85-01). Radiation Therapy Oncology Group. JAMA 1999;281:1623–7.

204. Forastiere AA, Heitmiller RF, Kleinberg L. Multimodality therapy for esophageal cancer. Chest 1997;112:195S–200S.

205. Bamias A, Hill ME, Cunningham D, et al. Epirubicin, cisplatin, and protracted venous infusion of 5-fluorouracil for esophagogastric adenocarcinoma: response, toxicity, quality of life, and survival. Cancer 1996;77:1978–85.

206. Webb A, Cunningham D, Scarffe JH, et al. Randomized trial comparing epirubicin, cisplatin, and fluorouracil versus fluorouracil, doxorubicin, and methotrexate in advanced esophagogastric cancer. J Clin Oncol 1997;15:261–7.

207. Ponec RJ, Kimmey MB. Endoscopic therapy of esophageal cancer. Surg Clin North Am 1997;77:1197–217.

208. Urba SG, Turrisi AT. Split-course accelerated radiation therapy combined with carboplatin and 5-fluorouracil for palliation of metastatic or unresectable carcinoma of the esophagus. Cancer 1995;75:435–9.

209. Hejna M, Kornek GV, Schratter-Sehn AU, et al. Effective radiochemotherapy with cisplatin and etoposide for the management of patients with locally inoperable and metastatic esophageal carcinoma. Cancer 1996;78: 1646–50.

210. Rice TW, Boyce GA, Sivak MV. Esophageal ultrasound and the preoperative staging of carcinoma of the esophagus. J Thorac Cardiovasc Surg 1991;101:536–44.

211. Dittler HJ, Siewert JR. Role of endoscopic ultrasonography in gastric carcinoma. Endoscopy 1993;25:162–6.

212. Streitz JM Jr, Ellis FH Jr, Gibb SP, et al. Adenocarcinoma in Barrett's esophagus. A clinicopathologic study of 65 cases. Ann Surg 1991;213:122–5.

6

Squamous Cell Carcinoma of the Esophagus

MARK K. FERGUSON, MD

ETIOLOGY AND EPIDEMIOLOGY

Squamous cell cancers represent the single most common malignancy of the esophagus worldwide. Social and environmental factors contribute substantially to its development. In Western society, alcohol consumption increases the risk of squamous cell cancer 10 to 25 times, and cigarette smoking has also been linked to an increased incidence of squamous cell cancer.[1,2] Combined cigarette use and alcohol consumption can increase the risk of squamous cell cancer up to 100-fold.[3] In the rest of the world, dietary and nutritional factors play an important role in the high incidence of squamous cell cancer of the esophagus. Risks include ingestion of nitrosamines, contamination of food by specific fungi, and factors such as the temperature of ingested fluids and the presence of mechanical irritants to the esophagus, such as silica and crushed seeds.[4,5] Squamous cell cancers are associated with chronic injury to the esophagus due to caustic ingestion, stasis of foodstuffs in patients with achalasia, and possibly gastroesophageal acid reflux disease.[6–10] The only familial abnormality that is associated with squamous cancer of the esophagus is tylosis A, which carries a 25 percent lifetime risk.[11] Human papillomavirus (HPV) is present in up to 50 percent of patients with squamous cell cancer of the esophagus and is more common in areas in which these tumors are endemic.[12,13]

Endemic areas for squamous cell cancer of the esophagus are the northern littoral in Iran; Linxian, China; and regions of South Africa, where the incidences are as high as 150 cases per 100,000 population.[10] In the United States, the incidence rate of squamous cell cancers is about 3 per 100,000 population, which translates to a new incidence of about 12,000 cases and nearly 12,000 deaths from squamous cell esophageal cancer in 1998.[14,15] Men are more commonly affected than are women, and the highest incidence occurs during the sixth through eighth decades of life (Figure 6–1).

DIAGNOSIS

The diagnosis of esophageal cancer is suspected on the basis of typical symptoms such as progressive dysphagia, odynophagia, and regurgitation. Weight loss occurs prior to diagnosis in about 50 percent of people. Chest pain may be present due to local invasion, ulceration within the esophagus, or obstructive effects with accompanying spasm. Locally advanced disease may lead to hoarseness due to recurrent laryngeal nerve involvement, malignant esophagorespiratory fistula, or cough due to irritation of the airways. Cytologic surveillance techniques for diagnosis of early-stage cancers have been used with success in regions in which squamous cell cancers are endemic. However, unlike recommendations for premalignant lesions such as Barrett's esophagus, surveillance endoscopy is not routinely indicated for possible squamous cell cancer of the esophagus because it is difficult to identify individuals in Western society who are at high risk. Possible high-risk categories include patients with achalasia, tylosis A, a history of caustic ingestion, and a history of squamous cell cancer of the head and neck.

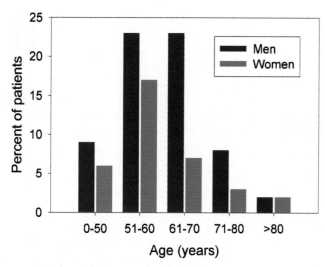

Figure 6–1. Distribution of squamous cell cancers of the esophagus according to age and sex.

Once an esophageal cancer is suspected, the primary method of diagnosis is flexible upper gastrointestinal endoscopy, which permits a clinical (visual) diagnosis and allows the collection of specimens for histology and cytology. Rigid esophagoscopy may be considered to permit larger and deeper biopsies if flexible endoscopic techniques fail to provide a diagnosis. A clinical diagnosis may be made on the basis of upper gastrointestinal contrast radiography, which is also important for providing information regarding the location of the tumor relative to the airways and the degree of obstruction caused by the tumor.

STAGING

Computed tomography (CT) of the chest and abdomen is the standard technique for staging squamous cell cancer of the esophagus. Although it is not very accurate for assessing tumor (T) status, CT is good for determining resectability with regard to local invasion. The overall accuracy of CT in assessing aortic invasion exceeds 90 percent; for assessing airway invasion, the overall accuracy approaches 90 percent.[16–21] Lymph node involvement is not accurately determined by CT because of variations in the normal size of lymph nodes in the mediastinum and abdomen and because nodal enlargement does not necessarily occur when metastatic spread develops.[21–25] Computed tomog-

raphy is useful for detecting distant organ metastases to the lung, liver, adrenal glands, and kidneys. The overall accuracy of metastasis (M) status assessment exceeds 90 percent.[16,20,22,24,26,27]

Squamous cell cancers of the esophagus typically occur adjacent to the major airways in the upper and middle thoracic esophagus. Computed tomography sometimes shows impingement upon the airways, displacement of the airways, or actual tumor invasion; the latter is the only reliable radiographic sign of airway involvement. Patients who are considered potential candidates for resection should undergo bronchoscopy to evaluate the airways for possible local invasion if the primary tumor abuts the trachea or a mainstem bronchus. The accuracy of predicting airway invasion with bronchoscopy exceeds 90 percent.[28]

Endoscopic ultrasonography (EUS) is rapidly becoming a standard technique for evaluating T and node (N) status in patients with squamous cell cancer of the esophagus. Up to 30 percent of patients have tumors that are sufficiently obstructing that standard EUS probes are unable to be passed into the distal esophagus and stomach, limiting the staging value of the examination. The accuracy of EUS increases as T status becomes more advanced, from 60 percent for T1 tumors to 98 percent for T4 tumors, and the overall accuracy is 80 percent.[21,29–34] The accuracy of EUS for T staging after the administration of neoadjuvant chemotherapy decreases to 45 percent due primarily to overstaging.[35–38] The accuracy of N staging by EUS is about 75 percent, which decreases to 50 percent after neoadjuvant therapy.[23,32–40]

Positron emission tomography (PET) was introduced as a modality for staging esophageal cancer in the mid-1990s. It is not useful for T staging, and its accuracy for N staging is about 60 percent, which is somewhat less than that of EUS. The accuracy of staging distant metastatic disease is over 90 percent; in about 20 percent of patients, sites of metastatic disease are identified that were unsuspected after standard staging tests such as CT.[41–43]

Laparoscopy and thoracoscopy have been used since the early 1980s and early 1990s, respectively, for staging esophageal cancer. Laparoscopy, sometimes with intraoperative ultrasonography, has been shown to be useful in the assessment of patients with adenocarcinomas but has not proven useful for staging squamous cell cancers of the esophagus, likely due to the fact that adenocarcinomas are generally located more distally in the esophagus, a location from which intra-abdominal spread of disease is more likely. In contrast, thoracoscopy has been shown to have an accuracy of 90 percent in regional nodal staging of squamous cell cancers of the esophagus.[25,44] Given the time required to perform the procedure and the need for postoperative hospitalization, whether thoracoscopy will prove cost-effective for staging squamous cell cancer of the esophagus remains to be determined.

In some centers, ultrasonography has proven useful in the evaluation of cervical and supraclavicular lymph nodes in patients with squamous cell cancer of the esophagus. Up to 30 percent of patients have clinically unsuspected nodal metastases, the identification of which may have important implications for the selection of therapy. The overall accuracy of neck ultrasonography is about 90 percent.[45,46] Needle aspiration under ultrasonographic guidance for cytology improves the yield of this valuable technique.[47]

There is no generally accepted algorithm for staging squamous cell cancer of the esophagus, but general guidelines can be suggested. All patients should undergo upper gastrointestinal endoscopy, chest radiography, contrast radiography of the esophagus and stomach, and CT of the chest and abdomen. Bronchoscopy is performed for patients who are potential surgical candidates and whose tumors abut the major airways. Endoscopic ultrasonography is particularly useful in patients who are suspected of having T4 disease on the basis of CT findings since information from EUS will assist in the selection of proper therapy. Because EUS provides regional staging information that is better than that of CT, it may also have practical value in selecting between transthoracic and other surgical approaches to resection. Bone scintigraphy is performed if there is a clinical suspicion of bone metastases. The role of PET has not yet been determined.

THERAPY

Options for treating squamous cell cancer of the esophagus include potentially curative therapies (resection, chemoradiotherapy, and trimodality therapy) and palliative therapy for patients with advanced-stage disease. Chapter 8 deals with combined-modality therapy, and Chapter 9 focuses on palliative treatment options. This chapter describes surgical approaches to squamous cell cancer of the esophagus and provides information related to neoadjuvant treatment and postoperative adjuvant therapies.

Pretreatment Assessment

Aggressive therapies such as resection or neoadjuvant chemoradiotherapy followed by resection require that a careful pretreatment assessment be performed to determine the patient's risk for such treatment. Evaluation includes a careful history and physical examination with special attention to cardiopulmonary status. The patient's age, weight, history of recent weight loss, nutritional status, performance status, hepatic dysfunction, renal dysfunction, and recent tobacco or alcohol abuse all contribute to treatment-related morbidity. Operative mortality is related to nutritional status, performance status, and the frequency with which an operation is performed in an institution.[48–51]

Surgery

Approaches to Resection

The optimal approach to resection for squamous cell carcinoma of the esophagus is dictated by the location of the tumor, the natural history of the cancer, and the personal preferences of the surgeon. Most such tumors are located in the upper and middle thoracic esophagus. An open transthoracic approach provides the best exposure for complete dissection of these neoplasms from surrounding structures, including the major airways and aorta (Figure 6–2). A thoracotomy also permits a complete nodal dissection when indicated. In contrast, a transhiatal approach is relatively contraindicated for tumors located in the middle and upper thoracic esophagus, except in the hands of the most experienced surgeons (Figure 6–3). The theoretic advantages of decreased postoperative morbidity and shortened time under anesthesia are offset by the increased risk of major vascular or airway injury and by the increased chance of an incomplete resection.

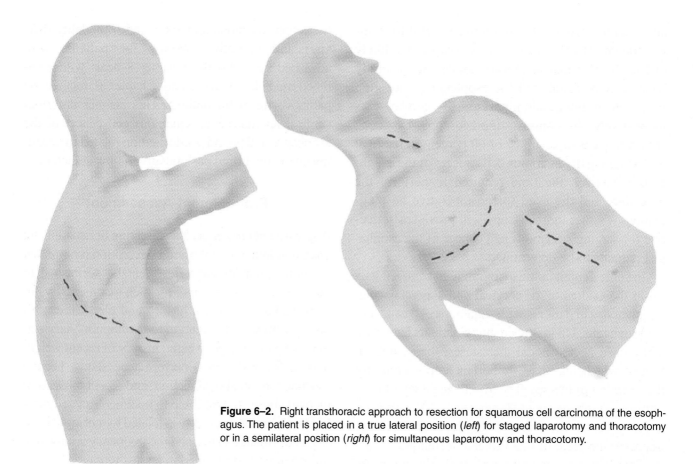

Figure 6–2. Right transthoracic approach to resection for squamous cell carcinoma of the esophagus. The patient is placed in a true lateral position (*left*) for staged laparotomy and thoracotomy or in a semilateral position (*right*) for simultaneous laparotomy and thoracotomy.

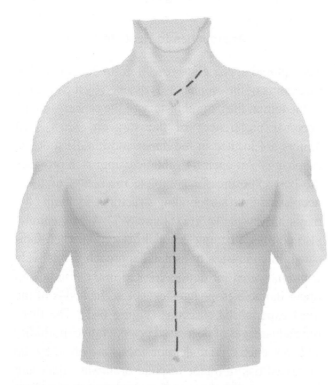

Figure 6–3. Transhiatal approach for esophagectomy.

Another approach to intrathoracic esophageal tumors is an operation performed exclusively through a left thoracotomy (Figure 6–4). This may be appropriate for selected patients who have squamous cell cancers of the distal third of the esophagus, but if the tumor is located more proximally, the arch of the aorta prevents adequate exposure for a complete dissection.

The patient's age and comorbid factors also play a role in determining the optimal approach to resection. Patients who are elderly or who have important medical problems and are marginal candidates for resection may benefit from a reduced duration of anesthesia. In such cases (particularly when the goal of the operation is primarily palliative), the surgeon may choose to perform the operation in the most expeditious manner possible. This often translates to a transhiatal approach. In contrast, some surgeons think that patients with relatively early-stage tumors benefit from a more aggressive operation, in which case an open and extended resection is theoretically indicated.

It is not possible to demonstrate the superiority of either the open transthoracic technique or the transhi-

Minimally invasive techniques have been introduced recently for the management of esophageal cancers, in an effort to minimize surgical trauma and decrease length of hospital stay. They combine thoracoscopic resection with an open or laparoscopic approach for the abdominal portion of the operation (Figure 6–5). The early experience with thoracoscopic esophagectomy for cancer suggests that operative morbidity and mortality, as well as postoperative length of stay, are similar to those of open operations.[59–64]

Malignancies of the cervical esophagus or at the thoracic inlet are the most difficult to manage because of problems with access and exposure and because of implications regarding the need for extended resections including the larynx. Options for resection include a limited cervical dissection, which preserves the intrathoracic esophagus, or a complete esophagectomy with an open cervical dissection and removal of the remaining esophagus, using a transhiatal approach (Figure 6–6). Additional exposure of the upper thoracic esophagus may be obtained by using a partial sternotomy.[65]

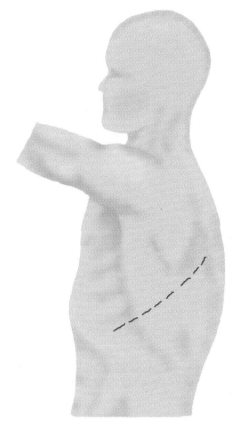

Figure 6–4. Exclusive left thoracotomy for resection of distal esophageal squamous cell cancer.

atal technique. Regardless of which approach is used, cardiopulmonary function suffers similar perturbations in the early postoperative period.[52] At institutions reporting results of both procedures, there has been little difference between the two in either postoperative morbidity or mortality (Table 6–1).[53–57] Other than a higher incidence of cervical anastomotic leaks among patients undergoing transhiatal resection, a meta-analysis demonstrated no apparent advantage for either technique with regard to other morbidities, operative mortality, or 5-year survival.[58]

Extent of Local Resection

A primary determinant of long-term survival after esophagectomy is whether an R0 (no residual gross or microscopic tumor) resection is accomplished. Opinion differs as to how to best achieve this goal. Most surgeons perform a so-called standard esophagectomy as a curative procedure. The extent of resection includes at least a 5-cm margin of esophagus proximal and distal to the gross extent of tumor, the soft tissues that surround the esophagus, and regional lymph nodes in the vicinity of the tumor (Figures 6–7 and 6–8). Longer proximal and distal

			Transthoracic Resection		Transhiatal Resection	
Lead Author	**Ref. No.**	**Year**	**Morbidity**	**Mortality**	**Morbidity**	**Mortality**
Moon	53	1992	10/24	3/24	27/63	8/63
Pac	54	1993	76/120	13/120	88/118	8/118
Tilanus	55	1993	—	13/152	—	7/141
Putnam	56	1994	101/179	13/179	23/42	2/42
Gluch	57	1999	—	2/33	—	3/65
Total			187/323 (57.9%)	44/508 (8.7%)	138/223 (61.9%)	28/429 (6.5%)

Table 6–1. STUDIES OF THE RELATIONSHIP OF OPERATIVE APPROACH TO POSTOPERATIVE MORBIDITY AND MORTALITY AFTER ESOPHAGECTOMY

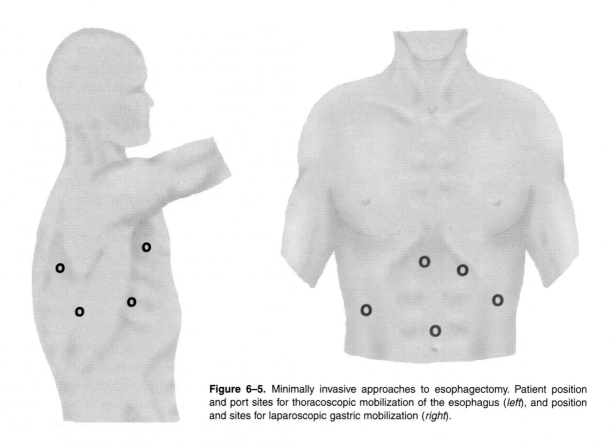

Figure 6–5. Minimally invasive approaches to esophagectomy. Patient position and port sites for thoracoscopic mobilization of the esophagus (*left*), and position and sites for laparoscopic gastric mobilization (*right*).

margins do not affect local recurrence or long-term survival rates.[66,67] However, squamous cell cancers are multifocal in up to 20 percent of patients, suggesting that under most circumstances, a near-total esophagectomy should be performed if the patient is to be rendered disease free.[68,69]

Because of concerns regarding the completeness of local resection obtained during a standard esophagectomy, radical en bloc esophagectomy was

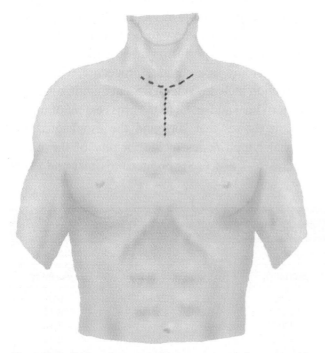

Figure 6–6. Options for approaching squamous cell cancers of the cervical esophagus or those located at the thoracic inlet.

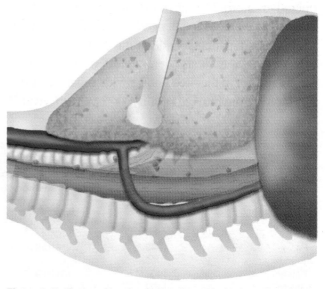

Figure 6–7. Extent of local resection for a standard esophagectomy approached through a right thoracotomy.

Squamous Cell Carcinoma of the Esophagus

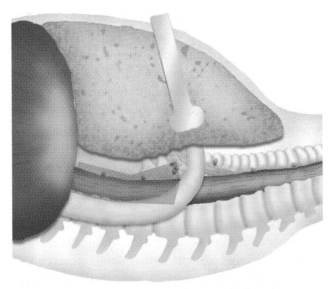

Figure 6–8. Extent of local resection for a standard esophagectomy approached through a left thoracotomy for a distal esophageal squamous cell cancer.

introduced in the late 1960s. The extent of radical soft tissue resection varies among surgeons. In the most aggressive dissection, tissues removed include the pericardium, a rim of diaphragm, bilateral pleura, the azygos vein, and the thoracic duct within 10 cm of the primary tumor (Figure 6–9). A true en bloc dissection is not possible for tumors of the upper thoracic and cervical esophagus. No randomized studies exist that permit comparison of results from en bloc esophagectomy and standard esophagectomy in similar patient groups. In patients with early-stage cancer (T1 N0 M0, stage I) the 5-year survival rates are similar for the two operations.[70–74] Patients with regionally advanced disease may experience improved long-term survival after en bloc esophagectomy, as opposed to standard esophagectomy. However, the groups of patients with regionally advanced disease that have been reported in retrospective studies are dissimilar with regard to age and year of operation, making it impossible to draw definitive conclusions regarding the effect different types of operation have on survival.[75,76]

Extent of Lymph Node Dissection

The typical lymph node dissection for patients undergoing a standard and potentially curative esophagectomy includes regional nodes adjacent to

the primary tumor, as well as subcarinal, left gastric artery, lesser gastric curvature, and celiac artery lymph nodes (Figure 6–10). There is concern that this extent of lymphadenectomy may not provide complete staging information because routine dissection of cervical lymph nodes in patients with squamous cell cancer of the esophagus reveals unsuspected nodal involvement in up to 30 percent of patients.[77–79] This has led some surgeons to recommend that patients routinely undergo an extended, or three-field, lymphadenectomy.

Extended lymphadenectomy consists of a complete lymph node dissection in the three regions that are typically affected by squamous cell cancers: the upper abdomen, the mediastinum, and the lower neck (Figure 6–11). The results of this approach demonstrate up-staging of the cancer in up to 30 percent of patients. The three-field dissection causes an increased incidence of complications, including recurrent laryngeal nerve palsy, respiratory insufficiency, tracheal ischemia, pulmonary compromise, and anastomotic leak; in some reports, operative mortality is also increased.[80–82] No randomized studies have been performed to permit a direct comparison of the survival rates of the two types of lymph node dissection. Most retrospective reviews demonstrate no significant improvement in long-term survival resulting from the three-field dissection.[82–85]

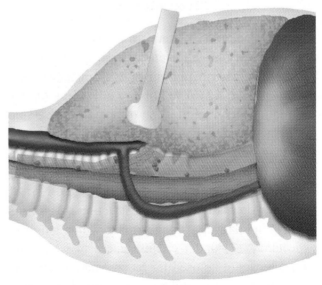

Figure 6–9. Extent of local resection for a radical en bloc esophagectomy.

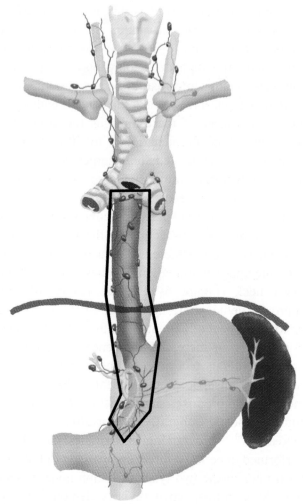

Figure 6–10. Extent of lymph node dissection for a standard esophagectomy.

Reconstruction

The most common method of re-establishing the continuity of the alimentary tract after esophagectomy is gastric pull-up and esophagogastrostomy (Figure 6–12). The primary advantage of this technique is its minimization of operative time due to the facts that no bowel mobilization is necessary and that only one anastomosis is required. The stomach also has the most reliable blood supply of any reconstructive organ, which limits the risk of necrosis. Alternatives for reconstruction are considered (1) in relatively young patients with a long life expectancy, (2) under circumstances in which the stomach cannot be used for reconstruction, and (3) in patients who undergo a limited cervical esophagectomy. The optimal alternative organ is the

colon, which is used in an isoperistaltic fashion, with the blood supply based on the ascending branch of the inferior mesenteric artery (Figure 6–13). The use of jejunum for a long-segment interposition is technically difficult, exposes the patient to an increased risk of necrosis of the interposition segment, and necessitates the loss of several additional feet of jejunum. A free jejunal graft, however, is an ideal organ for reconstructing the cervical esophagus after a limited resection. Composite reconstruction—combining a part of the stomach with a pedicled graft of colon or small bowel–may be considered if all other options are unavailable.

Because most patients with squamous cell cancer of the esophagus undergo a near-total esophagectomy, the anastomosis is performed either high in the right chest or in the neck. A cervical anastomosis reduces the incidence of acid reflux into the esophageal remnant. Also, if an anastomotic leak should occur, it is usually easy to manage simply by opening the cervical incision for drainage. In con-

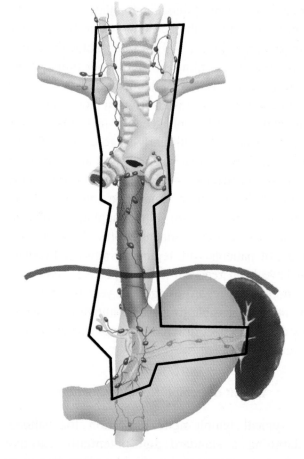

Figure 6–11. Extent of dissection for a three-field lymphadenectomy.

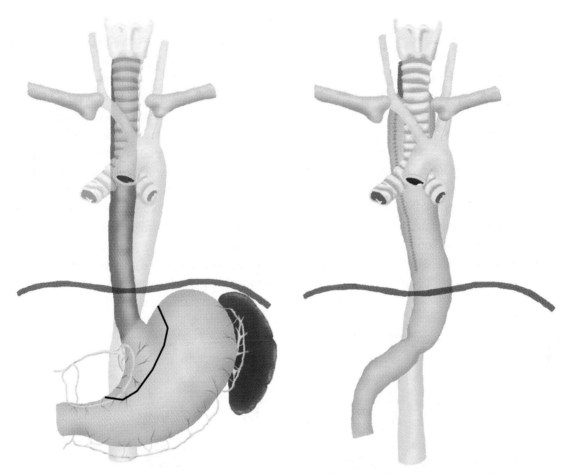

Figure 6–12. Extent of gastric resection (*left*) and position of the stomach after a gastric pull-up for esophageal reconstruction (*right*).

trast, leakage from an intrathoracic anastomosis exposes the patient to a high risk of systemic sepsis, and management of such a leak may be complex. The disadvantages of a cervical anastomosis include a substantially higher incidence of anastomotic leaks and subsequent stricture and recurrent laryngeal nerve injury. It is not known whether resection of the additional esophageal length enabled by a cervical anastomosis provides a survival advantage.[86–88]

The optimal route for reconstruction is unknown. The shortest route from the abdomen to the neck is through the posterior mediastinum (the bed of the resected esophagus) (Figure 6–14). The use of this route minimizes tension on the anastomosis if the length of the reconstructive organ is an issue. Placing the reconstructive organ in the posterior mediastinum also facilitates emptying.[89] However, the use of the posterior mediastinum may predispose to tumor infiltration if an incomplete resection is performed,

and postoperative irradiation may affect the function of the reconstructive organ when it is in this position. The primary alternative to reconstruction through the posterior mediastinal route is the substernal route (Figure 6–15). This is an important consideration when a staged reconstruction is performed, when there is gross contamination of the posterior mediastinum, and when high-dose postoperative irradiation is planned. However, the use of this route increases cardiopulmonary dysfunction in the early postoperative period, and prior sternotomy eliminates it as an option for reconstruction.

Postoperative Adjuvant Therapy

The rationale for recommending postoperative adjuvant therapy includes decreased local recurrence rates and improved long-term survival. Although such therapy is often recommended for patients with regionally advanced disease, there are few data that support the usefulness of this approach.

Postoperative radiotherapy theoretically permits the administration of a higher dose of radiation (50 to 70 Gy) than can be administered preoperatively although it is not certain that most patients will tolerate such a high dose when given in the early postoperative period. Postoperative radiotherapy increases the likelihood of anastomotic stricture, prolongs recovery from surgery, and worsens the quality of life.[90,91] The primary benefit of this therapy is to decrease the local recurrence rate, but it has no measurable positive influence on long-term survival.[90–92] In fact, there is some evidence that patients who undergo postoperative radiotherapy, compared to patients who have resection only, have a decreased median survival due to irradiation-induced mortality and the more rapid appearance of distant metastases.[90]

Chemotherapy as a postoperative adjuvant to resection is recommended in an effort to prevent the distant recurrence of disease in patients with regionally advanced or metastatic tumors. Single-agent therapy has shown poor response rates and provides no long-term survival benefits. Most recommendations are for cisplatin-based combination regimens. It is often difficult to complete a full course of intensive chemotherapy in patients who are recovering from esophagectomy, a fact that may have some bearing on the poor results of such treatment. Randomized studies have shown no long-term survival

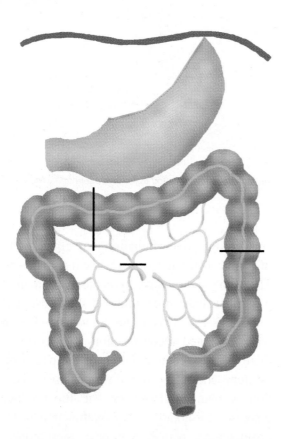

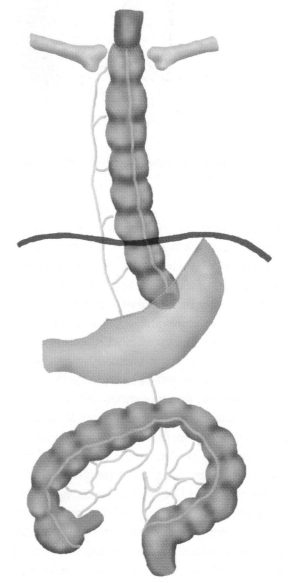

Figure 6–13. Left colon interposition for esophageal reconstruction based on the ascending branch of the inferior mesenteric artery (*left*) providing an adequate length of pedicled graft to reach to the cervical esophagus (*right*).

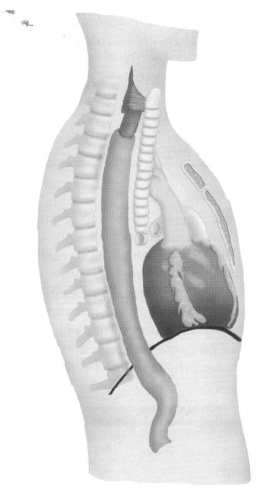

Figure 6–14. The posterior mediastinal route for esophageal reconstruction.

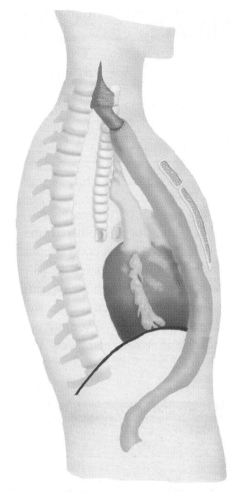

Figure 6–15. The substernal route for esophageal reconstruction.

benefit for patients undergoing resection followed by postoperative adjuvant chemotherapy, compared to resection alone.[93,94]

Because of the lack of success with postoperative adjuvant chemotherapy and radiotherapy, combined chemoradiotherapy has been used in an effort to improve local control of disease and to prevent distant recurrence. No randomized trials of postoperative chemoradiotherapy have been completed, and the potential advantages of neoadjuvant therapy make it unlikely that further information regarding this modality will be forthcoming.

Neoadjuvant Therapy

Interest in neoadjuvant therapy has been stimulated by both the high rate of local and distant failure in patients with squamous cell cancer of the esophagus treated by resection alone and the lack of efficacy of

postoperative adjuvant therapy. The potential advantages of neoadjuvant therapy include the improved likelihood of completing a full course of therapy and the possible down-staging of a tumor that may permit a more complete resection.

The preoperative administration of radiotherapy necessitates the use of a lower total dosage (30 to 50 Gy) than is permissible when radiotherapy is used as a single-modality agent or in a postoperative setting. Operative morbidity and mortality do not appear to be adversely affected by the use of neoadjuvant radiotherapy. Unfortunately, almost all randomized controlled studies fail to demonstrate any survival advantage for neoadjuvant radiotherapy when compared to resection alone (Table 6–2).[95–99] A meta-analysis of these data confirms these findings.[100]

Cisplatin-based combination chemotherapy regimens have been widely used in the management of

Table 6–2 RANDOMIZED CONTROLLED TRIALS EVALUATING PREOPERATIVE RADIATION THERAPY AS ADJUNCT TO SURGERY FOR ESOPHAGEAL CANCER

Lead Author	Ref. No.	Year	Dose (Gy)	Surgery Only		Surgery + Radiation	
				No. of Patients	5-Year Survival (%)	No. of Patients	5-Year Survival (%)
Launois	95	1981	40	57	11.5	67	9.5
Gignoux	96	1988	33	106	10.0	102	9.0
Wang	97	1989	40	102	30.0	104	35.0
Arnott	98	1992	20	86	17.0	90	9.0
Nygaard	99	1992	35	41	4.0*	48	18.0*

*3-year survival.

squamous cell cancer of the esophagus. Patients treated with neoadjuvant chemotherapy may have an increased incidence of postoperative septic and respiratory complications, compared to patients who undergo resection only, but this observation is not consistent among all published results. Neoadjuvant chemotherapy followed by resection provides no survival advantage when compared to resection alone (Table 6–3).[94,99,101–106]

The concurrent use of chemoradiotherapy has appeal because selected chemotherapeutic agents have radiosensitizing properties that may enhance the effects of radiotherapy. No prospective randomized studies demonstrate a survival advantage of neoadjuvant chemoradiotherapy followed by resection, compared to surgery alone, for patients with squamous cell cancer of the esophagus (Table 6–4).[107–109] Most studies show a survival benefit for patients who are

Table 6–3. RANDOMIZED CONTROLLED TRIALS OF NEOADJUVANT CHEMOTHERAPY FOR ESOPHAGEAL CANCER

Lead Author	Ref. No.	Year	Treatment	No. of Patients	Resectability (%)	Mortality (%)	Median Survival (mo)
Roth	101	1988	Cisplatin, bleomycin, vindesine + surgery	19	—	10	9
			Surgery	20	—	0	9
Nygaard	99	1992	Cisplatin, bleomycin + surgery	50	58	15	10
			Surgery	41	69	13	8
Schlag	102	1992	Cisplatin, 5-fluorouracil + surgery	21	69	—	6
			Surgery	24	79	—	8
Maipang	103	1994	Cisplatin, bleomycin, vinblastine + surgery	24	—	—	17
			Surgery	22	—	—	17
Ancona	104	1995	Cisplatin, 5-fluorouracil + surgery	35	78	7	—
			Surgery	43	86	5	—
Ando	94	1997	Cisplatin, vindesine + surgery	105	—	—	58
			Surgery	100	—	—	47
Law	105	1997	Cisplatin, 5-fluorouracil + surgery	73	95	9	13
			Surgery	74	89	8	17
Kelsen	106	1998	Cisplatin, 5-fluorouracil + surgery	213	76	7	15
			Surgery	227	89	6	16

Table 6–4. RANDOMIZED CONTROLLED TRIALS OF NEOADJUVANT CHEMOTHERAPY AND RADIATION THERAPY FOR SQUAMOUS CELL CANCER OF THE ESOPHAGUS

Lead Author	Ref. No.	Year	Preoperative Treatment	No. of Patients	Resectability (%)	Mortality (%)	Median Survival (mo)
LePrise	107	1994	Cisplatin, 5-fluorouracil + 20 Gy	41	85	9	10
			None	45	84	7	10
Bosset	108	1997	Cisplatin + 37 Gy	143	>80	4	19
			None	139	>80	13	19
Urba*	109	1997	Cisplatin, 5-fluorouracil + 45 Gy	50	—	—	18
			None	50	—	—	17

*Combines information from patients with either squamous cell cancer or adenocarcinoma of the esophagus.

found to have a complete pathologic response, suggesting that clinical research efforts should focus partly on identifying patients who are most likely to have a complete response.

REFERENCES

1. Yu MC, Garabrant DH, Peters JM, Mack TM. Tobacco, alcohol, diet, occupation, and carcinoma of the esophagus. Cancer Res 1988;48:3843–8.
2. Kjaereim K, Gaard M, Andersen A. The role of alcohol, tobacco, and dietary factors in upper aerodigestive tract cancers: a prospective study of 10,900 Norwegian men. Cancer Causes Controls 1998;9:99–108.
3. Castellsague X, Munoz N, De Stefani E, et al. Independent and joint effects of tobacco smoking and alcohol drinking on the risk of esophageal cancer in men and women. Int J Cancer 1999;82:657–64.
4. Craddock VM. Aetiology of oesophageal cancer: some operative factors. Eur J Cancer Prev 1992;1:89–103.
5. Kinjo Y, Cui Y, Akiba S, et al. Mortality risks of oesophageal cancer associated with hot tea, alcohol, tobacco, and diet in Japan. J Epidemiol 1998;8:235–43.
6. Isolauri J, Markkula H. Lye ingestion and carcinoma of the esophagus. Acta Chir Scand 1989;155:269–71.
7. Meijssen MA, Tilanus HW, van Blankenstein M, et al. Achalasia complicated by oesophageal squamous cell carcinoma: a prospective study in 195 patients. Gut 1992;33:155–8.
8. Sandler RS, Nyren O, Ekborn A, et al. The risk of esophageal cancer in patients with achalasia. JAMA 1995;274:1359–62.
9. Streitz JM Jr, Ellis FH Jr, Gibb SP, Heatley GM. Achalasia and squamous cell carcinoma of the esophagus: analysis of 241 patients. Ann Thorac Surg 1995;59:1604–9.
10. Sammon AM, Alderson D. Diet, reflux, and the development of squamous cell carcinoma of the oesophagus in Africa. Br J Surg 1998;85:891–6.
11. Maillefer RH, Greydanus MP. To B or not to B: is tylosis B truly benign? Am J Gastroenterol 1999;94:829–34.
12. Chang F, Syrjanen S, Wang L, Syrjanen K. Infectious agents in the etiology of esophageal cancer. Gastroenterology 1992;103:1336–48.
13. Bjorge T, Hakulinen T, Engeland A, et al. A prospective, seroepidemiological study of the role of human papillomavirus in esophageal cancer in Norway. Cancer Res 1997;57:3989–92.
14. Thomas RM, Sobin LH. Gastrointestinal cancer. Cancer 1995;75:154–70.
15. Landis SH, Murray T, Bolden S, Wingo PA. Cancer statistics, 1998. Ca Cancer J Clin 1998;48:6–29.
16. Thompson WM, Halvorsen RA, Foster WL Jr, et al. Computed tomography for staging esophageal and gastroesophageal cancer: reevaluation. AJR Am J Roentgenol 1983;141:951–8.
17. Lea JW IV, Prager RL, Bender HW Jr. The questionable role of computed tomography in preoperative staging of esophageal cancer. Ann Thorac Surg 1984;38:479–81.
18. Lehr L, Rupp N, Siewert JR. Assessment of resectability of esophageal cancer by computed tomography and magnetic resonance imaging. Surgery 1988;103:344–50.
19. Yasui A, Nimura Y, Hayakawa N. MRI and CT of intrathoracic esophageal carcinoma: radiological, surgical and histopathological correlation. Dis Esophagus 1990;3:13–20.
20. Takashima S, Takeuchi N, Shiozaki H, et al. Carcinoma of the esophagus: CT vs MR imaging in determining resectability. AJR Am J Roentgenol 1991;156:297–302.
21. Greenberg J, Durkin M, Van Drunen M, Aranha GV. Computed tomography or endoscopic ultrasonography in preoperative staging of gastric and esophageal tumors. Surgery 1994;116:696–702.
22. Quint LE, Glazer GM, Orringer MB. Esophageal imaging by MR and CT: study of normal anatomy and neoplasms. Radiology 1985;156:727–31.
23. Grimm H, Soehendra N, Hamper K, Maas R. Contribution of endosonography to preoperative staging in esophageal and stomach cancer. Chirurg 1989;60:684–9.
24. Maerz LL, Deveny CW, Lopez RR, McConnell DB. Role of computed tomographic scans in the staging of esophageal and proximal gastric malignancies. Am J Surg 1993;165:558–60.
25. Krasna MJ, Reed CE, Jaklitsch MT, et al. Thoracoscopic staging of esophageal cancer: a prospective, multiinstitutional trial. Ann Thorac Surg 1995;60:1337–40.
26. Watt I, Stewart I, Anderson D, et al. Laparoscopy, ultrasound and computed tomography in cancer of the oesophagus and gastric cardia: a prospective comparison for detecting intra-abdominal metastases. Br J Surg 1989;76:1036–9.
27. Block MI, Patterson GA, Sundaresan RS, et al. Improvement in staging of esophageal cancer with the addition of positron emission tomography. Ann Thorac Surg 1997;64:770–7.
28. Riedel M, Hauck RW, Stein HJ, et al. Preoperative bronchoscopic assessment of airway invasion by esophageal cancer. Chest 1998;113:687–95.
29. Takemoto T, Ito T, Aibe T, Okita K. Endoscopic ultrasonography in the diagnosis of esophageal carcinoma, with particular regard to staging it for operability. Endoscopy 1986;18:22–5.
30. Tio TL, Coene PPLO, Luiken GJHM, Tytgat GN. Endosonography in the clinical staging of esophageal carcinoma. Gastrointest Endosc 1990;36:S2–10.
31. Botet JF, Lightdale CJ, Zauber AG, et al. Preoperative staging of esophageal cancer: comparison of endoscopic US and dynamic CT. Radiology 1991;181:419–25.
32. Ziegler K, Sanft C, Zeitz M, et al. Evaluation of endosonography in TN staging of oesophageal cancer. Gut 1991;32:16–20.
33. Peters JH, Hoeft SF, Heimbucher J, et al. Selection of patients for curative or palliative resection of esophageal cancer based on preoperative endoscopic ultrasonography. Arch Surg 1994;129:534–9.
34. Altorki NK, Snady H, Skinner DB. Endosonography for cancer of the esophagus and cardia: is it worthwhile? Dis Esophagus 1996;9:198–201.
35. Isenberg G, Chak A, Canto MI, et al. Endoscopic ultrasound in restaging of esophageal cancer after neoadjuvant chemoradiation. Gastrointest Endosc 1998;48:158–63.
36. Bowrey DJ, Clark GWB, Roberts SA, et al. Serial endoscopic ultrasound in the assessment of response to chemoradiotherapy for carcinoma of the esophagus. J Gastrointest Surg 1999;3:462–7.
37. Laterza E, de Manzoni G, Guglielmi A, et al. Endoscopic ultrasonography in the staging of esophageal carcinoma

after preoperative radiotherapy and chemotherapy. Ann Thorac Surg 1999;67:1466–9.

38. Zuccaro G Jr, Rice TW, Goldblum J, et al. Endoscopic ultrasound cannot determine suitability for esophagectomy after aggressive chemoradiotherapy for esophageal cancer. Am J Gastroenterol 1999;94:906–12.

39. Tio TL, Cohen P, Coene PP, et al. Endosonography and computed tomography of esophageal carcinoma. Gastroenterology 1989;96:1478–86.

40. Rice TW, Boyce GA, Sivak MV. Esophageal ultrasound and the preoperative staging of carcinoma of the esophagus. J Thorac Cardiovasc Surg 1991;101:536–44.

41. Luketich JD, Schauer PR, Meltzer C, et al. Role of positron emission tomography in staging esophageal cancer. Ann Thorac Surg 1997;64:765–9.

42. Kole AC, Plukker JT, Nieweg OE, Vaalburg W. Positron emission tomography for staging of oesophageal and gastroesophageal malignancy. Br J Cancer 1998;78:521–7.

43. Rankin SC, Taylor H, Cook GJ, Mason R. Computed tomography and positron emission tomography in the pre-operative staging of oesophageal carcinoma. Clin Radiol 1998;53:659–65.

44. Krasna MJ, Flowers JL, Attar S, McLaughlin J. Combined thoracoscopic/laparoscopic staging of esophageal cancer. J Thorac Cardiovasc Surg 1996;111:800–7.

45. Tachimori Y, Kato H, Watanabe H, Yamaguchi H. Neck ultrasonography for thoracic esophageal carcinoma. Ann Thorac Surg 1994;57:1180–3.

46. Natsugoe S, Yoshinaka H, Shimada M, et al. Fukumoto T, Takao S, Aikou T. Assessment of cervical lymph node metastasis in esophageal carcinoma using ultrasonography. Ann Surg 1999;229:62–6.

47. van Overhagen H, Lameris JS, Zonderland HM, et al. Ultrasound and ultrasound-guided fine needle aspiration biopsy of supraclavicular lymph nodes in patients with esophageal carcinoma. Cancer 1991;67:585–7.

48. Law SYK, Fok M, Wong J. Risk analysis in resection of squamous cell carcinoma of the esophagus. World J Surg 1994;18:339–46.

49. Chan K-H, Wong J. Mortality after esophagectomy for carcinoma of esophagus: an analysis of risk factors. Dis Esophagus 1990;3:49–53.

50. Ferguson MK, Martin TR, Reeder LB, Olak J. Mortality after esophagectomy: risk factor analysis. World J Surg 1997;21:599–604.

51. Patti MG, Corvera CU, Glasgow RE, Way LW. A hospital's annual rate of esophagectomy influences the operative mortality rate. J Gastrointest Surg 1998;2:186–92.

52. Jacobi CA, Zieren HU, Muller JM, Pichlmaier H. Surgical therapy of esophageal carcinoma: the influence of surgical approach and esophageal resection on cardiopulmonary function. Eur J Cardiothorac Surg 1997;11:32–7.

53. Moon MR, Schulte WJ, Haasler GB, Condon RE. Transhiatal and transthoracic esophagectomy for adenocarcinoma of the esophagus. Arch Surg 1992;127:951–5.

54. Pac M, Basoglu A, Kocak H, et al. Transhiatal versus transthoracic esophagectomy for esophageal cancer. J Thorac Cardiovasc Surg 1993;106:205–9.

55. Tilanus HW, Hop WCJ, Langenhorst BLAM, van Lanschot JJ. Esophagectomy with or without thoracotomy. J Thorac Cardiovasc Surg 1993;105:898–903.

56. Putnam JB Jr, Suell DM, McMurtry MJ, et al. Comparison of three techniques of esophagectomy within a residency training program. Ann Thorac Surg 1994;57:319–25.

57. Gluch L, Smith RC, Bambach CP, Brown AR. Comparison of outcomes following transhiatal or Ivor Lewis esophagectomy for esophageal carcinoma. World J Surg 1999;23:271–6.

58. Rindani R, Martin CJ, Cox MR. Transhiatal versus Ivor Lewis oesophagectomy: is there a difference? Aust N Z J Surg 1999;69:187–94.

59. Akaishi T, Kaneda I, Higuchi N, et al. Thoracoscopic en bloc total esophagectomy with radical mediastinal lymphadenectomy. J Thorac Cardiovasc Surg 1996;112:1533–40.

60. Dexter SPL, Martin IG, McMahon MJ. Radical thoracoscopic esophagectomy for cancer. Surg Endosc 1996;10:147–51.

61. Roberston GS, Lloyd DM, Wicks AC, Veitch PS. No obvious advantages for thoracoscopic two-stage oesophagectomy. Br J Surg 1996;83:675–8.

62. Kawahara K, Maekawa T, Okabayashi K, et al. Video-assisted thoracoscopic esophagectomy for esophageal cancer. Surg Endosc 1999;13:218–23.

63. Law S, Fok M, Chu KM, Wong J. Thoracoscopic esophagectomy for esophageal cancer. Surgery 1997;122:8–14.

64. Peracchia A, Rosati R, Fumagalli U, et al. Thoracoscopic dissection of the esophagus for cancer. Int Surg 1997;82:1–4.

65. Fujita H, Kakegawa T, Yamana H, et al. Total esophagectomy versus proximal esophagectomy for esophageal cancer at the cervicothoracic junction. World J Surg 1999;23:486–91.

66. Tam PC, Cheung HC, Ma L, et al. Local recurrences after subtotal esophagectomy for squamous cell carcinoma. Ann Surg 1987;205:189–94.

67. Tsutsui S, Kuwano H, Watanabe M, et al. Resection margin for squamous cell carcinoma of the esophagus. Ann Surg 1995;222:193–202.

68. Mizobuchi S, Kato H, Tachimori Y, et al. Multiple primary carcinoma of the oesophagus. Surg Oncol 1993;2:249–53.

69. Pesko P, Rakic S, Milicevic M, et al. Prevalence and clinicopathologic features of multiple squamous cell carcinoma of the esophagus. Cancer 1994;73:2687–90.

70. Skinner DB, Little AG, Ferguson MK, et al. Selection of operation for esophageal cancer based on staging. Ann Surg 1986;204:391–401.

71. Siewert JR, Roder JD. Lymphadenectomy in esophageal cancer surgery. Dis Esophagus 1992;5:91–7.

72. Orringer MB, Marshall B, Sterling MC. Transhiatal esophagectomy for benign and malignant disease. J Thorac Cardiovasc Surg 1993;105:265–77.

73. Vigneswaran WT, Trastek VF, Pairolero PC, et al. Transhiatal esophagectomy for carcinoma of the esophagus. Ann Thorac Surg 1993;56:838–46.

74. Lieberman MD, Shriver CD, Bleckner S, Burt M. Carcinoma of the esophagus. Prognostic significance of histologic type. J Thorac Cardiovasc Surg 1995;105:130–8.

75. Hagen JA, Peters JH, DeMeester TR. Superiority of extended en bloc esophagogastrectomy for carcinoma of the lower esophagus and cardia. J Thorac Cardiovasc Surg 1993;106:850–9.

76. Altorki N, Girardi L, Skinner DB. Esophagectomy improves survival for stage III esophageal cancer. J Thorac Cardiovasc Surg 1997;114:948–56.

77. Akiyama H, Tsurumaru M, Udagawa H, Kajiyama Y. Systematic lymph node dissection for esophageal cancer—effective or not? Dis Esophagus 1994;7:2–13.

78. Altorki NK, Skinner DB. Occult cervical nodal metastases in esophageal cancer: preliminary results of three-field lymphadenectomy. J Thorac Cardiovasc Surg 1997;113:540–4.

79. van de Ven C, De Leyn P, Coosemans W, et al. Three-field lymphadenectomy and pattern of lymph node spread in T3 adenocarcinoma of the distal esophagus and gastro-esophageal junction. Eur J Cardiothorac Surg 1999;15:769–73.

80. Nishihira T, Mori S, Hirayama K. Extensive lymph node dissection for thoracic esophageal carcinoma. Dis Esophagus 1992;5:79–89.

81. Peracchia A, Ruol A, Bardini R, et al. Lymph node dissection for cancer of the thoracic esophagus: how extended should it be? Dis Esophagus 1992;5:69–78.

82. Fujita H, Kakegawa T, Yamana H, et al. Mortality and morbidity rates, postoperative course, quality of life, and prognosis after extended radical lymphadenectomy for esophageal cancer. Ann Surg 1995;222:654–62.

83. Akiyama H, Tsurumaru M, Udagawa H, Kajiyama Y. Radical lymph node dissection for cancer of the thoracic esophagus. Ann Surg 1994;220:364–73.

84. Lerut T, Coosemans W, De Leyn P, et al. Reflections on three field lymphadenectomy in carcinoma of the esophagus and gastroesophageal junction. Hepatogastroenterology 1999;46:717–25.

85. Tabira Y, Okuma T, Kondo K, Kitamura N. Indications for three field dissection followed by esophagectomy for advanced carcinoma of the thoracic esophagus. J Thorac Cardiovasc Surg 1999;117:239–45.

86. Chasseray VM, Kiroff GK, Buard JL, Launois B. Cervical or thoracic anastomosis for esophagectomy for carcinoma. Surg Gynecol Obstet 1989;169:55–62.

87. Lam TCF, Fok M, Cheng SWK, Wong J. Anastomotic complications after esophagectomy for cancer. J Thorac Cardiovasc Surg 1992;104:395–400.

88. Ribet M, Debrueres B, Lecomte-Houcke M. Resection for advanced cancer of the thoracic esophagus: cervical or thoracic anastomosis? J Thorac Cardiovasc Surg 1992;103:784–9.

89. Gawad KA, Hosch SB, Bumann D, et al. How important is the route of reconstruction after esophagectomy: a prospective randomized study. Am J Gastroenterol 1999;94:1490–6.

90. Fok M, Sham JST, Choy D, et al. Postoperative radiotherapy for carcinoma of the esophagus: a prospective, randomized controlled study. Surgery 1993;113:138–47.

91. Zieren HU, Muller JM, Jacobi CA, et al. Adjuvant postoperative radiation therapy after curative resection of squamous cell carcinoma of the thoracic esophagus: a prospective randomized study. World J Surg 1995;19:444–9.

92. Teniere P, Hay J-M, Fingerhut A, Fagniez PL. Postoperative radiation therapy does not increase survival after curative resection for squamous cell carcinoma of the middle and lower esophagus as shown by a multicenter controlled trial. French University Association for Surgical Research. Surg Gynecol Obstet 1991;173:123–30.

93. Pouliquen X, Levard H, Hay J-M, et al. 5-Fluorouracil and cisplatin therapy after palliative surgical resection of squamous cell carcinoma of the esophagus. Ann Surg 1996;223:127–33.

94. Ando N, Iizuka T, Kakegawa T, et al. A randomized trial of surgery with and without chemotherapy for localized squamous carcinoma of the thoracic esophagus: the Japan Clinical Oncology Group study. J Thorac Cardiovasc Surg 1997;114:205–9.

95. Launois B, Delarue D, Campion JP, Kerbaol M. Preoperative radiotherapy for carcinoma of the esophagus. Surg Gynecol Obstet 1981;153:690–2.

96. Gignoux M, Roussel A, Paillot B, et al. The value of preoperative radiotherapy in esophageal cancer: results of a study by the EORTC. Recent Results Cancer Res 1988;110:1–13.

97. Wang M, Gu XZ, Yin WB, et al. Randomized clinical trial on the combination of preoperative irradiation and surgery in the treatment of esophageal carcinoma: report on 206 patients. Int J Radiat Oncol Biol Phys 1989;16:325–7.

98. Arnott SJ, Duncan W, Kerr GR, et al. Low dose preoperative radiotherapy for carcinoma of the oesophagus: results of a randomized clinical trial. Radiother Oncol 1992;24:108–13.

99. Nygaard K, Hagen S, Hansen HS, et al. Pre-operative radiotherapy prolongs survival in operable esophageal carcinoma: a randomized, multicenter study of pre-operative radiotherapy and chemotherapy. The Second Scandinavian Trial in Esophageal Cancer. World J Surg 1992;16:1104–10.

100. Arnott SJ, Duncan W, Gignoux M, et al. Preoperative radiotherapy in esophageal carcinoma: a meta-analysis using individual patients data (Oesophageal Cancer Collaborative Group). Int J Radiat Oncol Biol Phys 1998;41:579–83.

101. Roth JA, Pass HI, Flanagan MM, et al. Randomized clinical trial of preoperative and postoperative adjuvant chemotherapy with cisplatin, vindesine, and bleomycin for carcinoma of the esophagus. J Thorac Cardiovasc Surg 1988;96:242–8.

102. Schlag PM. Randomized trial of preoperative chemotherapy for squamous cell cancer of the esophagus. Chirirgische Arbeitsgemeinschaft fuer Onkologie der Deutschen Gesellschaft fuer Chirurgie Study Group. Arch Surg 1992;127:1446–50.

103. Maipang T, Vasinanukorn P, Petpichetchian C, et al. Induction chemotherapy in the treatment of patients with carcinoma of the esophagus. J Surg Oncol 1994;56:191–7.

104. Ancona E, Ruol A, Chiarion-Sileni V, et al. Studio prospettico randomizzato di chemioterapia neoadjuvante versus sola chirurgia nel cancro operabile (T$_{2–3}$, ogni N, M$_0$) dell'esophago. Acta Chir Ital 1995;51:308–17.

105. Law S, Fok M, Chow S, et al. Preoperative chemotherapy versus surgical therapy alone for squamous cell carcinoma of the esophagus: a prospective randomized trial. J Thorac Cardiovasc Surg 1997;114:210–7.

106. Kelsen DP, Ginsberg R, Pajak TF, et al. Chemotherapy followed by surgery compared with surgery alone for localized esophageal cancer. N Engl J Med 1998;339:1979–84.

107. Le Prise E, Etienne PL, Meunier B, et al. A randomized study of chemotherapy, radiation therapy, and surgery versus surgery for localized squamous cell carcinoma of the esophagus. Cancer 1994;73:1779–84.

108. Bosset J-F, Gignoux M, Triboulet J-P, et al. Chemoradiotherapy followed by surgery compared with surgery alone in squamous-cell cancer of the esophagus. N Engl J Med 1997;337:161–7.

109. Urba S, Orringer M, Turrisi A, et al. A randomized trial comparing surgery to preoperative concomitant chemoradiation plus surgery in patients with resectable esophageal cancer: updated analysis. Proc Am Soc Clin Oncol 1997;16:A983.

7

Techniques of Esophageal Resection

MITCHELL C. POSNER, MD

Although the primacy of resection as the sole curative modality for esophageal cancer has been challenged, surgery (either alone or as a component of a combined-modality approach) remains an effective means of achieving palliation or a long-term disease-free state. Considerable energy has been expended on defining the optimal surgical approach to extirpate an esophageal tumor. It suffices to say that although each technical approach has its proponents and detractors, there is no sound evidence to suggest that one technique is superior to any other when the outcome end points are disease-free or overall survival.[1,2] These techniques include transhiatal esophagectomy, transthoracic (Ivor Lewis) esophagectomy, three-field lymphadenectomy, and minimally invasive esophagectomy. Each approach has advantages and disadvantages (described in Chapters 5 and 6). The surgeon should perform whichever procedure he or she is most comfortable with (from both a technologic and oncologic standpoint) that yields results that meet accepted standards. However, the surgeon should be facile with all of the above techniques and should individualize the surgical procedure on the basis of patient's performance status and on both the location and extent of the tumor. This chapter focuses on the technical details of the aforementioned esophageal resection procedures and addresses preoperative and postoperative considerations in the management of this challenging cohort of patients.

PREOPERATIVE EVALUATION AND STAGING

A complete history and physical examination is the initial step in the preoperative evaluation of a patient with esophageal cancer. The history should focus on known predisposing factors to esophageal malignancy (tobacco use, alcohol intake, reflux symptoms, surveillance or management of Barrett's esophagus, and prior head and neck malignancy), evidence of cardiorespiratory compromise, and previous thoracic or abdominal surgery. Prior procedures, including those on the stomach (anti-reflux procedures, resection) or colon, may have considerable impact on the reconstructive conduit (stomach or colon) chosen to re-establish alimentary continuity. In addition to the findings on routine physical examination that could precipitate additional preoperative testing or intraoperative monitoring, attention should be focused on signs and findings associated with unresectable or metastatic disease. These include hoarseness secondary to recurrent laryngeal nerve involvement, cervical or supraclavicular lymphadenopathy, pleural effusions, and new onset of bone pain.

Liquid oral contrast examination of the esophagus and stomach may be helpful for visualizing tumor extent with regard to length of involvement and degree of obstruction; however, in the era of flexible endoscopy, this is no longer a prerequisite. Esophagogastroduodenoscopy with biopsy is routinely performed and not only provides a tissue diagnosis but also is able to accurately determine the degree of esophageal and gastric involvement. As well, it has the potential to alleviate dysphagia (at least temporarily) via esophageal dilatation. All patients should undergo computed tomography (CT) of the chest, abdomen, and pelvis as a means of ruling out metastatic disease and obtaining other locoregional staging information. As suggested in Chapter 5, endoscopic ultrasonography is now an accepted component of preoperative clinical staging; in addition to being complementary to CT, it allows the sampling of regional lymphadenopathy. Endoscopic ultrasonography is especially useful for stratifying patients being treated in clinical trials. Pretreatment thoracoscopy and laparoscopy can provide accurate staging information, but this author does not routinely perform them before initiating preoperative chemoradiotherapy. All patients who are considered to be candidates for curative resection undergo laparoscopy at the time of the intended resection, to spare patients with distant disease from a potentially morbid procedure. In the absence of symptoms, a bone scan is not obtained, and bronchoscopy is reserved for those patients with lesions in the middle or upper esophagus. Positron emission tomography (PET) has great promise as a staging tool, but further investigation is required before its routine use can be advocated.

Therapeutic Approach

Due to the dismal results of resection alone, combined-modality therapy continues to be explored in an attempt to improve outcomes. Therefore, resection frequently follows chemotherapy, radiation therapy, or chemoradiotherapy as a component of a multimodality approach to patients with esophageal cancer. Although conclusive evidence regarding the benefit of induction therapy prior to resection is lacking, there is also little to suggest that the technique of esophageal resection should be altered following neoadjuvant therapy, and conflicting data exist regarding increased morbidity and mortality associated with resection in the setting of a combined-modality approach. These issues are addressed in Chapters 5, 6, and 8 and will not be discussed here.

PREOPERATIVE AND PERIOPERATIVE MANAGEMENT

All patients who are to undergo esophagectomy benefit from a comprehensive preoperative teaching program not only to prepare them for the intended surgery but also to educate them in regard to what to anticipate in the immediate postoperative period and in regard to the short- and long-term effects of the procedure. At this author's center, dedicated nursing personnel instruct the patients in pre- and postoperative pulmonary exercise, and patients are informed of the potential need for postoperative ventilatory support and possible supplemental enteral nutrition and are acquainted with the alterations in their dietary habits that may be necessitated by esophageal replacement. All patients undergo mechanical bowel preparation, and if colon interposition is entertained as a reconstructive option (albeit an unusual occurrence), oral antibiotics are also administered. In patients treated with esophagectomy without preoperative chemoradiotherapy, there is no demonstrable benefit from preresection parenteral or enteral nutritional support, which is therefore not routinely recommended. Patients receiving induction chemoradiotherapy prior to esophagectomy and who are unable to maintain nutritional status because of dysphagia may well benefit from either enteral or parenteral nutritional support during the preoperative phase of their treatment. All patients have an enteral feeding tube placed during surgery in case they are unable to sustain adequate oral intake during the initial postoperative period. Patients do not routinely require enteral nutritional support following esophagectomy.

Perioperative antibiotic prophylaxis against oral and gastrointestinal flora is routinely administered, and sequential compression stockings are placed to prevent deep venous thrombosis.

This author prefers that a thoracic epidural catheter be placed for optimal postoperative analgesia. A double-lumen endotracheal tube is not necessary. The right neck is the preferred site for the placement of a central venous access catheter. The right arm is left out at 90° for venous and arterial access.

OPERATIVE TECHNIQUE

Transhiatal Esophagectomy

With the patient placed supine on the operating table, the left arm is tucked to the side once all boney prominences have been padded. The head is turned to the right, extended, and stabilized with an O-ring padded foam protector. The skin is prepped with Betadine solution, from the left ear to the pubis and laterally to the midaxillary lines.

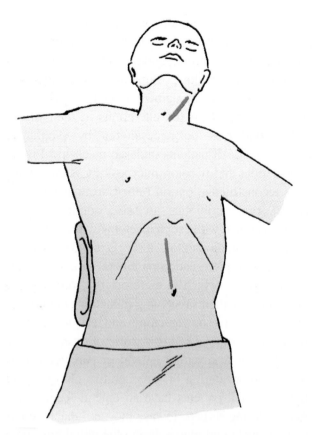

Figure 7–1. Transhiatal esophagectomy is performed through an upper midline incision and a left cervical incision.

An upper midline incision is made from the xiphoid process to the umbilicus (Figure 7–1), and wide exposure is provided with a self-retaining table-fixed retractor with the retractors hugging the right and left costal margins, lifting cephalad and toward their respective shoulders (Figure 7–2). The abdomen is thoroughly explored, and biopsies are performed on all suspicious nodules; the specimens are sent for frozen-section analysis as any evidence of metastatic disease will abort the intended procedure. The ligamentum teres is ligated and divided, both the falciform and left triangular ligaments are divided, and the left lateral segment of the liver is retracted upward and to the right. Attention is then directed to the greater curvature of the stomach, where division of the greater omentum outside the right gastroepiploic artery (which must be identified and protected throughout the procedure) is commenced. Injury to the right gastroepiploic vessels is avoided by maintaining a safe distance of at least 2 cm inferior to the vessels until the termination of the right gastroepiploic artery. The left gastroepiploic vessels and short gastric vessels are then encountered and may be ligated just outside the border of

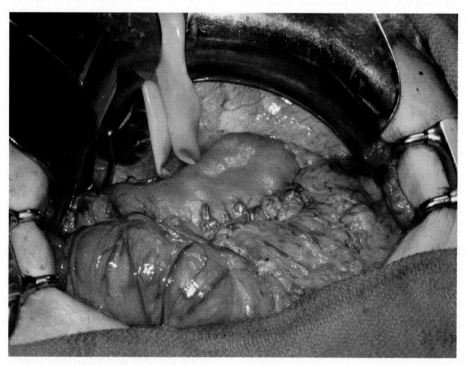

Figure 7–2. Exposure to the upper abdomen is obtained with a self-retaining retractor secured to the operating table, with retraction under both costal margins. A Penrose drain is in view at the gastroesophageal junction.

the greater curvature. The dissection is continued until all anteriorly based short gastric vessels are ligated and divided.

In the avascular plane overlying the caudate lobe of the liver, the gastrohepatic omentum is divided along the liver edge, cephalad to the crus of the diaphragm. If a replaced left hepatic artery is identified, this should be preserved. Dissection is then carried along the lesser curvature inferiorly until the right gastric vessels (which should be safeguarded) are encountered. The surgeon then dissects the remainder of the gastrocolic omentum from the greater curvature of the stomach, identifying and palpating the right gastroepiploic vessels and ensuring their preservation as dissection proceeds to the taking off of the right gastroepiploic vessels from the gastroduodenal artery. A generous Kocher maneuver is then performed to the border of the superior mesenteric vessels, and the hepatic flexure is taken down, thereby allowing full mobilization of the pylorus so that it may reach to the esophageal hiatus. At this time, either a pyloroplasty or pyloromyotomy is performed to limit gastric stasis secondary to vagal interruption.

A common hepatic, celiac-axis, proximal splenic, and left gastric lymphadenectomy is then performed, whereby all lymphatic and nodal tissue is swept up with the specimen prior to the division of the left gastric vessels. The stomach is then retracted anteriorly and superiorly, allowing both the coronary vein and left gastric artery to be ligated and divided at their origins. The remaining posterior gastric vessels are divided, and all lymphatic and nodal tissue is swept off of the crus of the diaphragm and abdominal aorta. At this point in time, the peritoneum overlying the esophagus and esophageal hiatus is incised, the gastroesophageal junction is encircled with finger dissection, and then an umbilical tape or Penrose drain (which will be used for traction as the esophagus is mobilized from the mediastinum) is secured around the distal esophagus (Figure 7–3). The esophageal hiatus is widened by dividing the crus of the diaphragm, with the cautery following the ligation of the inferior phrenic vein. This allows excellent exposure to the lower mediastinum up to the level of the carina. The initial dissection of the distal esophagus can now be undertaken (Figure 7–4) under direct vision; this includes a periesophageal and mediasti-

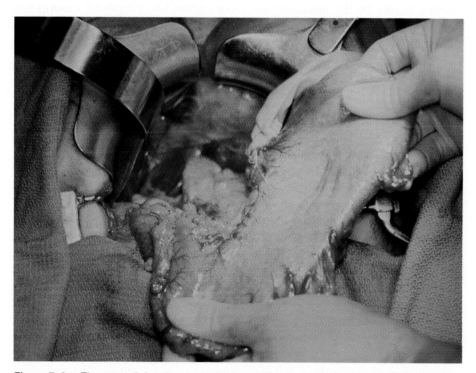

Figure 7–3.   The stomach has been completely mobilized, and its blood supply is based on the right gastroepiploic artery and right gastric artery. A Penrose drain secured around the gastroesophageal junction is used for traction as the esophagus is mobilized from the mediastinum.

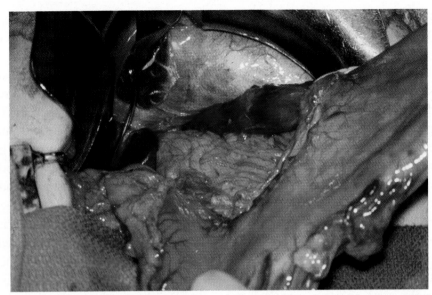

Figure 7–4. Dissection of the distal esophagus is initiated under direct vision, with all periesophageal tissue and mediastinal lymph nodes swept with the specimen up to the carina.

nal lymph node dissection that could incorporate the periesophageal soft tissue, pleura, and pericardium if such is the surgeon's preference. All attachments are circumferentially divided with the cautery between hemoclips up to the level of the carina.

The cervical component of the procedure is begun by making an incision approximately 6 to 7 cm long at the anterior border of the sternocleidomastoid muscle from just above the suprasternal notch (Figure 7–5). Following the division of the platysma muscle with the cautery, the dissection is carried down along the medial border of the sternocleidomastoid muscle, and the omohyoid muscle is incised. The dissection is continued medial to the left carotid artery and left internal jugular vein, dividing the middle thyroid vein to gain entrance to the prevertebral space. Blunt self-retaining Wheitlander retractors are then used to retract the sternocleidomastoid muscle, carotid artery, and internal jugular vein laterally and the thyroid and trachea medially. The cervical esophagus is then encircled with careful blunt and sharp dissection, maintaining

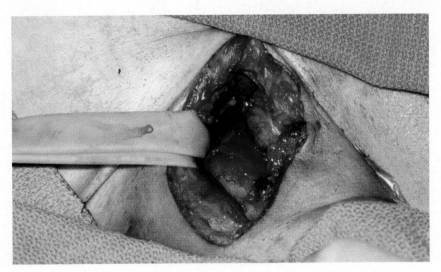

Figure 7–5. The cervical incision along the anterior border of the sternocleidomastoid muscle provides exposure to the cervical esophagus. Dissection is carried along the medial aspect of the internal jugular vein and carotid artery to the prevertebral space.

the dissection on the adventitia of the esophagus to avoid injury to the recurrent laryngeal nerve in the tracheoesophageal grove (Figure 7–6). With upward and superior traction on the Penrose drain, blunt dissection is continued circumferentially almost to the level of the carina (Figure 7–7).

The mediastinal component of the procedure is now addressed. With caudal traction on umbilical tape that has been secured to the gastroesophageal junction, a hand is placed through the open hiatus, posteriorly between the esophagus and the aorta, and the esophagus is bluntly freed from its posterior attachments. This maneuver is continued until the cervical portion of the dissection is reached by confirming that a finger placed through the cervical wound into the posterior mediastinum is able to be palpated by the other hand placed through the diaphragmatic hiatus and into the posterior mediastinum. Anteriorly, the hand placed through the transabdominal incision must hug the anterior wall of the esophagus, slip under the carina, and carefully free the esophagus from the membranous trachea until the cervical dissection is encountered. During this maneuver, periods of extreme hypotension can occur that respond well to volume resuscitation and limiting compression of the heart that may require the dissection to be stopped for short periods of time. The lateral attachments to the esophagus are then usually hooked with the index finger and, with the use of a long "sweetheart" retractor

placed into the mediastinum, divided between large hemoclips with the cautery (Figure 7–8). The most superior of these attachments are often divided "blindly" by finger dissection circumferentially and by a combination of a pushing and pulling of the final periesophageal attachments.

Now that the entire esophagus is free from its attachments, the cervical and upper mediastinal esophagus is mobilized into the cervical wound. A long 1-inch Penrose drain is placed on the esophagus, and both are divided, with the GIA stapler effectively securing the Penrose drain to the distal divided esophagus. The stomach, with the attached esophagus, is now brought through the abdominal wound, to lie on a moist lap pad (Figure 7–9). The attached Penrose drain has been drawn through the posterior mediastinum and will be used to help transpose the gastric tube through the mediastinum to the cervical incision. Selecting the highest point of the stomach (Figure 7–10), a gastric tube is formed by multiple firing of the GIA stapler (Figure 7–11), preserving the greater curvature and its blood supply and opening the lesser curvature angle to provide the greatest length possible (Figure 7–12). In so doing, the specimen will consist of the esophagus and its contained tumor and a considerable portion of the fundus cardia and lesser curvature (with the appropriate lymphadenectomy specimen), securing an adequate margin beyond the tumor edge (Figure 7–13). The right gastric vessels are pre-

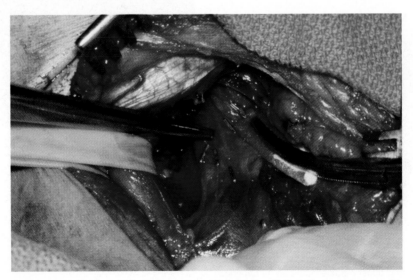

Figure 7–6. The cervical esophagus is encircled with a ¼-inch Penrose drain, avoiding dissection in the tracheoesophageal groove where the recurrent laryngeal nerve resides (forceps).

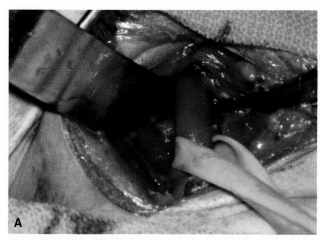

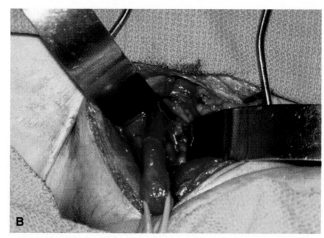

Figure 7–7.   *A,* Traction on the cervical esophagus allows for blunt dissection almost to *B,* the level of the tracheal bifurcation.

served, and care is taken not to oversew the staple line (Figure 7–14). The abdominal end of the Penrose drain is now secured to the posterior wall of the stomach with 3-0 silk sutures. The lesser-curvature suture is left long, and the suture along the greater curvature (the short gastric vessel side) is cut short so that the orientation of the transposed gastric tube can be easily identified and maintained. With very gentle traction on the cervical end of the Penrose drain, the gastric tube is placed through the esophageal hiatus by hand and gingerly pushed upward through the posterior mediastinum to the cervical incision. In doing so, a good 6 to 8 cm of stomach wall will be easily mobilized into the cervical field. The Penrose-drain sutures

to the posterior wall of the stomach are now inspected to ensure proper orientation and to confirm that there is no twisting of the gastric conduit. The sutures are then cut, and the Penrose drain is removed.

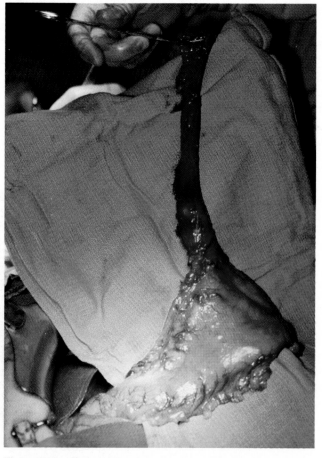

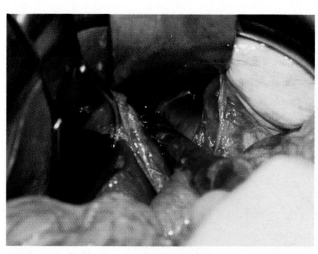

Figure 7–8.   With the crus of the diaphragm divided anteriorly, wide exposure to the mid- and upper mediastinum can be obtained with the use of long Harrington retractors; however, the area just posterior and superior to the carina requires blunt dissection without direct visualization.

Figure 7–9.   The cervical esophagus is divided, and the esophagus and stomach are delivered through the abdominal wound. The tumor can be seen bulging in the distal esophagus.

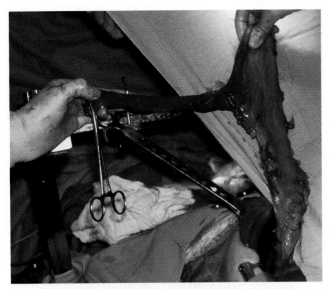

Figure 7–10. The highest point on the stomach is identified and will serve as the most superior tip of the gastric tube.

An automatic purse-string suture applier is then placed on the cervical esophagus, and the excess cervical esophagus is excised (Figure 7–15). Either a 28- or 25-mm EEA circular stapling device anvil is placed in the cervical esophagus, and the purse-string suture is tied (Figure 7–16). Through an anterior gastrotomy, the shaft of the EEA circular stapling device is inserted into the gastric tube, and the trocar is brought through the posterior gastric wall. The circular stapling device is then attached to the anvil, and the device is closed and fired, forming an esophagogastrostomy. The stapling device is removed, and the anvil is checked for two complete "donuts" of tissue; the proximal esophageal donut is sent to pathology as the final proximal margin. Through the anterior gastrotomy, the anastomosis can be inspected for bleeding and completeness. The excess gastric tube proximal to the anastomosis including the anterior gastrotomy is then excised with a linear stapling device (TA-60 with 4.8-mm staples). An endoscope is then passed transorally through the cricopharygeus to the anastomosis, and air is insufflated, with the anastomosis submerged under saline to detect any air leaks that need to be secured with 3-0 silk sutures. The gastric tube is also inspected for viability and to ensure that there has been no unrecognized twisting of the transposed stomach. Two 3-0 silk sutures are used to secure the gastric tube to the surrounding available tissue (but

not to the prevertebral fascia). A nasogastric (NG) tube is passed through the anastomosis, to lie just above the esophageal hiatus. The platysma is closed with a series of interrupted 3-0 absorbable sutures, and the skin is closed with skin staples (Figure 7–17). No drain is placed in the cervical field.

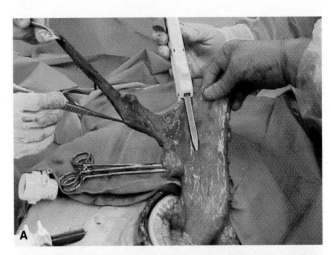

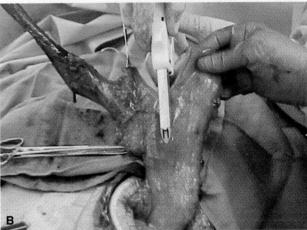

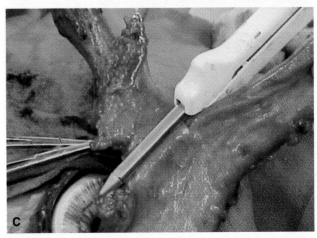

Figure 7–11. *A, B,* and *C,* The linear stapler is used to lengthen the lesser-curvature side of the gastric tube and to complete the resection.

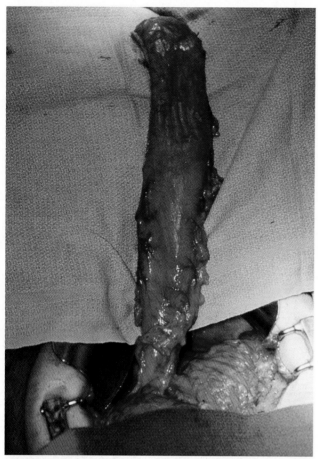

Figure 7–12. The gastric tube will serve as the reconstructive conduit.

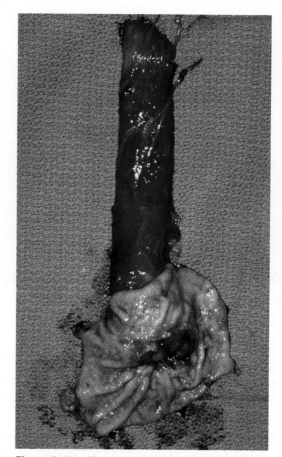

Figure 7–13. The specimen, with the tumor protruding through the gastroesophageal junction, is shown with an adequate proximal and distal margin.

Shifting attention to the abdominal compartment, the surgeon secures the stomach to the diaphragmatic hiatus with two 3-0 silk sutures. A needle catheter feeding jejunostomy is placed, and the abdominal wound is closed.

Transthoracic Esophagectomy

The standard transthoracic approach—a combined midline laparotomy and right thoracotomy (Ivor Lewis esophagectomy)—is described here (Figure

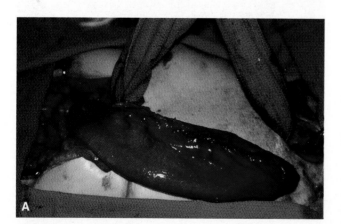

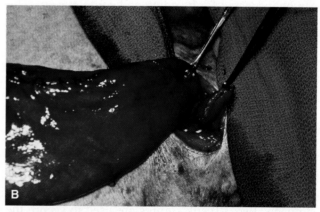

Figure 7–14. The gastric conduit provides adequate length to the cervical incision through the posterior mediastinum for a tension-free anastomosis. *A*, The gastric conduit on the anterior chest wall. *B*, Relationship to the cervical esophagus.

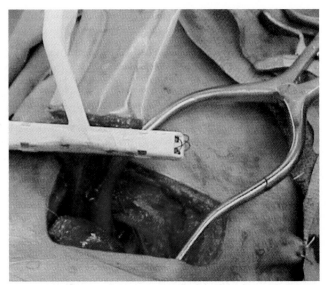

Figure 7–15. The automatic purse-string device is applied to the cervical esophagus.

7–18). The abdominal component of the transthoracic esophagectomy is identical to the abdominal phase of the transhiatal esophagectomy described above. Mobilization of the distal esophagus and stomach, lymphadenectomy, pyloromyotomy, and needle catheter feeding jejunostomy are performed, and the abdominal wound is closed prior to repositioning the patient for the mediastinal dissection. The patient is placed in a left lateral decubitus position, and a right lateral thoracotomy is performed, the thoracic cavity being entered through the fifth or sixth intercostal

space. As opposed to the transhiatal approach, a double-lumen endotracheal tube allows single-lung ventilation and provides ideal exposure to the esophagus and surrounding mediastinal structures. The azygos vein is divided with the endo-GIA vascular stapler (2 mm). The mediastinal pleura is incised along the entire length of the esophagus; the esophagus is encircled, and traction is applied as the dissection proceeds (Figure 7–19). The lymphadenectomy should include mediastinal lymph nodes from stations 2 and 4 (upper and lower paratracheal nodes from the intersection of the caudal margin of the innominate artery to the azygos vein), 3 (posterior mediastinal nodes above the tracheal bifurcation), 7 (subcarinal lymph nodes), and 8 (middle and lower periesophageal nodes from the tracheal bifurcation to the inferior pulmonary vein and extending inferiorly to the gastroesophageal junction to meet the abdominal dissection). The proximal esophagus is divided as far superior to the tumor edge as is possible (preferably with a 5-cm margin) with the GIA stapler. The gastroesophageal junction and stomach are then pulled through the esophageal hiatus and into the chest, ensuring that there is no twisting of the stomach that is to serve as the reconstructive conduit. The stomach is then divided with the GIA stapler, incorporating the lesser-curvature lymph nodes. The specimen is sent to pathology to confirm negative proximal and distal margins. If a stapled anastomosis

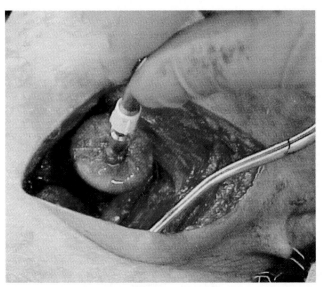

Figure 7–16. The 25-mm EEA anvil in the cervical esophagus, with purse-string suture tied.

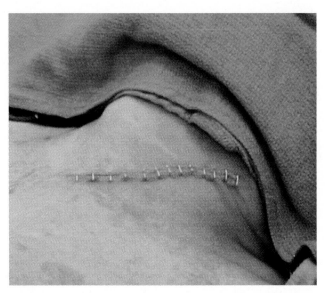

Figure 7–17. The cervical incision is closed with a skin-stapling device.

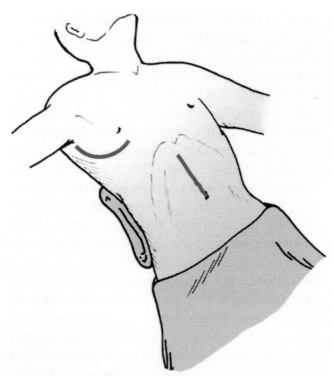

Figure 7–18. The thoracic and upper abdominal incisions for the Ivor Lewis esophagectomy.

stomach. An angled and straight 28F chest tube is placed, and the thoracotomy is closed.

If there is concern regarding an adequate proximal margin or if there is aversion to an intrathoracic anastomosis, the anastomosis can be performed in the cervical region, as previously described. If this decision is made prior to operation, one would start with a thoracotomy first and then reposition the patient for the abdominal and cervical portion of the procedure. If this decision is made intraoperatively following closure of the thoracotomy, the patient is repositioned for the cervical dissection.

Three-Field Lymphadenectomy

For those who adhere to the advantages of the radical esophagectomy, three-field lymph node dissection has been described and advocated by some authors because 30 percent of patients with midesophageal and lower esophageal cancers may have cervical lymph node involvement.[3] Whether this represents systemic disease or locoregional spread that can be addressed by a more radical procedure is not discussed here. Instead, the technique of the cervical component of lymph node dissection is briefly described. (The abdominal and mediastinal components have already been described.)

A U-shaped incision just above the suprasternal notch provides exposure to the bilateral lymph node stations to be dissected (Figure 7–20). The plane just

is preferred, the technique described in the previous section on the transhiatal technique is applicable as outlined. Alternatively, a hand-sewn anastomosis can be performed in an end-to-side fashion in two layers or (as this author prefers) with a single layer of interrupted 3-0 silk sutures. A nasogastric tube is then passed beyond the anastomosis, to lie in the distal

Figure 7–19. Transthoracic view of the mediastinal dissection, demonstrating traction on the thoracic esophagus as the periesophageal soft tissue and mediastinal lymph nodes are resected with the esophageal specimen.

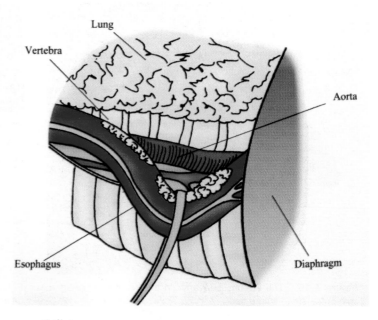

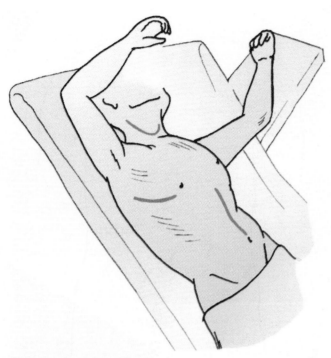

Figure 7–20. The cervical, thoracic, and abdominal incisions required for radical three-field lymphadenectomy.

deep to the platysma muscle is entered, and a flap is raised superiorly (as is done in a thyroid or parathyroid procedure). The boundaries of the dissection are superior to the middle thyroid vein, inferior to the pleura, and lateral to the spinal accessory nerve. The sternocleidomastoid muscle will be retracted either medially or laterally, depending on the point of dissection, and the division of the clavicular head usually facilitates this maneuver. The strap muscles are divided inferiorly as necessary to improve access to the lymph node basins to be dissected. The omohyoid muscle is divided with a cautery, and the deep external and lateral cervical lymph node basins are dissected from the pleura, from the posterior scalene muscles, and along the lateral border of the internal jugular vein. The thyrocervical trunk and its branches (as well as the phrenic, vagus, and spinal accessory nerves) are all preserved. The thoracic duct is divided at its proximal point of drainage into the venous system. Attention is then directed to the deep internal cervical lymph nodes around the internal jugular vein and medial to the common carotid artery. The recurrent laryngeal nerve must be identified and preserved. The dissection of the deep internal cervical nodes that run along the course of the recurrent laryngeal nerve is an extension of the level-two lymph nodes previously dissected during the thoracic component of the radical lymphadenectomy procedure.

Minimally Invasive Esophagectomy

A number of approaches to achieving a minimally invasive esophagectomy have been described, including combined thoracoscopic and laparoscopic esophagectomy, thoracoscopic esophagectomy with open gastric mobilization, laparoscopic gastric mobilization with minithoracotomy, laparoscopic transhiatal esophagectomy, and hand-assisted laparoscopic transhiatal esophagectomy. The largest experience to date has been reported for the combined thoracoscopic and laparoscopic approach, which are described in detail elsewhere.[4] This author's center has adopted the hand-assisted laparoscopic transhiatal esophagectomy, which is described below. The actual and theoretic advantages of this approach are that (1) there is no need for repositioning, (2) there is no need for single-lung ventilation, (3) tumor palpation achieves adequate distal margins, and (4) there is a shallow learning curve, and the procedure therefore has wide applicability to the surgical community.

The patient is placed in the supine position, with the left arm at the patient's side and the right arm at 90° as described for the open transhiatal approach. Although lithotomy is often used in laparoscopic approaches to foregut surgery, this author does not feel it is necessary in this situation. The patient is prepped and draped in a routine fashion (Figure 7–21). A periumbilical trocar is placed to the left of the linea alba, through the rectus muscle just cephalad (approximately 2 cm) to the umbilicus (Figure 7–22). A 30° laparoscope is passed through the periumbilical port. Next, three additional trocars are placed in the right hemiabdomen. The liver retractor port is placed as close to and as lateral to the costal margin as possible. This position allows the fulcrum of the retractor to elevate the left lobe of the liver while remaining outside the operative field. The next two trocars are placed in position to facilitate dissection along the greater curvature of the stomach. These are the working hands of the surgeon; they should be

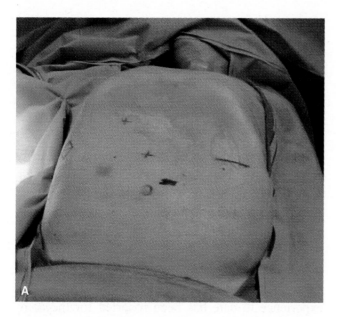

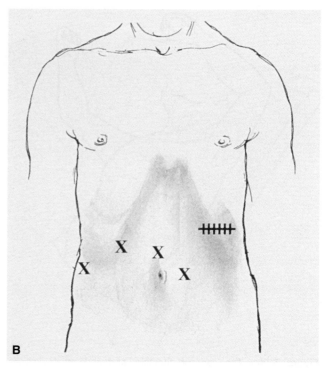

Figure 7–21.   *A,* Intraoperative photograph of port placement sites and left upper quadrant incision for hand-assisted laparoscopic transhiatal esophagectomy. *B,* Drawing of the port sites and left upper quadrant incision.

placed low enough to facilitate access to the duodenal sweep, to accomplish a wide Kocher maneuver. The trocar closest to the midline should not obscure the camera view into the mediastinum. The site of the incision through which the hand will be introduced into the peritoneal cavity is then selected in the left hemiabdomen, with the abdomen insufflated (Figure 7–23). The incision should be placed 2 to 3 cm below the costal margin, with its center in the projection of the lateral border of the rectus abdominus muscle. A

5- to 6-cm transverse incision is made and then extended into the anterior rectus sheath, and the rectus abdominus muscle is retracted medially. Next, a vertical incision is made in the posterior rectus sheath underneath the rectus muscle, and the peritoneum is entered. A number of devices have been designed to allow the introduction of the surgeon's hand into the

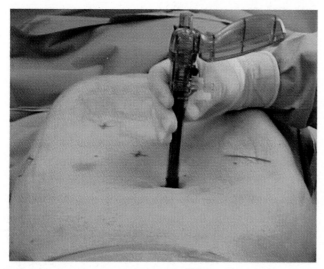

Figure 7–22.   Placement of a periumbilical port.

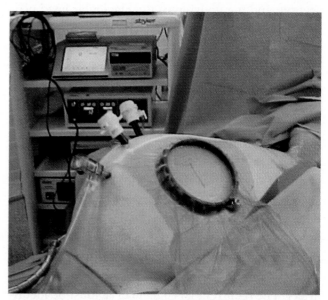

Figure 7–23.   With the abdomen insufflated and the port sites in place, the base of the Pneumo-sleeve® is placed prior to the left upper quadrant incision.

peritoneal cavity while allowing for retraction of the abdominal wound and maintenance of the pneumoperitoneum. These devices include the Pneumosleeve®, which requires a sterile sleeve apparatus over the routine gown and gloving, and the Gelport®, which requires no additional sleeve apparatus (Figure 7–24). The beauty of the hand-assisted laparoscopic transhiatal esophagectomy is that it exactly mimics the open technique and thus almost completely eliminates the learning curve and requires no extraordinary laparoscopic expertise (but it does require the prerequisite expertise in esophageal resection). Following visual identification and palpation of the right gastroepiploic artery, the gastrocolic omentum is divided with a harmonic scalpel. The gastrohepatic ligament is likewise divided (with the harmonic scalpel) up to the crus of the diaphragm and inferiorly to the right gastric artery, which is preserved. A wide Kocher maneuver is then performed, and the hepatic flexure is taken down, ensuring easy identification and preservation of the takeoff of the right gastroepiploic artery from the gastroduodenal artery. The stomach is then retracted cephalad and anteriorly, to divide any posterior attachments between the pancreas and the stomach, and the left gastric vessels are isolated (Figure 7–25). These vessels are then divided with the endo-GIA vascular stapler. All lymphatic and nodal tissue is swept up with the specimen. The peritoneum overlying the gastroesophageal junction is then divided, and the esophageal hiatus is opened

with the harmonic scalpel. A Penrose drain is then doubly looped around the gastroesophageal junction and is secured tightly with a 2-0 endostitch. This is then brought through the abdominal wall inferiorly to provide caudal traction for the mediastinal dissection (Figure 7–26). The hand-facilitated mediastinal dissection is undertaken (with the harmonic scalpel) up to the level of the carina (Figure 7–27). An attempt is made to perform a pyloromyotomy, which is facilitated with the placement of a lighted bougie introduced transorally through the esophagus and the stomach and into the duodenum through the pylorus. This author and colleagues have found this to be a technically difficult exercise and frequently have converted to a pyloroplasty, performed in the usual manner by making a longitudinal incision from the duodenum and through the pyloric muscle to the stomach and then closing the incision transversely with interrupted 3-0 endostitches. The cervical component of the dissection is an exact duplicate of that described for the open technique. The remainder of the mediastinal attachments are then bluntly divided by finger dissection, with a hand introduced through the abdominal port. The cervical esophagus is divided as described previously, and the specimen is brought through the left upper abdominal incision. The gastric tube is formed exactly as described for the open technique, allowing palpation of the tumor for an adequate margin. The Penrose drain from the cervical incision to the abdominal incision is then

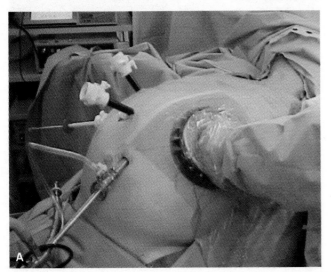 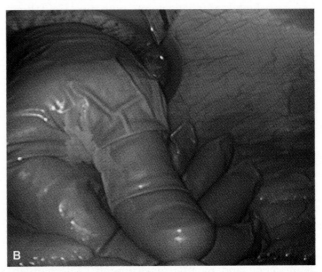

Figure 7–24. *A*, External view of the hand being placed through the left upper quadrant incision for hand-assisted laparoscopic transhiatal esophagectomy. *B*, Intra-abdominal view of the hand within the peritoneal cavity.

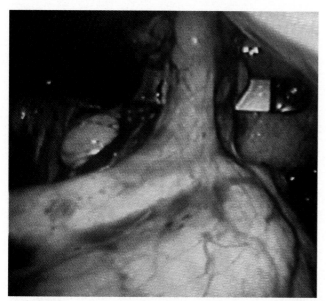

Figure 7–25.   Isolation of the left gastric vessels prior to division of the pedicle with endovascular GIA.

secured to the stomach. Once the pneumoperitoneum is again created, the gastric conduit is transferred from the abdomen through the mediastinum to the cervical incision under direct laparoscopic vision, thus ensuring proper orientation. The anastomosis is completed as described earlier. The fascia is closed, and the skin is approximated with a subcuticular closure (Figure 7–28).

Other Techniques

Siewert and colleagues described the technique of radical transhiatal esophagectomy with two-field lymphadenectomy.[5] This approach essentially combines the technique of transhiatal esophagectomy with that of radical en bloc esophagectomy, accepting the concept that most patients with distal esophageal tumors have regional lymph node spread to the abdominal and lower periesophageal lymph node basins, which are accessible through an abdominal and transhiatal approach. The diaphragm is opened widely, and the distal third of the esophagus is dissected and resected with the crus of the diaphragm and the pariental pleura bilaterally to achieve a normal tissue envelope around the tumor mass (Figure 7–29). The upper mediastinal dissection is facilitated by a special mediastinoscope and by microinstruments. Alternatively for tumors of the gastroesophageal junction, a total

gastrectomy or esophagogastrectomy via a transabdominal approach has also been described.

Reconstructive Techniques

The stomach is the preferred esophageal substitute, and the reconstructive technique has been outlined in detail in this chapter. Although it is most unusual that the stomach is deemed not to be a suitable conduit for the reconstruction, the surgeon must be prepared to use an alternative segment of intestine when it is required. The use of the colon as an esophageal substitute has been well described. The decision as to the preferred segment of colon (ie, right, transverse, or left) should be based on which vascular pedicle would provide the longest viable segment of colon. Therefore, test occlusion is used to confirm the viability of the segment to be transposed prior to division of the vascular pedicles (Figure 7–30). This

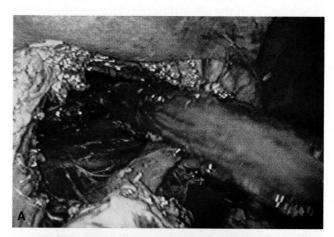

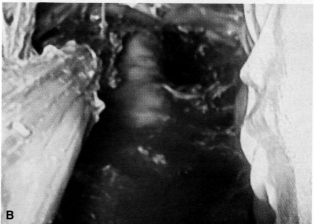

Figure 7–26.   *A,* Laparoscopic view of the initial distal esophageal dissection. *B,* Laparoscopic view of the mediastinal dissection. Note the relationship of the thoracic aorta to the dissected esophagus.

themselves at the cervical incision site and are easily managed by opening the cervical wound and administering local conservative wound care. If patients have an intrathoracic anastomosis, a contrast study is obtained, usually with dilute barium to avoid the catastrophic complications of meglumine diatrizoate

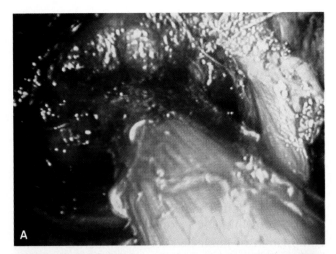

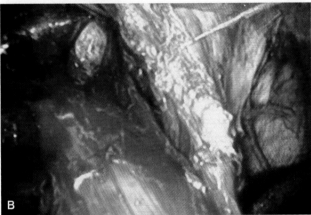

Figure 7–27. *A*, Laparascopic view of the carina. *B*, View of the carina, with periesophageal lymph nodes dissected with the specimen.

author prefers the transverse colon and the technique described by Akiyama.[6]

POSTOPERATIVE CARE

Although not mandatory at this author's center, mechanical ventilatory support is routinely continued until the first postoperative morning, when the patient is usually extubated with ease. Deep venous thrombosis prophylaxis with sequential compression stockings is continued until the patient is fully ambulatory. Early ambulation and pulmonary toilet is encouraged as with any major surgical procedure. The NG tube that was placed during the operation is secured and adjusted to low continuous suction until bowel function returns; it is then removed, and metoclopramide is initiated. A contrast study to examine anastomotic competency following cervical anastomosis is not routinely done since developing leaks will declare

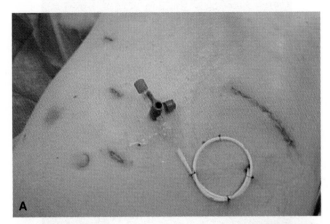

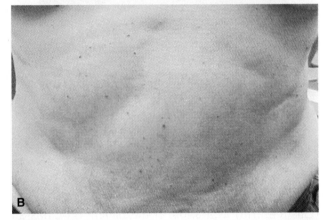

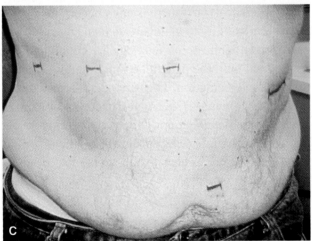

Figure 7–28. *A*, Closure of the abdominal incisions. The feeding jejunostomy is in place. *B*, View of the abdominal incisions 6 weeks after hand-assisted laparoscopic esophagectomy. *C*, Blue ink highlights the incisions.

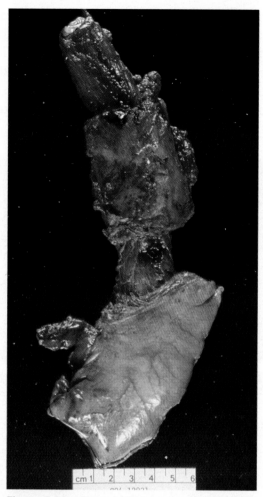

Figure 7–29. The resected specimen after radical transhiatal esophagectomy, demonstrating pleura and normal tissue enveloping the tumor mass.

(Gastrografin) aspiration. If the patient develops an anastomotic leak or if there is any concern regarding the patient's ability to maintain adequate nutrition via oral intake, jejunostomy feedings are begun and are maintained until the patient no longer requires nutritional supplementation. The patient is instructed in a postgastrectomy diet (six small meals per day) and is advised to maintain an upright position during meals and for 1 hour following meals. The patient should have his or her head elevated above the feet when in the recumbent position.

Postoperative Complications

As with any major surgical procedure, intraoperative or postoperative hemorrhage can occur. However, since most of the mediastinal dissection during trans-

hiatal esophagectomy is done under direct vision, blood loss during the procedure now averages between 500 and 700 cc. This author's center has had one injury to the azygous vein, which required an anteriolateral thoracotomy to repair. Although experience is limited at present, blood loss during a hand-assisted laparoscopic transhiatal esophagectomy is between 100 and 200 cc. A number of complications commonly associated with esophagectomy should be discussed. It should be noted that there are no large randomized trials of transhiatal versus transthoracic esophagectomy although a compilation of published series comparing the two procedures[7] does provide some insight into the relative rates of morbidity and mortality associated with the two procedures (Table 7–1).

Recurrent Laryngeal Nerve Paresis/Palsy

Recurrent laryngeal nerve paresis occurs in approximately 10 percent of patients undergoing transhiatal esophagectomy. The complication can be minimized by avoiding sustained mechanical retraction and minimizing dissection in the tracheoesophageal

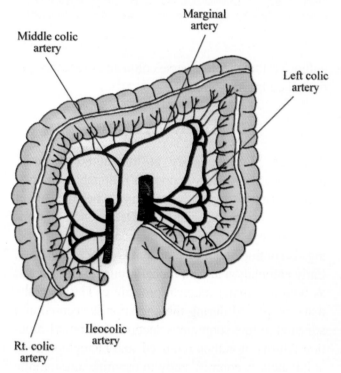

Figure 7–30. Sites for test occlusion of the vascular pedicle to determine the most viable segment of colon to be used as an esophageal substitute during colon interposition. (Rt. = right.)

Table 7–1. MORBIDITY AND MORTALITY OF TRANSHIATAL VERSUS TRANSTHORACIC ESOPHAGECTOMY FOR ESOPHAGEAL CANCER*

Morbidity/Mortality	THE (n = 2,675) (%)	TTE (n = 2,808) (%)
Postoperative morbidity		
Pulmonary	24.0	25.0
Cardiovascular	12.4	10.5
Wound infection	8.8	6.2
Anastomotic leak	16.0	10.0
Anastomotic stricture	28.0	16.0
RLN injury	11.2	4.8
Postoperative mortality	6.3	9.5

*From 14 published series, 1986 to 1996.
THE = transhiatal esophagectomy; TTE = transthoracic esophagectomy;
RLN = recurrent laryngeal nerve; n = sample size.

groove. At this author's center, blunt self-sustaining retractors are placed into the substance of the thyroid medially to avoid injury to the recurrent laryngeal nerve, and all retraction in the area of the tracheoesophageal groove is done with either a finger or a soft Kittner sponge on a Kelly clamp. It is crucial to maintain the dissection directly on the adventitia of the esophagus when encircling it to also avoid injury to the contralateral (right) recurrent laryngeal nerve. Most injuries to the nerve result in hoarseness, are temporary, and resolve without any intervention. However, dysphagia and aspiration can be troublesome, even if temporarily; therefore, avoidance of the injury is the best "treatment." Permanent palsy may require surgical correction.

Anastomotic Leaks

Anastomotic leaks occur in approximately 10 to 15 percent of patients. The rate of anastomotic leaks following cervical anastomosis is higher than with an intrathoracic anastomoses because of the potentially compromised blood supply to (and impeded venous outflow from) the top of the gastric tube. In addition, despite all efforts to avoid trauma to the cephalad portion of the gastric tube, trauma can and does occur. In this author's experience, the use of stapled anastomoses appears to have decreased the rate of anastomotic leaks. Almost all cervical anastomotic leaks can be managed with conservative care that includes opening the wound at the bedside and changing the dressing twice daily. If the drainage from the cervical wound is copious, this author does not hesitate to perform endoscopy and dilatation of the anastomosis or the pylorus to facilitate antegrade drainage and gastric emptying to facilitate closure. Oral intake is not discouraged, even with a cervical anastomotic leak. An intrathoracic anastomotic leak is a much more serious event that requires adequate chest drainage, antibiotics, and prolonged parenteral or enteral nutritional support.

One devastating complication is necrosis of the proximal gastric tube, which is heralded by foul-smelling cervical drainage and requires takedown of the anastomosis, creation of a cervical esophageal fistula, and placement of a gastrostomy tube into the remaining gastric stump. If the patient survives this extreme insult, gastrointestinal continuity can be reconstituted with either a colonic interposition or a small-bowel free flap.

Anastomotic Stricture

Anastomotic stricture is a relatively common complication following transhiatal esophagectomy and is more likely if an anastomotic leak occurs. Single or (more likely) multiple dilatations may be required to eliminate symptoms of dysphagia. This author normally uses progressive savary dilatations under fluoroscopic control.

Chylothorax

Injury to the thoracic duct can occur, especially with a locally advanced tumor of the distal esophagus. Excessive or increased chest tube drainage (as opposed to a decrease in chest tube output) following the 2nd postoperative day should alert the surgeon to this potential complication. Triglyceride levels can be obtained from the fluid draining from the chest tube; high-fat jejunostomy feedings will yield a milky fluid from the chest tube, which is diagnostic. Although conservative measures such as total parenteral nutrition can lead to closure of a chylous leak, it is much more expeditious to proceed with ligation of the divided thoracic duct, either via thoracoscopy or by a minithoracotomy. Early closure of a chylous leak may avoid prolonged nutritional depletion.

Postresection Follow-Up

The vast majority of recurrences will occur in the first 2 years post resection, and therefore, this author schedules office visits for esophagectomy patients every 3 months for the 1st 2 years and then every 6 months thereafter. A focused history and examination are performed at each visit, but no routine blood work is obtained. Computed tomography of the chest, abdomen, and pelvis and upper endoscopy can be obtained on a yearly basis, or imaging and invasive studies can be dictated by symptoms or by physical findings. Since the treatment of recurrence or metastatic disease is unlikely to prolong life, there is negligible gain in performing routine diagnostic studies (unless the patient is on a clinical trial) to detect an "early" recurrence prior to the development of symptoms.

REFERENCES

1. Chu KM, Law SY, Fok M, Wong J. A prospective randomized comparison of transhiatal and transthoracic resection for lower-third esophageal carcinoma. Am J Surg 1997; 174:320–4.
2. Goldminc M, Maddern G, Le Prise E, et al. Oesophagectomy by a transhiatal approach or thoracotomy: a prospective randomized trial. Br J Surg 1993;80:367–70.
3. Akiyama H, Tsurumaru M, Udagawa H, Kajiyama Y. Radical lymph node dissection for cancer of the thoracic esophagus. Ann Surg 1994;220:364–72.
4. Luketich JD, Schauer PR, Christie NA, et al. Minimally invasive esophagectomy. Ann Thorac Surg 2000;70:906–11.
5. Bumm R, Feussner H, Bartels H, et al. Radical transhiatal esophagectomy with two-field lymphadenectomy and endodissection for distal esophageal adenocarcinoma. World J Surg 1997;21:822–31.
6. Akiyama H. Surgery for cancer of the esophagus. Baltimore: Williams and Wilkins; 1990.
7. Rindani R, Martin CJ, Cox MR. Transhiatal versus Ivor-Lewis oesophagectomy: is there a difference? Aust N Z J Surg 1999;69:187–94.

8

Multimodality Therapy for Carcinoma of the Esophagus

ANN M. MAUER, MD
RALPH R. WEICHSELBAUM, MD

Approximately 12,000 people in the United States are diagnosed annually with carcinoma of the esophagus.[1] Although carcinoma of the esophagus is an uncommon malignancy within the Western world, it represents a major cause of cancer-related mortality worldwide. In the United States, the incidence of adenocarcinoma of the esophagus and proximal stomach is rising at an annual rate exceeding that of any other malignancy.[2] As a result, adenocarcinoma has recently replaced squamous cell carcinoma as the predominant esophageal carcinoma in the United States.[3]

The outcomes from esophageal carcinoma are stage related where survival decreases sharply with increasing stage for both squamous cell and adenocarcinoma histologies. The two histologies do not appear to differ in prognosis.[4] The low overall 5-year survival rate of 20 percent and the short median survival of 12 months illustrate the poor prognosis associated with esophageal carcinoma.[5] These unfavorable outcomes may be attributed to the early dissemination of tumor cells into the submucosal network and lymph nodes, as well as the absence of a serosal wall to limit local invasion. The majority of patients with localized esophageal carcinoma present with large primary tumors, extensive regional lymphadenopathy, or clinically occult metastases. In these patients, the failure to cure or to prolong survival occurs because of the inability to eradicate residual disease at the primary site and because of early systemic tumor dissemination. By the time symptoms develop from the primary tumor, micro-scopic or gross disease is often present within regional lymph nodes or at distant metastatic sites. Autopsy reports have confirmed the high prevalence of occult metastases at the time of presentation.[6,7]

Cancer of the esophagus is staged according to the tumor-node-metastasis (TNM) classification system[8] (Table 8–1). The management of esophageal cancer depends on the clinical stage. For disease limited to local and regional sites (T1 to T3, any N, M0, stages I to III), therapy is usually delivered with curative intent; however, when systemic metastases are present, the goal of treatment is the palliation of symptoms. The two potentially curative therapeutic approaches for the management of local and regional disease are (a) surgery alone and (b) concurrent chemotherapy and radiation. Primary therapy for patients with early-stage disease includes surgery when feasible. For more advanced local and regional disease, various treatment approaches have been investigated, including surgery alone, surgery plus postoperative radiotherapy, preoperative combined-modality therapy, radiation therapy alone, and chemoradiotherapy alone. Metastatic disease is managed with palliative therapies, which may include systemic chemotherapy or local treatments such as radiotherapy, brachytherapy, expansile stents, laser therapy, or photodynamic therapy.

This chapter discusses the individual modalities of surgery, radiation therapy, and chemotherapy as used in the management of the patient with esophageal cancer. The chapter will examine the primary treatment of localized nonmetastatic disease via surgical and nonsurgical approaches. The rationale for combined-modality treatment will be followed by a discussion of trials exploring the use of combined-modality therapy.

DIAGNOSTIC EVALUATION

The management and survival of the patient with esophageal carcinoma is dependent on the stage at the time of diagnosis. Computed tomography (CT) and endoscopic ultrasonography are routinely used to assess tumor penetration into the esophageal wall (Figures 8–1 to 8–3). Whereas features seen on CT scans may reliably predict local tumor invasion into adjacent structures, CT does not predict the depth of microscopic invasion for the determination of T stage. Computed tomography may also demonstrate enlarged lymph nodes that are suspicious for metastatic disease. The major use of CT is in the detection of distant metastatic disease; however, 30 to 60 percent of distant metastases may be radiographically occult. Endoscopic ultrasonography offers improved resolution of the esophageal wall and provides a more accurate assessment of tumor wall invasion and T stage.[9] This technique allows the identification of lymph nodes in greater detail than

with CT; however, it does not accurately differentiate non-tumor-bearing nodes from tumor-bearing nodes (Figure 8–4). Fine-needle aspiration of suspicious nodes can be done with the guidance of endoscopic ultrasonography. Barium esophagography provides information regarding the length of the primary tumor and the presence of synchronous lesions (Figure 8–5). Bronchoscopy should be performed to exclude synchronous primary lesions because the rate of second malignancy within the aerodigestive tract is high for individuals with squamous cell carcinoma. For individuals with cancers involving the cervical esophagus, rigid bronchoscopy is required to exclude the presence of a tracheoesophageal fistula. Bone scanning is indicated only for individuals with clinical findings or laboratory abnormalities suggestive of bone metastases. A number of other imaging techniques are available for staging esophageal cancer. Laparoscopy and positron emission tomography may aid in the detection of systemic tumor dissemination, but their use is still considered investigational.[10–12] As the current methods available for staging are limited, these newer techniques may provide more accurate staging information and a better determination of appropriate treatment.

SURGICAL THERAPY

For patients with esophageal carcinoma that is clinically limited to the local area (T1-3N0-1M0), two modalities exist: surgery and radiotherapy. For localized resectable esophageal tumors, surgical therapy is the standard of care. The selection of patients for surgical resection is based on various factors, including preoperative clinical staging, anatomic considerations, and the medical fitness of the patient. In about 30 to 60 percent of patients with local and regional disease, curative resection is not feasible because of extensive primary tumor. In one series, surgical staging demonstrated that invasion into the periesophageal tissues was evident in 38 percent of patients and that lymph node metastases were present in 41 percent of patients at the time of resection.[13] In other clinical circumstances, surgical exploration reveals hepatic metastases or peritoneal disease, precluding resection. The preoperative

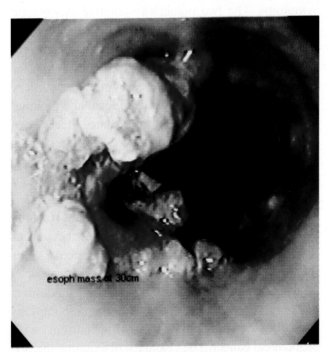

esoph mass at 30cm

Figure 8–1. Adenocarcinoma of the esophagus. Endoscopic view shows a fungating tumor mass.

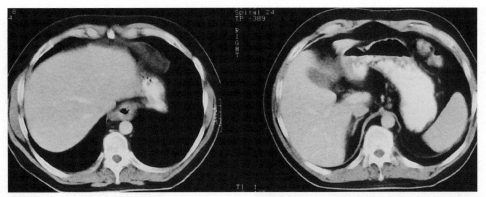

Figure 8–2. Adenocarcinoma in the same patient shown in Figure 8–1. Computed tomography (CT) scan on the left reveals circumferential thickening at the level of the gastroesophageal junction. This CT scan also demonstrates a 1-cm celiac-axis lymph node.

assessment should also evaluate for cardiac and pulmonary disorders (as well as nutritional status) that could contribute to surgical morbidity and mortality and that might negate attempts at resection.

Surgery may be curative for patients with stage I or IIA esophageal carcinoma. Long-term survival is uncommon for patients with regional lymph node metastases or histologically positive resection margins. Five-year survival rates following primary surgical resection are reported as less than 10 percent in literature reviews and retrospective analyses.[14,15] In more recent randomized trials, overall survival rates of up to 35 percent are noted at 5 years.[14,16] The retrospective analyses included all patients, and randomized trials excluded patients with unfavorable characteristics. Therefore, the observed survival differences may be the result of patient selection. Another reason for the apparent improvement in survival may be related to the decline in postoperative mortality over the past three decades. Whereas early series reported

postoperative mortality rates of up to 30 percent, more contemporary series from experienced surgical centers noted mortality rates in the range of 5 to 12 percent.[17–19] Another possible explanation for this improvement in survival is that the more accurate diagnostic imaging that has been available in recent years has resulted in clinical up-staging.

Resection of the esophagus can be accomplished by various surgical approaches that differ in the type of incision, the extent of resection, the conduit for reconstruction, and the method of reanastomosis. The most common approaches are the Ivor Lewis esophagectomy, which uses a right thoracotomy and laparotomy with an intrathoracic esophagogastric anastomosis, and the transhiatal esophagectomy, which involves resection through the esophageal hiatus and thoracic inlet via a cervical incision, with the anastomosis performed in the neck. These surgical techniques have not been directly compared in a randomized trial, and none appear to offer a survival

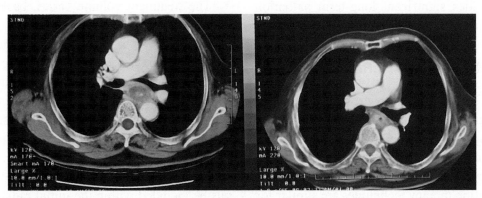

Figure 8–3. The CT scans show the same lesion before (*left*) and after (*right*) therapy with chemotherapy and radiation. This patient had a pathologic complete response to combined-modality therapy.

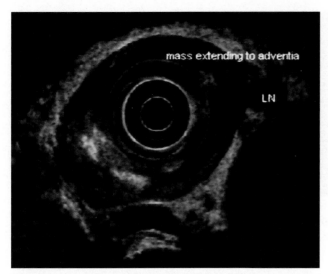

Figure 8–4. Adenocarcinoma of the gastroesophageal junction. Endoscopic ultrasonography reveals a mass extending into the adventitia. Also seen is a periesophageal lymph node.

benefit.[14] The surgical management of esophageal cancer is discussed in detail in Chapters 5, 6 and 7.

Although the majority of patients develop distant metastases following surgery, local failure occurs frequently. The rates of local failure following surgery are available from autopsy data and postoperative reviews.[6,7,20] In the surgical control arm of the recent Gastrointestinal Intergroup trial, INT 0113, the local failure rate following surgical resection was 31 percent for patients who underwent an R0 resection.[16] Of the patients who received an R0 resection in this trial, 50 percent developed distant metastases. Thus, the poor prognosis of patients with esophageal cancer appears to be the result of the limitations of local therapy in controlling the primary tumor and the high risk of distant metastases. Despite these shortcomings, definitive surgical resection provides significant long-term palliation of dysphagia in 80 to 90 percent of patients.[21,22]

RADIATION THERAPY

Radiotherapy has been used in the management of local and regional esophageal cancer as primary curative therapy, as postoperative therapy, and as combined-modality therapy. Many of the principles of radiotherapy are valid for each of these uses. In addition, radiation therapy techniques are similar for curative-intent situations in which therapy is deliv-

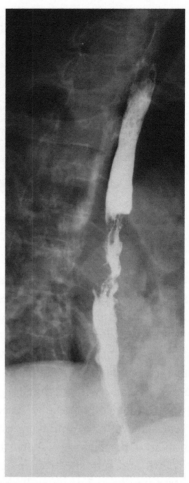

Figure 8–5. Squamous cell carcinoma. Barium swallow demonstrates a narrowing of the esophagus, with mucosal destruction.

ered as primary therapy or as part of a combined-modality approach. The overall goal of radiation therapy is to provide irradiation of the gross tumor as well as areas of possible microscopic involvement, while limiting the radiation dosage to adjacent structures such as the lung, heart, and spinal cord.

The treatment volume varies, based on the size and primary location of the tumor and regional lymph nodes. It is well described that esophageal cancer may be associated with multicentric disease or submucosa "skip" metastases sometimes found at a considerable distance from the primary tumor.[23] This finding offers support for the use of generous cephalad and caudal treatment margins of at least 5 to 6 cm above and below the tumor. Some groups have recommended that the entire thoracic esophagus be included within the initial radiation portal on the basis of a pilot study from Wayne State University that investigated radiotherapy with chemotherapy as curative therapy.[24] That study used an initial target volume with a longitudinal margin of 5 cm until several patients developed marginal recurrences; the trial was then modified to include irradiation of the entire esophagus for the first 30 Gy, followed by a boost of 20 Gy to the tumor plus 5 cm. Further support for the inclusion of the total esophagus in the initial target volume came from Elkon and colleagues, who reported on the sites of recurrence following curative radiotherapy. They noted that esophageal recurrences outside of the treatment field occurred in patients with clinical stage I disease despite treatment portals that included a 5-cm margin of apparently normal esophagus.[25] Based on several postoperative staging studies that indicate a high rate of lymph node involvement for this malignancy, regional lymph nodes should be included in the initial target volume.[23,26] Carcinoma of the upper esophagus is characterized by metastasis to the lower deep cervical lymph nodes at an early stage.[23] For tumors of the cervical esophagus, the treatment field usually extends from the laryngopharynx to the junction of the upper and middle two-thirds of the esophagus and includes the anterior cervical, superior mediastinal, and supraclavicular lymph nodes. For tumors of the lower two-thirds of the esophagus, treatment of the supraclavicular nodes is debated. For lower esophageal tumors, treatment of the celiac lymph nodes also warrants consideration.

Primary tumor volume may be ascertained through endoscopy, esophageal ultrasonography, barium swallow studies, CT, and magnetic resonance imaging. Double-contrast barium esophagography is useful for determining the length of the primary tumor. Portal arrangements are based on the location of the primary tumor and are best determined using three-dimensional simulation. With CT simulation, bulky tumors or lymph nodes that are not visualized well by conventional simulation techniques can be incorporated into the design of radiation portals. Some centers also have begun to use positron emission tomography for the determination of portal volumes. Generally, a combination of anteroposterior and oblique or lateral fields is used to minimize the dose to normal tissues.

Megavoltage photons are used for the treatment of esophageal cancer. The total dose and fractionation schema depend on whether the radiotherapy is being delivered alone or in combination with chemotherapy. Curative-intent single-modality radiotherapy requires at least 6,000 to 6,500 cGy administered in 180- to 200-cGy fractions. Although no dose regimen has been proven to be superior, available data suggest that the tumor response may be enhanced with increased radiotherapy dose. For large tumors, doses above 6,500 cGy are probably necessary to eradicate disease. In trials of radiotherapy administered with concurrent chemotherapy as definitive therapy, a similar fraction size has been used, but the cumulative dose was generally lower, in the range of 5,000 to 6,480 cGy. For chemoradiotherapy delivered in the preoperative setting, the total dose administered generally does not exceed 5,000 cGy. The dose to the spinal cord should not exceed 4,500 cGy in 180- to 200-cGy fractions. Maximum doses to the heart and lungs vary, based on the volume of tissue within the irradiated field. In general, when substantial volumes of lung are included, the dose to the lung should not exceed 2,000 cGy.

Stage	Primary Tumor (T)	Regional Lymph Nodes* (N)	Distant Metastasis (M)
Table 8–1. TUMOR-NODE-METASTASIS CLASSIFICATION OF ESOPHAGEAL CANCER			
0	TIS (carcinoma in situ)	N0	M0
I	T1 (invasion of lamina propria or submucosa)	N0	M0
IIA	T2 (invasion of muscularis propria)	N0	M0
	T3 (invasion of adventitia)	N0	M0
IIB	T1	N1	M0
	T2	N1	M0
III	T3	N1	M0
III	T4 (invasion of adjacent structures)	Any N	M0
IV	Any T	Any N	M1

*For cervical esophagus, regional lymph nodes include cervical and supraclavicular nodes only. For thoracic esophagus, regional lymph nodes include thoracic nodes only. For abdominal esophagus and gastroesophageal junction, celiac lymph nodes are considered regional.

The toxicity of radiation is a function of the total dose, fraction size, field size, and technique used. If the patient has undergone surgery or has received chemotherapy, these factors may influence the toxicity encountered. Results of acute toxicities commonly encountered include skin irritation, fatigue, nausea, esophagitis, leukopenia, and thrombocytopenia. The most frequent late complication following radiotherapy is esophageal stricture, which may occur as a complication of radiation therapy or which may result from local tumor recurrence. Other less common late complications include pneumonitis, pericarditis, and myelitis.

There are numerous reports of the results of external beam radiotherapy alone as primary therapy with curative intent for localized esophageal carcinoma.[27–30] Several reports published since 1979 are summarized in Table 8–2. These studies report 5-year survival rates of < 10 percent and indicate that single-modality radiotherapy is inadequate for the management of localized esophageal cancer. Among these reports of single-modality radiotherapy, the most favorable outcomes were noted in patients who received radiation for tumors with diameters of 5 cm or less.[29,30] Although the pattern of failure was not well described in most of these reports, Beatty and colleagues noted a predominant local pattern of failure, with 80 percent of the patients developing a local recurrence after radical radiotherapy.[29] Overall, the survival statistics reported for these series on radical radiotherapy are similar to those reported by Earlam and Cunha-Melo from their review of 49 manuscripts describing the outcomes of 8,489 patients treated with radiation therapy alone. Earlam and Cunha-Melo summarized survival rates after

radiation therapy alone as 8 percent at 2 years and 6 percent at 5 years.[31] Because of patient selection biases, direct comparisons between radiotherapy and surgical series are not meaningful. Curative radiotherapy is often offered to poor-prognosis patients with unfavorable tumor characteristics such as advanced tumor stage and positive lymph nodes or with medical comorbidities that make them unfit for surgery. Two prospective randomized trials comparing surgery and radiotherapy as primary therapy were initiated in the United States and Europe but were never completed due to poor accrual.[32]

As described above, it is clear that local and regional failure is common after radical radiotherapy. Accelerated-fraction radiotherapy and brachytherapy have been investigated as strategies for improving local control. In theory, an accelerated course of radiotherapy may be beneficial for patients with rapidly growing tumors with short doubling times. One possible way to reduce the overall treatment time is to administer radiotherapy for 6 to 7 days per week instead of the usual 5 days per week. Alternatively, the fraction size may be decreased to 140 to 160 cGy and the therapy administered twice daily. Several studies have demonstrated the feasibility of accelerated radiotherapy in patients with locally advanced esophageal cancer.[33,34] Further study is required to determine the optimal schedule of therapy and whether this approach improves local control and overall survival with acceptable levels of toxicity.

Brachytherapy involves the intraluminal placement of a radioactive source and allows the selective delivery of the radiation dose to the primary tumor while protecting the adjacent structures and normal tissues. Brachytherapy has been used alone in the

Table 8–2. TRIALS OF RADICAL RADIATION THERAPY FOR LOCAL AND REGIONAL CANCER OF THE ESOPHAGUS							
Lead Author (Reference No.)	Histology	Total Dose (Gy)	n	Stage	2 yr	3 yr	5 yr
Beatty (29)	SCC	40–60	146	Local/regional	20	—	0
Van Andel (27)	SCC, AC	60–66 (split course)	115	Local/regional	5	—	1
Newaishy (30)	SCC	50–55	444	Local/regional	18	—	9
De-Ren (28)	SCC	50–79	681	I (n = 3)	—	80	80
				II (n = 177)	—	34	22
				III (n = 501)	—	7	6

AC = adenocarcinoma; SCC = squamous cell carcinoma; n = number of subjects in sample.

palliative setting or after external beam radiation therapy. This therapy is characterized by the duration of treatment as well as the absorbed-dose rate and on this basis is referred to as "high dose rate" or "low dose rate." Several retrospective analyses[35–38] and two prospective randomized studies [39,40] comparing external beam radiotherapy with or without a brachytherapy boost reported improved local control, swallowing function, and survival in patients receiving brachytherapy. Although it remains to be proven that such a boost improves survival and local control, it may be of benefit in select patients. Guidelines for the use of brachytherapy in patients with carcinoma of the esophagus have beeen developed by the American Brachytherapy Society.[41] In the curative intent setting, therapy should be limited to tumors less than 10 cm in diameter. Contraindications to brachytherapy boost include cervical esophagus location, tracheal or bronchial involvement, and stenosis that cannot be bypassed. Brachytherapy should follow external beam radiation and should not be given concurrently with chemotherapy because concurrent administration may result in an increased incidence of complications.

External beam radiation provides effective palliation of dysphagia when used alone as primary therapy, but the relief is of short duration, and the long-term survival rate is a dismal 6 percent at 5 years.[31,42] In view of recent randomized trials showing the superiority of chemoradiation to radiation alone, single-modality radiation therapy is used infrequently as primary therapy for esophageal cancer. In the curative-intent setting, the use of radiation therapy alone is reserved for individuals who are medically unfit for chemoradiotherapy or who refuse such therapy. The dismal statistics afforded by primary surgical resection or radiotherapy are the result of the poor local control achieved with these approaches and the development of distant disease prior to or following primary local therapy. The low survival rates achieved with either of these single-modality therapies have prompted the investigation of multimodality therapy for locally advanced esophageal cancer.

Preoperative Radiotherapy

In theory, preoperative radiotherapy may increase the rate of curative-intent resection and improve local control. Table 8–3 summarizes the results of five randomized trials that addressed the benefits of preoperative radiotherapy in patients with local and regional esophageal cancer. Four of these randomized studies failed to demonstrate an impact on overall survival for patients who received preoperative radiotherapy.[43–46] One study reported improved survival with preoperative radiotherapy; however, the difference did not reach statistical significance, and some patients in this study also received chemotherapy.[47] Several studies reported a slightly higher rate of resection in the group that received preoperative therapy, and others noted decreased resectability in the radiotherapy group although none of these trends were statistically significant. In some cases, the treatment-related mortality rate for patients who received preoperative

Lead Author (Reference No.)	Histology	n	Total Dose (Gy/time)	Operable	Resectable	Operative Mortality (%)	Local Failure (%)	Resected 5-Year Survival (%)	3-Year Overal Survival (%)	5-Year Survival (%)
Launois (45)	SCC	57	—	46 (81%)	33 (58%)	11	NR	11.5	NR	NR
		67	39–45/8–12 d	62 (93%)	47 (71%)	14	NR	9.5	NR	NR
Gignoux (46)	SCC	106	—	106 (100%)	87 (82%)	19	33	10	NR	9
		102	33/12 d	97 (95%)	75 (74%)	24	21	16	NR	10
Mei (43)	NR	102	—	102 (100%)	87 (85%)	6	13	33	NR	30
		104	40/4 wk	104 (100%)	97 (93%)	5	4	37	NR	35
Nygaard (47)	SCC	50	—	41 (82%)	28 (68%)	13	NR	NR	9	NR
		58	35/4 wk	48 (83%)	26 (54%)	11	NR	NR	21	NR
Arnott (44)	SCC/AC	86	—	81 (94%)	62 (72%)	8	NR	NR	NR	17
		90	20/10 d	84 (93%)	67 (74%)	10	NR	NR	NR	9

Table 8–3. PREOPERATIVE RADIOTHERAPY: RANDOMIZED TRIALS

SCC = squamous cell carcinoma; AC = adenocarcinoma; NR = not reported; n = numbber of subjects in sample.

radiotherapy was higher than it was for patients who received surgery alone, and this rate exceeded 20 percent in several trials.[45,46] A meta-analysis (by the Oesophageal Cancer Collaborative Group) of these five randomized trials also failed to demonstrate conclusively that preoperative radiotherapy improves survival.[48] Therefore, preoperative therapy cannot be recommended outside of a clinical trial.

Postoperative Radiotherapy

Postoperative radiotherapy has also been studied as a measure to decrease the risk of local and regional recurrence and improve survival. Kasai and colleagues completed a retropective analysis that compared the outcomes of patients who received surgery and postoperative radiostherapy to the neck and mediastinum and the outcomes of patients who underwent surgery alone.[49] The authors reported a trend for improved 5-year survival as well as low local and regional failures in the node-negative group that received postoperative radiotherapy as part of this nonrandomized trial.

The potential benefits of postoperative radiotherapy were further studied in two prospective randomized studies by Teniere and colleagues and Fok and colleagues that are summarized in Table 8–4.[50,51] Neither study demonstrated an improvement in overall 5-year survival with the addition of radiotherapy; however, in the study by Teniere and colleagues, the rates of locoregional failure were lower in the group that received postoperative radiotherapy.[50] Although this difference reached statistical significance, the benefit was evident only in the subset of patients who were node negative. Fok and colleagues reported a high rate of therapy-related complications: 37 percent of patients in the radiotherapy arm developed complications such as gastritis or gastrointestinal bleeding, and 8 percent experienced treatment-related mortality.[51] On the basis of these randomized trials, there is no role for preoperative radiotherapy in the management of local and regional cancer of the esophagus, and the only possible role for postoperative radiotherapy is in the setting of positive margins.

COMBINED-MODALITY THERAPY

The treatment of esophageal carcinoma with radiotherapy or surgery alone has yielded unsatisfactory cure rates and has not resulted in a major impact on survival. Various multimodality approaches have been investigated in an effort to gain better local control and to manage the systemic disease in high-risk patients. These treatment approaches include preoperative combined-modality therapy or combined-modality therapy without surgical resection. Multiple phase II studies that have investigated various combinations of chemotherapy, radiotherapy, and surgery have indicated that multimodality therapy is tolerable. The survival times reported for these combined-modality trials are longer than those reported from most series of surgery or radiotherapy alone. Based on this suggested improvement, a number of randomized trials to determine whether combined-modality therapy is truly associated with improved outcomes have been completed. A second objective of these studies was to compare the toxicities of combined-modality therapy and single-modality therapy.

EXPERIENCE WITH CHEMOTHERAPY

Chemotherapy as a single modality has largely been used for the palliation of patients with recurrent or metastatic esophageal cancer. A number of cytotoxic

Table 8–4. POSTOPERATIVE RADIOTHERAPY: RANDOMIZED TRIALS							
Lead Author (Reference No.)	Cell Type	n	Total Dose (Gy)	Local/Regional Recurrence	Distant Recurrence	Median Survival (mo)	Overall 5-Year Survival (%)
Fok (51)	SCC	30	—	4 (13%)	9 (30%)	21.2	NR
	AC	30	49/350 fr	3 (10%)	12 (40%)	15.3	NR
Teniere (50)	SCC	119	—	15%	NR	NR	19
		102	45–55	30%*	NR	NR	19

SCC = squamous cell carcinoma; AC = adenocarcinoma; NR = not reported; fr = fraction; n = number of subjects in sample.
*Statistically significant difference in rate of local recurrence in patients without lymph node involvement ($p < .02$).

agents have been studied in regard to esophageal cancer, and most trials have evaluated their efficacy in patients with locally advanced or metastatic disease. The majority of these trials enrolled patients with squamous cell carcinomas; however, more recent trials have included patients with adenocarcinomas. Several reviews have described the results of trials of single-agent chemotherapy in patients with esophageal cancer.[52] Selected trials of single-agent chemotherapy are summarized in Table 8–5. Early reports came from phase I studies that enrolled a subset of patients with esophageal cancer or from phase II trials with broad eligibility criteria and in which many of the patients had received several prior chemotherapy agents. More recent phase II trials have enrolled patients who received limited chemotherapy or no prior chemotherapy. Response is defined as a shrinkage of measurable tumor lesions by 50 percent or greater. In these trials, single agents yielded modest objective response rates of 15 to 35 percent in the metastatic setting; higher response rates were seen in cases of localized disease. In early phase II studies, several agents that produced response rates of 15 percent or greater were identified. Although a number of agents demonstrated activity in cancer of the esophagus, the duration of response produced with these agents was generally brief, on the order of 2 to 4 months. No prospective trials have addressed whether chemotherapy provides a survival benefit to patients with metastatic carcinoma of the esophagus.

As single agents, the antitumor antibiotics bleomycin, mitomycin-C, and doxorubicin demonstrated antitumor activity, with response rates ranging from 15 to 26 percent in patients with squamous cell carcinoma. The antimetabolites fluorouracil and methotrexate also showed modest single-agent activity in patients with squamous cell carcinoma, with response rates of 10 to 35 percent. In the fluorouracil trials, bolus and infusional drug administration schedules were studied.[53,54]

Several platinum agents have been evaluated in patients with metastatic esophageal cancer. Cisplatin,

Table 8–5. ACTIVE SINGLE-AGENT CHEMOTHERAPY DRUGS FOR UNRESECTABLE OR METASTATIC ESOPHAGEAL CANCER: SELECTED TRIALS					
Lead Author (Reference)	**Agent**	**n**	**Histology**	**Response Rate**	**Response Duration**
Bonadonna (118)	Bleomycin	10	SCC	2 (20%)	NR
Tancini (119)	Bleomycin	29	SCC	4 (14%)	1–2 mo
Kolaric (120)	Bleomycin	15	SCC	4 (26%)	2.6 mo*
Whittington (121)	Mitomycin	7	NR	1 (14%)	NR
Engstrom (122)	Mitomycin	24	SCC	10 (42%)	12 wk*
Kolaric (120)	Doxorubicin	13	SCC	5 (38%)	3 mo
Ezdinli (53)	Doxorubicin	20	SCC	1 (5%)	13 wk
Lokich (54)	5-FU	13†	SCC/AC	11 (85%)	NR*
Ezdinli (53)	5-FU	26	SCC	4 (15%)	5–16 wk
Ezdinli (53)	Methotrexate	26	SCC	3 (12%)	8–15 wk
Advani (123)	Methotrexate	41†	SCC	20 (49%)	NR
Davis (124)	Cisplatin	17	SCC	1 (6%)	NR
Ravry (55)	Cisplatin	26	SCC	4 (15%)	1–12 mo
Panettiere (56)	Cisplatin	35	SCC	9 (26%)	3 mo*
Engstrom (122)	Cisplatin	24	SCC	6 (25%)	16 wk
Miller (57)	Cisplatin	15†	SCC	11 (73%)	NR
Kantarjian (58)	Cisplatin	12	AC	1 (8%)	NR
Sternberg (59)	Carboplatin	30	SCC	2 (7%)	7–16 mo*
Mannell (60)	Carboplatin	11	SCC	1 (9%)	NR
Bezwoda (64)	Vindesine	52	SCC	14 (27%)	26 wk
Conroy (65)	Vinorelbine	46	SCC	7 (15%)	21 wk*
Ajani (66)	Paclitaxel	18	SCC	5 (28%)	17 wk*
		32	AC	11 (34%)	
Einzig (68)	Docetaxel	41	AC	7 (17 %)	3–19 mo
Lin (71)	Irinotecan	21	AC	3 (14%)	NR
Enzinger (70)	Irinotecan	38	AC	15%	NR

AC = adenocarcinoma; 5-FU = 5-fluorouracil; n = number of subjects in sample; NR = not reported; SCC = squamous cell carcinoma.
*Median duration.
†Some patients were treated in preoperative setting.

administered by various schedules and doses, produced response rates of 15 to 26 percent in patients with metastatic squamous cell carcinoma.[55,56] More favorable antitumor activity was noted in a trial reported by Miller and colleagues, who used high-dose cisplatin to treat patients with nonmetastatic locally advanced squamous cell carcinoma.[57] In one small trial, cisplatin produced a low response rate in patients with adenocarcinoma of the esophagus.[58] Several phase II trials that investigated the activity of carboplatin in squamous cell carcinoma and adenocarcinoma cases found only limited antitumor activity for both histologic subtypes.[59–61]

The vinca alkaloid vindesine was studied in several phase II trials and demonstrated reproducible antitumor activity in cases of squamous cell carcinoma.[62–64] Vinorelbine, a newer plant alkaloid, has been also studied for treatment of squamous cell carcinoma. In a trial by the European Organization for Research and Treatment of Cancer, vinorelbine produced reponses in 20 percent of untreated patients.[65] The taxanes paclitaxel and docetaxel, which act at the level of the microtubules to produce cell-cycle arrest, have also been investigated. Ajani and colleagues have completed a phase II trial of paclitaxel as a single agent with filgrastim support in patients with untreated metastatic esophageal cancer.[66] Response activity was noted in 34 percent of adenocarcinoma patients and in 28 percent of patients with squamous cell carcinoma. A small trial investigating paclitaxel in patients with previously treated metastatic disease failed to demonstrate activity.[67] When evaluated as part of an Eastern Cooperative Oncology Group trial, docetaxel produced a response rate of 17 percent in patients with previously untreated metastatic esophageal or gastric adenocarcinoma.[68]

Etoposide, an inhibitor of type II topoisomerase, demonstrated a response rate of 19 percent in one trial.[69] The type I topoisomerase inhibitor irinotecan has been evaluated in untreated patients with unresectable adenocarcinoma. In a trial (by Enzinger and colleagues) of irinotecan administered weekly, 15 percent of patients achieved a partial response.[70] Lin and colleagues also observed activity for irinotecan administered at the same schedule and dose in patients with adenocarcinoma, many of whom had prior exposure to chemotherapy.[71]

Most of the drugs described above have been further studied in combination chemotherapy regimens. Results from selected phase II trials of multidrug regimens are summarized in Table 8–6. Overall, cisplatin-based combinations appear to be the best studied and demonstrate the most favorable reponse activity. Although early data suggest that tumors with squamous cell histology may be more responsive to chemotherapy,[72] it remains unclear whether a response difference exists. The response rates for cisplatin-based combination therapies range from 30 to 60 percent, and those results suggest that cisplatin-based combinations may be superior to single agents. One randomized phase II study compared the survival outcomes achieved with single-agent therapy to those achieved by combination therapy.[73] In this trial, 92 patients with locally advanced or metastatic esophageal cancer were randomized to receive either cisplatin with continuously infused fluorouracil every 3 weeks or cisplatin every 3 weeks. The response rates were 35 percent for the two-drug regimen and 19 percent for single-agent cisplatin. The median survival was 33 weeks for cisplatin/fluorouracil and 28 weeks for cisplatin alone. Treatment-related toxicity was more frequently encountered with the combination therapy: there were seven treatment-related deaths in the combination arm and no toxic deaths in the cisplatin-only arm. This phase II trial was not sufficiently powered to determine whether combination chemotherapy confers a survival benefit over single-agent chemotherapy.

The above-described phase II trials investigating chemotherapy for esophageal cancer vary considerably in their eligibility criteria, and the results are therefore difficult to compare directly. From these trials, it is evident that single-agent chemotherapy for patients with metastatic esophageal cancer produces modest response rates and brief response durations. Combination chemotherapy regimens appear to produce more favorable response rates; however, it is clear that agents that are more active are needed for the management of this disease.

Preoperative Chemotherapy

In theory, preoperative chemotherapy may eradicate micrometastatic disease and down-stage local disease to facilitate surgical resection. A potential advantage of preoperative chemotherapy is that the patient is best able to tolerate it early in the course of therapy, prior to a major resection. Another advantage is that the primary tumor response to chemotherapy may be assessed, and this information may be used to make decisions regarding the use of postoperative chemotherapy. One disadvantage of preoperative chemotherapy is that approximately half of the patients who receive it will not experience significant shrinkage of the primary tumor; they therefore derive no apparent benefit, and their surgery is delayed, increasing the potential risk for metastatic disease. In addition, a theoretic drawback is that early systemic therapy may allow the emergence of chemotherapy-resisitant cells.

A number of single-arm pilot studies have investigated preoperative chemotherapy for esophageal cancer. Selected phase II trials that investigated various preoperative combination chemotherapy regimens are summarized in Table 8–7. Some of the more recent trials have also included a course of postoperative chemotherapy. Collectively, these trials demonstrated the feasibility of this approach

when the majority of patients were able to undergo surgical resection after preoperative therapy. The rates of resection range from 47 to 90 percent, and the definition of resection appears to vary between series. The low rates of operative mortality encountered in these trials also suggest that preoperative chemotherapy does not adversely affect surgical outcome. On the basis of an apparent improvement in survival with this approach when compared with data from past surgical series, a series of phase III trials were undertaken to determine the true benefit of preoperative chemotherapy. These trials were designed to test the hypothesis that when compared with surgery alone, preoperative chemotherapy improves the outcomes of resection rate, disease-free survival, and overall survival.

Five phase III trials undertaken to compare preoperative chemotherapy to surgery alone are summarized in Table 8–8. One trial conducted by Roth and colleagues at the M.D. Anderson Cancer Center enrolled 39 patients to surgery alone or to two cycles of preoperative chemotherapy with cisplatin, bleomycin, and vindesine, followed by surgery and 6 months of postoperative chemotherapy with cisplatin

Table 8–6. ACTIVE COMBINATION CHEMOTHERAPY REGIMENS FOR UNRESECTABLE OR METASTATIC ESOPHAGEAL CANCER: SELECTED STUDIES					
Lead Author (Reference)	Combination Regimen	n	Histology	Response Rate	Response Duration
Coonley (125)	CDDP, bleomycin	18	SCC	3 (17%)	6 mo*
Kelsen (126)	CDDP, vindesine, bleomycin	24	SCC	8 (33%)	7 mo*
Dinwoodie (127)	CDDP, vindesine, bleomycin	27	SCC	7 (29%)	< 3 mo
Advani (123)	CDDP, MTX	42†	SCC	32 (76.2%)	12 mo*
Vogl (128)	CDDP, bleomycin, MTX	10	SCC	5 (50%)	6 mo*
De Besi (129)	CDDP, bleomycin, MTX	31	SCC	8 (26%)	5 mo*
Vogl (130)	CDDP, bleomycin, MTX, MGBG	14	SCC	9 (64%)	5 mo*
Kelsen (131)	CDDP, vindesine, MGBG	20	SCC	8 (40%)	3 mo
Chapman (132)	CDDP, vinblastine, MGBG	36	SCC	4 (11%)	6–24 wk
Gisselbrecht (133)	CDDP, 5-FU, doxorubicin	21	SCC	7 (33%)	3–22+ mo
DeBesi (134)	CDDP, 5-FU, allopurinol	37	SCC	13 (35%)	9 mo*
Iizuka (135)	CDDP, 5-FU	39	SCC	14 (36%)	3.5 mo*
Lovett (136)	Carboplatin, vinblastine	16	SCC	0 (0%)	NR
Kelsen (137)	Paclitaxel, CDDP	3	SCC	1 (33%)	> 4 mo
		17	AC	9 (53%)	
Petrasch (138)	Paclitaxel, CDDP	20	SCC + AC	8 (40%)	8 mo*
Ilson (139)	Paclitaxel, CDDP, 5-FU	30	SCC	15 (50%)	5.9 mo*
		30	AC	14 (47%)	5.7 mo*
Lokich (140)	Paclitaxel, CDDP, etoposide	22†	SCC + AC	22 (100%)	NR
Ilson (141)	Irinotecan/CDDP	35	SCC + AC	20 (57%)	4.2 mo*

AC = adenocarcinoma; CDDP = cisplatin; 5-FU = 5-fluorouracil; MGBG = mitoguanzone; MTX = methotrexate; NA = not available; NR = not reported; SCC = squamous cell carcinoma.
*Median duration.
†Some patients were treated in the preoperative setting.

Table 8–7. PHASE II TRIALS OF PREOPERATIVE CHEMOTHERAPY FOR ESOPHAGEAL CANCER

Lead Author (Reference)	Histology	Regimen	n	Operative Rate	Resection	Response	Pathologic Complete Response	Surgical Mortality	3-Year Survival	Median Survival (mo)
Kelsen (126)	SCC	CDDP, bleomycin, vindesine	45	34 (76%)	28 (62%)	28 (62%)	3 (9%)	2 (6%)	NR	16.2
Coonley (125)	SCC	CDDP, bleomycin	43	34 (80%)	26 (60%)	6 (14%)	0	4 (11%)	NR	11
Schlag (142)	SCC	CDDP, bleomycin, vindesine	42	40 (95%)	36 (90%)	17 (40%)	2 (5%)	4 (11%)	21%	15
Forastiere (143)	SCC/AC	CDDP, vinblastine, MGBG	29*	25 (86%)	80%*	12 (44%)	1 (3%)	0	21%	14
Carey (144)	SCC	CDDP, 5-FU	24*	22 (92%)	19 (79%)	14 (58%)	1 (5%)	1 (5%)	NR	6.7, 20.4†
Hilgenberg (145)	SCC	CDDP, 5-FU	35*	31 (88%)	27 (77%)	20 (57%)	1 (4%)	1 (4%)	54%	NR
Carey (146)	AC	CDDP, 5-FU	15*	11 (73%)	9 (60%)	6 (40%)	0	1 (7%)	NR	18.5
Kies (147)	SCC	CDDP, 5-FU	26*	14 (54%)	10 (38%)	11 (42%)	0	0	NR	17.8
Ajani (148)	AC	CDDP, 5-FU, etoposide	35*	32 (91%)	25 (71%)	17 (49%)	1 (3%)	NR	42%	23

SCC = squamous cell carcinoma; AC = adenocarcinoma; NR = not reported; CDDP = cisplatin; MGBG = mitoguanzone; 5-FU = 5-fluorouracil; n = number of subjects in sample.
*Some patients received postoperative chemotherapy or radiotherapy.
†Nonresponders and responders, respectively.

Table 8–8. RANDOMIZED TRIALS OF PREOPERATIVE CHEMOTHERAPY FOR ESOPHAGEAL CANCER

Lead Author (Reference)	Histology	Regimen	n	Operative Rate	Resection	Pathologic Complete Response	Surgical Mortality (%)	3-Year Survival (%)	Median Survival (mo)
Roth (74)	SCC	Surgery	20	19 (95%)	NS	—	0	NR	9
		CDDP/bleomycin/vindesine × 2 cycles, surgery, postoperative CDDP/vindesine × 6 mo*	19	17 (89%)	NS	6%	12	NR	9
Schlag (75)	SCC	Surgery	42	42 (100%)	33 (79%)	—	10	NR	10
		CDDP/5-FU × 3 cycles, surgery	34	27 (79%)	19 (56%)	NR	19	NR	10
Nygaard (47)	SCC	Surgery	50	41 (82%)	28 (68%)	—	13	9	NR
		XRT 3,500 cGy followed by surgery	58	48 (83%)	26 (54%)	NR	11	21	NR
		CDDP/bleomycin × 2 cycles, surgery	56	50 (89%)	29 (58%)	NR	15	3	NR
		Sequential CDDP/bleomycin × 2 cycles, then XRT 3,500 cGy, followed by surgery	53	47 (89%)	31 (66%)	NR	24	17	NR
Kelsen (16)	SCC/AC	Surgery	227	217 (96%)	205 (90%)	—	6	23	16.1
		CDDP/5-FU × 3 cycles, surgery, postoperative CDDP/5-FU × 2 cycles*	213	171 (80%)	162 (76%)	3%	6	26	14.9
Kok (77)	SCC	Surgery	74	73 (98%)	63 (85%)	—	NR	NR	11.0
		CDDP/5-FU × 2–4 cycles, surgery	74	68 (92%)	63 (85%)	NR	NR	NR	18.5
									(p = .002)

SCC = squamous cell carcinoma; AC = adenocarcinoma; NR = not reported; CDDP = cisplatin; 5-FU = 5-fluorouracil; XRT = radiotherapy; n = number of subjects in sample.
*Regimen also included postoperative chemotherapy.

and vindesine.[74] Although a 47 percent overall response rate and a 6 percent complete response rate were noted after preoperative chemotherapy, there was no difference in median survival or resectability between the two treatment groups. Chemotherapy was complicated by two treatment-related deaths and two postoperative deaths.

Schlag and colleagues studied 46 patients randomized to immediate surgery or to preoperative chemotherapy with cisplatin and fluorouracil for two cycles, then surgery.[75] The preoperative chemotherapy produced a response rate of 47 percent and was associated with considerable toxicity. There was no difference in the surgical resectability or median survival between treatment groups, but the chemotherapy group had higher postoperative mortality. Based on this interim analysis, the study was terminated before reaching its accrual goals.

Nygaard and colleagues randomized 186 patients to one of four treatment arms: surgery alone; preoperative chemotherapy and surgery; preoperative radiotherapy and surgery; and preoperative chemotherapy plus sequential radiotherapy, then surgery.[47] The preoperative chemotherapy consisted of two cycles of cisplatin and bleomycin. In a pooled subgroup analysis, there was no significant difference in survival for groups with or without chemotherapy. Three-year survival rates for the preoperative chemotherapy-plus-surgery arm and for the surgery arm were not significantly different (9% and 3%, respectively). When the preoperative-chemotherapy and preoperative-chemoradiation groups were compared with the preoperative-radiotherapy and surgery-alone groups, there was also no difference in survival. Several patients enrolled in the chemotherapy arms developed respiratory failure that was presumed to be secondary to bleomycin.

All three of these small randomized studies of preoperative chemotherapy were powered to detect only very large survival differences and were therefore considered inconclusive. Results of the US Gastrointestinal Intergroup study INT 113 (RTOG 89-11), a large phase III study comparing preoperative chemotherapy followed by surgery to surgery alone, have been reported.[16] The preoperative-treatment group received three cycles of cisplatin and fluorouracil, followed by surgery. Patients who had sta-

ble disease or responding disease following the preoperative therapy received two additional cycles of chemotherapy postoperatively. This study enrolled 467 patients with squamous cell carcinoma or adenocarcinoma. The preoperative cisplatin and fluorouracil appeared tolerable, and no increase in operative morbidity or mortality was reported in the preoperative-therapy group. There were no significant differences in median survival between the groups (14.9 months for preoperative chemotherapy and 16.1 months for surgery only). In addition, survival did not vary with histologic subtype. The frequency of first failure at a distant site was slightly higher in the surgery group than in the chemotherapy group (50% and 41%, respectively, $p = .21$). Although the regimen used as preoperative therapy is believed to be effective, one possible reason for the negative result is that inadequate amounts of therapy were administered. Only two-thirds of patients received the intended three cycles of preoperative therapy, and only a fraction of the patients received any postoperative therapy.

The preliminary results of a randomized trial investigating preoperative chemotherapy were recently reported by the British Medical Research Council Upper GI Tract Cancer Group.[76] This trial compared surgery alone to two courses of cisplatin and 5-fluorouracil (5-FU) followed by surgery. Over 800 patients with squamous cell carcinoma, adenocarcinoma, or undifferentiated carcinoma were enrolled in this trial. About two-thirds of the patients had adenocarcinomas. The preoperative chemotherapy proved tolerable, and the rates of postoperative complication were 38 percent for the chemotherapy arm and 41 percent for the surgery-alone arm. Overall survival was statistically better in the group that received preoperative chemotherapy (hazard ratio of 0.77, $p = .002$). The median survival was 17.4 months compared with 13.4 months for patients undergoing surgery alone, and the 2-year survival rates were 45 percent and 33 percent, respectively. There was no difference in treatment effect according to histology.

A smaller trial on preoperative chemotherapy was reported in abstract form by Kok and colleagues from the Netherlands.[77] In this study, 160 patients with squamous cell carcinoma of the esophagus were randomized to receive cisplatin/etoposide for two to four cycles, followed by esophagectomy or esophagectomy alone. Preliminary analysis of this trial indicated a significant survival difference: median survival was 18.5 months in the preoperative-chemotherapy arm and was 11 months in the surgery-alone arm ($p = .002$).

There has been one prospective randomized study that compared the preoperative modalities of radiotherapy and chemotherapy.[78] Ninety-six patients with operable squamous cell carcinoma were randomized to receive either two cycles of cisplatin, vindesine, and bleomycin or radiation (55 Gy) before a planned surgical procedure. Patients with tumors classed as T3 and any N or with unresectable tumors received postoperative crossover therapy of radiation given to patients receiving preoperative chemotherapy and vice versa. The objective response rates to preoperative therapy, the resection rates, and the operative mortality were similar for both modalities. There was no difference in the pattern of failure, based on the preoperative therapy. This finding suggests that the chemotherapy regimen used was ineffective in managing occult systemic disease and offers support for the investigation of new and more effective chemotherapy regimens in the preoperative setting. Because of the crossover design, it was not possible to analyze survival on the basis of the preoperative therapy delivered.

Several trials have addressed the possibility that chemotherapy following a potentially curative resection might improve survival outcomes. These trials have failed to demonstrate a benefit from postoperative chemotherapy. A recent trial by Ando and colleagues from Japan randomized patients with squamous cell carcinoma to esophageal resection only or to resection followed by combination chemotherapy with cisplatin and fluorouracil.[79] Preliminary analysis of this large trial of 242 patients revealed no statistically significant difference in overall survival (51% for the control group and 61% for the chemotherapy group). An improvement in 5-year disease-free survival for the group that received chemotherapy (46% vs 58%, $p = .05$) was noted.

In summary, several phase II and III trials have demonstrated that preoperative chemotherapy results in high overall response rates in the range of 45 to 65 percent; however, complete pathologic responses are less common. Several randomized trials have indicated no survival benefit from preoperative chemotherapy. However, a preliminary report of a larger randomized trial with a more powerful analysis indicated improved survival outcomes with the addition of chemotherapy to surgery. This trial offers support for the continued investigation of preoperative chemotherapy in randomized trials. At the present time, surgery alone is the standard of care for patients for whom surgical resection is part of the treatment plan.

Concomitant Chemotherapy and Radiotherapy (Chemoradiotherapy)

The simultaneous or concomitant administration of a chemotherapeutic agent with radiation therapy has been investigated in a number of advanced malignancies, including head and neck cancer, lung cancer, and anal carcinoma, as well as in esophageal carcinoma. The goal of concomitant chemoradiotherapy is to improve local control by overcoming radioresistance and to decrease systemic failure rates by eradicating distant micrometastases.[80,81]

Radiation and chemotherapy can interact theoretically in four different ways, as described by Steel and Peckham.[82] The first is the independent action of each treatment modality, or "spatial cooperation." Radiotherapy produces tumor reduction within the localized radiation field whereas chemotherapy exerts its effect against systemic disease that may be occult. The second mode of interaction is "toxicity independence," in which the chemotherapeutic agent and the radiation produce different or "nonoverlapping" toxicities. This property allows the two modalities to be administered safely and simultaneously at sufficient doses to produce an antitumor effect and preserve normal tissues. The theoretic outcome of the first two mechanisms is additive antitumor activity without interaction of the two modalities. The third mechanism postulates the protection of normal tissues by the chemotherapeutic agent's allowing of higher doses of radiation. Based on this postulate, increased efficacy would result only if the tumor were not radioprotected as well.

Finally, there can be a direct interaction between the chemotherapeutic agent and radiation, in which the drug enhances, sensitizes, or potentiates the effect of radiation on tumor tissue.

Various mechanisms of interaction between chemotherapy and radiation therapy have been proposed.[80,81] These interactions may result from the differential effects of chemotherapy and radiation on the cell population, based on certain features such as tumor cell hypoxia or cell-cycle specificity. Another interaction may result from decreased tumor cell repopulation following fractionated radiation due to chemotherapy. For example, certain chemotherapeutic agents may inhibit the repair of radiation-induced damage. Radiation sensitization may also result from cell-cycle synchronization or from the recruitment of tumor cells into a more radioresponsive cell-cycle phase. For example, paclitaxel produces arrest in the G_2-M phase of the cell cycle, the phase in which tumor cells are most sensitive to radiation. The interaction of the chemotherapy and radiation therapy may result in increased toxicity to human tissues. Therefore, acute toxicity may preclude the administration of chemotherapy at doses considered sufficient to provide systemic activity. Clearly, acute toxicity is dependent on the chemotherapy agents used and their schedule of administration. The most common acute toxicities of chemoradiation are esophagitis and hematologic depression. Since an effective chemoradiotherapy regimen will exploit the complex interactions to balance efficacy and tolerability, clinical trials must include end points of survival, treatment morbidity, and quality of life.

Combined Chemoradiotherapy as Curative Therapy

There are several potential advantages to the use of chemoradiation for esophageal cancer. When the two modalities are combined, both systemic and locoregional disease are addressed simultaneously at the earliest possible time. Another advantage is that a number of chemotherapy agents used in the management of esophageal cancer act as radiation sensitizers, and combining the two modalities may produce an additive effect locoregionally within the irradiated field. The disadvantage of this approach is that some chemoradiotherapy regimens may produce significant toxicity that can be life threatening or that can impair quality of life.

The initial studies of chemoradiation for esophageal cancer were undertaken at Wayne State University, where treatment was modeled after experience with concurrent radiation therapy and chemotherapy in anal carcinoma. These studies demonstrated that chemoradiation could produce complete responses in esophageal cancer, with an apparent benefit in survival.[83,84] Several phase II trials were later undertaken to further investigate the feasibility and tolerability of concurrent chemotherapy and radiation therapy for cancer of the esophagus. These trials incorporated a number of chemotherapy agents known to demonstrate activity in esophageal cancer; many (such as fluorouracil, cisplatin, and mitomycin) were also known to produce radiosensitization. The results of several early pilot studies of combined chemotherapy and radiotherapy are summarized in Table 8–9. Overall, the median survival times for patients enrolled in

Table 8–9. PHASE II TRIALS OF CHEMORADIOTHERAPY FOR ESOPHAGEAL CANCER

Lead Author (Reference)	Histology	Regimen	Radiotherapy (Gy)	n	Response Rate (%)	Median Survival (mo)	2-Year Survival (%)
Leichman (149)	SCC	5-FU/CDDP, mitomycin/bleomycin	5,000	20	NR	22	NR
Coia (85)	SCC/AC	5-FU, mitomycin	5,000–6,000	90	NR	Stage I, II: 18 Stage III: 9 Stage IV: 7	Stage I, II: 44
John (87)	SCC/AC	5-FU, mitomycin/CDDP	4,140–5,040	30	77	11	29
Seitz (86)	SCC	5-FU/CDDP	4,000	35	71	17 (Stage I, II: 28)	41

SCC = squamous cell carcinoma; AC = adenocarcinoma; NR = not reported; CDDP = cisplatin; 5-FU = 5-fluorouracil; n = number of subjects in sample.
*Regimen also included postoperative chemotherapy.

these studies were favorable (in the range of 9 to 22 months), and the toxicity appeared manageable although increased over radiotherapy alone. Coia and colleagues used fluorouracil and mitomycin together with 5,000 to 6,000 cGy of concurrent radiation therapy for all stages of squamous cell carcinoma.[85] They reported median survival times of 18 months and 5-year actuarial survival rates of 18 percent for patients with stage I and II disease. Results were less favorable for patients with stage III and IV disease, who had median survival times of 9 and 7 months, respectively. The dominant pattern of failure was distant; 72 percent of the patients developed systemic metastases, and 48 percent failed locally. Seitz and colleagues reported a trial of 35 patients with squamous cell carcinoma who received fluorouracil and cisplatin with concomitant split-course radiotherapy.[86] The median survival of stage I and II patients was 28 months. John and colleagues reported results with a regimen of infusional 5-FU, cisplatin, and mitomycin, administered with concurrent radiation at doses of 4,140 to 5,040 cGy.[87] After completion of the chemoradiation, three cycles of maintenance chemotherapy with methotrexate, fluorouracil, and leucovorin were delivered. The regimen demonstrated significant activity, with a 77 percent clinical complete-response rate.

These pilot trials indicated the feasibility of combining chemotherapy with chest radiation where the reported response activity and survival rates compared favorably to historical series. The toxicity encountered in these early trials was manageable but greater than what would be expected with radiation therapy alone. Later, it was shown that concurrent radiation and chemotherapy promotes the early restoration of swallowing and the long-term maintenance of swallowing function. A retrospective analysis by Coia and colleagues assessed the initial and long-term swallowing function of individuals who received concurrent chemoradiation.[88] They noted an initial improvement in dysphagia in more than 90 percent of patients, with a median time to improvement of 2 weeks. The majority of patients also experienced normal or near-normal swallowing at 3 years following treatment. The authors concluded that the regimen of chemotherapy and radiation offered superior swallowing function when compared to radiation therapy alone.

Four randomized studies comparing concurrent chemoradiation to radiation therapy alone as curative therapy for patients with locally advanced esophageal carcinoma are summarized in Table 8–10. A small randomized study reported from the National Cancer Institute of Brazil compared a regimen of concurrent fluorouracil, mitomycin, and bleomycin with radiation therapy (5,000 cGy) to radiation therapy (5,000 cGy) alone.[89] There was no significant difference in survival rates between the

Table 8–10. RANDOMIZED TRIALS OF CHEMORADIATION VERSUS RADIATION AS DEFINITIVE THERAPY FOR ESOPHAGEAL CANCER						
Lead Author (Reference)	Histology	Regimen	n	Median Survival (mo)	3-Year Overall Survival (%)	5-Year Overall Survival (%)
Smith (92)	SCC	XRT 4,000 cGy, then surgery or additional XRT 2,000 cGy	60	9.2	8	—
		Concurrent 5-FU/mitomycin × 2 cycles and XRT 4,000 cGy, then surgery or additional XRT 2,000 cGy	59	14.8*	13	—
Herskovic (93, 94)	SCC/AC	XRT 6,400 cGy	62	9.0	—	0
		Concurrent CDDP/5-FU and XRT 5,000 cGy	61	14.1**	—	27**
Araujo (89)	SCC	XRT 5,000 cGy	31	—	—	6
		Preoperative concurrent mitomycin/5-FU/bleomycin and XRT 5,000 cGy, then surgery	28	—	—	16
Slabber (90)	SCC	XRT 4,000 cGy (split course)	36	4.8	NR	—
		Preoperative concurrent CDDP/5-FU and XRT 4,000 cGy (split course)	34	5.7****	NR	—

SCC = squamous cell carcinoma; AC = adenocarcinoma; NR = not reported; CDDP = cisplatin; 5-FU = 5-fluorouracil; XRT = radiotherapy; n = number of subjects in sample.
*p = .03; **p = .0001; ***p = .16; ****p = .42.

treatment groups. Due to the small number of patients studied in this trial, the power was too low to detect any but a very large difference between the treatment arms. Esophagitis and myelosuppression were more severe in the combined-modality arm.

A trial conducted by Slabber and colleagues in South Africa also used a split course of radiation therapy in their small randomized trial comparing chemoradiation and radiation alone.[90] This trial randomized 70 patients with T3 N0–1 M0 squamous cell cancers of the esophagus to radiotherapy alone given as a split course of 4,000 cGy over 4 weeks or to combined-modality therapy of split-course radiation (4,000 cGy) with cisplatin (15 mg/m^2 daily) and continuous-infusion 5-FU (600 mg/m^2 daily) on days 1 to 5 and days 29 to 33. The treatment was described as well tolerated in both groups. There was no difference in median survival for the two groups although the low radiation dose delivered in both arms was suboptimal.

A study conducted by the Eastern Cooperative Oncology Group randomized 119 patients with squamous cell carcinoma to fluorouracil, cisplatin, and mitomycin with radiation (4,000 cGy) or radiation alone (4,000 cGy).[91,92] Chemotherapy included mitomycin-C (10 mg/m^2) administered on day 2 and continuous-infusion fluorouracil (1,000 mg/m^2 daily) administered on days 2 through 5 and days 28 to 31. Individuals in either treatment arm were allowed surgical resection after the radiation therapy; those who did not have surgery received an additional 2,000 cGy of radiotherapy. Twenty-three patients from each treatment arm underwent surgical resection; 7 patients (5 from the combined-modality arm and 2 from the radiotherapy arm) had a complete pathologic response documented at resection. Analysis of this trial showed a significant difference in median survival in favor of the combined-modality arm (14.8 months vs 9.2 months). Although the trial was not purely nonsurgical, the trend to improved survival was evident regardless of whether surgical resection was undertaken.

The Radiation Therapy Oncology Group conducted a randomized phase III study (RTOG 85-01) comparing combined chemoradiotherapy and radiotherapy alone in 123 patients with T1–3 N0–1 M0 squamous cell carcinoma or adenocarcinoma of the

thoracic esophagus (not including the cervical esophagus).[93, 94] The predominant tumor histology in this trial was squamous cell carcinoma. It is not clear what percentage of the patients enrolled in this trial was potentially resectable. The chemoradiation arm included two courses of chemotherapy concomitant with radiation therapy to a cumulative dose of 5,000 cGy, followed by two additional courses of the same chemotherapy. The chemotherapy regimen consisted of cisplatin (75 mg/m^2 on day 1) and fluorouracil (1,000 mg/m^2 daily on days 1 through 4), administered every 4 weeks during radiotherapy and then every 3 weeks after radiotherapy. The radiotherapy-alone arm included 6.4 weeks of therapy, to a cumulative dose of 6,400 cGy. Patients were treated surgically only for recurrences or complications. Systemic toxicity was greater in the multimodality arm. In the combined arm, 64 percent of patients experienced severe or life-threatening side effects, including esophagitis in 33 percent, nausea and vomiting in 8 percent, and hematologic toxicity in 46 percent. There were 2 treatment-related deaths in the multimodality arm. Patients who received radiotherapy alone had a 28 percent incidence of severe or life-threatening side effects. The most common acute toxicity with radiotherapy alone was esophagitis (in 18% of patients). There was no significant difference in long-term swallowing function between the two treatment arms. The initial report and an update of RTOG 85-01, with all cases followed to 5 years, demonstrated a survival advantage for concurrent chemoradiation. At 5 years, 30 percent of the patients in the chemoradiation group were alive, compared to 0 percent of patients in the radiotherapy-alone arm. Analysis of the failure rates at 2 years showed a lower rate of local failure (45% vs 59%) and a decreased incidence of systemic metastases (37% vs 21%) in the chemoradiation therapy arm when compared to the radiation-only arm. This study provides strong evidence that concurrent chemoradiation is superior to radiotherapy alone for patients with esophageal cancer, especially squamous cell carcinoma, who are managed without surgical resection. This trial also indicates greater but acceptable toxicities with combined-modality therapy. On the basis of these observations, this chemoradiation regimen has been accepted as a standard therapy for those individuals with localized esophageal cancer who require nonsurgical therapy.

In an attempt to improve the local and regional control achieved with chemoradiation in the RTOG 85-01 trial, a phase II trial (INT 0122) was designed to determine whether intensifiying the chemotherapy and increasing the doses of radiation therapy given concurrently with chemotherapy could provide benefit. In the INT 0122 trial, the RTOG 85-01 regimen was modified as follows: the 5-FU continuous infusion was increased from 4 to 5 days; the total number of cycles of chemotherapy was increased from four to five cycles; three full cycles of preoperative chemotherapy were added prior to combined chemoradiation; and the radiation dose was increased from 5,000 to 6,480 cGy.[95,96] Although the incidence of severe toxicity and survival for the INT 0122 trial was similar to that for the RTOG 85-01 study, the incidence of treatment-related mortality from preoperative 5-FU/cisplatin followed by combined-modality therapy was high, at 9 percent. Minsky and colleagues concluded that the intensive preoperative approach of the INT 0122 trial did not appear to offer a benefit when compared with conventional doses and techniques of combined-modality therapy.

The INT 0123 trial was initiated in follow up to the INT 0122 trial and was designed to test the hypothesis that increasing the doses of radiation therapy given concurrently with chemotherapy could provide benefit. In this trial, the chemoradiation arm from the RTOG 85-01 trial served as the control arm. The experimental arm used a chemotherapy regimen identical to the control arm, with radiation therapy doses of 6,480 cGy. When an interim analysis of the INT 0123 trial indicated inferior survival in the experimental arm, the trial was terminated early. Based on this trial, which indicates the poor tolerance to external beam radiation doses of > 6,500 cGy when delivered concurrently with chemotherapy, this approach remains investigational.

Other approaches to intensifying the radiation therapy delivered in combination with chemotherapy include accelerated fractionation and brachytherapy. Several series have investigated the incorporation of brachytherapy into the combined-modality approach. A phase II trial reported by Calais and colleagues indicated the feasibility and tolerance of external beam radiation plus concurrent chemotherapy and esophageal brachytherapy as definitive therapy for patients with unresectable carcinoma of the esophagus.[97] Treatment included three cycles of chemotherapy with fluorouracil, mitomycin, and cisplatin with concurrent external beam radiotherapy (6,000 cGy) followed by high-dose-rate brachytherapy (500 cGy per week for 2 weeks). At a median follow-up of 39 months, the 3- and 5-year actuarial survival rates were 27 percent and 18 percent, respectively. Eleven percent of the patients developed late-occurring toxicity, and one patient died from treatment-related toxicity. Two patients (4%) developed fistulas, although tumor progression was noted in both cases. Post-treatment swallowing function was noted as "good" in 75 percent of patients. The local failure rate was 43 percent. Overall, the results of this trial were comparable to those of other trials of curative chemoradiation.

The Radiation Therapy Oncology Group conducted a phase I/II trial (RTOG 92-07) to investigate the addition of brachytherapy to the combined-modality regimen used in the RTOG 85-01 trial.[98,99] Treatment included 50 Gy of external beam radiation given as 25 fractions over 5 weeks, followed 2 weeks later by esophageal brachytherapy given at either a high dose rate or a low dose rate. Of the initial 49 eligible patients, only 24 (49%) completed the entire course of therapy. This therapy produced an initial complete-response rate of 74 percent and an estimated 3-year survival rate of 29 percent. Severe toxicity was documented in 59 percent of patients and consisted of hematologic and gastrointestinal side effects. Life-threatening or fatal toxicity was encountered in 24 percent and 10 percent of patients on the brachytherapy and control arms, respectively. Esophageal strictures were fatal in 3 patients. Comparison of the response rates, pattern of failure, and survival rates resulting with the RTOG 92-07 regimen with the results from the RTOG 85-01 trial suggests that a brachytherapy boost provides little benefit over external beam radiation plus chemotherapy. Based on the high rate of esophageal stricture and the absence of clear benefit in terms of tumor response, local control, and survival rates, the regimen was not felt worthy of further investigation. The current guidelines of the American Brachytherapy Society do not recommend the use of concurrent brachytherapy and chemotherapy.[41]

Preoperative Chemoradiation

Several phase II trials of preoperative chemoradiotherapy for carcinoma of the esophagus have been conducted, and selected pilot studies of concurrent chemoradiation are summarized in Table 8–11. Many of these studies report high rates of pathologic response and survival results that compare favorably with historical controls. There is, nevertheless, toxicity with this combined-modality approach. On the basis of these phase II studies, several randomized trials comparing preoperative chemoradiation followed by surgery with surgery alone were undertaken. The results of these trials are summarized in Table 8–12.

One of the randomized trials investigated sequential chemoradiotherapy followed by surgery versus surgery alone in patients with squamous cell carcinoma. In the study reported by LePrise and colleagues, the multimodality therapy included a course of chemotherapy with cisplatin and fluorouracil, followed first by radiotherapy and then by a second course of cisplatin and 5-FU chemotherapy before surgery.[100] In this trial, the chemotherapy doses and the cumulative radiotherapy dose (2,000 cGy) were low. A total of 86 patients were enrolled, and there was no difference in 1- or 3-year survival rates.

The trial reported by Bosset and colleagues randomized 297 patients with stage I or II squamous cell carcinoma to surgery alone or to preoperative combined therapy.[101] Concurrent chemoradiotherapy was delivered as two 1-week courses separated by several weeks: cisplatin (80 mg/m^2) each week and radiotherapy in five daily fractions of 3.7 Gy. The chemoradiation group experienced longer disease-free survival and a higher frequency of curative resection. However, the postoperative mortality rate was higher with combined-modality therapy, and there was no difference in survival between the two groups. This study was criticized for the use of single-agent chemotherapy and the low cumulative radiation dose.[101]

Urba and colleagues reported a small phase III study of surgery alone versus trimodality therapy.[102–104] Of the 100 patients enrolled, 75 percent had adenocarcinoma and 25 percent had squamous cell carcinoma. The preoperative chemotherapy included a 21-day continuous infusion of 5-FU,

Table 8–11. PHASE II TRIALS OF PREOPERATIVE CHEMORADIOTHERAPY FOR CARCINOMA OF THE ESOPHAGUS

Lead Author (Reference)	Histology	Regimen	Radiotherapy (Gy)	n	Operative Rate	Resection Rate	Pathologic Complete Response	Surgical Mortality	Median Survival (mo)	Long-Term Survival (%)
Franklin (83)	SCC	Mitomycin, 5-FU	3,000	30	23 (77%)	23 (77%)	9 (39%)	4 (17%)	9*	NR
Leichman (149)	SCC	CDDP, 5-FU	3,000	21	19 (90%)	15 (71%)	7 (37%)	5 (27%)	18	NR
Poplin (150)	SCC	CDDP, 5-FU	3,000	113	71 (63%)	55 (49%)	18 (25%)	8 (11%)	12	3 yr:16
Seydel (151)	SCC	CDDP, 5-FU	3,000*	41	27 (66%)	26 (63%)	8 (30%)	1 (4%)	13	3 yr:8
Forastiere (108, 109)	SCC/AC	5-FU, CDDP, vinblastine	3,750 or 4,500	43	41 (95%)	36 (84%)	10 (24%)	1 (2%)	32 (AC), 23 (SCC)	5 yr AC: 34, 5 yr SCC: 31
Naunheim (152)	SCC/AC	CDDP, 5-FU	3,000 or 3,600	47	39 (83%)	34 (72%)	8 (21%)	1 (3%)	23	3 yr:40
Urba (153)	AC	CDDP, 5-FU	4,900 (350 cGy, 14 fx)	24	19 (83%)	19 (83%)	2 (11%)	1 (6%)	11	NR
Bates (110)	SCC/AC	CDDP, 5-FU	4,500	35	35 (100%)	33 (94 %)	18 (51%)	3 (9%)	25.8	3 yr: 41
Stahl (154)	SCC/AC	CDDP/etoposide/cisplatin†	4,000	72	49 (68%)	48 (67%)	16 (33%)	7 (15%)	17	2 yr: 33yr
Forastiere (155)	SCC/AC	CDDP, 5-FU	4,400	50	47 (94%)	45 (90%)	19 (40%)	0	31	2 yr: 58
Posner (156)	SCC/AC	CDDP, 5-FU, α-interferon	4,000	44	37 (94%)	36 (90%)	10 (24%)	3 (8%)	27	2 yr: 52

SCC = squamous cell carcinoma; AC = adenocarcinoma; NR = not reported; CDDP = cisplatin; 5-FU = 5-florouracil; fx = fractions; n = number of subjects in sample.
*Postoperative radiotherapy (2,000 Gy) was administered if pathologic complete response was not evident at resection.
†Regimen also included preoperative or postoperative chemotherapy.

Table 8–12. RANDOMIZED TRIALS OF PREOPERATIVE CHEMORADIOTHERAPY WITH SURGERY VERSUS SURGERY ALONE

Lead Author (Reference)	Histology	Regimen	n	Resection Rate	Pathologic Complete Response (%)	Surgical Mortality (%)	3-Year Survival (%)	Median Survival (mo)
Bosset (101)	SCC	Surgery	139	112 (81%)	—	3.6	25	18.6
		Concurrent CDDP × 2 cycles and XRT 3,750 cGy, then surgery	143	94 (69%)	26	12.3*	27	18.6
Walsh (105)	AC	Surgery	55	55 (100%)	—	3.6	6	11
		Concurrent CDDP/5-FU × 2 cycles and XRT 4,000 cGy, then surgery	58	55 (90%)	25	8.5	32**†	16**†
Urba (102–104)	SCC/AC	Surgery	50	NR	—	NR	16	17.6
		Concurrent CDDP/5-FU/vinblastine and XRT 4,500 cGy, then surgery	50	NR	28	NR	32***	16.9
Le Prise (100)	SCC	Surgery	45	42 (93%)	—	7.0	13.8	NR
		Sequential CDDP/5-FU × 2 cycles, then XRT 2,000 cGy followed by surgery	41	35 (85%)	10	8.5	19.2	NR

SCC = squamous cell carcinoma; AC = adenocarcinoma; NR = not reported; CDDP = cisplatin; 5-FU = 5-fluorouracil; XRT = radiotherapy; n = number of subjects in sample.
*p = .012; **p = .01; ***p = .15.
†Statistically significant difference.

combined with cisplatin and vinblastine. The concurrent radiotherapy was administered in 150-cGy fractions twice daily, to a total dose of 4,500 cGy. Three-year survival rates were 16 percent for the surgery alone and 30 percent for the multimodality arms (p = .15). This study was sufficiently powered to detect a large survival difference between the treatment groups and was designed on the assumption that combined-modality therapy would provide a doubling in median survival. Although there was no statistically significant survival difference between treatment arms, this trial did not have the ability to assess more subtle survival differences.

A randomized study by Walsh and colleagues compared surgery alone to multimodality therapy in 113 patients with esophageal adenocarcinoma.[105] Multimodality therapy included two courses of chemotherapy (fluorouracil, 15 mg/kg daily for 5 days, and cisplatin, 75 mg/m² on day 7) in weeks 1 and 6. Radiotherapy was administered, beginning with the first course of chemotherapy, for 15 fractions over 3 weeks, to a cumulative dose of 4,000 cGy. The chemoradiotherapy regimen was reportedly well tolerated; 10 percent of the patients experienced severe toxicity. A comparison of the treatment groups revealed a survival advantage for the multimodality group, with 3-year survival rates of 32 percent for the multimodal group and 6 percent for the surgery-alone group (p = .01). The 25 percent

rate of complete pathologic response following chemotherapy and radiation was comparable to that of other reported multimodality regimens. The pattern of failure was not reported for this study. A flaw of this study was the lack of pretreatment CT, which may have led to an imbalance in treatment assignments. Also criticized were the poor survival results obtained in the surgery-alone arm.

Thus, to date, one small phase III trial comparing concurrent chemoradiation plus surgery to surgery alone has demonstrated a statistically significant survival benefit from multimodality therapy. The other three randomized trials failed to demonstrate any survival benefit although the trial undertaken by Bosset and colleagues did report a decline in local failure. One explanation for the difference in outcomes between these randomized studies is that the studies by Bosset and colleagues and by LePrise and colleagues used sequential chemotherapy and radiation, which may provide suboptimal local control when compared with simultaneous chemoradiation.[100,101] In the study by Bosset and colleagues, the rate of perioperative mortality was high and may have negated the benefit from chemoradiotherapy. Interestingly, the positive trial was limited to patients with adenocarcinoma histology although this factor is not likely to explain why chemoradiation provided benefit. Since each of these randomized trials of preoperative chemoradiotherapy had design flaws and was small in size with low power, none of the trials are definitive. In 1994, a phase III trial comparing trimodality therapy to surgery alone was undertaken by the Cancer and Leukemia Group B with the support of the United States Gastrointestinal Intergroup to determine whether preoperative chemoradiation improves survival and quality of life. Because of the widespread use of trimodality therapy in the medical community, accrual to this trial was poor and warranted its recent closure.

The relative contribution of surgical resection to the multimodality approach is not known. For surgical resection to be beneficial, it must improve local control and survival as well as quality of life. Work by Gill and colleagues attempted to evaluate whether surgery following chemoradiation improves survival.[106] Their study suggested that if improved local and regional control occurs following chemoradiotherapy with or without surgery, a change in the pattern of relapse will result and will place more patients at risk of developing systemic metastases. A retrospective analysis reported by Denham and colleagues also indicated that the enhanced local control achieved with chemoradiation may not result in a survival advantage because distant metastases become the predominant and life-threatening pattern of failure.[107] The findings of these retrospective analyses are supported by the long-term results of the Wayne State University trial (published by Coia and colleagues), which indicated that the majority of patients who had recurrences following chemoradiation developed metastatic disease with or without local and regional failure.[85] From this series, it appeared that chemoradiation altered the failure pattern from local failure to one dominated by distant failure and that surgery would not have improved long-term survival. Investigators of several phase II and III trials of preoperative chemoradiation have reported that patients obtaining a pathologic complete response following chemoradiotherapy have more favorable outcomes.[107,108] This finding also suggests that if local control is achieved with chemoradiation and if systemic disease is absent or eradicated with chemotherapy, then surgical resection may not be a necessary component of the multimodality approach.

Results from a trial of preoperative chemoradiation followed by esophagectomy (published by Forastiere and colleagues) indicated that patients with complete pathologic tumor response and those with residual tumor present at esophagectomy could achieve long-term survival beyond 5 years.[108,109] Bates and colleagues also reported a prospective trial of preoperative chemoradiation, in which 25 percent of patients with residual tumor in the surgical specimen achieved long-term survival.[110] A University of Pittsburgh trial examining the necessity of esophagectomy following chemoradiotherapy also confirmed the finding of long-term survival in patients with residual disease present at resection.[111] These trials suggest that esophagectomy after concurrent radiotherapy and chemotherapy contributes to the local control of disease and provides survival benefit in a subset of patients. There are several possible explanations for the difference in outcomes noted in these trials and in the Wayne State trial. One potential factor is the difference in the intensity of the chemoradiation regimens used at each center. The University of Michigan regimen appeared more intensive, with preoperative chemotherapy plus radiation therapy twice daily. The cumulative radiation dose used in the Wayne State study was considerably lower than that used in the study reported by Forastiere and colleagues. A retrospective analysis by Kavanagh and colleagues compared patterns of failure for various multimodality approaches with and without surgery.[112] Their analysis indicated that multimodality treatment that included surgery resulted in improved local control and did not change the rates of distant metastasis or survival. This lack of survival benefit was attributed to the high rate of surgical mortality in the group of patients who underwent surgical resection. The question of whether surgical resection is an essential component of local therapy following chemoradiation can only be addressed by a randomized trial comparing trimodality therapy that includes surgery to chemoradiotherapy without surgery. To date, there has been no randomized comparison of chemoradiation without surgery to surgery with chemoradiation.

Two studies have attempted to determine whether a post-treatment evaluation can predict the presence of residual disease. Bates and colleagues investigated whether esophagogastroduodenoscopy (EGD) with biopsy was predictive of complete pathologic response following chemoradiation.[110] They concluded that analysis of preoperative endoscopic biopsy specimens did not reliably predict the presence of residual disease, based on the finding that 41 percent of patients whose preoperative biopsy specimen was negative for tumor had residual tumor in the resection specimen. Reports by Mallery and colleagues indicated that postpreoperative endoscopic ultrasonography (EUS) does not reliably predict the reponse to therapy.[113] Another study showed that EUS following combined-modality therapy predicted survival for patients with adenocarcinoma but not for those with squamous cell carcinoma.[114]

CONCLUSION

The treatment and prognosis of cancer of the esophagus depend on the extent of disease at the time of presentation. For patients with early-stage localized tumors, surgery is the standard treatment. Whether any benefit can be gained by the addition of other treatment modalities has not been determined. For patients with locally or regionally advanced disease, treatment approaches using multimodality therapy have produced encouraging results. Two trials that compared preoperative combined-modality therapy to surgery alone indicated survival benefits with the combined-modality approach, but this needs further confirmation. In the non-operative setting, randomized trials have indicated that chemotherapy plus radiotherapy is superior to radiotherapy alone. Thus, the standard of care for patients with unresectable nonmetastatic cancer of the esophagus is combined chemotherapy and radiation. Investigations to determine the optimal chemotherapeutic agents, radiotherapy fractionation schedules, and sequence of treatment modalities are currently being undertaken.

While the outcomes of patients with carcinoma of the esophagus appear to be improving with the use of multimodality therapy, this disease continues to be associated with a poor prognosis, and current treatments are limited by the lack of effective locoregional and systemic therapy. Clearly, the development of systemic therapies that possess better systemic activity and greater radiosensitization is needed. Based on data from recent phase II trials indicating the activity of new cytotoxic agents such as paclitaxel, docetaxel,

and irinotecan in metastatic esophageal cancer, these agents are being incorporated into combined-modality regimens.[115–117] Equally important is the development of novel agents and targeted therapies for the management of this disease. As more is understood about the details of carcinogenesis in this malignancy, new therapeutic strategies might be targeted at interrupting the various pathways that are important for malignant development. The investigation of newer agents and novel approaches through well-designed clinical trials remains critical.

REFERENCES

1. Greenlee RT, Murray T, Bolden S, Wingo PA. Cancer statistics, 2000. CA Cancer J Clin 2000;50:7–33.
2. Blot WJ, Devesa SS, Kneller RW, Fraumeni JF Jr. Rising incidence of adenocarcinoma of the esophagus and gastric cardia. JAMA 1991;265:1287–9.
3. Blot WJ. Esophageal cancer trends and risk factors. Semin Oncol 1994;21:403–10.
4. Klimstra DS. Pathologic prognostic factors in esophageal carcinoma. Semin Oncol 1994;21:425–30.
5. Daly JM, Karnell LH, Menck HR. National Cancer Data Base report on esophageal carcinoma. Cancer 1996;78: 1820–8.
6. Anderson LL, Lad TE. Autopsy findings in squamous-cell carcinoma of the esophagus. Cancer 1982;50:1587–90.
7. Bosch A, Frias Z, Caldwell WL, Jaeschke WH. Autopsy findings in carcinoma of the esophagus. Acta Radiol Oncol Radiat Phys Biol 1979;18:103–12.
8. Fleming ID, Cooper JS, Henson DE, et al. AJCC cancer staging manual. Philadelphia: Lippincott-Raven; 1997. p. 65–8.
9. Lightdale CJ. Staging of esophageal cancer. I: endoscopic ultrasonography. Semin Oncol 1994;21:438–46.
10. Luketich JD, Schauer PR, Meltzer CC, et al. Role of positron emission tomography in staging esophageal cancer. Ann Thorac Surg 1997;64:765–9.
11. O'Brien MG, Fitzgerald EF, Lee G, et al. A prospective comparison of laparoscopy and imaging in the staging of esophagogastric cancer before surgery. Am J Gastroenterol 1995;90:2191–4.
12. Heath EI, Kaufman HS, Talamini MA, et al. The role of laparoscopy in preoperative staging of esophageal cancer. Surg Endosc 2000;14:495–9.
13. Moertel CG. Carcinoma of the esophagus: is there a role for surgery? The case against surgery. Am J Dig Dis 1978;23: 735–6.
14. Roth JA, Putnam JB Jr. Surgery for cancer of the esophagus. Semin Oncol 1994;21:453–61.
15. Earlam R, Cunha-Melo JR. Oesophageal squamous cell carcinoma: I. A critical review of surgery. Br J Surg 1980; 67:381–90.
16. Kelsen DP, Ginsberg R, Pajak TF, et al. Chemotherapy followed by surgery compared with surgery alone for localized esophageal cancer. N Engl J Med 1998;339:1979–84.

17. Katlic MR, Wilkins EW Jr, Grillo HC. Three decades of treatment of esophageal squamous carcinoma at the Massachusetts General Hospital. J Thorac Cardiovasc Surg 1990;99:929–38.

18. Millikan KW, Silverstein J, Hart V, et al. A 15-year review of esophagectomy for carcinoma of the esophagus and cardia. Arch Surg 1995;130:617–24.

19. Fok M, Law SY, Wong J. Operable esophageal carcinoma: current results from Hong Kong. World J Surg 1994; 18:355–60.

20. Sugimachi K, Inokuchi K, Kuwano H, et al. Patterns of recurrence after curative resection for carcinoma of the thoracic part of the esophagus. Surg Gynecol Obstet 1983;157:537–40.

21. Ellis FH Jr, Gibb SP, Watkins E Jr. Esophagogastrectomy. A safe, widely applicable, and expeditious form of palliation for patients with carcinoma of the esophagus and cardia. Ann Surg 1983;198:531–40.

22. Sugimachi K, Maekawa S, Koga Y, et al. The quality of life is sustained after operation for carcinoma of the esophagus. Surg Gynecol Obstet 1986;162:544–6.

23. Miller C. Carcinoma of the esophagus and gasric cardia. Br J Surg 1962;49:507–22.

24. Herschovic A, Leichman L, Lattin P, et al. Chemo/radiation with and without surgery in the thoracic esophagus: the Wayne State experience. Int J Radiat Oncol Biol Phys 1988;15:655–62.

25. Elkon D, Lee MS, Hendrickson FR. Carcinoma of the esophagus: sites of recurrence and palliative benefits after definitive radiotherapy. Int J Radiat Oncol Biol Phys 1978;4:615–20.

26. Akiyama H, Tsurumaru M, Kawamura T, Ono Y. Principles of surgical treatment for carcinoma of the esophagus: analysis of lymph node involvement. Ann Surg 1981;194:438–46.

27. van Andel JG, Dees J, Dijkhuis CM, et al. Carcinoma of the esophagus: results of treatment. Ann Surg 1979;190:684–9.

28. De-Ren S. Ten-year follow-up of esophageal cancer treated by radical radiation therapy: analysis of 869 patients. Int J Radiat Oncol Biol Phys 1989;16:329–34.

29. Beatty JD, DeBoer G, Rider WD. Carcinoma of the esophagus: pretreatment assessment, correlation of radiation treatment parameters with survival, and identification and management of radiation treatment failure. Cancer 1979;43:2254–67.

30. Newaishy GA, Read GA, Duncan W, Kerr GR. Results of radical radiotherapy of squamous cell carcinoma of the oesophagus. Clin Radiol 1982;33:347–52.

31. Earlam R, Cunha-Melo JR. Oesophageal squamous cell carcinoma: II. A critical view of radiotherapy. Br J Surg 1980;67:457–61.

32. Earlam R. An MRC prospective randomised trial of radiotherapy versus surgery for operable squamous cell carcinoma of the oesophagus. Ann R Coll Surg Engl 1991; 73:8–12.

33. Powell ME, Hoskin PJ, Saunders MI, et al. Continuous hyperfractionated accelerated radiotherapy (CHART) in localized cancer of the esophagus. Int J Radiat Oncol Biol Phys 1997;38:133–6.

34. Girinsky T, Auperin A, Marsiglia H, et al. Accelerated fraction-

35. Hyden EC, Langholz B, Tilden T, et al. External beam and intraluminal radiotherapy in the treatment of carcinoma of the esophagus. J Thorac Cardiovasc Surg 1988;96: 237–41.

36. Hishikawa Y, Kurisu K, Taniguchi M, et al. High-dose-rate intraluminal brachytherapy (HDRIBT) for esophageal cancer. Int J Radiat Oncol Biol Phys 1991;21:1133–5.

37. Hishikawa Y, Kurisu K, Taniguchi M, et al. High-dose-rate intraluminal brachytherapy for esophageal cancer: 10 years experience in Hyogo College of Medicine. Radiother Oncol 1991;21:107–14.

38. Hareyama M, Nishio M, Kagami Y, et al. Intracavitary brachytherapy combined with external-beam irradiation for squamous cell carcinoma of the thoracic esophagus. Int J Radiat Oncol Biol Phys 1992;24:235–40.

39. Sur RK, Singh DP, Sharma SC, et al. Radiation therapy of esophageal cancer: role of high dose rate brachytherapy. Int J Radiat Oncol Biol Phys 1992;22:1043–6.

40. Kharadi MY, Qadir A, Khan FA, Khuroo MS. Comparative evaluation of therapeutic approaches in stage III and IV squamous cell carcinoma of the thoracic esophagus with conventional radiotherapy and endoscopic treatment in combination and endoscopic treatment alone: a randomized prospective trial. Int J Radiat Oncol Biol Phys 1997; 39:309–20.

41. Gaspar LE, Nag S, Herskovic A, et al. American Brachytherapy Society (ABS) consensus guidelines for brachytherapy of esophageal cancer. Clinical Research Committee, American Brachytherapy Society, Philadelphia, PA. Int J Radiat Oncol Biol Phys 1997;38:127–32.

42. Nishimura Y, Ono K, Tsutsui K, et al. Esophageal cancer treated with radiotherapy: impact of total treatment time and fractionation. Int J Radiat Oncol Biol Phys 1994; 30:1099–105.

43. Mei W, Xian-Zhi G, Weibo Y, et al. Randomized clinical trial on the combination of preoperative irradiation and surgery in the treatment of esophageal carcinoma: report on 206 patients. Int J Radiat Oncol Biol Phys 1989;16:325–7.

44. Arnott SJ, Duncan W, Kerr GR, et al. Low dose preoperative radiotherapy for carcinoma of the oesophagus: results of a randomized clinical trial. Radiother Oncol 1993;24:108–13.

45. Launois B, Delarue D, Campion JP, Kerbaol M. Preoperative radiotherapy for carcinoma of the esophagus. Surg Gynecol Obstet 1981;153:690–2.

46. Gignoux M, Roussel A, Paillot B, et al. The value of preoperative radiotherapy in esophageal cancer: results of a study of the E.O.R.T.C. World J Surg 1987;11:426–32.

47. Nygaard K, Hagen S, Hansen HS, et al. Pre-operative radiotherapy prolongs survival in operable esophageal carcinoma: a randomized, multicenter study of pre-operative radiotherapy and chemotherapy. The second Scandinavian trial in esophageal cancer. World J Surg 1992;16:1104–9.

48. Arnott SJ, Duncan W, Gignoux M, et al. Preoperative radiotherapy in esophageal carcinoma: a meta-analysis using individual patient data (Oesophageal Cancer Collaborative Group). Int J Radiat Oncol Biol Phys 1998;41:579–83.

49. Kasai M, Mori S, Watanabe T. Follow-up results after resection of thoracic esophageal carcinoma. World J Surg 1978;2:543–51.

50. Teniere P, Hay JM, Fingerhut A, Fagniez PL. Postoperative radiation therapy does not increase survival after curative resection for squamous cell carcinoma of the middle and lower esophagus as shown by a multicenter controlled trial. French University Association for Surgical Research. Surg Gynecol Obstet 1991;173:123–30.

51. Fok M, Sham JS, Choy D, et al. Postoperative radiotherapy for carcinoma of the esophagus: a prospective, randomized controlled study. Surgery 1993;113:138–47.

52. Enzinger PC, Ilson DH, Kelsen DP. Chemotherapy in esophageal cancer. Semin Oncol 1999;26(5 Suppl 15):12–20.

53. Ezdinli EZ, Gelber R, Desai DV, et al. Chemotherapy of advanced esophageal carcinoma: Eastern Cooperative Oncology Group experience. Cancer 1980;46:2149–53.

54. Lokich JJ, Shea M, Chaffey J. Sequential infusional 5-fluorouracil followed by concomitant radiation for tumors of the esophagus and gastroesophageal junction. Cancer 1987;60:275–9.

55. Ravry MJ, Moore MR, Omura GA, et al. Phase II evaluation of cisplatin in squamous carcinoma of the esophagus: a Southeastern Cancer Study Group trial. Cancer Treat Rep 1985;69:1457–8.

56. Panettiere FJ, Leichman LP, Tilchen EJ, Chen TT. Chemotherapy for advanced epidermoid carcinoma of the esophagus with single-agent cisplatin: final report on a Southwest Oncology Group study. Cancer Treat Rep 1984;68:1023–4.

57. Miller JI, McIntyre B, Hatcher CR Jr. Combined treatment approach in surgical management of carcinoma of the esophagus: a preliminary report. Ann Thorac Surg 1985;40:289–93.

58. Kantarjian H, Ajani JA, Karlin DA. Cis-diaminodichloroplatinum (II) chemotherapy for advanced adenocarcinoma of the upper gastrointestinal tract. Oncology 1985;42:69–71.

59. Sternberg C, Kelsen D, Dukeman M, et al. Carboplatin: a new platinum analog in the treatment of epidermoid carcinoma of the esophagus. Cancer Treat Rep 1985;69:1305–7.

60. Mannell A, Winters Z. Carboplatin in the treatment of oesophageal cancer. S Afr Med J 1989;76:213–4.

61. Queisser W, Preusser P, Mross KB, et al. Phase II evaluation of carboplatin in advanced esophageal carcinoma. A trial of the Phase I/II Study Group of the Association for Medical Oncology of the German Cancer Society. Onkologie 1990;13:190–3.

62. Kelsen DP, Bains M, Cvitkovic E, Golbey R. Vindesine in the treatment of esophageal carcinoma: a phase II study. Cancer Treat Rep 1979;63:2019–21.

63. Bedikian AY, Valdivieso M, Bodey GP, Freireich EJ. Phase II evaluation of vindesine in the treatment of colorectal and esophageal tumors. Cancer Chemother Pharmacol 1979;2:263–6.

64. Bezwoda WR, Derman DP, Weaving A, Nissenbaum M. Treatment of esophageal cancer with vindesine: an open trial. Cancer Treat Rep 1984;68:783–5.

65. Conroy T, Etienne PL, Adenis A, et al. Phase II trial of vinorelbine in metastatic squamous cell esophageal carcinoma. European Organization for Research and Treatment of Cancer Gastrointestinal Treat Cancer Cooperative Group. J Clin Oncol 1996;14:164–70.

66. Ajani JA, Ilson DH, Daugherty K, et al. Activity of taxol in patients with squamous cell carcinoma and adenocarcinoma of the esophagus. J Natl Cancer Inst 1994;86:1086–91.

67. Xiao H, O'Reilly E, Ilson D, et al. A phase II trial of 96 hour paclitaxel in patients with previously treated esophageal cancer. Proc Am Soc Clin Oncol 1998;17:306a.

68. Einzig AI, Neuberg D, Remick SC, et al. Phase II trial of docetaxel (Taxotere) in patients with adenocarcinoma of the upper gastrointestinal tract previously untreated with cytotoxic chemotherapy: the Eastern Cooperative Oncology Group (ECOG) results of protocol E1293. Med Oncol 1996;13:87–93.

69. Harstrick A, Bokemeyer C, Preusser P, et al. Phase II study of single-agent etoposide in patients with metastatic squamous-cell carcinoma of the esophagus. Cancer Chemother Pharmacol 1992;29:321–2.

70. Enzinger PC, Kulke MH, Clark JW, et al. Phase II trial of CPT-11 in previously untreated patients with advanced adenocarcinoma of the esophagus and stomach. Proc Am Soc Clin Oncol 2000;19:315a.

71. Lin L, Hecht JR. A phase II trial of irinotecan in patients with advanced adenocarcinoma of the gastroesophageal (GE) junction. Proc Am Soc Clin Oncol 2000;19:289a.

72. Ilson DH, Kelson DP. Chemotherapy in esophageal cancer. Anticancer Drugs 1993;4:287–99.

73. Bleiberg H, Conroy T, Paillot B, et al. Randomised phase II study of cisplatin and 5-fluorouracil (5-FU) versus cisplatin alone in advanced squamous cell oesophageal cancer. Eur J Cancer 1997;33:1216–20.

74. Roth JA, Pass HI, Flanagan MM, et al. Randomized clinical trial of preoperative and postoperative adjuvant chemotherapy with cisplatin, vindesine, and bleomycin for carcinoma of the esophagus. J Thorac Cardiovasc Surg 1988;96:242–8.

75. Schlag P. Randomized trial of preoperative chemotherapy for squamous cell cancer of the esophagus. Arch Surg 1992;127:1446–50.

76. Clark PI. Medical research council randomised trial of surgery with or without pre-operative chemotherapy in resectable cancer of the oesophagus (MRC Upper GI Tract Cancer Group) Eur Soc Med Oncol 2000;11 Suppl 4:4.

77. Kok TC, von Lanschot J, Sirsman PD, et al. Neoadjuvant chemotherapy in operable esophageal carcinoma: final report of a phase III multicenter randomized controlled trial [abstract]. Proc Am Soc Clin Oncol 1997;16:277a.

78. Kelsen DP, Minsky B, Smith M, et al. Preoperative therapy for esophageal cancer: a randomized comparison of chemotherapy versus radiation therapy. J Clin Oncol 1990;8:1352–61.

79. Ando N, Iizuka T, Ide H, et al. A randomized trial of surgery alone vs surgery plus postoperative chemotherapy with cisplatin and 5-fluorouracil for localized squamous cell carcinoma of the thoracic esophagus: the Japan Clinical Oncology Group Study (JCOG 9204). Proc Am Soc Clin Oncol 1999;18:269a.

80. Vokes EE, Weichselbaum RR. Concomitant chemoradiotherapy: rationale and clinical experience in patients with solid tumors. J Clin Oncol 1990;8:911–34.

81. Vokes EE. Interactions of chemotherapy and radiation. Semin Oncol 1993;20:70–9.

82. Steel GG, Peckham MJ. Exploitable mechanisms in combined radiotherapy-chemotherapy: the concept of additivity. Int J Radiat Oncol Biol Phys 1979;5:85–91.

83. Franklin R, Steiger Z, Vaishampayan G, et al. Combined modality therapy for esophageal squamous cell carcinoma. Cancer 1983;51:1062–71.

84. Steiger Z, Franklin R, Wilson RF, et al. Eradication and palliation of squamous cell carcinoma of the esophagus with chemotherapy, radiotherapy, and surgical therapy. J Thorac Cardiovasc Surg 1981;82:713.

85. Coia LR, Engstrom PF, Paul AR, et al. Long-term results of infusional 5-FU, mitomycin-C and radiation as primary management of esophageal carcinoma. Int J Radiat Oncol Biol Phys 1991;20:29–36.

86. Seitz JF, Giovannini M, Padaut-Cesana J, et al. Inoperable nonmetastatic squamous cell carcinoma of the esophagus managed by concomitant chemotherapy (5-fluorouracil and cisplatin) and radiation therapy. Cancer 1990;66:214–9.

87. John MJ, Flam MS, Mowry PA, et al. Radiotherapy alone and chemoradiation for nonmetastatic esophageal carcinoma. A critical review of chemoradiation. Cancer 1989;63:2397–403.

88. Coia LR, Soffen EM, Schultheiss TE, et al. Swallowing function in patients with esophageal cancer treated with concurrent radiation and chemotherapy. Cancer 1993;71:281–6.

89. Araujo CM, Souhami L, Gil RA, et al. A randomized trial comparing radiation therapy versus concomitant radiation therapy and chemotherapy in carcinoma of the thoracic esophagus. Cancer 1991;67:2258–61.

90. Slabber CF, Nel JS, Schoeman L, et al. A randomized study of radiotherapy alone versus radiotherapy plus 5-fluorouracil and platinum in patients with inoperable, locally advanced squamous cancer of the esophagus. Am J Clin Oncol 1998;21:462–5.

91. Sischy B, Ryan L, Haller D, et al. Interim report of EST1282 phase III protocol for the evaluation of combined modalities in the treatment of patients with carcinoma of the esophagus. Proc Am Soc Clin Oncol 1990;9:105a.

92. Smith TJ, Ryan LM, Douglass HO Jr, et al. Combined chemoradiotherapy vs. radiotherapy alone for early stage squamous cell carcinoma of the esophagus: a study of the Eastern Cooperative Oncology Group. Int J Radiat Oncol Biol Phys 1998;42:269–76.

93. Herskovic A, Martz K, al-Sarraf M, et al. Combined chemotherapy and radiotherapy compared with radiotherapy alone in patients with cancer of the esophagus. N Engl J Med 1992;326:1593–8.

94. al-Sarraf M, Martz K, Herskovic A, et al. Progress report of combined chemoradiotherapy versus radiotherapy alone in patients with esophageal cancer: an intergroup study. J Clin Oncol 1997;15:277–84.

95. Minsky BD, Neuberg D, Kelsen DP, et al. Neoadjuvant chemotherapy plus concurrent chemotherapy and high-dose radiation for squamous cell carcinoma of the esophagus: a preliminary analysis of the phase II intergroup trial 0122. J Clin Oncol 1996;14:149–55.

96. Minsky BD, Neuberg D, Kelsen DP, et al. Final report of Intergroup Trial 0122 (ECOG PE-289, RTOG 90-12): phase II trial of neoadjuvant chemotherapy plus concurrent chemotherapy and high-dose radiation for squamous

cell carcinoma of the esophagus. Int J Radiat Oncol Biol Phys 1999;43:517–23.

97. Calais G, Dorval E, Louisot P, et al. Radiotherapy with high dose rate brachytherapy boost and concomitant chemotherapy for stages IIB and III esophageal carcinoma: results of a pilot study. Int J Radiat Oncol Biol Phys 1997;38:769–75.

98. Gaspar LE, Qian C, Kocha WI, et al. A phase I/II study of external beam radiation, brachytherapy and concurrent chemotherapy in localized cancer of the esophagus (RTOG 92-07): preliminary toxicity report. Int J Radiat Oncol Biol Phys 1997;37:593–9.

99. Gaspar LE, Winter K, Kocha WI, et al. A phase I/II study of external beam radiation, brachytherapy, and concurrent chemotherapy for patients with localized carcinoma of the esophagus (Radiation Therapy Oncology Group Study 9207): final report. Cancer 2000;88:988–95.

100. Le Prise E, Etienne PL, Meunier B, et al. A randomized study of chemotherapy, radiation therapy, and surgery versus surgery for localized squamous cell carcinoma of the esophagus. Cancer 1994;73:1779–84.

101. Bosset JF, Gignoux M, Triboulet JP, et al. Chemoradiotherapy followed by surgery compared with surgery alone in squamous-cell cancer of the esophagus. N Engl J Med 1997;337:161–7.

102. Urba S, Orringer M, Turrisi A, et al. A randomized trial comparing transhiatal esophagectomy (THE) to preoperative concurrent chemoradiation (CT/XRT) followed by esophagectomy in locoregional esophageal carcinoma (CA). Proc Am Soc Clin Oncol 1995;14:1995.

103. Urba S, Orringer M, Turrisi A, et al. A randomized trial comparing surgery (S) to preoperative concomitant chemoradiation plus surgery in patients (pts) with resectable esophageal cancer (CA): updated analysis [abstract]. Proc Am Soc Clin Oncol 1997;16:277a.

104. Urba SG, Orringer MB, Turrisi A, et al. Randomized trial of preoperative chemoradiation versus surgery alone in patients with locoregional esophageal carcinoma. J Clin Oncol 2001;19:305–13.

105. Walsh TN, Noonan N, Hollywood D, et al. A comparison of multimodal therapy and surgery for esophageal adenocarcinoma. N Engl J Med 1996;335:462–7.

106. Gill PG, Denham JW, Jamieson GG, et al. Patterns of treatment failure and prognostic factors associated with the treatment of esophageal carcinoma with chemotherapy and radiotherapy either as sole treatment or followed by surgery. J Clin Oncol 1992;10:1037–43.

107. Denham JW, Burmeister BH, Lamb DS, et al. Factors influencing outcome following radio-chemotherapy for oesophageal cancer. The Trans Tasman Radiation Oncology Group (TROG). Radiother Oncol 1996;40:31–43.

108. Forastiere AA, Orringer MB, Perez-Tamayo C, et al. Preoperative chemoradiation followed by transhiatal esophagectomy for carcinoma of the esophagus: final report. J Clin Oncol 1993;11:1118–23.

109. Forastiere AA, Orringer MB, Perez-Tamayo C, et al. Concurrent chemotherapy and radiation therapy followed by transhiatal esophagectomy for local-regional cancer of the esophagus. J Clin Oncol 1990;8:119–27.

110. Bates BA, Detterbeck FC, Bernard SA, et al. Concurrent radi-

ation therapy and chemotherapy followed by esophagectomy for localized esophageal carcinoma. J Clin Oncol 1996;14:156–63.

111. Kane JM 3rd, Shears LL, Ribeiro U, et al. Is esophagectomy following upfront chemoradiotherapy safe and necessary? Arch Surg 1997;132:481–5.

112. Kavanagh B, Anscher M, Leopold K, et al. Patterns of failure following combined modality therapy for esophageal cancer, 1984–1990. Int J Radiat Oncol Biol Phys 1992;24:633–42.

113. Mallery S, DeCamp M, Bueno R, et al. Pretreatment staging by endoscopic ultrasonography does not predict complete response to neoadjuvant chemoradiation in patients with esophageal carcinoma. Cancer 1999;86:764–9.

114. Chak A, Canto MI, Cooper GS, et al. Endosonographic assessment of multimodality therapy predicts survival of esophageal carcinoma patients. Cancer 2000;88:1788–95.

115. Meluch AA, Hainsworth JD, Gray JR, et al. Preoperative combined modality therapy with paclitaxel, carboplatin, prolonged infusion 5-fluorouracil, and radiation therapy in localized esophageal cancer: preliminary results of a Minnie Pearl Cancer Research Network phase II trial. Cancer J Sci Am 1999;5:84–91.

116. Heath EI, Burtness BA, Heitmiller RF, et al. Phase II evaluation of preoperative chemoradiation and postoperative adjuvant chemotherapy for squamous cell and adenocarcinoma of the esophagus. J Clin Oncol 2000;18:868–76.

117. Mauer AM, Haraf DC, Ferguson MK, et al. Docetaxel-based combined modality therapy for locally advanced carcinoma of the esophagus and gastric cardia. Proc Am Soc Clin Oncol 2000;19:954a.

118. Bonadonna G, De Lena M, Monfardini S, et al. Clinical trials with bleomycin in lymphomas and in solid tumors. Eur J Cancer 1972;8:205–15.

119. Tancini G, Bajetta E, Bonadonna G. [Bleomycin alone and in combination with methotrexate in the treatment of carcinoma of the esophagus (author's transl)]. Tumori 1974;60:65–71.

120. Kolaric K, Maricic Z, Dujmovic I, Roth A. Therapy of advanced esophageal cancer with bleomycin, irradiation and combination of bleomycin with irradiation. Tumori 1976;62:255–62.

121. Whittington RM, Close HP. Clinical experience with mitomycin C (NSC-26980). Cancer Chemother Rep 1970;54:195–8.

122. Engstrom PF, Lavin PT, Klaassen DJ. Phase II evaluation of mitomycin and cisplatin in advanced esophageal carcinoma. Cancer Treat Rep 1983;67:713–5.

123. Advani SH, Saikia TK, Swaroop S, et al. Anterior chemotherapy in esophageal cancer. Cancer 1985;56:1502–6.

124. Davis S, Shanmugathasa M, Kessler W. cis-Dichlorodiammineplatinum(II) in the treatment of esophageal carcinoma. Cancer Treat Rep 1980;64:709–11.

125. Coonley CJ, Bains M, Hilaris B, et al. Cisplatin and bleomycin in the treatment of esophageal carcinoma. A final report. Cancer 1984;54:2351–5.

126. Kelsen D, Hilaris B, Coonley C, et al. Cisplatin, vindesine, and bleomycin chemotherapy of local-regional and advanced esophageal carcinoma. Am J Med 1983;75:645–52.

127. Dinwoodie WR, Bartolucci AA, Lyman GH, et al. Phase II

evaluation of cisplatin, bleomycin, and vindesine in advanced squamous cell carcinoma of the esophagus: a Southeastern Cancer Study Group Trial. Cancer Treat Rep 1986;70:267–70.

128. Vogl SE, Greenwald E, Kaplan BH. Effective chemotherapy for esophageal cancer with methotrexate, bleomycin, and cis-diamminedichloroplatinum II. Cancer 1981;48:2555–8.

129. De Besi P, Salvagno L, Endrizzi L, et al. Cisplatin, bleomycin and methotrexate in the treatment of advanced oesophageal cancer. Eur J Cancer Clin Oncol 1984;20:743–7.

130. Vogl SE, Camacho F, Berenzweig M, Ruckdeschel J. Chemotherapy for esophageal cancer with mitoguazone, methotrexate, bleomycin, and cisplatin. Cancer Treat Rep 1985;69:21–3.

131. Kelsen DP, Fein R, Coonley C, et al. Cisplatin, vindesine, and mitoguazone in the treatment of esophageal cancer. Cancer Treat Rep 1986;70:255–9.

132. Chapman R, Fleming TR, Van Damme J, Macdonald J. Cisplatin, vinblastine, and mitoguazone in squamous cell carcinoma of the esophagus: a Southwest Oncology Group Study. Cancer Treat Rep 1987;71:1185–7.

133. Gisselbrecht C, Calvo F, Mignot L, et al. Fluorouracil (F), adriamycin (A), and cisplatin (P) (FAP): combination chemotherapy of advanced esophageal carcinoma. Cancer 1983;52:974–7.

134. De Besi P, Sileni VC, Salvagno L, et al. Phase II study of cisplatin, 5-FU, and allopurinol in advanced esophageal cancer. Cancer Treat Rep 1986;70:909–10.

135. Iizuka T, Kakegawa T, Ide H, et al. Phase II evaluation of cisplatin and 5-fluorouracil in advanced squamous cell carcinoma of the esophagus: a Japanese Esophageal Oncology Group Trial. Jpn J Clin Oncol 1992;22:172–6.

136. Lovett D, Kelsen D, Eisenberger M, Houston C. A phase II trial of carboplatin and vinblastine in the treatment of advanced squamous cell carcinoma of the esophagus. Cancer 1991;67:354–6.

137. Kelsen D, Ginsberg R, Bains M, et al. A phase II trial of paclitaxel and cisplatin in patients with locally advanced metastatic esophageal cancer: a preliminary report. Semin Oncol 1997;24(6 Suppl 19):S19–81.

138. Petrasch S, Welt A, Reinacher A, et al. Chemotherapy with cisplatin and paclitaxel in patients with locally advanced, recurrent or metastatic oesophageal cancer. Br J Cancer 1998;78:511–4.

139. Ilson DH, Ajani J, Bhalla K, et al. Phase II trial of paclitaxel, fluorouracil, and cisplatin in patients with advanced carcinoma of the esophagus. J Clin Oncol 1998;16:1826–34.

140. Lokich JJ, Sonneborn H, Anderson NR, et al. Combined paclitaxel, cisplatin, and etoposide for patients with previously untreated esophageal and gastroesophageal carcinomas. Cancer 1999;85:2347–51.

141. Ilson DH, Saltz L, Enzinger P, et al. Phase II trial of weekly irinotecan plus cisplatin in advanced esophageal cancer. J Clin Oncol 1999;17:3270–5.

142. Schlag P, Herrmann R, Raeth U, et al. Preoperative (neoadjuvant) chemotherapy in squamous cell cancer of the esophagus. Recent Results Cancer Res 1988;110:14–20.

143. Forastiere AA, Gennis M, Orringer MB, Agha FP. Cisplatin, vinblastine, and mitoguazone chemotherapy for epidermoid and adenocarcinoma of the esophagus. J Clin Oncol 1987;5:1143–9.

144. Carey RW, Hilgenberg AD, Wilkins EW, et al. Preoperative chemotherapy followed by surgery with possible postoperative radiotherapy in squamous cell carcinoma of the esophagus: evaluation of the chemotherapy component. J Clin Oncol 1986;4:697–701.

145. Hilgenberg AD, Carey RW, Wilkins EW Jr, et al. Preoperative chemotherapy, surgical resection, and selective postoperative therapy for squamous cell carcinoma of the esophagus. Ann Thorac Surg 1988;45:357–63.

146. Carey RW, Hilgenberg AD, Choi NC, et al. A pilot study of neoadjuvant chemotherapy with 5-fluorouracil and cisplatin with surgical resection and postoperative radiation therapy and/or chemotherapy in adenocarcinoma of the esophagus. Cancer 1991;68:489–92.

147. Kies MS, Rosen ST, Tsang TK, et al. Cisplatin and 5-fluorouracil in the primary management of squamous esophageal cancer. Cancer 1987;60:2156–60.

148. Ajani JA, Roth JA, Ryan B, et al. Evaluation of pre- and postoperative chemotherapy for resectable adenocarcinoma of the esophagus or gastroesophageal junction. J Clin Oncol 1990;8:1231–8.

149. Leichman L, Steiger Z, Seydel HG, Vaitkevicius VK. Combined preoperative chemotherapy and radiation therapy for cancer of the esophagus: the Wayne State University, Southwest Oncology Group and Radiation Therapy Oncology Group experience. Semin Oncol 1984;11:178–85.

150. Poplin E, Fleming T, Leichman L, et al. Combined therapies for squamous-cell carcinoma of the esophagus, a Southwest Oncology Group Study (SWOG-8037). J Clin Oncol 1987;5:622–8.

151. Seydel HG, Leichman L, Byhardt R, et al. Preoperative radiation and chemotherapy for localized squamous cell carcinoma of the esophagus: a RTOG Study. Int J Radiat Oncol Biol Phys 1988;14:33–5.

152. Naunheim KS, Petruska P, Roy TS, et al. Preoperative chemotherapy and radiotherapy for esophageal carcinoma. J Thorac Cardiovasc Surg 1992;103:887–93.

153. Urba SG, Orringer MB, Perez-Tamayo C, et al. Concurrent preoperative chemotherapy and radiation therapy in localized esophageal adenocarcinoma. Cancer 1992;69:285–91.

154. Stahl M, Wilke H, Fink U, et al. Combined preoperative chemotherapy and radiotherapy in patients with locally advanced esophageal cancer. Interim analysis of a phase II trial. J Clin Oncol 1996;14:829–37.

155. Forastiere AA, Heitmiller RF, Lee DJ, et al. Intensive chemoradiation followed by esophagectomy for squamous cell and adenocarcinoma of the esophagus. Cancer J Sci Am 1997;3:144–52.

156. Posner MC, Gooding WE, Landreneau RJ, et al. Preoperative chemoradiotherapy for carcinoma of the esophagus and gastroesophageal junction. Cancer J Sci Am 1998;4:237–46.

9

Palliation of Esophageal Cancer

HANS GERDES, MD
MARK K. FERGUSON, MD

Esophageal cancer is a progressive and debilitating disease that most often results in significant impairment in the ability to swallow solid food and (at times) liquids. Because of its often prolonged latent phase, many patients present with significant weight loss. For 50 to 60 percent of patients, metastatic disease or locally advanced disease is found at the time of diagnosis. Curative surgical resection, therefore, is not an option for most, and the primary focus of treatment becomes the palliation of symptoms and the prolongation of survival.

The growth pattern of esophageal cancer usually results in circumferential involvement of the esophageal wall, with constriction and reduction of the esophageal lumen (Figures 9–1 and 9–2). There is a loss of distensibility and the experience of dysphagia to solid food in 80 to 96 percent of patients.[1] Many ignore the initial signs, adjusting their intake to pureed foods or liquids while denying the severity of their dysphagia. At times, however, this may lead to sudden presentation with food bolus impaction (Figure 9–3). Patients eventually lose weight while their dysphagia progresses to include liquids and ultimately their own saliva. The time course is variable; at presentation, many patients admit to at least several months of dysphagia. The common finding of weight loss in about 42 to 46 percent of patients is indicative of the chronicity of disease in many.[1] Pain in up to 20 percent of patients may indicate distension of the proximal esophagus with meals or infiltration into surrounding structures. Cough with drinking or eating is potentially a sign of tracheoesophageal fistula, which fortunately occurs only in 1 to 13 percent of patients.[1] In the setting of such clinical features, the approach to palliation generally focuses on methods for re-expanding the esophageal lumen or providing an alternative source of nourishment.

This chapter focuses on the available methods of palliating symptoms associated with esophageal cancer. Since dysphagia and weight loss represent the most common symptoms, discussion will primarily center on approaches to achieving esophageal luminal patency, relieving dysphagia and pain, and providing adequate nutritional support. As no method has yet been shown to be superior, each method will be presented individually, with available data.

To better understand dysphagia and success in palliation, clinicians and investigators should attempt to quantify the severity of dysphagia by using the scale proposed by Mellow and Pincus (Table 9–1).[2] This is a simple and reproducible method that can be assessed at all clinic visits and that provides a clear picture of the status of the patient's symptoms. This classification helps to focus the palliative approach to the symptoms and also permits quantification of the success in palliation. A one-point improvement in dysphagia grade may result in a patient being able to tolerate a liquid diet; reductions of two or three points clearly indicate measurable improvements, permitting comparison between modalities.

Currently available methods of palliating dysphagia associated with esophageal cancer include endoscopic approaches, surgery, radiation therapy, and chemotherapy. As a result of technologic advances and the persistently high morbidity and mortality associated with surgery, there has been a trend toward endoscopic therapy as the primary

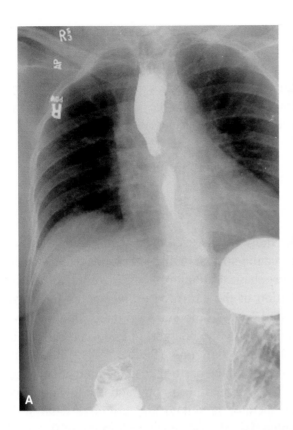

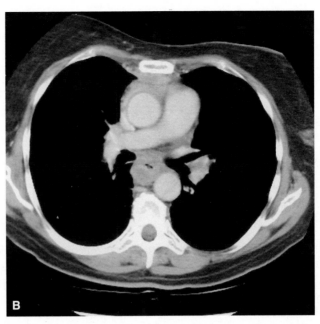

Figure 9–1. *A,* Barium radiograph of a patient with an obstructing midesophageal carcinoma, demonstrating constriction of the esophageal lumen and dilation of the proximal esophagus. *B,* Computed tomography scan of the same patient in *A.* Note the circumferential thickening of the midesophageal wall.

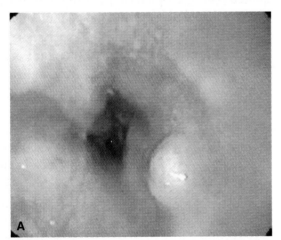

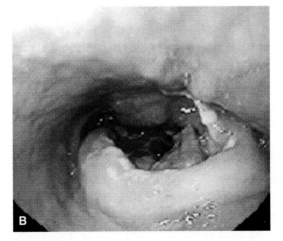

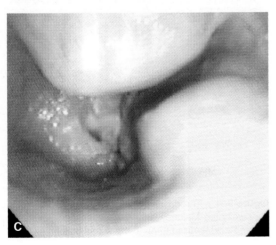

Figure 9–2. *A,* Endoscopic photograph of an esophageal cancer with an infiltrative growth pattern. *B,* An ulcerating polypoid mass of the esophagus. *C,* A distal esophageal mass, with mediastinal lymph nodes impinging on the esophageal wall proximal to the mass.

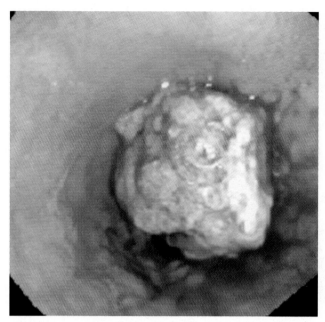

Figure 9–3. Endoscopic photograph of food bolus impaction in a patient with a distal esophageal mass.

approach over the past 10 years. Radiation therapy continues to offer effective results for some, and the introduction of new and somewhat effective chemotherapy drugs has rekindled an interest in its palliative use. In the interest of completeness, available approaches and data to support the current recommendations will be presented.

ENDOSCOPIC THERAPY

Endoscopic methods of dysphagia palliation can be classified into mechanical methods, tumor ablative methods, and nutritional palliation methods. While each approach has its merit, few trials exist comparing them to each other or to surgical or radiologic methods of palliation. The palliative management of each patient with esophageal cancer needs to be individualized. It is our opinion that no one method can be offered to all patients as success rates vary

according to the individual patient's needs and expectations, the location and extent of disease, and the patient's cultural beliefs in regard to food and nutrition. The approaches described here provide the clinician with a choice of methods, each with acceptable efficacy and safety profiles.

Mechanical Methods

Esophageal Dilation

The most widely used mechanical method of endoscopic therapy for malignant esophageal obstruction is esophageal dilation. This involves the forceful dilation of the narrowed esophagus by using wire-guided olives, mercury-weighted dilators, wire-guided polyvinyl bougies, or endoscopically guided hydrostatic balloons (Figure 9–4). This simple approach can be performed at the time of endoscopy, with or without fluoroscopy, and is safely done when the operator is skilled and exercises caution. The quoted risk of esophageal perforation of 0.1 percent is lower than that seen with the dilation of achalasia; however, this is in the hands of experts.[3]

Several suggestions in the literature are felt to increase the safety and efficacy of esophageal dilation.[4] These include carefully planning the procedure with evaluation of the anatomy prior to dilation, and dilating slowly during multiple sessions, over several weeks if necessary. The use of fluoroscopy and endoscopy during the dilation (especially dilation with wire-guided dilators) ensures the proper placement of the guide wire and the alignment of the

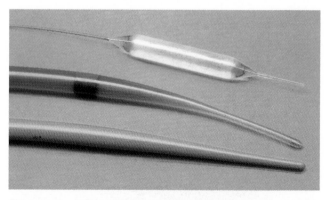

Figure 9–4. Three types of esophageal dilators (from top, a mercury-weighted Maloney dilator, a wire-guided Savary-Guilliard dilator, and a water-filled through-the-scope balloon dilator).

Table 9–1. DYSPHAGIA GRADING	
Grade	Symptom
0	Able to eat normal diet
1	Able to eat some solid food
2	Able to eat semisolids only
3	Able to swallow liquids only
4	Unable to swallow anything, including saliva

dilators, reducing the risk of false passages and ensuring a good result. This is especially true in very bulky obstructing tumors, where the lumen may follow an angulated or tortuous path not readily apparent when the scope is unable to pass. A gradual approach with a stepwise increase in the diameter of the dilators and with the dilation limited to three bougies beyond the point of resistance during each session is recommended.

The long-term success of dilation in the management of obstructing esophageal cancer is poor because the presence of the tumor results in rapid reocclusion of the esophageal lumen. Sparse data exist for long-term results, but personal experiences demonstrate that the duration of palliation is 3 to 4 weeks at best.[5] Therefore, this procedure is ideally used as a temporizing measure, such as for a patient undergoing chemotherapy or chemoradiation and experiencing severe dysphagia and dehydration. We have found it particularly useful in managing patients undergoing neoadjuvant chemoradiation prior to curative resection. With this approach, a reduction in tumor size from the antitumor therapy is often seen within 2 to 3 weeks of the initiation of treatment. Dilation can also be used to permit passage of the scope during the performance of other therapeutic interventions such as laser ablation or percutaneous gastrostomy, and it certainly is an important maneuver in the placement of esophageal stents.

Esophageal Stenting

Plastic Esophageal Stents. Multiple devices and techniques for the insertion of esophageal stents have been developed over the years. The original method involved the forceful insertion of rubber tubes during laparotomy or thoracotomy, using the "pull-through" technique.[6] This permitted the palliation of dysphagia in patients with unresectable esophageal cancer but was associated with a high mortality rate of 10 to 29 percent.[4]

The oral pulsion technique later described in the 1960s led to greater ease of insertion with reduced complication rates but met with mixed reviews in the United States because it required specialized technical skills and the use of general anesthesia and because it had a persistently high rate of major complications.[7] A multitude of plastic stent designs evolved over the years, but the Celestin and Atkinson tubes became popular with thoracic surgeons; these tubes can be rapidly inserted under rigid esophagoscopic control with the Nottingham introducer, providing excellent palliation of dysphagia (Figure 9–5, A). Due to the perceived need for general anesthesia and the high complication rates, most gastrointestinal endoscopists avoided the plastic stents

One variation of these stents that is similar to the Celestin tube design has been adopted by some gastroenterologists. Available as a kit with a simplified insertion design, the stent is fitted over a polyvinyl bougie of the Savary-Guilliard type and is pushed into place over a guide wire under fluoroscopic guidance, much like Savary dilation (see Figure 9–5, B). Boyce suggests that with stepwise sequential dilations over days or weeks, palliation could safely be achieved by the insertion of these plastic stents, without the need for general anesthesia.[4] This method provides a patent lumen of 10 to 12 mm, with a lower reported perforation risk of 2 percent and no deaths.[4] However, experience with plastic stents varies around the world, with some studies showing higher complication rates[6–10] (Table 9–2).

The critical requirements for safe insertion of plastic esophageal stents are careful selection of patients and careful radiographic and endoscopic evaluation of patient strictures prior to attempted stent placement. Patients should have adequate dilation of the stricture, preferably several days in advance of intubation with the stent. Finally, it is critical to have a well-designed mechanism for the smooth and accurate delivery of the stent into the stricture lumen, with minimal lateral deviation and trauma.[4]

Once the stent is successfully placed, radiographic confirmation should be obtained, with barium or Gastrografin contrast to demonstrate appropriate bridging of the stricture and to verify the absence of perforation. Patients with these types of esophageal prostheses must be carefully instructed to avoid firm or fibrous foods such as beef or chicken, to chew their food slowly and thoroughly, and to consume carbonated beverages with meals. This helps to reduce the risk of food impaction within the stent. Despite careful counseling, delayed problems with these stents are common, so patients

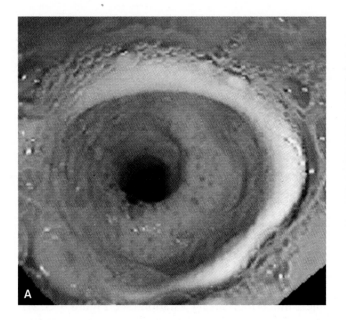

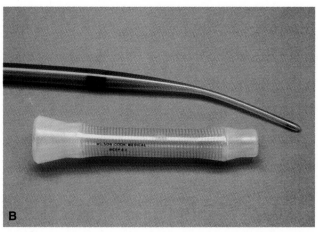

Figure 9–5. *A,* Endoscopic photograph of an esophageal Atkinson tube in a patient with a proximal esophageal cancer. *B,* Celestin-type Wilson Cook plastic esophageal stent, shown with a guiding 10-mm Savary-Guilliard dilator.

should be followed closely and should be instructed to present themselves immediately upon the onset of new symptoms.

Expandable Metal Esophageal Stents. The newly available expandable metal esophageal stents have improved the ability of gastroenterologists and surgeons to palliate patients with obstructing esophageal cancer (Figure 9–6). While many designs and brands exist, all share a thin wire-guided introducer, easy release, and relatively atraumatic insertion (Figures 9–7 and 9–8). By virtue of such design, these metal stents can be easily inserted in a patient under conscious sedation, with minimal pre-insertion dilation of the tumor stricture (Figure 9–9). These stents have inherent radial expansile properties that permit them to maintain outward pressure on the tumor, providing long-term luminal patency and stability (Figures 9–10 and 9–11). The sleek design of their introducers results in reduced morbidity and mortality associated with insertion.

Initial experiences with the four types of expandable metal stents demonstrated high success rates with low morbidity. The ease of insertion and rapid palliation resulted in great enthusiasm for their use. In a prospective randomized comparison between conventional Celestin-type stents and expandable metal stents, Knyrim and colleagues demonstrated equal technical success and improvement in dysphagia and in Karnofsky performance status with the insertion of plastic or expandable metal stents in patients with obstructing esophageal cancer but demonstrated an improved safety profile with the expandable metal stents.[12] The tumor strictures treated with plastic stents required dilation to 20 mm prior to insertion whereas those receiving expandable metal stents required dilation to only 10 mm. Patients receiving plastic stents had longer hospital stays (12.5 vs 5.4 days) and a higher complication rate (9% vs 0%), with three perforations, one case of pneumonia, and five stent migrations. Other prospective studies subsequently demonstrated similar results with other metal stent designs and confirmed the efficacy and increased safety of expandable metal stents[13,14] (Table 9–3).

Table 9–2. COMPLICATIONS OF PLASTIC ESOPHAGEAL STENTS						
		Immediate Complications (%)			Late Complications (%)	
Study (Reference)	Year	Perforation	Bleeding	Death	Migration	Obstruction
Jager et al (8)	1979	8	1.5	2	22	17.5
Siefert et al (9)	1983	11.5	0	3.8	11.5	11.5
Chavy et al (10)	1986	14	5	4	16	16

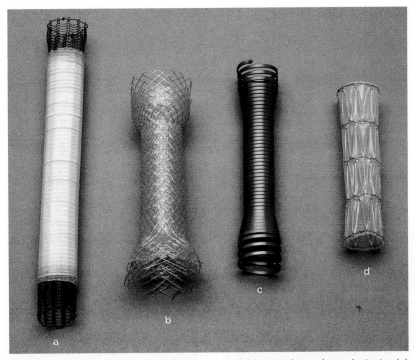

Figure 9–6. Four brands of available expandable metal esophageal stents: (*a*) Ultraflex® stent (Microvasive); (*b*) Wallstent® (Schneider); (*c*) EsophaCoil® (InStent); (*d*) Gianturco Z® stent (Wilson Cook).

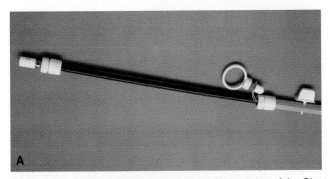

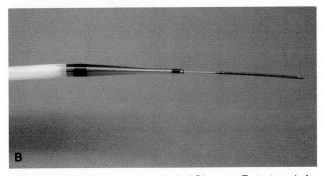

Figure 9–7. *A,* Back end of the introducer for insertion of the Gianturco Z® stent. *B,* Insertion tip and preloaded Gianturco Z stent ready for insertion, with a Savary-type guide wire passing through it.

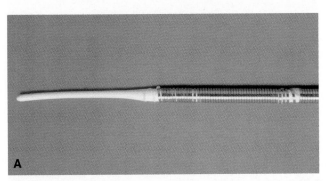

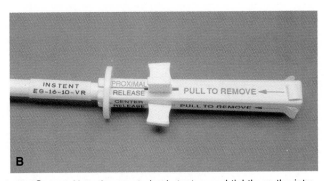

Figure 9–8. *A,* Tip of the deployment device for insertion of the EsophaCoil® stent. Note the constrained stent wound tightly on the introducer. *B,* Back end of the EsophaCoil introducer, demonstrating the lever for release of the proximal end of the stent.

However, the enthusiasm for the metal stents has been somewhat tempered by reports of stents slipping into the stomach during insertion (Figure 9–12, A) and high migration rates in patients undergoing radiation therapy or chemotherapy.[14] The occlusion of stents by tumor ingrowth and overgrowth has also been reported (see Figure 9–12, B), as has recurrent food bolus impaction caused by overzealous consumption of solid food. Despite these issues, these stents have gained widespread

acceptance because of their ease of use and the resultant rapid improvement in dysphagia. When initially approved by the United States Food and Drug Administration (USFDA), expandable metal esophageal stents were constructed of bare meshes of stainless steel or nitinol. Not surprisingly, this design was associated with a high rate of tumor ingrowth causing reocclusion and recurrent dysphagia, often within 2 to 3 months. They have since been modified by the application of a plastic or sili-

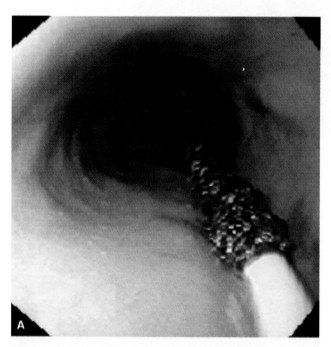

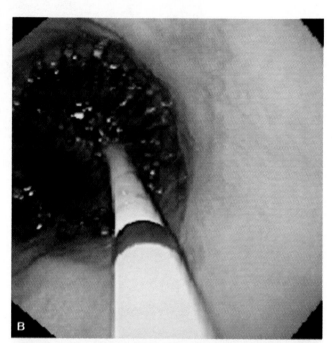

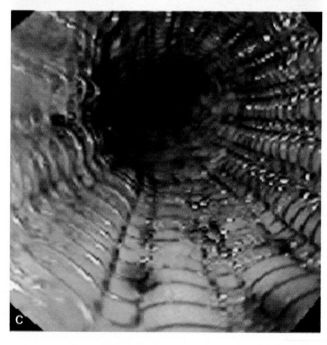

Figure 9–9. Endoscopic photograph of the first-generation Ultraflex® stent being deployed. The blue gelatin coating is gradually melted by body temperature or by the instillation of warm water. *B, C,* Gradual expansion of the Ultraflex stent® eventually fully expanded within the esophagus.

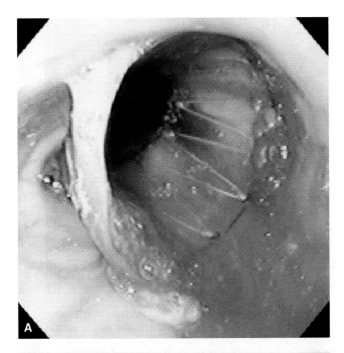

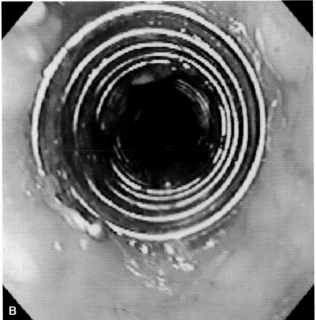

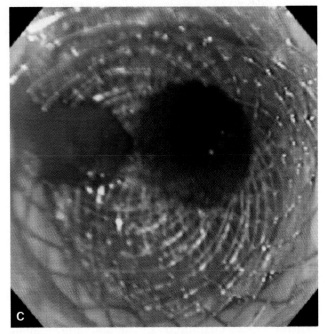

Figure 9–10. *A,* Endoscopic photograph of a newly placed Gianturco Z® stent. Notice the large luminal diameter of the expanded stent. *B,* Endoscopic photograph of a newly inserted EsophaCoil® stent. *C,* Endoscopic photograph of a newly inserted Wallstent®. Note the flare at the top of all the stents.

cone membrane around the body of the stent, resulting in a prolongation of the effective period of palliation due to the inhibition of tumor ingrowth (see Figure 9–12, B). This new design also permitted the use of these stents to seal esophageal leaks caused by tracheoesophageal fistulization or traumatic esophageal perforations[15–17] (Figure 9–13).

When initially designed as bare wire meshes, expandable stents were considered permanent devices because they became embedded in the grow-

ing tumor. With the application of membrane coatings, the stents have become more slippery and prone to migration upon insertion or subsequently (see Figure 9–12, A). This has forced some users to devise methods of retrieving the dislodged stents.[18,19] No guidelines have been provided by any of the manufacturers thus far, but concerns about the potential of pyloric or small-bowel obstruction caused by dislodged stents exist. There is at least one published report of a dislodged stent becoming embedded in

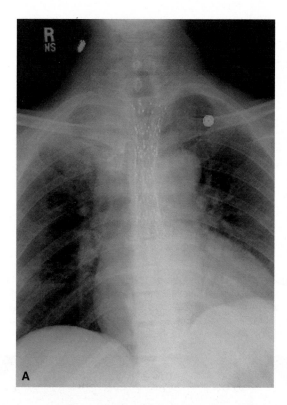

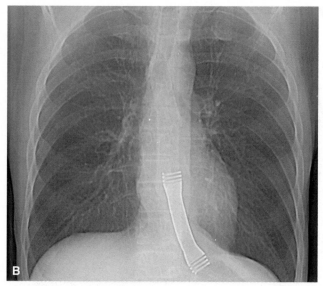

Figure 9–11. *A,* Chest x-ray of a newly inserted Gianturco Z® stent in a patient with an obstructing proximal esophageal cancer with an esophagopleural fistula. Barium radiography revealed complete sealing of the fistula (see Figure 9–13). *B,* Chest radiograph from a patient who has just had an EsophaCoil® stent inserted for treatment of an obstructing esophagogastric-junction tumor.

the rectum and requiring surgical removal,[20] and we have had one case of small-bowel obstruction caused by a migrated esophageal stent (unpublished data).

The removal of malpositioned or dislodged stents is technically difficult and potentially hazardous for the patient and should therefore not be attempted, except by endoscopists with experience with foreign body retrieval. A few limited reports of endoscopic removal of dislodged stents with and without the use of overtubes and with the use of snares and/or graspers have been published.[18,19] We have found the removal of dislodged stents from the stomach to be simple and safe with Microvasive Ultraflex® stents, Wilson Cook Gianturco Z® stents, and Instent EsophaCoil® stents but much more difficult and dangerous with Schneider Wallstents®.

We recommend that Ultraflex and Gianturco Z stents that have migrated to the stomach be grasped at their midpoint, using a strong snare to crimp the stent, forming a waist. The stent is then easily pulled out relatively atraumatically. The use of an overtube can reduce trauma to the esophagus but is not necessary since the stents are relatively soft. For the removal of dislodged EsophaCoil stents, however, we do recommend the use of a long overtube that either reaches the stomach or at least reaches the top of the obstructing tumor. The free end of the stent should be grasped with the use of a strong snare and then pulled with steady traction to permit the stent to uncoil into the overtube. There is much tension with the uncoiling of this stent; therefore, when the proximal portion exits the overtube hemostat clamps

Table 9–3. COMPLICATIONS OF PLASTIC AND EXPANDABLE METAL ESOPHAGEAL STENTS											
		Immediate Complications (%)						Late Complications (%)			
		Perforation		Bleeding		Death		Migration		Obstruction	
Study (Reference)	Year	Metal	Plastic	Metal	Plastic	Metal	Plastic	Metal	Plastic	Metal	Plastic
Knyrim et al (12)	1993	0	14	0	0	0	14	0	24	33	33
DePalma et al (13)	1996	0	15	0	5	0	16.6	0	15	31	25
Siersema et al (14)	1998	3	11	8	13	3	11	8	0	16	24

should be used to grasp the stent to prevent it from recoiling. Continuous steady traction will ultimately result in full uncoiling and removal of the stent.

Although four brands of metal stents are currently available (see Figure 9–6), each has variations in design, which result in differences in performance on insertion and function. In our experience, all are simple to insert, all provide good palliation of dysphagia, and all are associated with similar early and late complication rates. There are no data to suggest that any brand is superior, so we recommend that clinicians familiarize themselves with the use of one brand, according to individual preference or availability. Although not scientifically proven, it is our opinion that Ultraflex stents are easiest to insert, EsophaCoil stents and Wallstents are ideal in the setting of very fibrotic and tight tumor strictures, and the Gianturco Z stent with the DUA anti-reflux valve is ideal for stenting tumors that cross the esophagogastric (EG) junction. Tracheoesophageal fistulas associated with obstructing esophageal tumors are well sealed by any one of the covered metal stents.

Endoscopic Tumor Ablation

Several endoscopic methods of tumor ablation have been developed over the past 20 years. These include thermal methods, such as bicap cautery and high-energy neodymium (Nd):YAG laser; chemical methods, including the use of sclerosants such as absolute alcohol; and the newly approved photodynamic therapy approach, which makes use of a photosensitizing drug (Photofrin) followed by its activation with low-energy monochromatic laser light.

Bicap Tumor Probe

Thermal tumor ablation can be achieved through the use of cautery devices or high-energy laser. Following the initial development of endoscopic bicap probes for treating bleeding ulcers, larger tumor probes that could be positioned within an obstructing tumor were developed.[21] Electrical energy is delivered, heating the surface of the tumor and causing necrosis, with a delayed slough of several millimeters of tumor tissue. Although limited in depth of tissue destruction, this technique has been used by some to partially relieve tumor obstruction of the esophagus. Some data exist for this modality, but it has not been met with widespread enthusiasm.[21]

High-Energy Laser

Greater experience exists with high-energy lasers, particularly the Nd:YAG laser, which causes heating

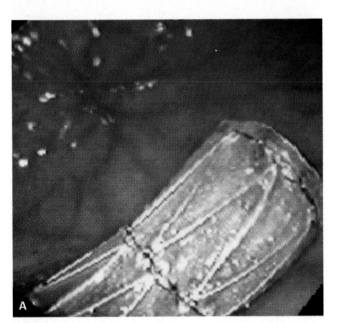
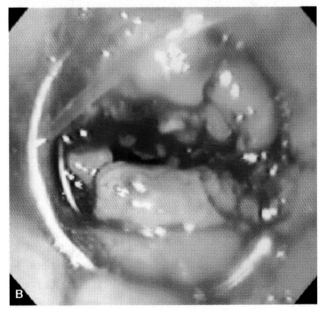

Figure 9–12.   Endoscopic photograph of a Gianturco Z® stent that has slipped into the stomach immediately after deployment. With some effort, this stent was removed completely, and a new stent was inserted. *B,* Endoscopic photograph demonstrating tumor ingrowth at the top of an EsophaCoil® stent.

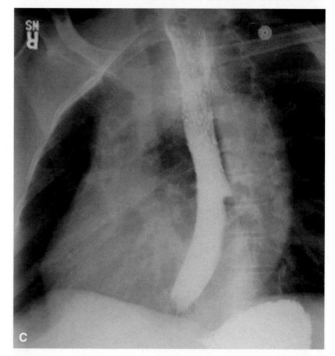

Figure 9–13. *A,* Barium radiography of a patient with proximal esophageal cancer demonstrates a tight stricture and leakage of barium into the chest cavity. *B,* Endoscopic photograph demonstrating the opening of the esophagopleural fistula. *C,* Barium radiograph of the same patient 1 day after insertion of a Gianturco Z® stent. There is complete sealing of the esophageal leak and relief of esophageal obstruction, permitting the patient to consume a regular diet.

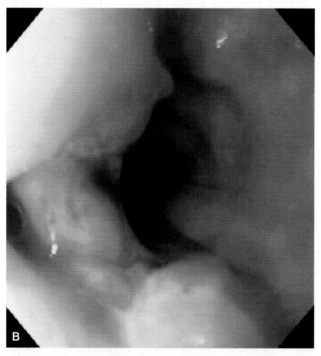

and vaporization of tumor tissue through the delivery of an intense beam of laser light.[22,23] This causes a burn that is deep enough to effectively and rapidly reconstitute the patency of the esophageal lumen. Most operators use noncontact quartz fibers to deliver the laser energy (Figure 9–14). The fibers are cooled either by water or by coaxial carbon dioxide (CO_2) and are easily passed through the suction channel of standard gastroscopes. The laser beam is aimed directly at the obstructing tumor from a distance of about 1 to 2 cm. With the laser set to maximum output, 60 to 100 watts of energy is delivered, producing both coagulation and vaporization. The entire luminal surface of the tumor can be treated by using to-and-fro motions, resulting in whitening and charring of the tumor surface. Patency (as evidenced by an improvement in the ability to pass the scope and by an improved dysphagia grade) can be

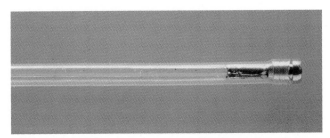

Figure 9–14. Tip of an endoscopic laser fiber used with a neodymium (Nd):YAG laser to treat obstructing esophageal tumors.

achieved immediately in some patients (Figure 9–15) and on the same day in many patients. For some patients, dysphagia improves within 24 to 48 hours following the resolution of edema and the sloughing of necrotic tumor tissue.

Initial studies of esophageal cancer treatment with Nd:YAG laser demonstrated success in palliating dysphagia in 70 to 80 percent of patients.[22,23] This translated to an ability to tolerate soft food in most patients and was associated with low morbidity and mortality as compared with the outcomes of the insertion of plastic esophageal stents. Patients with short bulky midesophageal tumors seemed to achieve the greatest benefit from Nd:YAG laser treatment whereas patients with long (> 8 cm) infiltrating tumors in the upper or lower esophagus did

less well.[23,24] The average duration of palliation with Nd:YAG laser tumor ablation is estimated at about 4 weeks. In a prospective comparison between Nd:YAG tumor ablation and intubation with an Atkinson tube, Loizou and colleagues demonstrated comparable success at palliating dysphagia; for patients with tumors crossing the cardia, however, stenting provided superior palliation, with fewer procedures.[25] For other patients, laser therapy provided a greater ability to eat solid food and was associated with a lower perforation rate.[25]

Photodynamic Therapy

Several years ago, many years of research finally culminated in the USFDA's approval of photodynamic therapy (PDT), a new local method of tumor ablation. This treatment takes advantage of the phenomenon that light can activate certain chemicals to destroy living cells. Porfimer sodium (Photofrin [Sanofi-Synthelabo, New York]) is currently the only photosensitizing compound approved by the USFDA. It is a purified mixture of hematoporphyrins, which are naturally occurring substances that are potent photosensitizers. When Photofrin-bearing tissue is exposed to light, a series of reac-

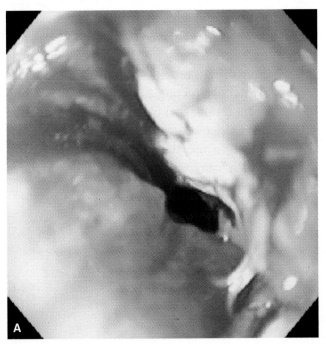

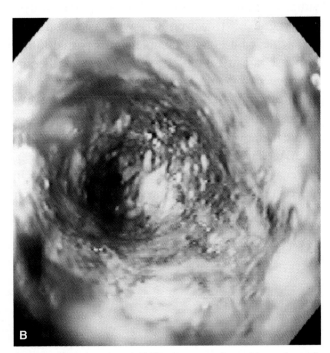

Figure 9–15. Endoscopic photograph of an obstructing esophageal tumor prior to laser treatment. *B,* The same esophageal tumor immediately upon completion of Nd:YAG laser treatment. Note the charred surface of the tumor and the increase in luminal diameter.

tions is initiated through the release of singlet oxygen and the formation of free radicals that cause intracellular injury and vascular changes. This cascade of events in the tumor tissue results in local tumor destruction equivalent to that of other tumor ablative methods.[26,27]

The drug Photofrin is administered systemically via intravenous injection. Within 24 to 48 hours after injection, porfimer sodium is thought to accumulate at higher concentrations in tumor tissue than in normal tissue. Esophageal tumors in patients receiving porfimer sodium can then be exposed to intense red light (wavelength of 630 nm) from a tunable dye laser at 400 to 2,000 mW of output (300 J/cm² of tumor treated), using diffusing fibers that are thin enough to pass through standard endoscopes (Figure 9–16). Two days after exposure to light, the patient is re-examined, with endoscopy revealing ischemic necrosis and sloughing of dead tumor tissue. Adherent necrotic tissue can be readily débrided with the passage of the endoscope, reducing the inner bulk of the tumor in a manner equivalent to that of the Nd:YAG laser but without the thermal effects (Figure 9–17).

In a national randomized study comparing Nd:YAG laser therapy to PDT using Photofrin for the palliation of obstructing esophageal cancer, the two treatments were shown to be equivalent in providing an improvement of one to two points in dysphagia grade.[28] However, PDT was easier to deliver and achieved a greater complete plus partial tumor response rate at 1 month than Nd:YAG laser therapy (32% vs 20%), with fewer adverse events requiring the termination of treatment sessions and with fewer major complications (eg, perforation). Photodynamic therapy also seemed to be more effective than Nd:YAG laser therapy in the treatment of longer, more angulated, and more infiltrating tumors. In other studies, PDT was shown to result in a greater improvement in Karnofsky performance status than Nd:YAG laser therapy and to provide a longer duration of response (84 days vs 57 days).[29] The major deterrents to the use of PDT, however, remain the high costs of the laser (approximately $100,000) and the drug (approximately $3,000 to 6,000 per dose) and the prolonged duration of photosensitivity of the eyes and skin, lasting as long as 4 to 6 weeks. For a patient with a limited long-term survival, quality of life is of great importance, so the inability to walk outdoors on a sunny day for 4 to 6 weeks after treatment is often unacceptable to the patient.

Endoscopic Methods of Nutritional Palliation

Despite the successful application of endoscopic tumor ablation or esophageal stent placement for relief of esophageal tumor obstruction, some patients continue to lose weight or become dehydrated due to poor oral intake. The anorexia associated with cancer often cannot be overcome by relieving esophageal obstruction. For such patients, the only alternative to starvation and dehydration is to direct gastric or enteral infusion of nutritional formulas and water. The techniques for endoscopic insertion of gastrostomies and jejunostomies have been well described[30–32] (Figure 9–18). While performed with ease in patients with an intact esophagus and stomach, percutaneous endoscopic gastrostomy (PEG) in a patient with esophageal cancer is mostly limited by the ability to advance the endoscope past the obstructing tumor.[33,34] In the setting of significant esophageal obstruction, prior dilation of the tumor stricture may be required. An alternative would be to use the thinner pediatric gastroscopes, which can pass relatively tight strictures without the added risk of esophageal dilation.

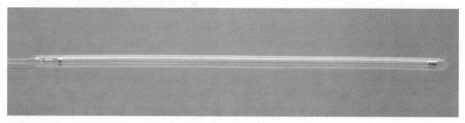

Figure 9–16.   Tip of a 5-cm cylindrical diffusing fiber used to deliver red laser light in the photodynamic therapy of obstructing esophageal tumors.

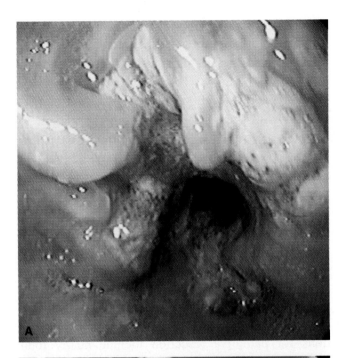

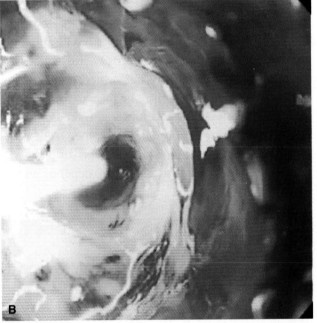

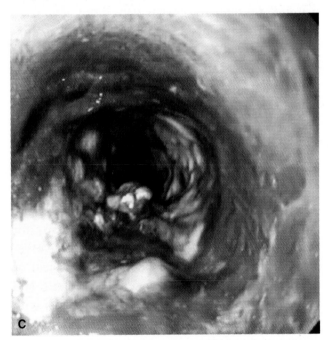

Figure 9–17. *A,* Endoscopic photograph of an obstructing esophageal mass prior to photodynamic therapy (PDT). *B,* Photodynamic therapy being delivered to the same tumor. *C,* Endoscopic photograph from the same patient, 2 days after PDT. Note the white and gray necrotic tumor and the increased luminal diameter.

Although more challenging, even patients who have had prior surgical alteration of the upper gastrointestinal tract can undergo direct percutaneous endoscopic jejunostomy (PEJ) with excellent palliative results and acceptable risk.[34,35] With the new enteroscopes or the thin pediatric colonoscopes, the proximal jejunum is easily reached with the patient under conscious sedation. In patients who have had prior gastric or esophageal resection, surgical scars can make the procedure more difficult. Despite this,

reaching a point in the jejunum that is amenable to transillumination is feasible and permits the placement of a direct PEJ. The original "pull" technique used in the insertion of standard PEG tubes can also be used. With this approach, a gastrostomy tube (15F to 21F) can be inserted directly into the jejunum, permitting the administration of standard nutritional formulas. Unlike in gastrostomies, however, the tolerance of the small bowel for hyperosmolar formulas is limited, so we recommend the use of iso-osmolar formulas that are administered at a slower rate, preferably with the aid of a pump. In our experience, such patients can be nutritionally palliated for long periods, with a complication rate of only 6 percent following direct PEJ.[37]

SURGERY

Prior to the introduction of the wide variety of palliative endoscopic techniques discussed above, surgical therapy was commonly used to provide symptomatic relief and to improve the quality of life in patients with incurable esophageal cancer. The use of surgical modalities for these indications is now appropriately quite limited. The postoperative pain, duration of recovery, and expense are difficult to justify. Moreover, surgical options expose patients to the risk of important complications and death, risks that are substantially greater than those associated with endoscopic modalities. Thus, surgical palliation is reserved for patients who are in excellent general health, for whom the life expectancy is greater than 1 year, and for whom other palliative modalities are contraindicated or have failed.

Resection

Resection is potentially curative for patients with stages I to III of disease and in whom an R0 resection is performed. Resection for this indication and the use of potentially curative surgical therapy for patients with stage IV disease (by virtue of involvement of metastatic lymph nodes in the cervical or celiac axis regions) are discussed in Chapter 6 and will not be further addressed here. In patients with stage IV disease, or for those with lesser stages of disease who undergo R1 or R2 resections, surgery is considered palliative. For the latter group of patients, it is rare that the palliative nature of such operations is known before well into the operation or before pathology results become available. In the unlikely instance in which it is known preoperatively that M1 disease exists or that a resection will be incomplete, surgery is performed with the knowledge that it is for palliative reasons only. The objectives in such a situation are relief of bleeding or dysphagia, control of locoregional disease, and prevention of local complications.

Appropriate selection of patients for resection is particularly important when the intent of the operation is palliative. The median survival for patients undergoing palliative resection is only 5 to 10 months, making it important that resection be performed with the goal of returning the patient to optimal performance status as quickly as possible.[36–41] This is made more difficult by the fact that the risks of nonfatal complications and mortality increase with more advanced stages of disease and are higher in patients for whom the intent of the operation is palliative.[42–45]

Relative contraindications to palliative resection include invasion of the aorta, airways, or vertebral bodies, distant organ metastases, poor performance status, significant cardiopulmonary disease, and life expectancy of less than 6 months. Specific indications for palliative resection include nearly total esophageal obstruction that is not amenable to laser therapy or stenting, persistent bleeding, perforation, and locally advanced primary tumors, with impending invasion of the aorta or airway. Resection for these indications is usually performed transthoracically by using an open technique because of the need to carefully dissect the primary tumor from surrounding structures. Local recurrence rates are higher when a transhiatal approach is used.[47] The choice of a right or left thoracotomy depends on the

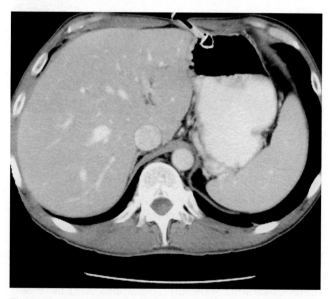

Figure 9–18. Computed tomography scan of a patient with obstructing esophageal cancer, demonstrating a percutaneous endoscopic gastrostomy (PEG) tube in the stomach for feeding.

location of the tumor and the potentially involved adjacent structures. Most palliative resections are performed through a right thoracotomy to provide optimal access to the entire esophagus as well as the proximal descending aorta and major airways (Figure 9–19). A left thoracotomy provides the best access to the lower thoracic esophagus, cardia, and distal thoracic aorta (Figure 9–20).

A careful assessment of resectability is performed, and an exploration of the chest and abdomen is undertaken before the resection is commenced. In contrast to approaches for potentially curative resections, there is little controversy about the appropriate extent of palliative esophagectomy. The tumor is excised with a small amount of surrounding tissue, obviously involved lymph nodes are removed, and reconstruction is performed with the stomach to limit operative time and minimize the

risk of postoperative complications. If the stomach is not available for reconstruction, a colon interposition is used, but the long-term survival rate for patients having colon interposition after palliative resection is substantially worse than for those undergoing a gastric pull-up.[45] Reconstruction may be performed through the bed of the resected esophagus (posterior mediastinum) although subsequent irradiation to this field may interfere with the functioning of the reconstructive organ. Alternatively, a substernal route may be used for reconstruction although this produces more cardiopulmonary compromise in the early postoperative period. A jejunostomy feeding tube is placed to provide enteral alimentation during the postoperative recovery period.

Complications after palliative resection include pneumonia, respiratory insufficiency, anastomotic leak, and other infection. About 50 percent of

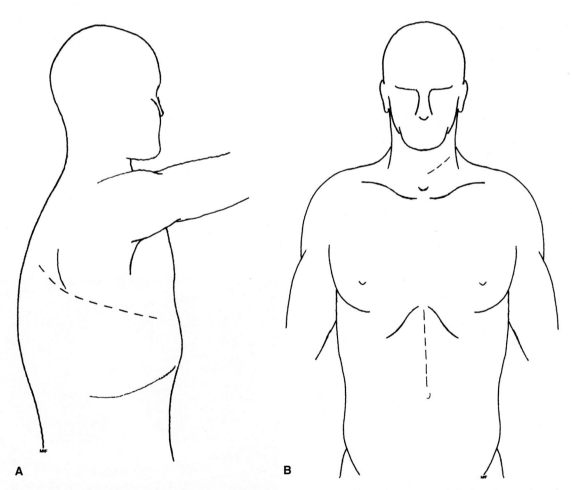

Figure 9–19.   Incisions for palliative esophagectomy via a modified Ivor Lewis approach. *A,* A right thoracotomy through the fifth intercostal space provides access to the thoracic esophagus. *B,* After completion of the intrathoracic portion of the operation, the patient is turned supine to permit gastric mobilization through a laparotomy, and a cervical anastomosis is eventually performed.

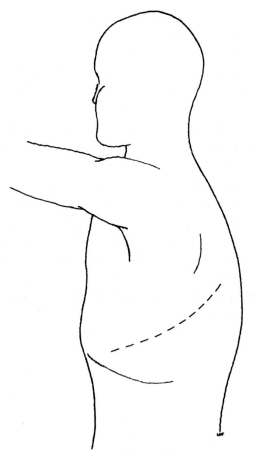

Figure 9–20. A left thoracotomy incision for palliative esophagectomy through the seventh or eighth intercostal space provides access to the lower esophagus and upper abdomen through a peripheral incision in the diaphragm.

patients can be expected to develop a nonfatal major complication. The mortality rate for palliative esophagectomy ranges from 10 to 20 percent.[36,37,40,46]

Bypass

Surgical bypass for unresectable esophageal cancer has been advocated as a method of restoring the continuity of the alimentary tract since the early twentieth century.[47] The fact that the operation was developed before the introduction of high-quality intraluminal prostheses accounts for its frequent use in the palliation of unresectable cancers prior to the final decade of the twentieth century. Among the common indications for bypass prior to that time were unresectable tumors that were complicated by an esophageal-airway fistula or that produced near total obstruction. The availability of intraluminal

prostheses to restore the patency of the esophageal lumen and to seal airway fistulae has greatly limited the use of esophageal bypass.

Current indications for esophageal bypass are limited to high-grade esophageal obstruction by an unresectable tumor not amenable to laser therapy or stenting (Figure 9–21), free perforation of an unresectable esophageal cancer, and an esophageal-airway fistula not amenable to stenting (Figure 9–22). The latter two situations occur occasionally when a fistula or perforation develops in an area of the esophagus other than where the tumor is located, preventing the successful use of a stent for sealing the communication. When contemplating this operation, one should note that the median survival for patients undergoing bypass is only 3 to 6 months.[45,48–55] Patients with an important clinical pneumonia resulting from an airway fistula are usually considered to be too ill to permit safe bypass surgery. Intervention, when appropriate, should take place prior to the development of frank pneumonia.

The operation is performed with the patient in a supine position. The stomach is mobilized, preserving the right gastroepiploic arcade as its main blood supply, and is divided from the esophagus just above the esophagogastric junction. The junction is resected to prevent ulceration of any residual squamous mucosa. The cervical esophagus is mobilized, and a substernal tunnel is created bluntly. The stomach is pulled up through the substernal tunnel and is anastomosed to the cervical esophagus in an end-to-side fashion (Figure 9–23). A feeding jejunostomy is

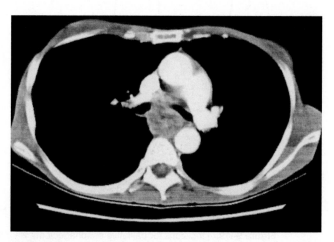

Figure 9–21. A possible indication for palliative bypass surgery is high-grade obstruction caused by an esophageal cancer that is not amenable to resection due to airway and aortic invasion.

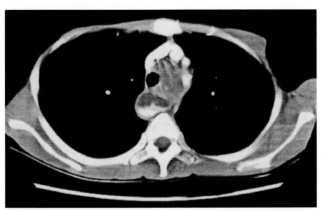

Figure 9–22. A possible indication for palliative bypass surgery is an esophagorespiratory fistula that is not amenable to stenting.

placed to permit enteral alimentation during the early postoperative recovery period.

The main controversies regarding the operative techniques center on the proper management of the proximal and distal ends of the esophagus. If an

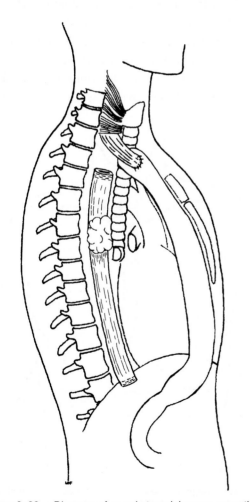

Figure 9–23. Diagram of a substernal bypass operation for a malignant esophagorespiratory fistula.

esophageal-airway fistula exists, the ends of the esophagus can be stapled, leaving the mucus produced by the esophagus to drain innocuously into the airway. For patients with perforation, a drain is placed through the proximal cut end of the esophagus and is brought out of the neck for long-term decompression of the thoracic esophagus. Patients who have esophageal obstruction pose a more challenging problem. Drainage with an indwelling tube is appropriate for the esophagus proximal to the obstruction, but this tube will not decompress the esophagus distal to the obstruction. If left undrained, the stapled end of the distal esophagus will open due to continued esophageal peristaltic activity, creating a fistula into the mediastinum, pleura, or peritoneal cavity. Under most circumstances, it is appropriate to consider anastomosing the distal esophageal segment to a Roux-en-Y limb of jejunum for decompression (Figure 9–24).

The nonfatal complication rate after palliative esophageal bypass exceeds 75 percent and is primarily due to pre-existing respiratory problems caused by esophageal-airway fistulas. Historically, the operative mortality rate ranged from 33 to 55 percent and was higher in patients with esophageal-airway fistulas.[48–50,54,56] Current operative mortality rates range from 15 to 30 percent.[55,57–60] Survival appears to be no better after palliative bypass surgery than after palliative radiation therapy.[61]

Esophagostomy and Enteral Feeding Tube

Esophageal exclusion by a combination of a cervical esophagostomy and an enteral feeding tube has been used for decades for the palliation of completely obstructing esophageal cancer and malignant esophagorespiratory fistula (Figure 9–25). The advantages of this treatment are minimization of pulmonary soilage by aspirated saliva, the ability to provide enteral nutrition, and low operative morbidity and mortality. Unfortunately, this technique provides little palliative benefit other than the prevention of pneumonia. The fact that the patient is unable to eat results in a very poor quality of life. Life expectancy is somewhat increased due to the prevention of pulmonary complications, but since regional disease is unaffected by the exclusion operation, tumor-related survival is not influenced. In addition, if a need arises for intraluminal therapy, the patient will not be eligible due to lack of access to the esophagus. Exclusion performed as the first stage of a two-stage operation may permit a carefully selected patient to recover from respiratory embarrassment due to a malignant esophagorespiratory fistula, making bypass surgery safe as the second stage.

OTHER PALLIATIVE MODALITIES

Radiation Therapy

Although radiation therapy has been used for decades as a potentially curative treatment for localized esophageal cancer, its role as an adjuvant to surgery or chemotherapy remains to be determined. An additional current role is in the palliation of unresectable obstructing esophageal tumors. Potential palliative effects include relief of dysphagia, control of pain due to local invasion, and prevention of esophagorespiratory fistulas. The only available data on the effectiveness of symptom palliation by radiation therapy concern the relief of dysphagia. Controversies exist regarding whether external beam radiotherapy should be combined with intraluminal brachytherapy and whether external beam radiotherapy is more effective when administered concomitantly with systemic chemotherapy.

External Beam Radiotherapy

External beam radiotherapy is an important method of palliation for high-grade obstruction caused by esophageal cancer. Indications for palliative external beam radiotherapy include unresectable regional disease and metastatic disease complicated by dysphagia. A palliative course of radiotherapy for optimal relief of symptoms consists of 50 to 60 Gy administered over 5 to 6 weeks. In symptomatic patients with very limited life expectancy, higher daily fractions can decrease the duration of therapy. Short courses of 30 Gy over 2 weeks may be indi-

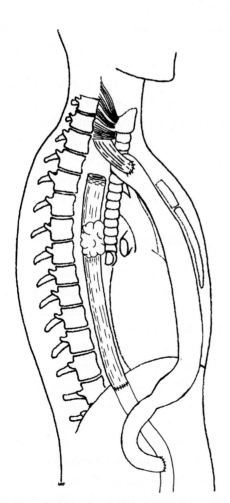

Figure 9–24. Diagram of a substernal bypass operation for obstructing esophageal cancer, showing the distal esophagus decompressed via a Roux-en-Y esophagojejunostomy.

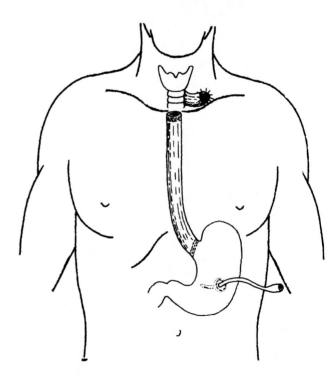

Figure 9–25. Diagram showing the technique for esophageal exclusion for the management of a malignant obstruction or a malignant esophagorespiratory fistula.

cated for patients who are terminal. Relief of dysphagia does not occur immediately, and several weeks are usually required for substantial benefit to become evident. Esophagitis may aggravate the symptoms of dysphagia in the interim. The likelihood of substantial symptomatic improvement at the conclusion of therapy is 70 to 90 percent. The duration of palliation is about 3 months.[62–65]

Brachytherapy

Endoluminal brachytherapy has been used for the palliation of esophageal cancer since the early 1900s. It has recently gained popularity as a means to achieve improved local tumor control and palliate obstructive symptoms, as opposed to external beam radiotherapy alone. The indications for brachytherapy are similar to those for external beam radiotherapy. In addition, brachytherapy can be used to palliate patients in whom treatment with external beam radiotherapy has failed. Guidelines for the palliative administration of brachytherapy suggest that it be used after limited-dose external beam radiotherapy (30 Gy).[66] In patients whose life expectancy is less than 3 months, external beam radiotherapy may be omitted. Treatments are administered at a high dose rate (10 to 14 Gy in one or two fractions) or a low dose rate (20 to 25 Gy in a single fraction at 0.4 to 1 Gy/h), depending on the radiation source and afterloading technology that are available. Relief of dysphagia is similar to that provided by external beam radiotherapy alone, but some quality-of-life advantage may be provided by the shortened course of treatment associated with brachytherapy.[61,67–70]

Combined Chemoradiotherapy

The suboptimal results provided by radiotherapy alone have stimulated the use of combined-modality therapy for palliative and potentially curative treatment of esophageal cancer. Results of the palliative use of chemoradiotherapy have not been widely reported, and there are few data regarding symptomatic relief from dysphagia in a truly palliative setting. Most multimodality therapies combine standard external beam radiotherapy with systemic agents (usually cisplatin or 5-fluorouracil) that act as

radiosensitizers to provide synergistic antitumor effects. Relief of dysphagia is experienced by 60 to 80 percent of patients, similar to the percentage of patients given dysphagia relief by radiation therapy alone.[71–73] There is no convincing evidence that other important palliative benefits are provided by multimodality therapy.[74,75] Due to the added toxicity, expense, and duration of therapy, combined-modality therapy currently has little to recommend it over radiation therapy alone. Currently, palliative multimodality therapy should be used only in an investigational setting.

REFERENCES

1. Roth J, Lichter AS, Putnam JB, Forastiere AA. Cancer of the esophagus. In: DeVita VT, Hellman S, Rosenberg SA, editors. Cancer: principle and practice of oncology. 4th ed. Philadelphia: JB Lippincott Co.; 1993. p. 776–817.
2. Mellow MH, Pinkas H. Endoscopic laser therapy for malignancies affecting the esophagus and gastroesophageal junction: analysis of technical and functional efficacy. Arch Intern Med 1985;145:1443–6.
3. Tulman AB, Boyce HW. Complications of esophageal dilation and guidelines for their prevention. Gastrointest Endosc 1981;27:229–34.
4. Boyce HW. Palliation of advanced esophageal cancer. Semin Oncol 1984;11:186–94.
5. Lundell L, Leth R, Lind T, et al. Palliative endoscopic dilatation in carcinoma of the esophagus and esophagogastric junction. Acta Chir Scand 1989;155:179–84.
6. Weisel W, Raine F, Watson RR, Frederick JJ. Palliative treatment of esophageal carcinoma: a method and its evaluation. Ann Surg 1959;149:207.
7. Earlam R, Cunha-Melo JR. Malignant oesophageal strictures: a review of techniques for palliative intubation. Br J Surg 1982;69:61–8.
8. den Hartog Jager FC, Bartelsman JF, Tytgat GN. Palliative treatment of obstructing esophagogastric malignancy by endoscopic positioning of a plastic prosthesis. Gastroenterology 1979;77:1008–14.
9. Siefert E, Reinhard A, Lutke A, Gail K. Palliative treatment of inoperable patients with carcinoma of the cardia region. Gastrointest Endosc 1983;1:6–7.
10. Chavy AL, Rougier PM, Piddeloup CH, et al. Esophageal prosthesis for neoplastic stenosis. Cancer 1986;57:1426–31.
11. Atkinson M, Ferguson R, Parker GC. Tube introducer and modified Celestin tube for use in palliative intubation of oesophagogastric neoplasms at fibreoptic endoscopy. Gut 1978;19:669–71.
12. Knyrim K, Wagner HJ, Bethge N, et al. A controlled trial of expansile metal stent for palliation of esophageal obstruction due to inoperable cancer. N Engl J Med 1993;329: 1302–7.
13. DePalma GD, diMatteo E, Romano G, et al. Plastic prosthesis versus expandable metal stents for palliation of inop-

erable thoracic carcinoma: a controlled prospective study. Gastrointest Endosc 1996;43:787–2.

14. Siersema FD, Hop WCJ, Dees J, et al. Coated self-expanding metal stents versus latex prostheses for esophagogastric cancer with special reference to prior radiation and chemotherapy: a controlled, prospective study. Gastrointest Endosc 1998;47:113–20.

15. Kozarek RA, Raltz S, Brugge WR, et al. Prospective multicenter trial of esophageal Z-stent placement for malignant dysphagia and tracheoesophageal fistula. Gastrointest Endosc 1996;44:562–7.

16. Raijman I, Siddique I, Ajani J, Lynch P. Palliation of malignant dysphagia and fistulae with coated expandable metal stents: experience with 101 patients. Gastrointest Endosc 1998;48:172–9.

17. Dumonceau JM, Cremer M, Lalmand B, Deviere J. Esophageal fistula sealing: choice of stent, practical management and cost. Gastrointest Endosc 1999;49:70–8.

18. Rollhauser C, Fleischer DE. Late migration of a self-expandable metal stent and successful endoscopic management. Gastrointest Endosc 1999;49:541–4.

19. May A, Gobner L, Feeb F, et al. Extraction of migrated self-expanding esophageal stents. Gastrointest Endosc 1999; 49:524–27.

20. Begbie S, Briggs G, Levi J. A late complication of palliative stenting of malignant oesophageal obstruction. Aust N Z J Med 1996;26:115.

21. Johnston JH, Fleischer D, Petrini J, Nord HJ. Palliative bipolar electrocoagulation therapy of obstructing esophageal cancer. Gastrointest Endosc 1987;33:349–53.

22. Fleischer D, Sivak MV. Endoscopic Nd:YAG laser therapy as palliation for esophagogastric cancer: parameters affecting initial outcome. Gastroenterology 1985;89:827–31.

23. Lightdale CJ, Zimbalist E, Winawer SJ. Outpatient management of esophageal cancer with endoscopic Nd:YAG laser. Am J Gastroenterol 1987;82:46–50.

24. Alderson D, Wright PD. Laser recanalisation versus endoscopic intubation in the palliation of malignant dysphagia. Br J Surg 1990;77:1151–3.

25. Loizou LA, Grigg D, Atkinson M, et al. A prospective comparison of laser therapy and intubation in endoscopic palliation for malignant dysphagia. Gastroenterology 1991; 100:1303–10.

26. Dougherty TJ, Kaufman JE, Goldfarb A, et al. Photoradiation therapy for the treatment of malignant tumors. Cancer Res 1978;38:2828–35.

27. McCaughan JS, Nims TA, Guy JT, et al. Photodynamic therapy for esophageal tumors. Arch Surg 1989;124:74–80.

28. Lightdale CJ, Heier SK, Marcon NE, et al. Photodynamic therapy with porfimer sodium versus thermal ablation therapy with Nd:YAG laser for palliation of esophageal cancer: a multicenter randomized trial. Gastrointest Endosc 1995;42:507–12.

29. Heier SK, Rothman KA, Heier LM, Rosenthal WS. Photodynamic therapy for obstructing esophageal cancer: light dosimetry and randomized comparison with Nd:YAG laser therapy. Gastroenterology 1995;109:63–72.

30. Gauderer MWL, Ponsky JL, Izant RJ. Gastrostomy without laparotomy: a percutaneous endoscopic technique. J Pediatr Surg 1980;15:872–5.

31. Ponsky JL, Gauderer MWL, Stellato TA. Percutaneous endoscopic gastrostomy: review of 150 cases. Arch Surg 1983;18:913–4.

32. Ponsky JL, Aszodi A. Percutaneous endoscopic jejunostomy. Am J Gastroenterol 1984;79:113–6.

33. Shike M, Berner YN, Gerdes H, et al. Percutaneous endoscopic gastrostomy and jejunostomy for long-term feeding in patients with cancer of the head and neck. Otolaryngol Head Neck Surg 1989;101:549–54.

34. Shike M, Wallach C, Likier H. Direct percutaneous endoscopic jejunostomies. Gastrointest Endosc 1991;37:62–5.

35. Shike M, Latkany L, Gerdes H, Block A. Direct percutaneous endoscopic jejunostomies for enteral feeding. Gastrointest Endosc 1996;44:536–40.

36. Segalin A, Little AG, Ruol A, et al. Surgical and endoscopic palliation of esophageal carcinoma. Ann Thorac Surg 1989;48:267–71.

37. Abe S, Nakamura T, Tachibana M, Yoshimura H. Surgical treatment of esophageal cancer: what is palliative resection? Dis Esophagus 1990;3:41–8.

38. Lerut TE, de Leyn P, Coosemans W, et al. Advanced esophageal carcinoma. World J Surg 1994;18:379–87.

39. Chak A, Canto M, Gerdes H, et al. Prognosis of esophageal cancers preoperatively staged to be locally invasive (T4) by endoscopic ultrasound (EUS): a multicenter retrospective cohort study. Gastrointest Endosc 1995;42:501–6.

40. Matsubara T, Ueda M, Nakajima T, et al. Can esophagectomy cure cancer of the thoracic esophagus involving the major airways? Ann Thorac Surg 1995;59:173–7.

41. Fockens P, Kisman K, Merkus MP, et al. The prognosis of esophageal carcinoma staged irresectable (T4) by endosonography. J Am Coll Surg 1998;186:17–23.

42. Nishi M, Hiramatsu Y, Hioki K, et al. Risk factors in relation to postoperative complications in patients undergoing esophagectomy or gastrectomy for cancer. Ann Surg 1988;207:148–54.

43. Chan K–H, Wong J. Mortality after esophagectomy for carcinoma of esophagus: an analysis of risk factors. Dis Esophagus 1990;3:49–53.

44. Elias D, Lasser P, Mankarios H, et al. Esophageal squamous cell carcinoma: the specific limited place of surgery defined by a prospective multivariate study of prognostic factors after surgical approach. Eur J Surg Oncol 1992;18:563–71.

45. Horvath OP, Lukacs L. Palliation of esophageal cancer: palliative resection and bypass surgery. Dis Esophagus 1996;9:117–22.

46. Ferguson MK. Esophageal perforation and caustic injury: management of perforated esophageal cancer. Dis Esophagus 1997;10:90–4.

47. Kirschner M. Ein neues Verfahren der Oesophagus plastik. Arch Klin Chir 1920;114:606–63.

48. Roeher HD, Horeyseck G. The Kirschner bypass operation— a palliation for complicated esophageal carcinoma. World J Surg 1981;5:543–6.

49. Wong J, Lam KH, Wei WI, Ong GB. Results of Kirschner operation. World J Surg 1981;5:547–52.

50. Conlan AA, Nicolaou N, Delikaris PG, Pool R. Pessimism concerning palliative bypass procedures for established malignant esophagorespiratory fistulas: a report of 18 patients. Ann Thorac Surg 1984;37:108–10.

51. Little AG, Ferguson MK, DeMeester TR, et al. Esophageal carcinoma with respiratory tract fistula. Cancer 1984;53: 1322–8.

52. Symbas PN, McKeown PP, Hatcher CR Jr, Vlasis SE. Tracheoesophageal fistula from carcinoma of the esophagus. Ann Thorac Surg 1984;38:382–6.

53. Burt M, Diehl W, Martini N, et al. Malignant esophagorespiratory fistula: management options and survival. Ann Thorac Surg 1991;52:1222–9.

54. Meunier B, Spiliopoulos Y, Stasik C, et al. Retrosternal bypass operation for unresectable squamous cell cancer of the esophagus. Ann Thorac Surg 1996;62:373–7.

55. Cantero R, Torres AJ, Hernando F, et al. Palliative treatment of esophageal cancer: self-expanding metal stents versus Postlethwait technique. Hepatogastroenterology 1999;46: 971–6.

56. Orringer MB, Sloan H. Substernal gastric bypass of the excluded thoracic esophagus for palliation of esophageal carcinoma. J Thorac Cardiovasc Surg 1975;70:836–51.

57. Hirai T, Yamashita Y, Mukaida H, et al. Bypass operation for advanced esophageal cancer—an analysis of 93 cases. Jpn J Surg 1989;19:182–8.

58. Muller JM, Erasmi J, Stelzner M, et al. Surgical therapy of esophageal carcinoma. Br J Surg 1990;77:845–57.

59. Voros A, Kiss J, Altorjay A. Late results of operations on esophagus and cardia tumors (1973–1990). In: Nabeya K, Hanaoka T, Nogami H, editors. Recent advances in diseases of the esophagus. Tokyo: Springer-Verlag; 1993. p. 644–50.

60. Fok M, Law SYK, Wong J. Operable esophageal carcinoma: results for Hong Kong. World J Surg 1994;18:355–60.

61. Iwasa M, Ohmori Y, Iwasa Y, et al. Effect of multidisciplinary treatment with high dose rate intraluminal brachytherapy on survival in patients with unresectable esophageal cancer. Dig Surg 1998;15:227–35.

62. Caspers RJ, Welvaart K, Verkes RJ, et al. The effect of radiotherapy on dysphagia and survival in patients with esophageal cancer. Radiother Oncol 1988;12:15–23.

63. Roussel A, Jacob JH, Haegele P, et al. Controlled clinical trial for the treatment of patients with inoperable esophageal carcinoma: a study of the EORTC Gastrointestinal Tract Cancer Cooperative Group. Recent Results Cancer Res 1988;110:21–9.

64. Whittington R, Coia LR, Haller DG, et al. Adenocarcinoma of the esophagus and esophago-gastric junction: the effects of single and combined modalities on the survival and pattern of failure following treatment. Int J Radiat Oncol Biol Phys 1990;19:593–603.

65. Petrovich Z, Langholz B, Formenti S, et al. Management of carcinoma of the esophagus: the role of radiotherapy. Am J Clin Oncol 1991;14:80–6.

66. Gaspar LE, Nag S, Herskovic A, et al. American Brachytherapy Society (ABS) consensus guidelines for brachytherapy of esophageal cancer. Int J Radiat Oncol Biol Phys 1997;38:127–32.

67. Caspers RJ, Zwinderman AH, Griffioen G, et al. Combined external beam and low dose rate intraluminal radiotherapy in oesophageal cancer. Radiother Oncol 1993;27:7–12.

68. Feldmann HJ, Grosu A, Molls M. Palliation of esophageal cancer: endoluminal brachytherapy. Dis Esophagus 1996; 9:90–7.

69. Datta NR, Kumar S, Nangia S, et al. A non-randomized comparison of two radiotherapy protocols in inoperable squamous cell carcinoma of the oesophagus. Clin Oncol 1998; 10:306–12.

70. Sur RK, Donde B, Levin VC, Mannell A. Fractionated high dose rate intraluminal brachytherapy in palliation of advanced esophageal cancer. Int J Radiat Oncol Biol Phys 1998;40:447–53.

71. Gill PG, Denham JW, Jamieson GG, et al. Patterns of treatment failure and prognostic factors associated with the treatment of esophageal carcinoma with chemotherapy and radiotherapy either as sole treatment or followed by surgery. J Clin Oncol 1992;10:1037–43.

72. Izquierdo MA, Marcuello E, Gomez de Segura G, et al. Unresectable nonmetastatic squamous cell carcinoma of the esophagus managed by sequential chemotherapy (cisplatin and bleomycin) and radiation therapy. Cancer 1993;71:287–92.

73. Urba SG, Turrisi AT III. Split-course accelerated radiation therapy combined with carboplatin and 5-fluorouracil for palliation of metastatic or unresectable carcinoma of the esophagus. Cancer 1995;75:435–9.

74. Minsky BD. Palliation of esophageal cancer: palliative external beam radiation therapy and combined modality therapy. Dis Esophagus 1996;9:86–9.

75. Slabber CF, Nel JS, Schoeman L, et al. A randomized study of radiotherapy alone versus radiotherapy plus 5-fluorouracil and platinum in patients with inoperable, locally advanced squamous cancer of the esophagus. Am J Clin Oncol 1998;21:462–5.

10

Epidemioloigy of Gastric Cancer

NUBIA MUÑOZ, MD, MPH

The most recent estimates of global cancer incidence indicate that stomach cancer was the second most frequent cancer in the world (after lung cancer) in 1990, with about 800,000 new cases diagnosed every year.[1] Steady declines in the rates have been observed everywhere in the last few decades, but the absolute number of new cases per year is increasing, mainly because of aging of the population.

The most recent available estimates of global cancer incidence indicate that stomach cancer was the second most frequent cancer in the world after lung cancer, with about 800,000 new cases (10% of all cancers) diagnosed in 1990, 60 percent of which occurred in developing countries.[1] Fatality rates are high (the overall mortality incidence is around 70 to 90% in most countries, except in Japan, where it is 40%), and as a cause of death, stomach cancer ranked second, worldwide.[2] Steady declines have been observed everywhere in the last few decades.

The exact causes of the decline of gastric cancer are not well understood, but the causes must include improvements in diet, better food storage (eg, refrigeration) and (possibly) the decline of *Helicobacter pylori* infection.[3,4]

In this chapter, the geographic distribution and recent trends of gastric cancer will be examined. With respect to its causes, priority will be given to dietary habits, *H. pylori* infection, and the implications of these factors for the prevention of this malignancy.

GEOGRAPHIC DISTRIBUTION

Around 1990, the estimated incidence rates of cancer of the stomach in men, standardized to the world population, ranged from below 10 per 100,000 in North America, northern Africa, and South and Southeast Asia to very high rates (> 40 per 100,000) in East Asia, most notably in Japan (78 per 100,000), the former Union of Soviet Socialist Republics (USSR), and China[5] (Figures 10–1 and 10–2).

Data from selected population-based cancer registries indicate that the highest rates (over 40 per 100,000 in males) are reported from Japan, China, the former USSR, and certain countries in Latin America. The lowest rates (< 15 per 100,000) are seen in North America (specifically, its white population), India, the Philippines, most African countries, some countries in western Europe, and Australia. Intermediate rates are seen elsewhere (Table 10–1). There is an approximate 15- to 20-fold difference in incidence between the rates of Japan and those of white populations of the United States and of the population of some African countries. Substantial variations in gastric cancer incidence also exist within countries; a good example is Italy, where male incidence rates around 1990 ranged from 36.3 per 100,000 in Florence to 13.2 per 100,000 in Ragusa[5] (see Table 10–1).

The mortality pattern is very similar to the incidence pattern, due to the high fatality rates.[2] In Latin America, the highest mortality rates in males are reported from Costa Rica and Chile, and the lowest are reported from Mexico and Cuba.[6]

Using the histologic classification originally proposed by Jarvi and Lauren, this author and colleagues[7] reviewed slides of gastric cancer cases from a variety of populations in Colombia, Mexico, Israel, Poland, the former Yugoslavia, and the

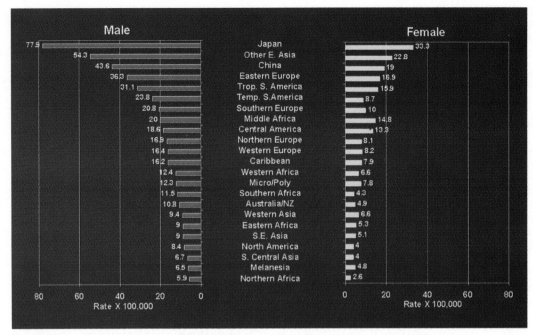

Figure 10–1. Estimated age-standardized incidence rates of stomach cancer, circa 1990.

United States. It was found that the intestinal type predominated in high-risk areas, especially in men and in older age groups, whereas the diffuse type was more frequent in low-risk areas and at younger ages.

TIME TRENDS

A steady decline in the incidence and mortality rates of gastric adenocarcinoma has been observed worldwide over the past several decades, but the

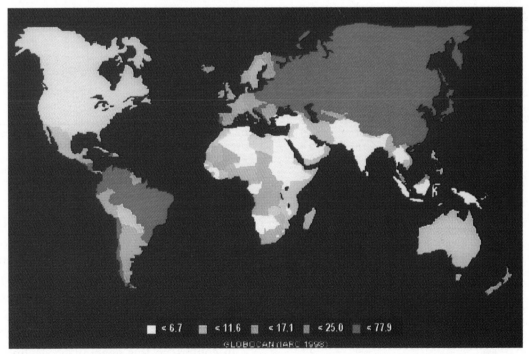

Figure 10–2. Age-standardized worldwide distribution of stomach cancer. (Trop. = tropical; Temp. = temperate; Micro/Poly = Micronesia and Polynesia; NZ = New Zealand.)

Table 10–1. AGE-STANDARDIZED ANNUAL INCIDENCE RATES OF STOMACH CANCER BY SEX, CIRCA 1990		
	Incidence per 100,000	
Tumor Registry	Men	Women
Western Europe		
Germany, Saarland	18.5	9.0
Netherlands, Eindhoven	17.0	7.4
Netherlands, Maastricht	15.4	6.5
Switzerland, Neuchatel	12.7	5.4
Switzerland, Vaud	10.4	4.2
France, Doubs	10.7	3.7
France, Calvados	13.4	4.8
France, Bas Rhin	12.2	4.9
France, Isère	11.8	4.7
France, Tarn	8.6	3.3
Northern Europe		
Iceland	20.2	10.4
Finland	16.6	9.2
UK, Scotland	17.7	7.5
UK, England and Wales	16.1	6.3
Norway	13.6	6.4
Ireland, southern	13.3	5.0
Sweden	10.7	5.4
Denmark	9.0	4.7
Southern Europe		
Slovenia	27.0	10.6
Spain, Basque country	24.2	9.6
Spain, Navarra	25.4	10.3
Spain, Murcia	15.1	7.3
Spain, Tarragona	13.5	6.2
Italy, Florence	36.3	15.9
Italy, Parma	33.7	14.7
Italy, Varese	26.6	12.7
Italy, Torino	17.3	8.7
Italy, Ragusa	13.2	6.4
Malta	11.2	6.0
Ex-USSR		
Belarus	46.8	20.1
Estonia	34.0	16.6
Latvia	31.1	14.1
Eastern Europe		
Poland, Lower Silesia	24.7	10.4
Poland, Cracow	21.5	8.0
Poland, Warsaw City	19.1	6.9
Croatia	28.1	11.5
Yugoslavia, Vojvodina	20.8	9.4
Slovakia	24.5	10.3
Czech Republic	19.5	9.2
Germany (ex-GDR)	20.1	10.5
North America		
USA, Los Angeles (Korean American)	35.5	16.2
USA, Los Angeles (Japanese American)	21.2	12.0
USA, Los Angeles (African American)	13.6	5.9
USA, Los Angeles (Hispanic)	18.8	6.9
USA, Los Angeles (White)	7.6	3.2
USA, C. Louisiana (African American)	14.4	5.5
USA, C. Louisiana (White)	6.0	2.2
USA, Connecticut (African American)	13.2	6.7
USA, Connecticut (White)	9.2	3.8
SEER, USA (African American)	14.5	5.9
SEER, USA (White)	7.5	3.1
Canada	10.6	4.5

Table 10–1. *continued*		
	Incidence per 100,000	
Tumor Registry	Men	Women
Latin America		
Costa Rica	51.5	22.7
Colombia, Cali	33.3	19.3
Brazil, Porto Alegre	27.9	8.9
Brazil, Goiania	19.2	10.6
Ecuador, Quito	32.2	19.5
Peru, Trujillo	31.1	20.1
Argentina, Concordia	24.2	9.9
Uruguay, Montevideo	19.3	9.0
Africa		
Mali, Bamako	19.6	11.1
Algeria, Setif	14.4	3.5
Zimbabwe, Harare (African)	13.8	18.4
Zimbabwe, Harare (European)	8.3	6.3
Uganda, Kyadondo	5.4	3.2
Asia		
Japan, Yamagata	95.5	40.1
Japan, Miyagi	82.7	32.8
Japan, Osaka	65.0	27.3
Korea, Kangwha	65.9	25.0
China, Shanghai	46.5	21.0
China, Tianjin	29.8	11.4
Hong Kong	19.4	9.5
Singapore (Chinese)	29.3	13.6
Singapore (Indian)	10.3	7.9
Singapore (Malay)	8.7	5.5
Philippines, Manila	11.1	6.4
India, Madras	15.9	7.0
India, Bombay	7.7	3.8
India, Trivandrum	6.8	2.5
Israel (Jewish)	13.0	6.2
Israel (Israeli born)	8.9	6.0
Kuwait (non-Kuwaiti)	10.1	2.3
Kuwait (Kuwaiti)	4.1	4.8
Oceania		
New Zealand (Maori)	27.9	13.7
New Zealand (non-Maori)	11.0	4.8
Australia, Victoria	11.7	4.9
Australia NSW	10.1	4.2

GDR = German Democratic Republic; NSW = New South Wales; SEER = Surveillance, Epidemiology, and End Results.
Adapted with permission from Parkin DM, Whelan SL, Ferlay J, et al. Cancer incidence in five continents. Vol. VII. IARC Scientific Publications, No. 143. Lyon: International Agency for Research on Cancer; 1997.

absolute number of new cases per year is increasing, mainly because of the growth and aging of the population.[8] Figure 10–3 shows time trends in the mortality rates for selected countries. Analysis of time trends by histologic type indicates that the decline in incidence is principally due to a decline in the intestinal type.[7]

In contrast to this generalized decline in gastric adenocarcinoma, an increase in the incidence of cardia adenocarcinoma has been reported in Canada and the United States (Figure 10–4), some European countries, and Australia.[9] In most areas, the increase in cardia cancer has been concomitant with an increase in adenocarcinoma of the esophagus. Although the reasons for this increase are not fully understood, it seems that changes in diagnostic and classification practices may account for only a small proportion of the increase in the United States but for a substantial proportion in other countries.[9]

Recent epidemiologic studies indicate that adenocarcinoma of the cardia and of the lower esophagus share common risk factors (eg, obesity, gastroesophageal reflux, and subsequent Barrett's esophagus) and that the increases in the prevalence of these risk factors might be possible explanations for the increased incidence of these tumors.[10]

AGE AND SEX DISTRIBUTION

Gastric cancer is extremely rare in individuals below the age of 30 years; thereafter, it increases rapidly and steadily and reaches the highest rates in the oldest age groups, both in males and females.

The intestinal type of gastric cancer rises faster with age than the diffuse type, and it is more frequent in males than in females.

In most populations, there is a twofold to threefold greater incidence in males as compared to females (see Table 10–1). This male predominance tends to be more evident in high-risk populations than in low-risk populations. This pattern is expected in view of the male predominance in the intestinal type in the high-risk areas and a sex ratio that is close to 1.0 in the low-risk areas.[7]

For cancer in the cardia, the sex ratio is higher (usually over 4.0) than for cancers in the distal stomach.

RISK FACTORS

Diet

Over 30 case-control studies and 6 cohort studies conducted all over the world have shown that diets high in fresh fruits and vegetables offer a remarkably consistent protection against the development of gastric cancer.[11]

Studies were carried out in a great variety of geographic locations, and each study differed with regard to the type and number of vegetable and fruit items elicited in the questionnaire. However, with only a few exceptions, negative associations were found with the high intake of most types of vegetables, most notably fruits (especially citrus fruit) and raw and *Allium* vegetables. The consistency of these studies is remarkable in view of the limitations of the questionnaire-based methods used to assess past diet.

A panel of experts recently reviewed all available epidemiologic and laboratory evidence on diet and

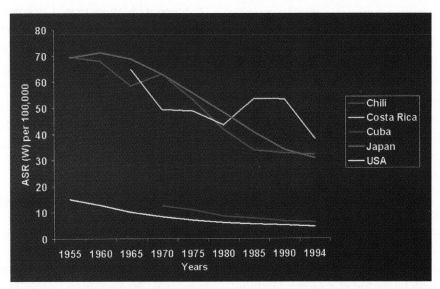

Figure 10–3. Stomach cancer mortality among males in five countries from 1955 to 1994. (ASR = age-standardized rates; W = world (standardized to the world population.)

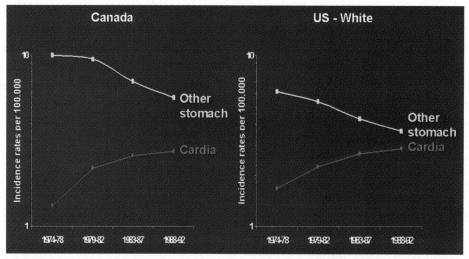

Figure 10–4.   North American time trends of cancer of the stomach and cardia.

gastric cancer. The following four levels of strength of scientific evidence of causal relationships were considered in their evaluation:

1. Convincing (when the evidence of a causal relationship is strong, consistent, and biologically plausible)
2. Probable (when the epidemiologic evidence is somewhat weaker and less consistent but the experimental evidence is supportive)
3. Possible (when the epidemiologic studies are generally supportive but limited in quality, quantity, or consistency)
4. Insufficient (when there are only a few studies and these are limited in quality and consistency)

The main conclusions of this panel can be summarized as follows:

• Evidence that diets high in vegetables and fruits decrease the risk of stomach cancer was convincing. Vegetables and fruits contain many compounds that may be responsible for the protective effect revealed by the epidemiologic studies. The most likely anticarcinogenic compounds are antioxidant vitamins. Several epidemiologic studies have shown a consistent protective effect associated with higher intakes of vitamin C and β-carotene. However, most of the evidence regarding vitamin E and stomach cancer suggests no relationship although a few studies have shown decreased risk with higher intakes of this vitamin.
• Evidence that the long-term use of refrigeration

to preserve food is associated with a reduced risk was also considered convincing. This effect is probably mediated through a concomitant decreased intake of salty food or a concomitant increased intake of raw vegetables or fruits.
• High salt intake is associated with an increased risk, probably via the induction of chronic gastritis. The evidence for an association with salt and the evidence suggesting that vitamin C reduces the risk of stomach cancer were considered probable.
• Evidence that a high intake of whole-grain cereals, green tea, and carotenoids reduces the risk of stomach cancer as well as evidence that a high intake of grilled or barbecued meat and starchy food is associated with an increased risk were considered possible. The association with starchy foods is possibly explained by the fact that these monotonous diets are poor in protective compounds.[11]
• Evidence indicating that fiber, selenium, and garlic decrease the risk of stomach cancer was considered insufficient, as was the suggestion that cured meats and *N*-nitrosocompounds increase the risk.

Helicobacter pylori Infection

Substantial evidence indicates that *Helicobacter pylori* is the main cause of chronic gastritis and peptic ulcer. The final proof of causation for these diseases was derived from a few human experiments showing that the ingestion of *H. pylori* causes acute gastritis[12] and from controlled intervention trials showing that *H. pylori* eradication has consistently led to the resolution of the gastritis and peptic ulcer.[13]

The epidemiologic evidence linking *H. pylori* to gastric cancer, although highly suggestive, is less straightforward. It is largely based on seroepidemiologic studies that have several methodological limitations.[14] However, an international working group convened by the International Agency for Research on Cancer (IARC) in 1994 considered the available evidence as sufficient to classify *H. pylori* as carcinogenic to humans,[15] and a National Institutes of Health (NIH) consensus panel that was convened in the same year concluded that the evidence linking *H. pylori* to gastric cancer was not conclusive and that further research was required.[16] Since then, additional epidemiologic studies have been reported, and these will be reviewed here together with the previous evidence.

Ecologic Studies

At least 12 ecologic studies have assessed the correlation between incidence or mortality rates of stomach cancer and the prevalence of *H. pylori* antibodies, with inconsistent results. Seven of them showed a statistically significant correlation,[17–23] and five did not.[24–28] Results from the above studies are not very helpful in assessing the association between *H. pylori* and gastric cancer. In addition to giving inconsistent and weak associations, no control for potential confounders was attempted in any but one of them. In the study carried out in 46 counties of rural China, the reported positive correlation remained after adjustment for dietary habits but was no longer statistically significant after adjustment for serum levels of certain micronutrients.[29] Moreover, a serious limitation of this study design was that gastric cancer

rates were compared with *H. pylori* prevalence rates in contemporaneous time periods whereas the relevant *H. pylori* prevalence rates are those that existed in the study populations several decades before the establishment of the cancer diagnosis.

Retrospective Case-Control Studies

Over a dozen retrospective case-control studies have been reported. The main limitation of this study design is that the prevalence of antibodies is measured at the time of the diagnosis of gastric cancer and thus might not reflect the relevant exposure (ie, *H. pylori* infection) that occurred many years before the development of cancer.

In most studies carried out in developed countries with low or intermediate rates of gastric cancer, the prevalence of *H. pylori* was higher among cases than among controls[30–35] (Table 10–2). The association was stronger in younger patients. In the Swedish study, the odds ratio increased with decreasing age at cancer diagnosis; the odds ratio was 9.3 (95% CI, 1.4 to 100.7) in patients under 60 years of age and 1.2 (95% CI, 0.4 to 3.0) in those over 70 years of age. In the most recent Finnish study[34] only patients under 45 years of age were included.

It should be noted that adjustment for major potential confounders (such as socioeconomic status and diet) was made in only one of these studies and that the significant association with *H. pylori* remained after the adjustment.[32] Thus, the argument that the weak associations observed in some studies[30,31,34] or the lack of association in others[33,35] could be due to confounding or to selection bias cannot be excluded. On the other hand, 6 of the 10 case-control studies carried out in populations at high risk for gastric cancer failed to show a significant association

Table 10–2. CASE-CONTROL STUDIES OF *HELICOBACTER PYLORI* IN COUNTRIES AT LOW RISK FOR GASTRIC CANCER

Country and Study (Reference)	Cases		Controls		
	No. Tested	% HP+	No. Tested	% HP+	OR (95% CI)
United States, Talley et al, 1991 (30)	37	65.0	252	38.0	2.8 (1.3–5.6)
Finland, Sipponen et al, 1992 (31)	54	70.4	83	51.8	2.2 (1.0–4.4)
Sweden, Hansson et al, 1993 (32)	112	80.4	103	61.2	2.6 (1.4–5.0)
Netherlands, Kuipers et al, 1993 (33)	116	77.0	116	79.0	0.9 (0.5–1.7)
Finland, Kokkola et al, 1996 (34)	50	72.0	50	43.0	3.3 (1.4–7.5)
Germany, Rudi et al, 1995 (35)	111	58.6	111	50.5	1.4 (0.7–2.5)

CI = confidence interval; HP+ = *Helicobacter pylori* positive; OR = odds ratio.

(Table 10–3).[36–45] Possible explanations for this lack of association could be the following:

- Misclassification of *H. pylori* status resulting from the use of inaccurate serologic assays. The *H. pylori* strains that are isolated from populations at low risk for gastric cancer and used as antigen sources in the commercial kits for serologic assays may be different from the *H. pylori* strains prevalent in populations at high risk for gastric cancer. One study conducted in Thailand supports this possibility.[46]
- It has been argued that *H. pylori* antibodies measured at the time of diagnosis of gastric cancer underestimate past exposure to *H. pylori* among cases. Because of the extensive areas of atrophy and intestinal metaplasia in the noncancerous mucosa of these patients, the intragastric environment may become unsuitable for *H. pylori* growth. The low bacterial load in these patients could lead to a low antibody response. However, there are no clear data in favor of this hypothesis.[47–49]
- It is possible that *H. pylori* prevalence has been measured accurately in some of the studies but that the very high prevalence in the general population or control groups makes the detection of a difference in risk between cases and controls difficult, except in extremely large studies.

Nested Case-Control Studies

The 10 nested case-control studies so far reported are summarized in Table 10–4. These studies are more informative because the *H. pylori* antibody levels were measured in sera collected years before the cancer diagnosis. Seven have been published in full, and three have been published as abstracts. A significant increased risk of gastric cancer was observed in five of the studies[50–54] and a nonsignificant increase in risk was found in the other five studies.[54–58]

In the study conducted among Japanese Americans living in Hawaii, the increased risk was observed for both intestinal and diffuse cancers, and the risk was stronger with increasing antibody titers and increasing intervals between serum collection and cancer diagnosis.[52] Based on the latter observation, it has been proposed that the lack of significant association reported in the studies from China and Taiwan[39,53] could be due to the shorter intervals between serum collection and cancer diagnosis in these studies. However, in the studies conducted in Finland, Japan, and Iceland, which had longer intervals between serum collection and cancer diagnosis, a nonsignificant increase in risk was also observed.[56–58] Thus, another possible explanation for the lack of association in these studies could be a misclassification of *H. pylori* exposure, resulting from the use of inaccurate serologic assays. Adjustments for major potential confounders (such as diet and socioeconomic status) were attempted in only 3 of these 10 studies.[51,53,56]

Intervention Studies

Several treatment regimens have been used to eradicate *H. pylori* infection, but the triple therapy including bismuth salts, amoxicillin, and clarithromycin is currently the regimen of choice. The disappearance of nonatrophic gastritis after the erad-

Table 10–3. CASE-CONTROL STUDIES OF *HELICOBACTER PYLORI* IN COUNTRIES AT HIGH RISK FOR GASTRIC CANCER

Country and Study (Reference)	Cases		Controls		
	No. Tested	% HP+	No. Tested	% HP+	OR (95% CI)
Japan, Igarashi et al, 1992 (36)	67	73.0	111	61.3	1.6 (0.8–3.1)
Italy, Miglio et al, 1992 (37)	64	53.0	64	54.0	1.0 (0.5–1.9)
Portugal, Estevens et al, 1993 (38)	80	70.0	80	81.0	0.6 (0.3–1.1)
Taiwan, Lin et al, 1993 (39)	148	62.2	276	72.8	0.6 (0.4–0.9)
Korea, Kang et al, 1992 (40)	28	89.0	30	67.0	4.2 (1.0–17.2)
Japan, Blaser et al, 1994 (41)	29	83.0	58	67.0	2.1 (1.5–4.3)
Japan, Asaka et al, 1994 (42)	213	88.3	214	74.6	2.6 (1.5–4.3)
Japan, Barreto-Zuñiga et al, 1997 (43)	55	82.0	75	60.0	3.0 (1.7–5.3)
Mexico, Lopez-Carrillo et al, 1997 (44)	109	87.2	177	82.5	1.4 (0.7–2.8)
Korea, Kim et al, 1997 (45)	160	60.0	160	51.9	1.4 (0.9–2.2)

CI = confidence interval; HP+ = *Helicobacter pylori* positive; OR = odds ratio.

| Location, Study (Reference) | Cases | | Controls | | Mean Follow-up (yr) | OR (95% CI) |
	No. Tested	% HP+	No. Tested	% HP+		
UK, Forman et al, 1991 (50)	29	69.0	111	46.6	6.0	2.8 (1.0–8.0)
California, USA, Parsonnet et al, 1991 (51)	109	84.4	109	60.6	14.2	3.6 (1.8–7.3)
Hawaii, USA, Nomura et al, 1991 (52)	109	94.5	109	76.1	13.5	6.0 (2.1–17.3)
Taiwan, Lin et al, 1993 (39)	29	69.0	220	59.0	3.1	1.6 (0.7–2.6)
Norway, Hansen et al, 1994 (55)	201	NA	603	NA	12.4	1.8 (1.2–2.6)
China, Webb et al, 1996 (53)	87	54.0	261	56.0	2.4	1.2 (0.5–1.5)
Finland, Aromaa et al, 1996 (56)	84	86.9	146	82.8	9.5	1.5 (0.7–3.2)
Japan, Watanabe et al, 1997 (57)	45	NA	255	NA	8.0	1.8 (0.6–5.7)
Sweden, Simán et al, 1997 (54)	46	78.0	184	50.0	5.7	3.9 (1.7–9.2)
Iceland, Tulinius et al, 1997 (58)	40	NA	240	NA	1.0–29.0	NS

Table 10–4. CASE-CONTROL *HELICOBACTER PYLORI* STUDIES NESTED WITHIN COHORTS

CI = confidence interval; HP+ = *Helicobacter pylori* positive; NA = not available; NS = not statistically significant; OR = odds ratio.

ication (by antibiotics) of *H. pylori* infection has been reported by several investigators.[12,59,60] However, the effect of this eradication on advanced precancerous lesions (ie, atrophic gastritis and intestinal metaplasia and dysplasia) is controversial.[61–65]

The effect of *H. pylori* eradication on early gastric cancer has been reported in a nonrandomized trial involving 132 *H. pylori*–infected patients from Japan. Endoscopic resection of the early gastric cancer was performed in all patients, and anti–*H. pylori* treatment was given to 65 patients (group A) but not to the other 67 patients (group B). All patients were observed for 2 years. Disappearance of the gastritis, a decrease in the severity of intestinal metaplasia, and no new gastric cancers were observed in group A. However, 6 patients (9%) in group B developed new gastric cancers after 3 years of follow-up.[66]

The intervention studies described above had several methodological limitations; all but one[58] were noncontrolled nonrandomized trials and had small sample sizes and short follow-up periods. In addition, misclassification of histologic diagnoses because of interobserver variation and/or sampling error was not taken into consideration.

Studies conducted by this author and colleagues in developing countries with a high prevalence of *H. pylori* infection and a high incidence of gastric cancer, such as Venezuela and Costa Rica, have shown that antibiotic regimens that are effective in eradicating *H. pylori* infection in developed countries give a low eradication rate in developing countries.[67,68] Primary prevention by effective vaccines against *H. pylori* may thus be the strategy of choice for the long-term control of gastric cancer in developing countries. Prophylactic vaccines (to prevent *H. pylori* infection) and therapeutic vaccines (to induce the regression of lesions) are under development.

Other Factors

Tobacco

There are 42 studies that have examined tobacco consumption as a risk factor for stomach cancer;[69] these comprise 12 cohort studies and 30 case-control studies. Ten of the cohort studies found a positive association between some aspect of tobacco use and gastric carcinoma whereas two did not find such an association. Eight of the cohort studies examined the presence of a dose-response relationship; three of these studies found a positive dose-response trend while the other five studies did not.

Of the 30 case-control studies, 19 found an association between some aspect of tobacco use and stomach cancer whereas 11 did not. Seventeen of the studies examined a dose-response relationship between the amount of tobacco consumed and gastric carcinoma risk. Of these, six studies reported that the dose-response trend was positive; in the other eleven studies, a dose-response trend was not found. Overall, these studies suggest that tobacco smoking has a role in gastric cancer.

In regard to mechanisms, the direct carcinogenic effect of ingested tobacco or tobacco smoke may include the development of precursor gastric lesions such as in gastritis, gastric peptic ulceration, and intestinal metaplasia. The indirect effects of inhaled tobacco smoke in gastric carcinogenesis may involve both the nitrosamines found in smoke and the endogenously formed nitrosamines in smokers.

Alcohol

Alcohol drinking is strongly related to cancers of the upper digestive tract, and relative-risk estimates for cancers of the oral cavity, pharynx, and esophagus are elevated by 10-fold or more among heavy drinkers as compared to nondrinkers. The risk pattern with alcohol drinking is clearly different for gastric cancer,[70] but some relation is biologically plausible. Alcohol could act as a contributory factor by causing chronic irritation of the gastric mucosa. Chronic gastritis, a disease that is thought to predispose to cancer of the stomach, is very common among alcoholics.

Occupation and Social Class

An inverse socioeconomic gradient has been observed in most populations; the rate in lower socioeconomic groups is two to three times higher than in the more affluent classes.[7] An excess risk has been linked to certain industries such as coal mining, fishing, and agriculture. Since occupations are clearly related to socioeconomic background, some of the excess risk observed might be attributable to patterns of lifestyle, such as dietary habits.

Genetic Factors

Although epidemiologic evidence indicates that environmental factors play a major role in gastric carcinogenesis, a role for genetic factors is suggested by the study of blood groups and determinants of chronic gastritis.[71] Individuals with type A blood have been known for decades to show an approximately 20 percent excess incidence of gastric cancer than those with types O, B, or AB blood. They also show a similar excess incidence of pernicious anemia. Some data suggest that type A blood may be particularly associated with the diffuse type of gastric cancer.[71] A genetic etiology has been reported for chronic atrophic gastritis, a precursor of gastric carcinoma.[72] Genetic segregation analysis showed mendelian transmission of a recessive auto-

somal gene, with penetrance dependent on age and the mother's chronic atrophic gastritic status. Of individuals with affected mothers, 48 percent were affected, compared to only 7 percent of those whose mothers did not have chronic atrophic gastritis.

Finally, a familial tendency to stomach cancer has long been suspected and has been repeatedly confirmed.[71,73,74] An estimated 10 percent of these tumors have an inherited familial component. Germline mutations in a gene encoding the cell adhesion protein E-cadherin (CDH1) lead to an autosomal dominant predisposition to diffuse gastric cancer.[75–76] Genetic abnormalities of the E-cadherin gene have also been reported in sporadic gastric cancers, especially those of the diffuse type.[77]

CONCLUSION AND PERSPECTIVES FOR PREVENTION

Geographic distribution, time trends, and the results of etiologic studies of stomach cancer are consistent in indicating a few major determinants of risk: insufficient fresh fruit and vegetable intake, excessive salt intake, gastric infection with *H. pylori*, and (possibly) genetic factors. Recent population-based survival data show that even in Western countries, 5-year relative-survival rates for stomach cancer are very low (approximately 20%) and that improvement over time is small.[78] In the absence of widely available and effective screening programs, primary prevention by decreasing the exposure to identified risk factors or by increasing the protection against them might be the most effective way of controlling the disease. Despite clear improvements in the last decades, dietary modification and (possibly) vitamin supplementation remain the most important tools for the prevention of gastric cancer. However, no intervention trial on diet and stomach cancer is in progress, and none is planned. The main reasons for this are the logistic difficulties associated with changing the diet at a population level, especially in developing countries, and the tendency toward changes in the same direction in both the placebo group and the treatment group. This tendency occurs mainly in Eastern countries, in which a substantial proportion of the population takes vitamin supplements, and in developing countries that are undergoing rapid economic change that is influencing the food supply, such as China.

Two trials on the chemoprevention of precancerous lesions of the stomach are being completed in high-risk areas of Colombia and Venezuela, and a third one is being planned in low- and intermediate-risk areas in Europe. (The main features of these trials [in which the efficacy of anti–*H. pylori* treatment and antioxidant vitamins is being assessed] have been described in the literature.[79]) Recently reported results of the Colombian trial indicate that anti–*H. pylori* treatment and antioxidant vitamins may interfere with the precancerous process, mostly by increasing the rate of regression of precancerous lesions.[80]

Control of *H. pylori* infection by means of eradication or immunization is also likely to have great potential in the prevention of stomach cancer. Ongoing studies in Venezuela suggest that the prevention and/or eradication of *H. pylori* by vaccines that are currently under development is more promising than eradication of the bacteria by antibiotics.[81]

REFERENCES

1. Parkin DM, Pisani P, Ferlay J. Estimates of the worldwide incidence of 25 major cancers in 1990. Int J Cancer 1999; 80:827–41.

2. Pisani P, Parkin DM, Bray F, Ferlay J. Estimates of the worldwide mortality from 25 cancers in 1990. Int J Cancer 1999;83:18–29.

3. Howson CP, Hiyama T, Wynder EL. The decline in gastric cancer: epidemiology of an unplanned triumph. Epidemiol Rev 1986;8:1–27.

4. Muñoz N. Is *Helicobacter pylori* a cause of gastric cancer? An appraisal of the seroepidemiological evidence. Cancer Epidemiol Biomarkers Prev 1994;3:445–51.

5. Parkin DM, Whelan SL, Ferlay J, et al. J. Cancer incidence in five continents. Vol. VII. IARC Scientific Publications, No. 143. Lyon: International Agency for Research on Cancer; 1997.

6. La Vecchia C, Lucchini F, Negri E, et al. Trends in cancer mortality in the Americas, 1955-1989. Eur J Cancer 1993; 29A:431–70.

7. Muñoz N. Descriptive epidemiology of stomach cancer. In: Reed PI, Hill MJ, editors. Gastric carcinogenesis. Amsterdam, New York, Oxford: Excerpta Medica; 1988. p. 51–69.

8. Muñoz N, Franceschi S. Epidemiology of gastric cancer and perspectives for prevention. Salud Publica Mex 1997; 39:318–30.

9. Devesa SS, Blot WJ, Fraumeni JF Jr. Changing patterns in the incidence of esophageal and gastric carcinoma in the United States. Cancer 1998;83:2049–53.

10. Devesa SS, Fraumeni JF Jr. The rising incidence of gastric cardia cancer. J Natl Cancer Inst 1999;91:747–9.

11. World Cancer Research Fund. Food, nutrition and the prevention of cancer: a global perspective. Washington (DC): World Cancer Research Fund, American Institute for Cancer Research; 1997.

12. Marshall BJ, Armstrong JA, McGechie DB, Glancy RJ. Attempt to fulfill Koch's postulates for pyloric *Campylobacter*. Med J Aust 1985;142:436–9.

13. Valle J, Seppälä K, Sipponen P, Kosunen T. Disappearance of gastritis after eradication of *Helicobacter pylori*. A morphometric study. Scand J Gastroenterol 1991;26:1057–65.

14. Muñoz N, Pisani P. *Helicobacter pylori* and gastric cancer. Eur J Gastroenterol Hepatol 1994;6:1097–103.

15. International Agency for Research on Cancer. Monographs on the evaluation of the carcinogenic risks to humans. Vol. 61. Schistosomes, liver flukes and *Helicobacter pylori*. Lyon: International Agency for Research on Cancer; 1994.

16. NIH Consensus Conference. *Helicobacter pylori* in peptic ulcer disease. NIH Consensus Development Panel on *Helicobacter pylori* in Peptic Ulcer Disease. JAMA 1994; 272:65–9.

17. Correa P, Fox J, Fontham E, et al. *Helicobacter pylori* and gastric carcinoma: serum antibody prevalence in populations with contrasting cancer risks. Cancer 1990;66:2569–74.

18. Forman D, Sitas F, Newell DG, et al. Geographic association of *Helicobacter pylori* antibody prevalence and gastric cancer mortality in rural China. Int J Cancer 1990;46:608–11.

19. Eurogast Study Group. An international association between *Helicobacter pylori* infection and gastric cancer. Lancet 1994;341:1359–62.

20. Lin JT, Wang LY, Wang JT, et al. Ecological study of association between *Helicobacter pylori* infection and gastric cancer in Taiwan. Dig Dis Sci 1995;40:385–8.

21. Fraser AG, Scragg R, Melcalf D, et al. Prevalence of *Helicobacter pylori* infection in different ethnic groups in New Zealand children and adults. Aust N Z J Med 1996; 26:646–51.

22. Fock KM, Khor CJL, Goh KT, et al. Seroprevalence of *Helicobacter pylori* infection and the incidence of gastric cancer in a multi-ethnic population. Gut 1997;41 Suppl 1:A50.

23. Perez-Perez GI, Bhat N, Gaensbauer J, et al. Country-specific constancy by age in cagA+ proportion of *Helicobacter pylori* infections. Int J Cancer 1997;72:453–6.

24. Sierra R, Muñoz N, Peña AS, et al. Antibodies to *Helicobacter pylori* and papsinogen levels in children from Costa Rica: comparison of two areas with different risks for stomach cancer. Cancer Epidemiol Biomarkers Prev 1992;1:449–54.

25. Palli D, Decarli A, Cipriani F, et al. *Helicobacter pylori* antibodies in areas of Italy at varying gastric cancer risk. Cancer Epidemiol Biomarkers Prev 1993;2:37–40.

26. Fukao A, Komatsu S, Tsubono Y, et al. *Helicobacter pylori* infection and chronic atrophic gastritis among Japanese blood donors: a cross-sectional study. Cancer Causes Control 1993;4:307–12.

27. Tsugane S, Kabuto M, Imai H, et al. *Helicobacter pylori*, dietary factors, and atrophic gastritis in five Japanese populations with different gastric cancer mortality. Cancer Causes Control 1993;4:297–305.

28. Chen SY, Liu TY, Chen MJ, et al. Seroprevalences of hepatitis B and C viruses and *Helicobacter pylori* in a small,

isolated population at high risk of gastric and liver cancer. Int J Cancer 1997;75:776–9.

29. Kneller RW, Guo WD, Hsing AW, et al. Risk factors for stomach cancer in sixty-five Chinese counties. Cancer Epidemiol Biomarkers Prev 1992;1:113–8.

30. Talley NJ, Zinsmeister AR, Weaver A, et al. Gastric adenocarcinoma and *Helicobacter pylori* infection. J Natl Cancer Inst 1991;83:1734–9.

31. Sipponen P, Kosunen TU, Valle J, et al. *Helicobacter pylori* infection and chronic gastritis in gastric cancer. J Clin Pathol 1992;45:319-23.

32. Hansson LE, Engstrand L, Nyrén OL, et al. *Helicobacter pylori* infection: independent risk indicator of gastric adenocarcinoma. Gastroenterology 1993;105:1098–103.

33. Kuipers EJ, Gracia-Casanova M, Peña AS, et al. *Helicobacter pylori* serology in patients with gastric carcinoma. Scand J Gastroenterol 1993;28:433–7.

34. Kokkola A, Valle J, Haapiainen R, et al. *Helicobacter pylori* infection in young patients with gastric carcinoma. Scand J Gastroenterol 1996;31:643–7.

35. Rudi J, Muller M, von Herbay A, et al. Lack of association of *Helicobacter pylori* seroprevalence and gastric cancer in a population with low gastric cancer incidence. Scand J Gastroenterol 1995;30:958–63.

36. Igarashi H, Takahashi S, Ishiyama N, et al. Is *Helicobacter pylori* a causal agent in gastric carcinoma? Ir J Med Sci 1992;161 Suppl 10;69.

37. Miglio F, Miglio M, Mazzeo V, et al. Prevalence of *Helicobacter pylori* (HP) in patients with gastric carcinoma (GC). Ir J Med Sci 1992;161 Suppl 10:70.

38. Estevens J, Fidalgo P, Tendeiro T, et al. Anti-*Helicobacter pylori* antibodies prevalence and gastric adenocarcinoma in Portugal: report of a case-control study. Eur J Cancer Prev 1993;2:377–80.

39. Lin JT, Wang JT, Wu MS, et al. *Helicobacter pylori* infection in a randomly selected population, healthy volunteers, and patients with gastric ulcer and gastric adenocarcinoma. Scand J Gastroenterol 1993;28:1067–72.

40. Kang HC, Chung IS. *Helicobacter pylori* infection and gastric adenocarcinoma in Korea: prevalence and distribution of *Helicobacter pylori* in resected specimen of gastric cancer. J Cath Med Coll 1992;45:849–62.

41. Blaser MJ, Kobayashi K, Clover TL, et al. *Helicobacter pylori* infection in Japanese patients wtih adenocarcinoma of the stomach. Int J Cancer 1994;55:799–802.

42. Asaka M, Kimura T, Kato M, et al. Possible role of *Helicobacter pylori* infection in early gastric cancer development. Cancer 1994;73:2691–4.

43. Barreto-Zuñiga R, Maruyame M, Kato Y, et al. Significance of *Helicobacter pylori* infection as a risk factor in gastric cancer: serological and histological studies. J Gastroenterol 1997;32:289–94.

44. Lopez-Carrillo L, Fernandez-Ortega C, Robles-Diaz G, et al. [*Helicobacter pylori* infection and gastric cancer in Mexico. A challenge for prevention and population control]. Rev Gastroenterol Mex 1997;62:22–8.

45. Kim HY, Cho BD, Chang WK, et al. *Helicobacter pylori* infection and the risk of gastric cancer among the Korean population. J Gastroenterol Hepatol 1997;12:100–3.

46. Bodhidatta L, Hoge CW, Churmratanakul S, et al. Diagnosis of *Helicobacter pylori* infection in a developing country; comparison of two ELISAs and a seroprevalence study. J Infect Dis 1994;168:1549–53.

47. Liston R, Pitt MA, Banerjee AK. IgG ELISA antibodies and detection of *Helicobacter pylori* in elderly patients. Lancet 1996;347:269.

48. Testoni PA, Colombo E, Cottani L, et al. *Helicobacter pylori* serology in chronic gastritis with antral atrophy and negative histology for *Helicobacter*-like organisms. J Clin Gastroenterol 1996;22:182–5.

49. Muñoz N, Kato I, Peraza S, et al. Prevalence of precancerous lesions of the stomach in Venezuela. Cancer Epidemiol Biomarkers Prev 1996;5:41–6.

50. Forman D, Newell DG, Fullerton F, et al. Association between infection with *Helicobacter pylori* and risk of gastric cancer: evidence from a prospective investigation. BMJ 1991;302:1302–5.

51. Parsonnet J, Friedman GD, Vandersteen DP, et al. *Helicobacter pylori* infection and the risk of gastric carcinoma. N Engl J Med 1991;325:1127–31.

52. Nomura A, Stemmerman GN, Chyou PH, et al. *Helicobacter pylori* infection and gastric carcinoma among Japanese Americans in Hawaii. N Engl J Med 1991;325:1132–6.

53. Webb PM, Yu MC, Forman D, et al. An apparent lack of association between *Helicobacter pylori* infection and risk of gastric cancer in China. Int J Cancer 1996;67:603–7.

54. Simán JH, Forsgren A, Floren CH. Association between *Helicobacter pylori* and gastric carcinoma in the city of Malmo, Sweden. A prospective study. Gut 1997;41 Suppl 1:A45.

55. Hansen S, Vollset SE, Melby K, Vellum E. Strong association of previous *Helicobacter pylori* infection to distal gastric adenocarcinoma. Am J Gastroenterol 1994;89:1358.

56. Aromaa A, Kosunen TU, Knekt P, et al. Circulating anti-*Helicobacter pylori* immunoglobulin A antibodies and low serum pepsinogen I level are associated with increased risk of gastric cancer. Am J Epidemiol 1996;144:142–9.

57. Watanabe Y, Kurata JH, Mizuno S, et al. *Helicobacter pylori* infection and gastric cancer. A nested case-control study in a rural area of Japan. Dig Dis Sci 1997;42:1383–7.

58. Tulinius H, Ogmundsdottir H, Kristinsson KG, et al. A retrospective case-control study of *H. pylori* infection and subsequent gastric cancer in Iceland [abstract]. Proceedings of the IACR Annual Meeting; 1997 Nov 3–5; Abidjan, Ivory Coast [In press].

59. Rauws EAJ, Langenberg W, Houthoff HJ, et al. *Campylobacter pyloridis*-associated chronic active antral gastritis. A prospective study of its prevalence and the effects of antibacterial and antiulcer treatment. Gastroenterology 1988;94:33–40.

60. Genta RM, Lew GM, Graham DY. Changes in the gastric mucosa following eradication of *Helicobacter pylori*. Mod Pathol 1993;6:281–9.

61. Graham DY, Walsh JH, Schubert TT, et al. Short term treatment with ranitidine bismuth citrate (RBC) improves *H. pylori* gastritis in the antrum and corpus. Gut 1996;39 Suppl 2:A24.

62. Fossati D, Alvisi C, Frego R, et al. No change in intestinal metaplasia after *H. pylori* eradication. Gut 1996;39 Suppl 2:A104.

63. van der Hulst RWM, Rauws EAJ, Köycü B, et al. The influ-

ence of cure of *H. pylori* infection on the long term sequelae of gastritis: a prospective long term follow up study. Gut 1997; 41 Suppl 1:A54.

64. Pasztorova I, Chinyama C, Filipe MI, et al. Regression of gastric intestinal metaplasia after eradication of *Helicobacter pylori*: a prospective study. Gut 1997; 41 Suppl 1:A55.

65. Griffiths AE, Thursz MR, Walker MM. Do intestinal metaplasia and gastric atrophy reverse after *H. pylori* eradication? Gut 1997;41 Suppl 1:A48.

66. Uemura N, Mukai T, Okamoto S, et al. Effect of *Helicobacter pylori* eradication on subsequent development of cancer after endoscopic resection of early gastric cancer. Cancer Epidemiol Biomarkers Prev 1997;6:639–42.

67. Buiatti E, Muñoz N, Vivas J, et al. Difficulty in eradicating *Helicobacter pylori* in a population at high risk for stomach cancer in Venezuela. Cancer Causes Control 1994;5: 249–54.

68. Sierra R, Salas P, Mora-Zúñiga F, et al. Erradicación de *Helicobacter pylori* en una población de alto riesgo de cáncer gástrico. Acta Med Costarricense 1998;40:30–5.

69. Kune GA, Vitetta L. Smoking and tobacco as an aetiologic factor in gastric carcinoma. Gastrointest Cancer 1995;I:33–8.

70. Franceschi S, La Vecchia C. Alcohol and the risk of cancers of the stomach and colon-rectum. Dig Dis 1994;12:276–89.

71. Langman MJS. Genetic influences upon gastric cancer frequency. In: Reed PI, Hill MJ, editors. Gastric carcinogenesis. Amsterdam, New York, Oxford: Excerpta Medica; 1988. p. 81–6.

72. Bonney GE, Elston RC, Correa P, et al. Genetic association of gastric carcinoma: I. Chronic atrophic gastritis. Genet Epidemiol 1986;3:213–24.

73. Palli D, Galli M, Caporaso NE, et al. Family history and risk of stomach cancer in Italy. Cancer Epidemiol Biomarkers Prev 1994;3:15–8.

74. Zhao L, Blot WJ, Liu W-D, et al. Familial predisposition to precancerous gastric lesions in a high-risk area of China. Cancer Epidemiol Biomarkers Prev 1994;3:461–4.

75. Guilford P, Hopkins J, Harrawy J, et al. E-cadherin germline mutations in familial gastric cancer. Nature 1998;392:402.

76. Guilford P, Hopkins J, Grady W, et al. E-cadherin germline mutations define an inherited cancer syndrome dominated by diffuse gastric cancer. Hum Mutat. [In press]

77. Mayer B, Johnson JP, Leitl F, et al. E-cadherin expression in primary and metastatic gastric cancer: down-regulation correlates with cellular dedifferentiation and glandular disintegration. Cancer Res 1993;53:1690.

78. National Cancer Institute. Cancer statistics review 1973–1988. Bethesda (MD): Department of Health and Human Services (US); 1991. NIH Publication No.: 91–2789.

79. Muñoz N, Vivas J, Buiatti E, Oliver W. Chemoprevention trial on precancerous lesions of the stomach in Venezuela: summary of study design and baseline data. In: Stewart BW, McGregor D, Kleihues P, editors. Principles of chemoprevention. IARC Scientific Publications, No. 139. Lyon: International Agency for Research on Cancer; 1996. p. 125–33.

80. Correa P, Fontham ETH, Bravo JC, et al. Chemoprevention of gastric dysplasia: randomized trial of antioxidant supplements and anti-*Helicobacter pylori* therapy. J Natl Cancer Inst 2000;92:1881–8.

81. Buiatti E, Muñoz N, Vivas J, et al. Difficulty in eradicating *Helicobacter pylori* in a population at high risk for stomach cancer in Venezuela. Cancer Causes Control 1994; 5:249–54.

11

Pathology of Gastric Neoplasms

SHIH-FAN KUAN, MD, PHD

Gastric neoplasms continue to be a challenge for the surgeon and pathologist. When gastric neoplasms are compared with colonic neoplasms (a more common and well-studied type of malignancy), there are several features of gastric tumors that may account for the difficulties encountered regarding pathology. First, gastric tumors encompass a wide spectrum of pathology when compared to colonic tumors. Some tumors, such as gastrointestinal (GI) stromal tumors and endocrine cell hyperplasia, have an uncertain biologic behavior. Second, gastric tumors share similar nosology with colonic tumors (eg, hyperplastic polyps and adenomatous polyps), but these carry somewhat different clinical implications and pathologic features. Third, gastric cancers are less prevalent than colonic cancers. Therefore, the adenoma-carcinoma sequence and other possible precancerous lesions in the stomach are not as well studied as those in the colon. Finally, molecular pathology has recently elucidated the histogenesis and genetic defects of some interesting gastric tumors, such as GI stromal tumors and juvenile polyps. This chapter focuses on these unique features and on recent developments regarding gastric tumors. A classification of gastric tumors, based mostly on their histologic origins, is shown in Table 11–1.

GASTRIC POLYPS

Adenoma and Dysplasia

There are no generally accepted definitions of dysplasia and adenoma of the stomach.[1,2] Dysplasia is best defined as an unequivocal neoplastic epithelial alteration. Adenomas consist of nodules of dysplastic epithelium. However, not all dysplastic epithelia form circumscribed nodules. Dysplasia may be found in flat epithelium. In other words, two types of dysplasias are recognized: adenomatous and nonadenomatous dysplasia. The two types have identical histopathologies.

Adenomas are uncommon in the stomach, in contrast to colonic adenomas, which are more frequent. Gastric adenomas occur almost exclusively in the

Table 11–1. CLASSIFICATION OF GASTRIC POLYPS AND TUMORS
Gastric polyps
Adenoma and dysplasia
Hyperplastic polyp
Hamartomatous polyp
Juvenile polyp
Fundic gland polyp
Pancreatic heterotopia
Giant fold disease/hyperplastic gastropathy
Ménétrier's disease
Zollinger-Ellison syndrome
Extensive or diffuse neoplastic infiltrate
Epithelial tumors (adenocarcinoma)
Early gastric carcinoma
Advanced gastric carcinoma
Intestinal type
Diffuse type
Endocrine tumors
Endocrine hyperplasia
G-cell hyperplasia
ECL-cell hyperplasia
Carcinoid tumor
Mesenchymal tumors
Gastrointestinal stromal tumor (GIST)
Leiomyoma
Lipoma
Neurofibroma
Granular cell tumor
Glomus tumor
Malignant lymphoma

ECL = enterochromaffin-like.

antrum. Adenomas are frequently seen in two clinical settings: one setting is in patients with familial adenomatous polyposis, or Gardner's syndrome;[3] the other is associated with chronic atrophic gastritis.

In contrast to adenomas in the colon, most adenomas in the stomach are sessile or grow into flat mucosa; pure pedunculated adenoma is uncommon. Gastric adenoma has a tubular, villous, or mixed tubulovillous appearance in histology. Tubular adenomas tend to be sessile whereas villous and tubulovillous adenomas are more likely to be pedunculated (Figure 11–1, A). Two major microscopic variants are found in adenomas.[4] The intestinal type (the more common type) is composed of dysplastic epithelium arising in the intestinal metaplastic epithelium. Cytologically, these cells have large, elongated, and hyperchromatic nuclei arranged in pseudostratification (see Figure 11–1, B). Goblet cells, Paneth's cells, and endocrine cells can be seen occasionally. The gastric type (the less common type) is composed of dysplastic epithelium similar to the foveolar epithelium containing PAS(+) (period acid-Schiff-positive) apical neutral mucin. This type of dysplasia usually consists of round and basal nuclei, in contrast to the elongated and pseudostratified nuclei of the intestinal type of dysplasia.

The adenoma-carcinoma sequence in the stomach is not as well defined as that in the colon since the majority of gastric carcinomas do not arise from pre-existing adenomas. It is unlikely that these adenomas have been destroyed by the bulk of a gastric carcinoma because adenomas are also uncommon in early gastric carcinoma,[5] which should have a better preservation of the precursor lesion. The incidence of synchronous carcinomas associated with gastric adenomas varies from report to report[6,7] and depends on the size and duration of the adenoma. Most carcinoma-associated gastric adenomas are > 2 cm in diameter. It may take 10 to 15 years for a gastric adenoma to transform into carcinoma. Although limited data on its proper treatment have been published, it is reasonable that gastric adenoma should be completely excised by endoscopic or surgical resection.

Hyperplastic Polyps

The definition of hyperplastic polyps varies.[1,8] All definitions recognize the basic abnormality, namely, hyperplasia or expansion of the pit compartment. Thus, any mucosal polyp composed of too many pits or made up of elongated pits satisfies the definition of a hyperplastic polyp. Hyperplastic polyps are the most common polyps of the stomach, constituting 50 to 90 percent of all gastric polyps. About two-thirds of hyperplastic polyps occur in the antrum.

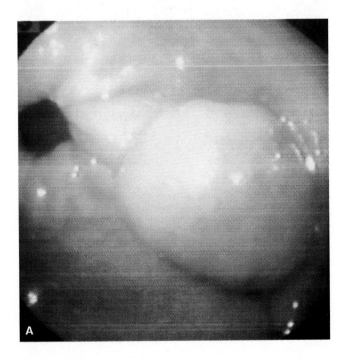
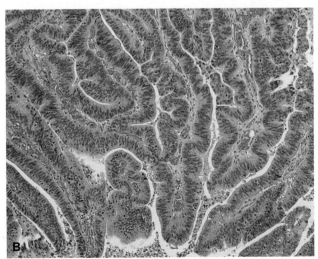

Figure 11–1. Villous adenoma of the stomach. *A,* Endoscopic view of a pedunculated adenoma at the antrum of the stomach. *B,* The histologic features are similar to those of villous adenoma of the colon. The epithelial cells contain enlarged, elongated, and hyperchromatic nuclei arranged in a pseudostratified pattern.

They tend to develop in association with atrophic gastritis and probably represent regenerative hyperplasia of the foveolar epithelium. *Helicobacter pylori* infection was found to be associated with hyperplastic polyp formation in a recent report.[9]

The gross appearance of hyperplastic polyps depends on their size, which ranges from 0.5 to 2.5 cm in diameter. The smaller polyps tend to be sessile whereas the larger ones may be pedunculated and lobulated (Figure 11–2, A). The basic histologic abnormalities involve the pits, which are elongated, branched, and distorted. The lengthening exaggerates the surface contours, producing coarse or irregular villi. The distortion takes several forms. Some of the elongated pits have a serrated or corkscrew configuration, others are cystic, and still others branch (see Figure 11–2, B). Superimposed on the pit changes are inflammatory changes. The malignant potential of hyperplastic polyps is low (0.4%); malignancy occurs mostly in polyps > 2 cm in diameter.[10] However, it is debatable whether hyperplastic polyps may simply share the same etiologic factors as gastric carcinomas or a precursor of the latter.

In addition to the above-mentioned ordinary hyperplastic polyps, three other variants of hyperplastic polyps are worthy of special mention. The first is focal foveolar hyperplasia,[11] which consists of small multiple sessile lesions that are frequently observed endoscopically and which may represent the early and miniature form of hyperplastic polyps. The second variant is inflammatory polyps at the gastroesophageal junction; these polyps are commonly associated with reflux esophagitis.[12] The third variant is hyperplastic polyps on the gastric side of gastroenteric anastomoses.[13] Hyperplastic polyps occur in approximately 10 percent of gastric remnants, especially after a Billroth II gastrojejunal anastomosis, usually 10 to 15 years after surgery.[14] Grossly, they are pedunculated polyps with lobulated and villiform surfaces (Figure 11–3). Histologically, some hyperplastic pits form cystic spaces and extend into the submucosa, a feature that has been

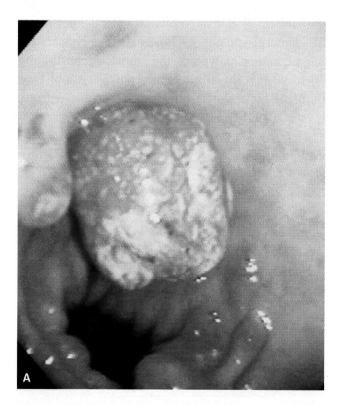

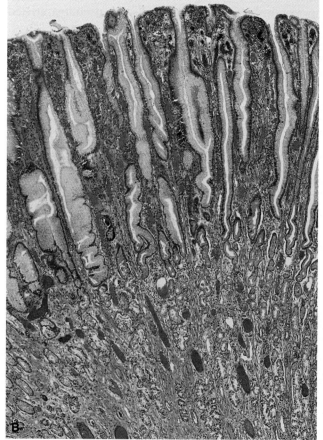

Figure 11–2. Hyperplastic polyp of the stomach. *A*, Endoscopic view of a pre-pyloric hyperplastic polyp that shows a lobulated surface. *B*, The hyperplasia involves the foveolar surface pit epithelium but not the deep mucous glands. Some of the elongated pits have a branched and corkscrewlike appearance.

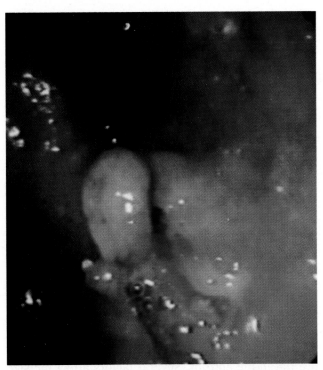

Figure 11–3. Endoscopic view of gastric stromal polypoid hyperplasia. Hyperplastic polyps developed 10 years after a Billroth II anastomosis. These polyps always occur on the gastric side of the anastomosis, sparing the enteric side.

described as gastritis cystica polyposa, gastric cystic polyposis, and stromal polypoid hypertrophic gastritis. Multiple factors may contribute to the pathogenesis of these polyps at gastroenterostomy sites. Chronic bile reflux, ischemia, or regeneration secondary to mucosal prolapse have all been proposed. Postanastomotic dysplasia and carcinoma may develop in these polyps.[15]

Hamartomatous Polyps (Peutz-Jeghers Syndrome)

Peutz-Jeghers syndrome (PJS) is an autosomal dominant inherited disorder that is characterized by gastrointestinal polyposis involving the colon, small bowel, and stomach, as well as mucocutaneous pigment deposition in the lips, gums, and buccal mucosa.[16] Gastric polyps occur in 25 to 49 percent of patients with PJS. They tend to develop in the antrum. Histologically, these polyps have cystically dilated pits separated by delicate fibrovascular stroma. An arborizing framework of smooth muscle is not as prominent as in their counterparts in the

intestine. Dysplasia and carcinoma have been reported in the stomach[17] but are more common in the small and large intestine. The genetic defect of PJS has recently been identified as LBK1/STK11 on chromosome segment 19p13.3, which encodes a serine/threonine kinase.[18]

Juvenile Polyps

Juvenile polyps are hamartomatous polyps that can occur in sporadic or familial form. Sporadic juvenile polyps tend to be single and are common in the colon. However, the familial form is usually multiple and also involves other locations of the GI tract, including the stomach and small intestine.[19] Juvenile polyposis is inherited as an autosomal dominant trait and is heterogeneous in genetic mutation. Recent studies have linked juvenile polyposis to mutations in the PTEN gene located on chromosome band 10q23 or in the SMAD4/DPC4 gene located on chromosome band 18q21.[20,21] SMAD4 is a key cytoplasmic protein in the signal transduction of transforming growth factor-β. Gastric juvenile polyps are characterized by cystically dilated glands surrounded by edematous and inflamed granulation-like stroma. Surface ulceration is common in these polyps. Patients with juvenile polyposis have an increased risk for colo-rectal cancer, gastric cancer, and pancreatic cancer.[22]

Fundic Gland Polyps

Fundic gland polyps are small sessile lesions that occur in the fundus of the stomach. Fundic gland polyps can be found in three different clinical settings: (1) in patients with familial adenomatous polyposis (FAP),[23] (2) in patients without FAP,[24] and (3) in association with the use of omeprazole.[25] There is evidence that both sporadic and FAP-associated fundic gland polyps overexpress transforming growth factor-α (TGF-α) and its receptor. There is also evidence that long-term treatment with omeprazole (a proton pump inhibitor) may be followed by the development of fundic gland polyps.[25]

Fundic gland polyps are small dome-shaped nodules with smooth surfaces (Figure 11–4, A). Usually, they are multiple, especially if they are associated with FAP. Regardless of the clinical setting, fundic gland polyps have a normal or shortened pit compartment that leads into an altered glandular compartment that contains cystic glands lined by parietal and chief cells (see Figure 11–4, B). Fundic gland polyps that are associated with omeprazole treatment are characterized by parietal cell hypertrophy with tonguelike projection into the cystically dilated lumens.[25] There is no increased risk of malignant change in fundic gland polyps in general although dysplasia has been reported in rare FAP-associated fundic gland polyps.

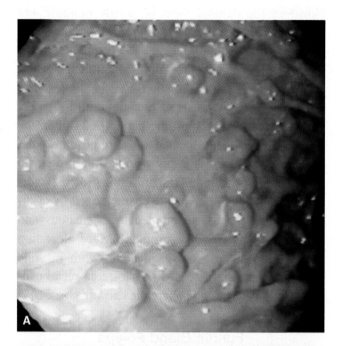

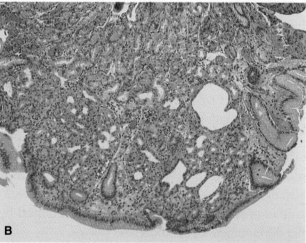

Figure 11–4. Fundic gland polyps. *A,* Endoscopic view demonstrates multiple small dome-shaped fundic gland polyps on the surface of the stomach. These polyps are located in the fundus and tend to fuse with gastric folds. *B,* Histologic study of a fundic gland polyp shows normal short pits with cystically dilated fundic glands.

Ectopic Pancreas (Pancreatic Heterotopia)

In pancreatic heterotopia, submucosal tumors, 1 to 2 cm in diameter, are found on the greater curvature of the antrum, forming a dome-shaped mass that protrudes into the lumen.[26] Central depression and umbilication are useful signs on endoscopic examination (Figure 11–5); however, they occur in only less than half of the cases. Because patients are usually asymptomatic, most of these tumors are incidental findings during surgery or autopsy. Any complications that occur in the pancreas, such as pancreatitis and pancreatic carcinoma, can also occur in the ectopic pancreas.

GIANT FOLD DISEASES (HYPERPLASTIC GASTROPATHIES)

Normal gastric folds are prominent in the fundus and are flat in the antrum. Several factors affect the size of these folds, including age and the degree of gastric distention. Giant folds are usually defined as large folds that persist even in the distended stomach. The precise definition depends on the methods of study. By radiologic or endoscopic measurement the general cut-off size is 1 cm in height or width.[27] Giant fold diseases are heterogeneous in their pathogenesis.

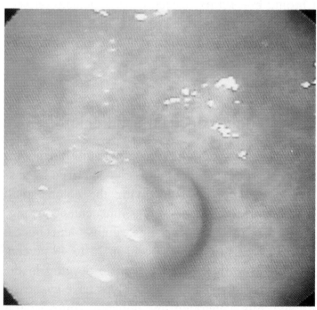

Figure 11–5. Endoscopic view of ectopic pancreas. Central depression and umbilication are characteristic findings in ectopic pancreas but are found only in less than half of the cases.

Some giant folds are accompanied by clinical symptoms whereas others are not. Giant folds may be caused by neoplastic or non-neoplastic processes; they may also occur as a variant of normal folds. The most common clinical conditions associated with gastric giant folds are Ménétrier's disease, Zollinger-Ellison syndrome, and diffuse neoplastic infiltrates.

Ménétrier's Disease

Ménétrier's disease is a syndrome that includes gastric giant folds, protein loss, and decreased gastric acid production.[28] Giant folds occur in the body and fundus, and the antrum appears normal (Figure 11–6, A). The etiology is unknown although there is evidence of excessive production of TGF-α in these patients. A Ménétrier disease–like condition has been observed in transgenic mice that overexpressed TGF-α.[29] Transforming growth factor-α is expressed in the normal surface epithelium and parietal cells of the gastric body mucosa but is absent in normal pit epithelium. It also appears in the hyperplastic pit epithelium in patients with Ménétrier's disease. Ménétrier's disease usually develops in adults at a mean age of 55 to 60 years. A self-limited Ménétrier disease–like condition in children is probably postinfectious, occurring especially after *Cytomegalovirus* infection.[30]

The typical histologic findings are florid pit hyperplasia accompanied by atrophy or loss of deep glands. The pits are unusually elongated and have a corkscrewlike appearance (see Figure 11–6, B). Surface edema is not uncommon, but inflammation is not a significant component. Histologic assessment was formerly limited by the difficulty of performing a full-thickness biopsy of the hyperplastic gastric mucosa.

The course of Ménétrier's disease is unpredictable. In adults, fully developed disease is usually progressive; however, the disease is generally benign and self-limited in children. Resection is indicated when hypoproteinemia leads to uncontrollable edema. A few patients may respond to H_2 (histamine) receptor blockers. A few cases of Ménétrier's disease are complicated by adenocarcinoma, but it is uncertain whether this is a precursor lesion for gastric cancer.

Zollinger-Ellison Syndrome

Zollinger-Ellison syndrome is characterized by multiple intractable peptic ulcers, which are usually duodenal, resulting from hypergastrinemia from a gastrin-producing tumor.[31] The tumors are most common in the pancreas but can also be seen in the duodenum. Pancreatic gastrinoma is a component of type I mul-

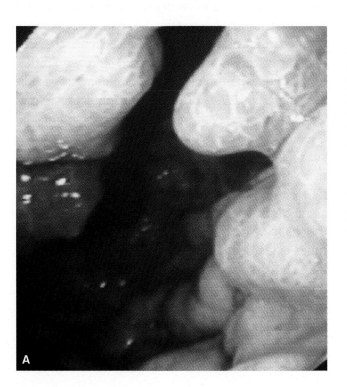

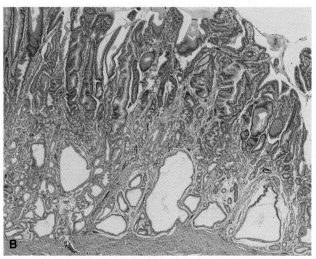

Figure 11–6. Ménétrier's disease. *A,* Endoscopic view shows grossly enlarged and knobby gastric folds. *B,* The elongated pits have serrated and corkscrew contours. Some pits may extend to the base of the mucosa and form cystic glands. The native mucosal glands at the base of the mucosa are atrophic because of the compression of the bulk of hypertrophic pits.

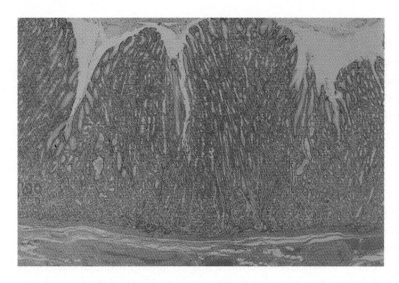

Figure 11–7.   Zollinger-Ellison syndrome (ZES). In contrast to Ménétrier's disease, a typical case of ZES has a normal thickness of the pit and a hyperplastic glandular component (caused by hypergastrinemia) that is composed mainly of an increased number of parietal cells.

tiple endocrine neoplasia syndrome (MEN-I).[32] Grossly, the fundic mucosal folds are enlarged and grow into a cobblestone pattern. Histologic features are characterized by hyperplasia and hypertrophy of parietal cells in the fundic mucosa, caused by the trophic effect of gastrin (Figure 11–7). Enterochromaffin-like endocrine cells of the body are also hyperplastic because of the stimulation of gastrin. In contrast to Ménétrier's disease, the pit compartment is generally normal in this syndrome. Hypertrophic hypersecretory gastropathy[33] is a normogastrinemic variant of giant fold disease that resembles Zollinger-Ellison syndrome. Patients with this syndrome have large folds that tend to have a particularly nodular appearance. Although they have hypersecretion of gastric acid and frequent peptic ulcers, they do not have pancreatic tumors or hypergastrinemia.

Diffuse Neoplastic Infiltrates

One of the classic gross findings in gastric lymphoma patients is that of fold enlargement. These large folds are usually coarse and irregular. Adenocarcinomas, especially the diffuse signet-ring cell type, can also produce giant folds.

MALIGNANT EPITHELIAL TUMORS: GASTRIC CARCINOMA

Gastric carcinoma is the second most common cancer in the world. Its incidence varies from country to country. In the United States, there has been a steady decline in the incidence of gastric cancer; the present rate is approximately 10 cases per 100,000. Nevertheless, it was estimated that approximately 21,500 new cases would be diagnosed in 2000.[34] There has also been a worldwide decline in the incidence of gastric cancer since 1930.[35] However, the poor prognosis for advanced gastric carcinomas (a 5-year survival of 16.3% in the United States) makes early diagnosis an important objective.

Carcinoma arising in the gastric cardia appears to have different etiologic factors and a different biologic behavior from distal noncardia carcinoma.[36] First, the incidence of cardia carcinoma has recently increased in many countries whereas the incidence of noncardia gastric carcinoma has decreased. Second, cardia carcinoma is associated more with reflux esophagitis whereas noncardia carcinoma is associated more with *Helicobacter pylori* infection. However, there are several controversies regarding the issue of cardia carcinoma. First, there is no consensus on the anatomic definition of the cardia. Second, there are no distinct morphologic features that separate cardia carcinoma from Barrett's carcinoma; some cardia cancers can grow upward into the distal esophagus whereas Barrett's carcinomas can sometimes extend below the junction, to involve the cardia. Third the recently described entities of cardia intestinal metaplasia and carditis (inflammation of the gastric cardia) raise the issue of their etiology and possible role in cardia carcinoma. Understanding of the pathogenesis of cardia carcinoma must await more clinicopathologic studies in the future.

The precancerous lesions of gastric cancer are not as well defined as those of colon cancers, in which an adenoma-carcinoma sequence has been widely accepted. Several prediposing conditions are associated with increased risk of cancer, including *H. pylori* infection, atrophic gastritis, subtotal gastrectomy, immunodeficiency syndrome, and Ménétrier's disease. Correa recognized a stepwise progression from normal epithelium to chronic gastritis, followed by intestinal metaplasia, dysplasia, and carcinoma.[37] Intestinal metaplasia has been associated with gastric carcinoma of the intestinal type in epidemiologic, prospective, and morphologic studies.[38] However, the overall incidence of cancer developing in patients with intestinal metaplasia is so low that routine biopsy is not justified for the screening of gastric cancer.

It is noteworthy that *H. pylori* has been declared as a group I carcinogen by the World Health Organization.[39] The strongest evidence of an association between *H. pylori* and gastric carcinoma comes from a series of prospective studies in which banked sera from blood donors were used.[40] Several reports indicated a significantly increased risk of gastric cancer in donors with positive serum antibodies for *H. pylori*, compared to age- and gender-matched controls with negative antibody titers.[41] Both intestinal and diffuse types of cancer have been linked to *H. pylori* infection. However, only noncardia cancers are associated with *H. pylori*.

Early Gastric Carcinoma

Based on the depth of invasion, gastric carcinoma can be divided into early gastric cancer and advanced gastric cancer. Early gastric carcinoma (EGC) is defined as a gastric carcinoma with invasion confined to the mucosa and submucosa, regardless of the presence or absence of lymph node metastases.[42] The concept of EGC is different from that of carcinoma in situ or gastric dysplasia, in which cancer cells have not penetrated the basement membrane and have no metastatic potential. Some patients with EGC may already have lymph node metastases. However, the overall "cure" rate by surgery for these patients is higher than for patients with advanced gastric carcinoma. In Japan, the 5-year survival of patients with EGC after resection is approximately 95 percent, compared to only 5 to 15 percent for all other gastric carcinomas.[43]

Early gastric carcinoma was first recognized in Japan, where the incidence of gastric carcinoma is high. In 1962, the Society for Gastrointestinal Endoscopy of Japan recognized three major gross morphologic types of EGC: protruded (type I), superficial (type II), and excavated (type III).[44] The superficial type is further divided into elevated (IIa), flat (IIb), and depressed (IIc) subtypes. This classification may help the endoscopist to identify subtle mucosal alterations. However, the correlation of gross findings with histology and prognosis is poor. The histologic types of EGC vary among different reports. In general, differentiated carcinomas (tubular or papillary) are more common in type I (protruded) EGC. Undifferentiated carcinomas (signet-ring cell, mucinous, and poorly differentiated) are found more often in the depressed groups (IIc and IIc+III) (Figure 11–8).

Advanced Gastric Carcinoma

There are several classification systems[45–47] for advanced gastric carcinoma, based on the gross morphology or histopathology (Table 11–2). The classifications based on gross morphology are less useful because of their low predictive value for patients' prognoses. The simplest and most widely used system is Lauren's classification,[45] which divides gastric carcinoma into two types: intestinal and diffuse (Table 11–3). The intestinal type is presumed to arise from intestinalized gastric mucosa and closely resembles ordinary colon cancer. Grossly, the tumors are usually nodular, polypoid, or fungating (Figure 11–9, A). Histologically, they are characterized by various extents of glandular formation and by frequent association with intestinal metaplasia (see Figure 11–9, B). The liver is the most common site of metastases. In contrast, the diffuse type is grossly ill defined and may have the appearance of a plaque or linitis plastica (which has the gross appearance of a leather bottle) (Figure 11–10, A). The histology is remarkable for isolated and poorly differentiated carcinoma or signet-ring cells (see Figure 11–10, B). Metastases are commonly found in the serosa or lymph nodes.

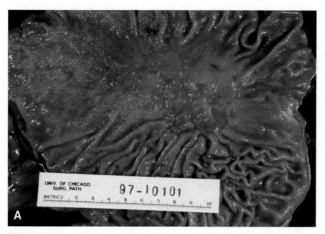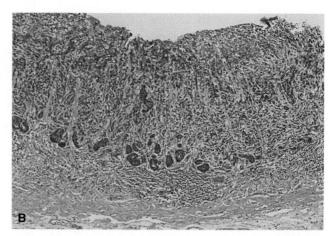

Figure 11–8. Early gastric carcinoma. *A,* Gross appearance of a resection specimen of type IIc early gastric carcinoma with a superficially depressed lesion in the greater curvature. *B,* Histologic study of the same case shows the infiltrating poorly differentiated carcinoma limited to the mucosal layer.

Borrmann's classification is widely used for describing the gross appearance of gastric carcinoma:[48] type I is a polypoid and fungating tumor, type II is a polypoid tumor with a central ulceration, type III is an ulcerated tumor with infiltrative margins, and type IV is the linitis plastica variety.

Gastric carcinoma usually emerges as a localized tumor and spreads to the adjacent structures by one of three modes: lymphatic invasion, hematogenous dissemination, and peritoneal extension. The most common mode is lymphatic metastasis to lymph nodes along the greater and lesser curvature of the stomach. Occasionally, supraclavicular nodes (Virchow's nodes) may be involved, via the thoracic duct. The liver is the most common site of hematogenous spread. The lungs and the central nervous system are not commonly involved by gastric cancer. Peritoneal spread can involve many locations in the abdominal cavity; however, the ovaries (Krukenberg's tumor)

and the rectal shelf (Blumer's tumor) are typically involved by peritoneal spread. Other sites of peritoneal extension include the pancreas, the transverse colon, and the undersurface of the diaphragm.

Pathologic Staging and Prognostic Factors for Gastric Carcinoma

The tumor-node-metastasis (TNM) system has become the principal method of staging gastric cancer. The extent of disease is determined by the following three components: (1) the primary tumor (T), which represents the depth of invasion through the gastric wall; (2) the regional lymph nodes (N), which include the lymph nodes along the lesser and greater curvature as well as the pancreatic and splenic areas; and (3) distant metastasis (M), which refers to spread to the liver, peritoneal surfaces, and nonregional lymph nodes, including the retropancreatic,

Table 11–2. CLASSIFICATION OF GASTRIC ADENOCARCINOMA	
Based on Gross Morphology	**Based on Histopathology**
Ming	Lauren
Expanding	Intestinal
Infiltrating	Diffuse
Stout	WHO
Fungating	Papillary
Ulcerating	Tubular
Superficial spreading	Mucinous
Diffusely infiltrating	Signet-ring

WHO = World Health Organization.

Table 11–3. COMPARISON OF INTESTINAL AND DIFFUSE TYPES OF GASTRIC CARCINOMA		
Characteristic	**Intestinal Type**	**Diffuse Type**
Gross appearance	Elevated, fungating	Depressed, infiltrating
Histology	Glandular	Isolated
Metastasis	Liver	Lymph nodes, serosa
Intestinal metaplasia	Almost 100%	Less common
Sex predominance	Male	Female
Age	Old	Young
5-year survival	~ 20%	< 10%
Etiology	Diet, enviroment, *Helicobacter pylori*	Unknown, genetic? (associated with blood group A)

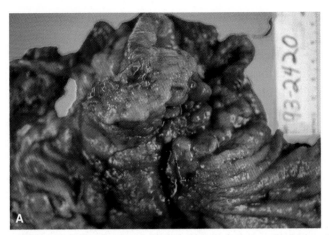
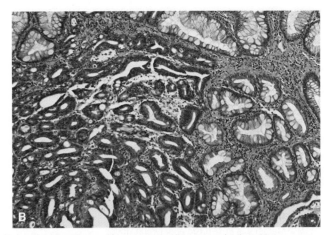

Figure 11–9. Advanced gastric carcinoma of the intestinal type. *A,* Resection specimen shows a protruding mass in the antrum, corresponding to Borrmann's type I adenocarcinoma. *B,* Histologic study of the same case shows gland-forming adenocarcinoma and adjacent intestinal metaplasia.

para-aortic, portal, retroperitoneal, and mesenteric nodes. In 1997, the American Joint Committee on Cancer (AJCC) published its fifth revised staging criteria for gastric carcinoma [49] (Tables 11–4 and 11–5). The major change in this current version is the reclassification of regional lymph node metastases (N) according to the number of positive nodes rather than the distance from the tumor edge to the lymph nodes, as proposed in a prior version.

The most useful prognostic factors are the depth of invasion and the spread to regional lymph nodes. The location and Borrmann's gross morphologic types are two other important prognostic factors. Distal gastric carcinoma has a more favorable prognosis than proximal cancer. Borrmann types I and II have a better prognosis than Borrmann types III and

IV, independent of the status of lymph node metastases. Both histologic type and grade have an impact on the prognosis. The intestinal type of gastric cancer classified by Lauren has a better prognosis than the diffuse type. Low-grade adenocarcinoma also has a better prognosis than high-grade cancer. The overall prognosis for gastric cancer is poor; the 5-year survival rate is less than 20 percent, even after "curative" surgery.

Various molecular markers, including oncogenes and tumor-suppressor genes, have been used to predict prognosis. For instance, amplification of the HER-2/neu gene seems to be a prognostic factor of metastatic potential.[50] However, the application of such molecular markers in clinical practice awaits further study.

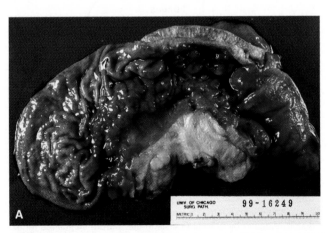
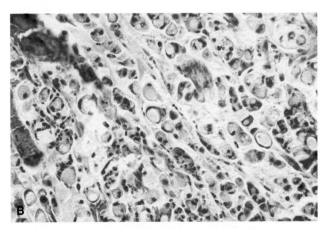

Figure 11–10. Advanced gastric carcinoma of the diffuse type. *A,* Resection specimen shows marked thickening of the wall, having the contour of a leather bottle (the so-called linitus plastica of Borrmann's type IV adenocarcinoma). *B,* Histologic study of the same case shows diffuse infiltration of isolated signet-ring cells, without any glandular formation.

Table 11–4. STAGING OF GASTRIC CARCINOMA: TUMOR-NODE-METASTASIS GROUPING*		

Primary tumor (T)
- Tx   Primary tumor cannot be assessed
- T0   No evidence of primary tumor
- Tis Carcinoma in situ (intraepithelial tumor without invasion of the lamina propria)
- T1   Tumor invades lamina propria or submucosa
- T2   Tumor invades muscularis propria or submucosa
- T3   Tumor penetrates serosa (visceral peritoneum) without invasion of adjacent structures
- T4   Tumor invades adjacent structures

Regional lymph nodes (N)
- Nx   Regional lymph node(s) cannot be assessed
- N0   No regional lymph node metastasis
- N1   Metastasis in 1–6 regional lymph nodes
- N2   Metastasis in 7–15 regional lymph nodes
- N3   Metastasis in > 15 regional lymph nodes

Distant metastasis (M)
- Mx   Distant metastasis cannot be assessed
- M0   No distant metastasis
- M1   Distant metastasis

*American Joint Committee on Cancer criteria, 1997.

ENDOCRINE TUMORS

Various types of endocrine cells are present throughout the entire GI tract. In the stomach, the two key endocrine cell types are gastrin-producing G cells and histamine-producing enterochromaffin-like (ECL) cells. G cells are located at the junction of the gastric pits and pyloric glands in the antrum whereas ECL cells are found between the parietal and chief cells in the fundus. In the normal stomach, gastrin is secreted by G cells in response to negative feedback by hydrochloric acid. Gastrin, in turn, drives the ECL cells to produce histamine, which is the main activator of acid secretion by parietal cells[51] (Figure 11–11).

Endocrine Cell Hyperplasia

In most cases, gastric endocrine cell hyperplasia is secondary to hypochlorhydria, with a small portion due to MEN-I syndrome.[52] Type A chronic atrophic gastritis (CAG) is the main cause of hypochlorhydria. Acid-suppressing drugs such as H_2 blockers or proton pump inhibitors can also induce endocrine cell hyperplasia in rodents and humans (although carcinoid tumor was reported only in rodents).

Two types of endocrine hyperplasia are associated with hypochlorhydria: G-cell hyperplasia of the antrum and ECL hyperplasia in the fundus.[53] Hypochlorhydria lifts the negative-feedback mechanism of hydrochloric acid and then induces G-cell hyperplasia. In turn, G cells cause ECL-cell hyperplasia, via hypergastrinemia.

Carcinoid Tumor

Gastric carcinoid tumor accounts for about 3 percent of all GI carcinoids. It has gained additional atten-

Table 11–5. STAGING OF GASTRIC CARCINOMA: STAGE GROUPING*			
Stage	**TNM Classifications**		
0	Tis	N0	M0
IA	T1	N0	M0
IB	T1	N1	M0
	T2	N0	M0
II	T1	N2	M0
	T2	N1	M0
	T3	N0	M0
IIIA	T2	N2	M0
	T3	N1	M0
	T4	N0	M0
IIIB	T3	N2	M0
IV	T4	N1	M0
	T1	N3	M0
	T2	N3	M0
	T3	N3	M0
	T4	N2	M0
	T4	N3	M0
	Any T	Any N	M1

TNM = tumor-node-metastasis.
*American Joint Committee on Cancer criteria, 1997.

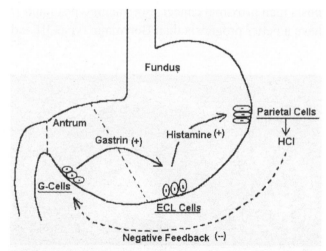

Figure 11–11. Schematic diagram of the control of gastric acid by G cells and enterochromaffin-like (ECL) cells in the normal stomach. Gastrin released by normal G cells in the antrum stimulates fundic ECL cells to release histamine, which stimulates the secretion of hydrochloric acid (HCl) by parietal cells. The intragastric acidity exerts a feedback inhibition on the gastrin release by G cells.

tion recently because of reports on experimentally induced rodent gastric carcinoid with long-term usage of gastric acid inhibitors such as omeprazole. Gastric carcinoid is heterogeneous and consists of three clinical subtypes,[54] as discussed below.

Carcinoid Associated with Type A Chronic Atrophic Gastritis with or without Pernicious Anemia

Type A chronic gastritis, presumably autoimmune in etiology, is caused by antibodies to parietal cells and intrinsic factor in a patient's serum.[55] The disease involves only the fundic mucosa, leading to glandular atrophy, achlorhydria, and eventually pernicious anemia in a majority of patients. The antral mucosa is intact; the antral G cells, without the negative feedback of hydrochloric acid, undergo hyperplasia, which results in the autonomous secretion of gastrin. Hypergastrinemia, in turn, causes ECL-cell hyperplasia and subsequent transformation into carcinoid tumor. The pathogenetic pathway is summarized in Figure 11–12. This is the most common variant, and it often has a benign course. Histologically, the lesions are usually small, multiple, and confined to the gastric mucosa (Figure 11–13, A). The fundic mucosa is atrophic, but the antrum is characterized

by G-cell hyperplasia (see Figure 11–13, B) clinically associated with hypergastrinemia. Lymph node or distant metastasis is uncommon. According to Rindi and colleagues,[54] this is a relatively benign tumor, and conservative therapies such as endoscopic removal or gastric resection (including the gastrin-producing mucosa) seem appropriate. Tumor regression has been reported after antrectomy, which removes the bulk of G cells.

Carcinoid Associated with Zollinger-Ellison Syndrome

Carcinoids associated with Zollinger-Ellison syndrome (ZES)[56] account for 8.6 percent of all gastric carcinoids and occur almost exclusively in patients with MEN-I syndrome. Unlike CAG-associated carcinoids, hypergastrinemia in ZES is associated with gastrinoma in the pancreas rather than G-cell hyperplasia in the antrum. Furthermore, the fundic mucosa is hypertrophic because of the trophic effect of gastrin. The pathogenetic pathway is summarized in Figure 11–14. Surgery should aim at the localization and excision of gastrinoma. The mere excision of gastrin-producing gastric mucosa does not halt the progression of carcinoid tumor.

Carcinoid Tumor of Sporadic Form

Carcinoid tumors of sporadic form are gastrin independent and are not associated with hypergastrinemia.[57] The fundic mucosa appears normal. Sporadic carcinoids account for about a quarter of all gastric carcinoids and have a worse prognosis than carcinoids associated with CAG or ZES. Patients usually have larger tumors and are in more advanced stage of disease. Therapy should be more aggressive in light of the malignant potential of this tumor. In addition to surgery, combined chemotherapy and radiation may be required for neuroendocrine carcinoma.

Hyperplasia-Dysplasia-Neoplasia Sequence of Gastric Carcinoids

The histogenesis of carcinoid tumors in most organs has not been established. Gastric carcinoids are the only carcinoid tumors with a well-documented

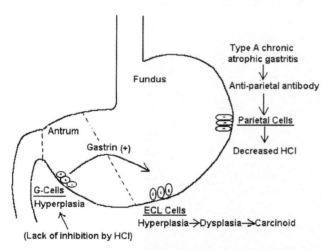

Figure 11–12. Schematic diagram of gastric carcinoid associated with type A chronic atrophic gastritis (CAG). In CAG, parietal cells have been destroyed by antiparietal antibody. The resulting hypochlorhydria removes the inhibitory feedback of hydrochloric acid (HCl) on G cells. Both G cells and enterochromaffin-like (ECL) cells become hyperplastic and autonomous in secreting gastrin and histamine, respectively. Long-term hyperplasia of ECL cells will transform into dysplasia and eventually into carcinoid tumor. Hyperplastic G cells rarely transform into carcinoid tumors.

hyperplasia-dysplasia-neoplasia sequence based on experimental and clinical observations. It was postulated that the lack of feedback inhibition by gastric acid (hypochlorhydria) is the common cause of G-cell hyperplasia resulting from various conditions, including atrophic gastritis with or without pernicious anemia, vagotomy, chronic administration of H_2 antagonists, or proton pump inhibitors. Hypergastrinemia secondary to G-cell hyperplasia causes ECL-cell hyperplasia in turn. Detailed histologic examination by Solcia and colleagues[58] has documented the progression of ECL-cell hyperpla-

sia to dysplasia and finally to microcarcinoid and invasive carcinoid.

MESENCHYMAL TUMORS

Gastrointestinal mesenchymal tumor is a broad term to cover tumors of heterogeneous cell lineage, including smooth-muscle, neural, adipose, vascular, or lymphatic origin; the remaining histologically uncommitted tumors are collectively named gastrointestinal stromal tumors (GISTs).[59,60] However, it has been found recently that these "traditional" GISTs show

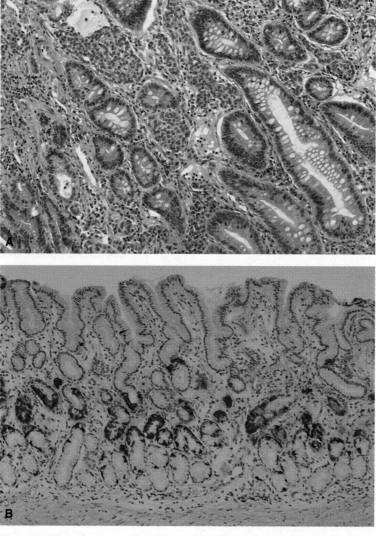

Figure 11–13. Gastric carcinoid associated with type A chronic atrophic gastritis. *A,* The fundic mucosa shows multiple nodules of carcinoid tumor arising from the base of the mucosa. Diffuse intestinal metaplasia and atrophy of deep fundic glands indicate a late stage of type A chronic atrophic gastritis. *B,* The antral mucosa shows G-cell hyperplasia secondary to hypochlorhydria, demonstrated by immunostaining for gastrin (*red color*).

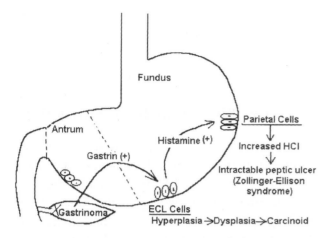

Figure 11–14. Schematic diagram of gastric carcinoid associated with Zollinger-Ellison syndrome (ZES). Gastrin-producing tumors in the pancreas cause hyperplasia of enterochromaffin-like (ECL) cells. Long-term hyperplasia of ECL cells is subject to the risk of malignant transformation into carcinoid tumor. The treatment of ZES should aim at the removal of the gastrinoma or a total gastrectomy. Antrectomy alone will not eliminate the risk of carcinoid tumor in the fundus. (HCl = hydrochloric acid.)

mutation of the c-kit proto-oncogene (CD117) and loss of DNA on chromosome arm 14q.[61] Because CD117 is positive only for mast cells and interstitial cells of Cajal (ICCs) in the GI tract, it was postulated that GISTs originate from ICCs and should be renamed interstitial cells of Cajal tumors.[62]

Gastrointestinal Stromal Tumor

Although GISTs can occur throughout the entire GI tract, the stomach is the most common site, accounting for 60 to 70 percent of all cases. These tumors occur predominantly in persons over 40 years of age, with an equal sex incidence. Benign GISTs outnumber malignant ones by a margin of 10:1. Although GISTs are rare in individuals under the age of 40 years, malignant GISTs occur more often in this age group.

Grossly, benign GISTs are usually sharply demarcated nodules 2 to 5 cm in diameter (Figure 11–15, A). Malignant GISTs are usually more than 10 cm in maximal diameter and often show mucosal ulceration and areas of necrosis and hemorrhage. Malignant GISTs often show spread of multiple tumor nodules into the surrounding omental or mesenteric soft tissue. However, GISTs do not disseminate to the regional lymph nodes. Microscopically, GISTs show

two histologic patterns: spindle cell (70%) and epithelioid cell (30%) (see Figure 11–15, B).

The histologic features that correlate best with development of recurrence and metastasis include mitotic activity, tumor size, and the presence of tumor necrosis. Gastrointestinal stromal tumors with the following histologic features are considered malignant: (1) mitotic counts higher than 5 mitoses/10 high-power fields; (2) size larger than 5 cm; and (3) large areas of necrosis, hemorrhage, hypercellularity, or atypia.[59]

Immunohistochemically, GISTs are typically positive for vimentin, CD34, and CD117/c-kit protein. A hematopoietic progenitor cell antigen, CD34 can occur in a wide variety of mesenchymal tumors of fibroblastic, lipomatous, and endothelial origin; CD117 is a more specific marker for a diagnosis of GIST[61] (see Figure 11–15, C). Patients with a mutation of the *c-kit* gene have more frequent recurrences and a higher mortality than those without the mutation.[63]

Leiomyoma

Leiomyomas are benign smooth-muscle tumors that are most commonly seen in the cardia. Grossly, the tumor is well circumscribed, with muscular proliferations demonstrating a whorled and elastic cross section.

Lipoma and Neurofibroma/ Neurofibromatosis

Lipomas are rare benign tumors that occur in the gastric submucosa. Small lipomas are ususally asymptomatic; however, some lipomas larger than 3 cm in diameter can cause ulceration, epigastric pain, bleeding, and gastric outlet obstruction. Grossly, lipomas are round well-defined submucosal nodules with a typical yellowish cross section. Histologically, the tumor consists of mature adipose tissue with no significant inflammation unless the mucosa is ulcerated.

Both von Recklinghausen's neurofibromatosis and type II multiple endocrine neoplasia (MEN-II) can affect the GI tract.[64] These lesions include mucosal neuromas and ganglioneuromas (in both syndromes) and plexiform neuromas (in von Recklinghausen's disease). However, the stomach is less frequently involved than the small intestine and the colon.

Granular Cell Tumor and Glomus Tumor

Granular cell tumors are proliferations of plump spindled or epithelioid cells, which are presumably Schwann cells in origin. The cytoplasm stains positively with periodic acid–Schiff stain (PAS) and S-100 protein. The tumors are located at the submucosa or muscularis propria of the stomach.

Glomus tumor is a rare vascular tumor that is presumed to arise from the normal structure of the glomus body. The tumor commonly occurs in the antrum as a solitary nodule in the muscularis propria. Histologically, the round and uniform tumor cells are surrounded by vascular space and can sometimes be mistaken for carcinoid tumors (Figure 11–16). The tumor cells are immunoreactive for smooth-muscle actin, vimentin, laminin, and type IV collagen. The tumors are mostly benign and solitary although a multiple glomus tumor with intravascular spread has been reported.[65]

LYMPHOPROLIFERATIVE DISORDERS

The GI tract is the most common site of primary extranodal non-Hodgkin's lymphoma, and more than 50 percent of all GI lymphomas arise from the stomach. However, the overall number is small, and gastric lymphomas account for less than 5 percent of all gastric tumors. There is no satisfactory classification of GI lymphomas at present.[66] Except for a few cases of T-cell lymphoma, the majority of gastric lymphomas are of B-cell origin. Approximately 90 percent of gastric lymphomas are of the diffuse type, and only 10 percent of them are of the follicular type. In a report in 1983, Isaacson and Wright

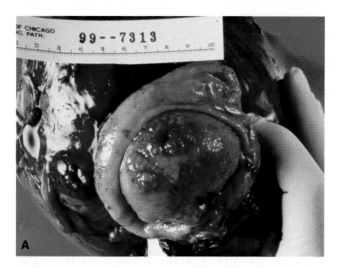

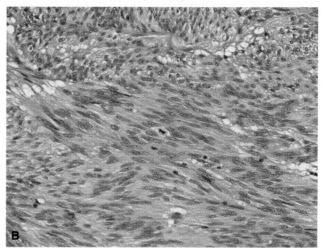

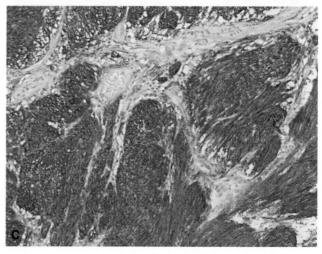

Figure 11–15. Gastrointestinal stromal tumor (GIST). *A,* Resection specimen of a case of GIST shows a large bulging tumor with surface erosion. Attached to this small segment of the stomach is the spleen, which has been partially infiltrated on the capsule. *B,* Histologically, the tumor consists of densely packed spindle cells with increased mitosis. *C,* Strongly stained tumor cells with antibody to CD117/c-kit protein (*brown color*) are a characteristic feature of GISTs.

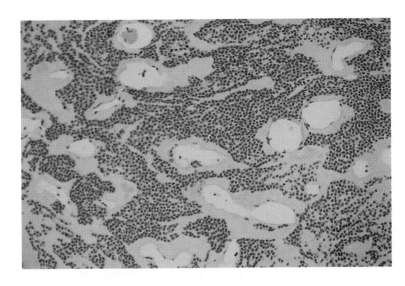

Figure 11–16. Glomus tumor. The glomus tumor has round and uniform tumor cells reminiscent of carcinoid tumor. The presence of a surrounding irregular vascular space is characteristic of glomus tumors rather than carcinoid tumors.

found that low-grade gastric lymphomas have histologic features more similar to mucosa-associated lymphoid tissue (MALT) than to nodal lymphoid tissue.[67] The term "MALT lymphoma" was suggested later for this group of lymphomas. Only MALT lymphoma is discussed in this chapter because it accounts for > 90 percent of all gastric lymphomas.

Mucoca-Associated Lymphoid-Tissue Lymphoma of the Stomach

Several patterns of gastric lymphoma are noted at endoscopic examination: ulceration, gastritis, poly-poid mass, and diffuse growth (Figure 11–17, A). In general, the gross appearance is related to the tumor grade. Low-grade lymphomas are usually superficial with focal ulceration whereas high-grade lymphomas show diffuse infiltration or nodular growth with extensive ulceration. The gastric antrum is the most common site of involvement, followed by the body and the cardia.

Low-grade MALT lymphomas are characterized by lymphoepithelial lesions, subepithelial plasma cells, and reactive lymphoid follicles. A lymphoepithelial lesion refers the intraepithelial migration of atypical lymphocytes (see Figure 11–17, B). These

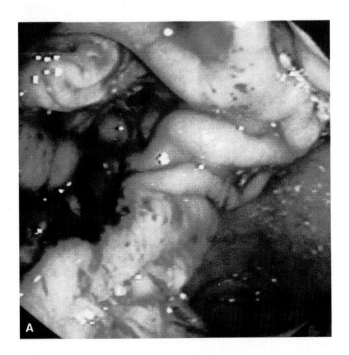

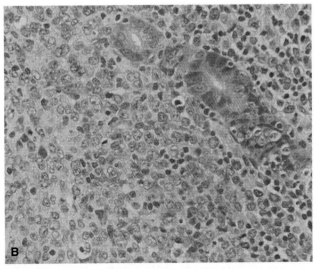

Figure 11–17. Malignant lymphoma. *A,* Endoscopic view of a gastric lymphoma shows giant gastric folds with a nodular appearance. *B,* Histologic study of a lymphoepithelial lesion shows a gastric gland infiltrated by large atypical lymphocytes.

atypical lymphocytes are of B-cell origin rather than being T cells, which make up a population of normal intraepithelial lymphocytes. Reactive lymphoid follicles are surrounded by neoplastic lymphocytes in the marginal zone.

The etiology of gastric lymphoma is not completely understood. Associations with *H. pylori* infection, immunodeficiency disorders, and autoimmune states such as celiac sprue have been reported. Wotherspoon and colleagues found *H. pylori* infection in 92 percent of patients with gastric lymphoma, compared with an infection rate of 50 percent to 60 percent in the general population.[68] Hussell and associates have shown that certain strains of *H. pylori* can stimulate the in vitro proliferation of gastric lymphoma cells.[69] This process is T-cell dependent and interleukin-2 related. Sigal hypothesized that *H. pylori* infection leads to chronic antigenic stimulation, which elicits a dense polyclonal lymphoid proliferation.[70] Persistent antigenic stimulation in conjunction with dietary mutagens eventually generates monoclonal lymphoid cells. Initially, some of these monoclonal lymphocytes may be antigen dependent and can respond to antibiotic treatment, which eliminates *H. pylori* infection and removes the antigenic stimulation.[71] Unlike the low-grade lymphomas in lymph nodes, MALT lymphomas tend to be localized in the stomach, without involving the bone marrow.

Low-grade MALT lymphoma can transform into a high-grade lymphoma. Microscopically, it is difficult to distinguish between a high-grade lymphoma of the MALT type and the nodal type unless the preceding low-grade disease (such as the presence of lymphoepithelial lesions and reactive follicles) is identified. This raises another issue in distinguishing primary gastric MALT lymphoma from a nodal lymphoma with secondary gastric involvement. The lack of Bcl-2 protein, CD5, and CD10, as well as the positive expression of KB61 in gastric MALT lymphoma, may help in the distinction.[72]

REFERENCES

1. Watanabe H, Jass JR, Sobin LH. Histological typing of oesophageal and gastric tumors. Berlin: Springer-Verlag; 1990.
2. Nakamura T, Nakano GI. Histopathological classification and malignant change in gastric polyps. J Clin Pathol 1985;38:754–64.
3. Iida M, Yao T, Itoh H, et al. Natural history of gastric adenomas in patients with familial adenomatosis coli/Gardner's syndrome. Cancer 1988;61:605–11.
4. Muratani M, Nakamura T, Nakano GI, Mukawa K. Ultrastructural study of two subtypes of gastric adenoma. J Clin Pathol 1989;42:352–9.
5. Hirato T, Ming SC. Early gastric carcinoma. In: Ming SC, Goldman H, editors. Pathology of the gastrointestinal tract. Philadelphia: WB Saunders; 1992. p. 570–82.
6. Hirato T, Okada M, Itabashi M. Histogenesis of human gastric cancer—with special reference to significance of adenoma as a precancerous lesion. In: Ming SC, editor. Precursors of gastric cancer. New York: Praeger; 1984. p. 233–52.
7. Kamiya T, Morishita T, Asakura H, et al. Long-term follow-up study of gastric adenoma and its relation to gastric protruded carcinoma. Cancer 1982;50:2496–503.
8. Elster K. Histologic classification of gastric polyps. In: Morson BC, editor. Pathology of the gastro-intestinal tract. Berlin: Springer-Verlag; 1976. p. 77–93.
9. Wauters GV, Ferrell L, Ostroff JW, Heyman MB. Hyperplastic gastric polyps associated with persistent *Helicobacter pylori* infection and active gastritis. Am J Gastroenterol 1990;85:1395–7.
10. Daibo M, Itabashi M, Hirota T. Malignant transformation of gastric hyperplastic polyps. Am J Gastroenterol 1987;82:1016–25.
11. Koch HK, Lecsh R, Cremer M, Oehlert W. Polyps and polypoid foveolar hyperplasia in gastric biopsy specimens and their precancerous prevaleance. Front Gastrointest Res 1979;4:183–91.
12. Rabin MS, Bremner CG, Botha JR. The reflux gastroesophageal polyp. Am J Gastroenterol 1980;73:451–3.
13. Jablokow VR, Aranha GV, Reyes CV. Gastric stomal polypoid hyperplasia: report of four cases. J Surg Oncol 1982;19:106–8.
14. Savage A, Jones S. Histological appearances of the gastric mucosa 15–27 years after partial gastrectomy. J Clin Pathol 1979;32:179–86.
15. Janunger KG, Domellof L. Gastric polyps and precancerous mucosal changes after partial gastrectomy. Acta Chir Scand 1978;144:293–8.
16. Entius MM, Westerman AM, van Velthuysen MLF, et al. Molecular and phenotypic markers of hamartomous polyposis syndromes in the gastrointestinal tract. Hepatogastroenterology 1999;46:661–6.
17. Halbert RE. Peutz-Jeghers syndrome with metastasizing gastric adenocarcinoma. Arch Pathol Lab Med 1982;106:517–20.
18. Hemminki A, Markie D, Tomlinson I, et al. A serine/threonine kinase gene defective in Peutz-Jeghers syndrome. Nature 1998;391:184–7.
19. Watanabe A, Nagashima H, Motoi M, Ogawa K. Familial juvenile polyposis of the stomach. Gastroenterology 1979;77:148–51.
20. Lynch ED, Ostermeyer EA, Lee MK, et al. Inherited mutations in PTEN that are associated with breast cancer, Cowden disease, and juvenile polyposis. Am J Hum Genet 1997;61:1254–60.
21. Howe JR, Roth S, Ringold JC, et al. Mutation in the

SMAD4/DPC4 gene in juvenile polyposis. Science 1998; 280:1086–8.

22. Sassatelli R, Bertoni G, Serra L, et al. Generalized juvenile polyposis with mixed pattern and gastric cancer. Gastroenterology 1993;104:910–5.

23. Watanabe H, Enjoji M, Yao T, Ohsato K. Gastric lesions in familial adenomatosis coli. Their incidence and histologic analysis. Hum Pathol 1978;9:269–83.

24. Iida M, Yao T, Watanabe H, et al. Fundic gland polyposis in patients without familial adenomatosis coli: its incidence and clinical features. Gastroenterology 1984;86:1437–42.

25. el-Zimaity HM, Jackson FW, Graham DY. Fundic gland polyps developing during omeprazole therapy. Am J Gastroenterol 1997;92:1858–60.

26. Lai EC, Tompkins RK. Heterotopic pancreas. Review of a 26 year experience. Am J Surg 1986;151:697–700.

27. Blakstone MO. Endoscopic interpretation. Normal and pathologic appearance of the gastro-intestinal tract. New York: Raven Press; 1984. p. 100–14.

28. Appelman HD. Menetrier's disease. In: Haggitt RC, Appelman HD, Riddell RH, editors. Diseases of the gastrointestinal tract. Chicago: ASCP Press; 1989. p. 25–30.

29. Takagi H, Jhappan C, Sharp R, Merlino G. Hypertrophic gastropathy resembling Menetrier's disease in transgenic mice overexpressing transforming growth factor α in the stomach. J Clin Invest 1992;90:1161–7.

30. Chouraqui JP, Roy CC, Brochu RP, et al. Menetrier's disease in children: report of a patient and review of sixteen other cases. Gastroenterology 1981;80:1042–7.

31. Creutzfeldt W, Arnold R, Creutzfelt C, Track NS. Pathomorphologic, biochemical, and diagnostic aspects of gastrinomas (Zollinger-Ellison syndrome). Hum Pathol 1975; 6:47–76.

32. Solcia E, Capella C, Fiocca R, et al. Gastric argyrophil carcinoidosis in patients with Zollinger-Ellison syndrome due to type I multiple endocrine neoplasia. A newly recognized association. Am J Surg Pathol 1990;14:503–13.

33. Tan DTD, Stempien SJ, Dagradi AE. The clinical spectrum of hypertrophic hypersecretory gastropathy. Report of 50 patients. Gastrointest Endosc 1971;18:69–73.

34. Greenlee RT, Murray T, Bolden S et al. Cancer statistics 2000. CA Cancer J Clin 2000;50:7–33.

35. Nobrega FT, Sedlack JD, Sedlack RE, et al. A decline in carinoma of the stomach: a diagnostic artifact? Mayo Clin Proc 1983;58:255–60.

36. Heidl G, Langhans P, Krieg V, et al. Comparative studies of cardia carcinoma and infracardial carcinoma. J Cancer Res Clin Oncol 1993;120:91–4.

37. Correa P. Human gastric carcinogenesis: a multistep and multifactorial process—first American Cancer Society award lecture on cancer epidemiology and prevention. Cancer Res 1992;52:6735–40.

38. Filipe MI, Munoz N, Matko I, et al. Intestinal metaplasia types and the risk of gastric cancer: a cohort study in Slovenia. Int J Cancer 1994;57:324–9.

39. World Health Organization. The evaluation of carcinogenic risks to humans. Monograph No. 61. Lyon, France: International Agency for Research on Cancer; 1994. p. 177–240.

40. Forman D, Newell DG, Fullerton F, et al. Association between infection with *Helicobacter pylori* and risk of gastric cancer: evidence from a prospective investigation. BMJ 1991;302:1302–5.

41. Parsonnet J. *Helicobacter pylori* and gastric adenocarcinoma. In: Parsonnet J, editor. Microbes and malignancy. New York: Oxford University Press; 1999. p. 372–408.

42. Mochizuki T. Method for histopathological examination of early gastric cancer. In: Murakami T, editor. Early gastric cancer. Gann Monogr Cancer Res, No. 11. Tokyo: University of Tokyo Press; 1971. p. 57–65.

43. Kidokoro T. Frequency of resection, metastasis, and five year survival rate of early gastric carcinoma in a surgical clinic. In: Murakami T, editor. Early gastric cancer. Gann Monogr Cancer Res, No. 11. Tokyo: University of Tokyo Press; 1971. p. 45–9.

44. Murakami T. Pathomorphological diagnosis. Definition and gross classification of early gastric cancer. In: Murakami T, editor. Early gastric cancer. Gann Monogr Cancer Res, No. 11. Tokyo: University of Tokyo Press; 1971. p. 53–5.

45. Lauren P. The two histological main types of gastric carcinoma: diffuse and so-called intestinal-type carcinoma. An attempt at a histo-clinical classification. Acta Pathol Microbiol Scand 1965;64:31–49.

46. Stout A. Pathology of carcinoma of the stomach. Arch Surg 1943;46:807–22.

47. Ming SC. Gastric carcinoma: a pathobiological classification. Cancer 1977;39:2475–85.

48. Borrmann R. Geschwulste des Magens und Duodenums. In: Henke F, Lubarsch O, editors. Handbuch der speziellen pathologischen Anatomie und Histologie. Berlin: Springer; 1926. p. 865.

49. American Joint Committee on Cancer. Stomach. In: Fleming ID, Cooper JS, Henson DE, et al, editors. AJCC cancer staging manual. 5th ed. Philadelphia: Lippincott-Raven; 1997. p. 71–6.

50. Brien TP, Depowski PL, Sheehan CE, et al. Prognostic factors in gastric cancer. Mod Pathol 1998;11:870–7.

51. Schubert ML. Control of gastric acid secretion. Curr Opin Gastroenterol 1992;8:895–906.

52. Freston JW, Borch K, Brand S, et al. Effect of hypochlorhydria and hypergastrinemia on structure and function of gastrointestinal cells. Dig Dis Sci 1995;40:50S–62S.

53. Modlin IM, Nangia AK. The pathobiology of the human enterochromaffin-like cell. Yale J Biol Med 1992;65: 775–92.

54. Rindi G, Luinetti O, Cornaggia M, et al. Three subtypes of gastric argyrophil carcinoid and the gastric neuroendocrine carcinoma: a clinicopathologic study. Gastroenterology 1993;104:994–1006.

55. Solcia E, Rindi G, Fiocca R, et al. Distinct patterns of chronic gastritis associated with carcinoid and cancer and their role in tumorigenesis. Yale J Biol Med 1992;65:793–804.

56. Lehy T, Cardiot G, Mignon M, et al. Influence of multiple endocrine neoplasia type 1 on gastric endocrine cells in patients with Zollinger-Ellison syndrome. Gut 1992;33: 1275–9.

57. Bordi C, Yu J-Y, Baggi MY, et al. Gastric carcinoids and their precursor lesions. A histologic and immunohistochemical study of 23 cases. Cancer 1991;67:663–72.

58. Solcia E, Fiocca R, Villani L, et al. Hyperplastic, dysplastic, and neoplastic enterochromaffin-like-cell proliferations

of the gastric mucosa: classification and histogenesis. Am J Surg Pathol 1995;19 Suppl 1:S1–7.

59. Miettinen M, Sarlomo-Rikala M, Lasota J. Gastrointestinal stromal tumors. Ann Chir Gynaecol 1998;87:278–81.

60. Miettinen M, Sarlomo-Rikala M, Lasota J. Gastrointestinal stromal tumors: recent advances in understanding of their biology. Hum Pathol 1999;30:1213–20.

61. Sarlomo-Rikala M, Kovatich AJ, Barusevicius A, Miettinen M. CD117: a sensitive marker for gastrointestinal stromal tumors that is more specific than CD34. Mod Pathol 1998;11:728–34.

62. Sircar K, Hewlett BR, Huizinga JD, et al. Interstitial cells of Cajal as precursors of gastrointestinal stromal tumors. Am J Surg Pathol 1999;23:377–89.

63. Taniguchi M, Nishida T, Hirota S, et al. Effect of c-kit mutation on prognosis of gastrointestinal stromal tumors. Cancer Res 1999;59:4297–300.

64. Petersen JM, Ferguson DR. Gastrointestinal neurofibromatosis. J Clin Gastroenterol 1984;6:529–34.

65. Haque S, Modlin IM, West AB. Multiple glomus tumors of the stomach with intravascular spread. Am J Surg Pathol 1992;16:291–9.

66. Isaacson PG. Lymphoma of mucosa-associated lymphoid tissue (MALT). Histopathology 1990;16:617–9.

67. Isaacson P, Wright DH. Malignant lymphoma of mucosa-associated lymphoid tissue: a distinct type of B-cell lymphoma. Cancer 1983;52:1410–6.

68. Wotherspoon AC, Ortiz-Hidalgo C, Falzon MR, Isaacson PG. Helicobacter pylori-associated gastritis and primary B-cell gastric lymphoma. Lancet 1991;338:1175–6.

69. Hussell T, Isaacson PG, Crabtree JE, Spencer J. The response of cells from low-grade B-cell gastric lymphomas of mucosa associated lymphoid tissue to Helicobacter pylori. Lancet 1993;342:571–4.

70. Sigal SH, Saul SH, Auerbach HE, et al. Gastric small lymphocytic proliferation with immunoglobulin gene rearrangement in pseudolymphoma versus lymphoma. Gastroenterology 1989;97:195–201.

71. Wotherspoon AC, Doglioni C, Diss TC, et al. Regression of primary low-grade B-cell gastric lymphoma of mucosa-associated lymphoid tissue after eradication of Helicobacter pylori. Lancet 1993;342:575–7.

72. Isaacson PG, Wotherspoon AC, Diss TC, Pan LX. Bcl-2 expression in lymphoma. Lancet 1991;337:175–6.

12

Diagnosis and Staging of Gastric Cancer

MARTIN R. WEISER, MD
KEVIN C. CONLON, MD, MBA

Worldwide, gastric cancer affects almost 800,000 individuals per year[1] and is most commonly seen in eastern Asia. In North America, adenocarcinoma of the stomach occurs less frequently. The clinical manifestations and physical findings of gastric cancer are nonspecific and overlap with benign disease, frequently resulting in a delay in diagnosis. As outcome is largely related to stage, patients in the United States, as a whole, have poor outcomes due to their late presentation.[2,3]

Surgical resection remains the treatment of choice. However, improvements in multimodal chemotherapy and radiotherapy have influenced treatment algorithms. This therapy can be administered prior to resection (neo-adjuvant or induction) or postoperatively. Increasing interest in the neo-adjuvant approach has required the development of accurate and cost-efficient preoperative staging. Currently, gastric cancer staging is based on the tumor-node-metastasis (TNM) system and relies on tumor depth, nodal spread, and distant metastases.

Endoscopy and biopsy are the most common method of initial diagnosis. Computed tomography is the most accepted radiologic modality for diagnosing advanced disease. Other methods for staging disease include endoscopic ultrasonography, magnetic resonance imaging, and positron emission tomography. Laparoscopy and laparoscopic ultrasonography are minimally invasive procedures that have recently become important components in the staging algorithm for gastric cancer patients. Inves-

tigational modalities include peritoneal-fluid cytology and molecular staging techniques.

DIAGNOSIS OF GASTRIC CANCER

Clinical Manifestations

Two-thirds of patients with gastric cancer in the United States will present with advanced disease.[4,5] Early symptoms, including nonspecific abdominal pain and dyspepsia, are usually ignored or treated with empiric antiulcer therapy. As the disease progresses, the symptoms become more pronounced and commonly include anorexia, weight loss, and nausea. In a review of more than 18,000 patients with gastric cancer by the American College of Surgeons, over half of the patients presented with weight loss and abdominal pain.[5] Nausea, anorexia, and dysphagia were noted in approximately 30 percent of patients, and melena was noted in 25 percent. Approximately 20 percent of patients had a prior history of gastric ulcer. Despite the nonspecific nature of the presenting symptoms, some complaints may suggest the location of the primary tumor. For instance, dysphagia is usually associated with tumors of the cardia or the gastroesophageal junction. Antral tumors can be associated with gastric-outlet obstruction, and early satiety is seen with a diffusely infiltrating tumor that produces a nondistensible gastric wall.

The majority of patients show no significant findings on examination, and the development of specific physical signs usually indicates metastatic disease. The presence of an intra-abdominal mass, hepatomegaly, or ascites is usually due to extensive and incurable disease. Other physical findings consistent with widely metastatic disease include a palpable umbilical mass (Sister Mary Joseph node), a palpable supraclavicular lymph node (Virchow's node), peritoneal implants in the pelvis (Blumer's shelf), and an ovarian mass (Krukenberg's tumor).

Diagnostic Modalities

In the United States, the majority of gastric cancers currently are diagnosed by endoscopy. Although less widely used today, the barium contrast study previously played an important role in the detection of stomach malignancies and remains a sensitive modality. In experienced hands, a double-contrast upper-gastrointestinal series will diagnose 99 percent of abnormalities and 96 percent of gastric malignancies.[6,7] The radiologic characteristics of gastric malignancy include rigidity or thickening of the gastric wall, prominent and irregular gastric rugae, large ulcers with irregular nodular margins and elevated borders, and intraluminal masses.[8] Figure 12–1 shows a lesion at the gastroesophageal junction.

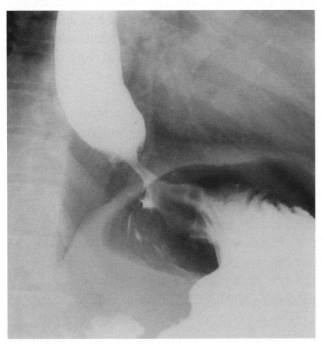

Figure 12–1. Esophagogram of a patient with a lesion at the gastroesophageal junction. Endoscopy and biopsy proved adenocarcinoma.

Endoscopy is used to confirm abnormalities seen by a contrast study and can visualize both early and advanced malignancies. Since the clinical manifestations of gastric cancer overlap with those of benign ulcer disease, the early use of endoscopy with biopsy is recommended in symptomatic patients. For this reason, most centers currently perform endoscopy as the initial diagnostic procedure.

The diagnostic accuracy of endoscopic biopsy appears to be related to the number of samples obtained, the location of the biopsy, and the histology of the cancer. In a series of over 200 patients with esophageal and gastric cancer, a diagnosis was made for 70 percent of patients after the first biopsy, 95 percent of patients after the fourth biopsy, and 98.9 percent of patients after seven biopsies.[9] The site examined also influences the accuracy of endoscopic biopsy; in a study by Hatfield and colleagues, diagnosing a malignancy was most successful if biopsy specimens were taken from the base and rim of an ulcerated lesion.[10] Winawer noted that the accuracy of the biopsy is related to histology. Fifty percent of diffusely infiltrating lesions were correctly identified on biopsy, compared to 92 percent of exophytic lesions.[11] The addition of brush cytology to biopsy increases the diagnostic yield of cancers located in the cardia and in stenotic lesions.[12]

Mass population screening with endoscopy is efficacious in regions with a high incidence of gastric cancer, such as Japan.[13] In Western countries, early endoscopy to confirm benign lesions and diagnose malignant disease is advocated although such use is probably not cost-effective in such low-risk populations. In a British prospective trial of symptomatic patients over 45 years of age, endoscopy diagnosed an abnormality in 75 percent of patients. High-risk premalignant disease was diagnosed in 493 (19%) of the 2,659 patients, and malignancy was found in 115 (4%).[14] The importance of diagnosing benign disease should not be underestimated. Recent studies have found an association between *Helicobacter pylori* infection and gastric cancer,[15,16] and some evidence suggests that treatment of *H. pylori* may have an impact on the progression to gastric cancer.

The measurement of serum tumor markers has not been useful in the diagnosis of gastric cancer. Although tumor markers such as carcinoembryonic antigen (CEA), CA19-9, CA72-4, and α-fetoprotein can be abnormally elevated in 15 to 60 percent of patients,[17–23] they are not specific for gastric cancer. Some authors have advocated the measurement of serum markers preoperatively since recurrence may be detected by a postoperative rise in these markers.[22] Currently, the use of serum markers is of research interest only.

PATHOLOGIC STAGING OF GASTRIC CANCER

Gastric malignancies are pathologically staged according to depth of invasion (T stage), number of lymph node metastases (N stage), and presence of distant disease (M stage). There is now an international agreement among the American Joint Committee on Cancer (AJCC), the Union Internationale Contre le Cancer (UICC), and the Japanese Research Society for Gastric Cancer (JRSFC) to use the TNM staging system (Tables 12–1 and 12–2).

In this system, tumors designated as T1 tumors invade the mucosa or submucosa, T2 tumors penetrate through the muscularis propria or subserosa, T3 tumors penetrate the serosa, and T4 tumors invade other structures. The 1997 edition of the AJCC cancer staging manual has adopted a new N stage definition based on the number of positive lymph nodes: N1 disease for 1 to 6 positive nodes, N2 for 7 to 15 positive nodes, and N3 for more than 15 positive nodes. The older 1992 classification system was based on a determination of the location of positive nodes and their distance from the primary tumor that was often subjective. The revised nodal staging system has been verified recently in the German Gastric Cancer Study.[24] This study concluded that the N classification, based on the number of positive nodes, was superior to the old 1992 classification system for estimating a prognosis and that it eliminated the subjectivity inherent in determining lymph node location and distance from the primary tumor. However, the new classification of N status relies on a systematic and reproducible approach to resecting and analyzing perigastric lymph nodes. The UICC and the AJCC suggest that to improve the quality of staging, at least 15 negative nodes be analyzed before the diagnosis of N0 is rendered.

PREOPERATIVE STAGING OF GASTRIC CANCER

The limited efficacy of adjuvant chemotherapy in gastric cancer has resulted in renewed interest in preoperative therapy. Patients who are found to have locally advanced disease (serosal invasion with nodal disease) and no evidence of distant metastases will often be treated with neoadjuvant chemotherapy followed by surgical resection (Figure 12–2). Preoperative staging is critical when selecting patients for this approach. At our institution, we currently rely on a combination of computed tomography, endoscopic ultrasonography, magnetic resonance imaging, and the selective use of laparoscopy and laparoscopic ultrasonography. Investigational techniques that have had preliminary success include positron

Table 12–1. TUMOR-NODE-METASTASIS CATEGORIES FOR GASTRIC CANCER

Primary Tumor
T1	Invasion of lamina propria into submucosa
T2	Invasion of muscularis propria/subserosa
T3	Invasion of serosa
T4	Invasion of adjacent structures

Regional Lymph Nodes
N0	No regional lymph node metastasis
N1	Metastasis in 1 to 6 regional lymph nodes
N2	Metastasis in 7 to 15 regional lymph nodes
N3	Metastasis in more than 15 regional lymph nodes

Distant Metastasis
M0	No distant metastasis
M1	Distant metastasis

Table 12–2. STAGING FOR GASTRIC CANCER*

Stage	Tumor	Node	Metastasis
0	T1s	N0	M0
IA	T1	N0	M0
IB	T1	N1	M0
	T2	N0	M0
II	T1	N2	M0
	T2	N1	M0
	T3	N0	M0
IIIA	T2	N2	M0
	T3	N1	M0
	T4	N0	M0
IIIB	T3	N2	M0
IV	T4	N1	M0
	T1–3	N3	M0
	T4	N2–3	M0
	Any	Any	M1

*American Joint Committee on Cancer classification.

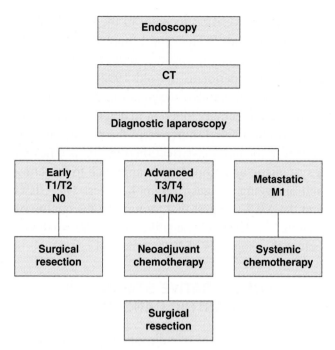

Figure 12–2. Memorial Sloan-Kettering Cancer Center staging and treatment algorithm for patients with gastric adenocarcinoma. (CT = computed tomography.)

emission tomography, peritoneal cytology, and molecular staging.

Computed Tomography

Computed tomography (CT) is the most frequently used radiologic staging modality for gastric cancer. Computed tomography detects intraluminal tumors, a thickened gastric wall, and direct invasion of the primary tumor into surrounding structures; it appears to be optimal for determining locally advanced and metastatic disease. Enlarged perigastric, celiac, or preaortic lymph nodes can be detected, as can liver, lung, or adrenal metastases.[8]

Luminal distension is key to the evaluation of the gastric wall. A wall thickness > 1 cm is considered abnormal when the stomach is well distended.[25] The use of water as a distending agent for the stomach, with bolus administration of intravenous contrast, improves the accuracy of CT for staging gastric cancer.[26,27] Antimotility agents can be given to reduce peristalsis and gastric emptying, which minimize motion artifact. With these techniques, the stomach appears as three layers: an inner layer that enhances and corresponds to the mucosa; a low-attenuation

intermediate layer that corresponds to the submucosa; and an outer layer of slightly higher attenuation, which corresponds to the muscularis and serosa.[28] Gastric cancer can be seen as an intraluminal mass or as a markedly thickened enhancing wall.[27] Figure 12–3 shows diffuse wall thickening in a nondistensible stomach with linitis plastica. Using helical and dynamic techniques with optimal gastric distension, CT detects approximately 90 percent of gastric cancer cases and accurately assesses wall invasion (T stage) in 40 to 80 percent of cases.[29–31] Computed tomography appears to be more useful in diagnosing locally advanced disease than early disease;[30–32] it will detect 95 to 100 percent of bulky advanced gastric cancers and will accurately determine tumor depth (T stage) in over 80 percent of these cases.[26–33] However, CT can have difficulty in determining tumor invasion of contiguous organs (ie, T4 tumor) since this modality cannot differentiate inflammation from tumor.[25] Several recent series have noted an improved accuracy for helical techniques in identifying invasion of the pancreas and colon.[34,35] Figure 12–4 shows a locally advanced gastric cancer with bulky disease at the lesser curve of the stomach and in the gastrohepatic ligament. In contrast to its ability to detect advanced lesions, CT detects only 25 to 50 percent of early gastric lesions and correctly stages wall invasion in 15 percent of these cases.[26,32,33]

Computed tomography has been relatively poor at staging lymph node metastases,[34] with an accuracy of between 25 percent and 70 percent reported in the literature.[26,30,31,35–37] Computed tomography

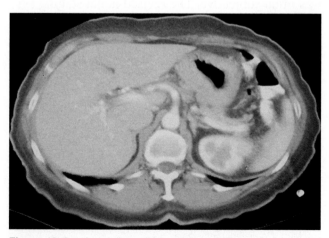

Figure 12–3. A nondistensible gastric wall shown by computed tomography indicates a diffusely infiltrating cancer.

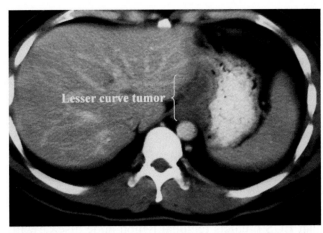

Figure 12–4. Computed tomography scan of a patient with a locally advanced tumor of the lesser curve of the stomach.

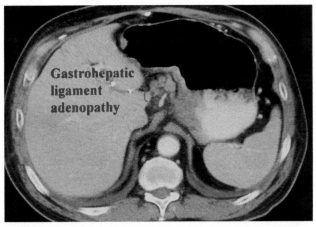

Figure 12–5. Computed tomography scan of a patient with a tumor of the lesser curve of the stomach. Computed tomography correctly identifies locally advanced disease with an enlarged lymph node in the gastrohepatic ligament.

mostly relies on nodal size to diagnose metastases. However, CT cannot differentiate inflammatory or reactive nodes from those with metastatic disease.[25] Fukuya and colleagues studied the efficacy of helical CT in detecting lymph nodes in gastric cancer patients;[38] CT detected only 1 percent of nodes < 5 mm in size, 45 percent of nodes between 5 and 9 mm, and over 70 percent of nodes > 9 mm in size. Lymph node size correlated with the potential for harboring metastatic disease. Over 80 percent of nodes > 14 mm in size seen by CT contained metastases. However, not all the metastases were found in enlarged lymph nodes. Metastatic cancer was noted in 5 percent of lymph nodes < 5 mm in size, 21 percent of nodes from 5 to 9 mm in size, and 23 percent of nodes from 10 to 14 mm in size. In this study, involved nodes were hyperdense, with a greater short-to-long axis ratio (ie, a rounder shape) than nodes without tumor. Overall, diagnosing lymph node metastases remains a challenge, especially in nodes < 15 mm in diameter. Figure 12–5 is an example of CT detecting a discrete enlarged lymph node in the gastrohepatic ligament. In general, it can be stated that CT will understage the extent of nodal disease.[31]

The strength of CT lies in its ability to diagnose distant metastatic disease.[30,32,34,35,39] Carcinomatosis with diffuse peritoneal seeding, malignant ascites, and adnexal and pelvic metastases are well demonstrated by CT.[25] Figure 12–6 shows an example of carcinomatosis and omental "caking." Computed tomography will accurately assess the liver for metas-

tases in 79 to 96 percent of gastric cancer cases.[35,37,40] However, small-volume metastatic disease in the peritoneal cavity and liver will be missed.[30,34,35,37,41–43]

Endoscopic Ultrasonography

Endoscopic ultrasonography (EUS) overcomes the two-dimensional limitation of conventional endoscopy and allows the evaluation of the gastric mucosa and underlying layers. In the normal stomach, EUS identifies five gastric wall layers: mucosa, submucosa, muscularis propria, subserosa, and serosa. Disruption of the normal ultrasonographic appearance of these layers determines the depth of invasion (Figure 12–7).

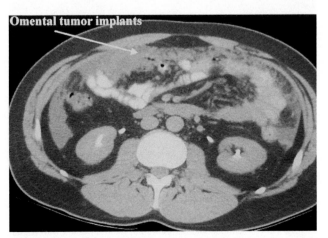

Figure 12–6. Computed tomography depicts metastatic gastric adenocarcinoma with omental carcinomatous implants.

The accuracy of EUS for determining the depth of the primary tumor ranges from 60 to 90 percent.[36,44–49] Endoscopic ultrasonography has difficulty differentiating inflammation and fibrosis from tumor, and this is the most common reason for misdiagnosis.[47,50–52] The ability to visualize tumor by EUS is related to the tumor's morphology and to the stage of disease. Endoscopic ultrasonography most accurately stages early well-differentiated polypoid cancers.[44] Difficulty arises in differentiating deep T2 tumors from superficial T3 cancers or in recognizing adjacent organ infiltration.[46,53] There is a tendency to overestimate the depth of penetration in cases of extensive perigastric adenopathy and fibrosis.[51]

Endoscopic ultrasonography is sensitive for diagnosing enlarged perigastric lymph nodes. It will detect 40 percent of nodes > 5 mm and 60 percent of nodes > 10 mm in size.[54] Large nodes detected by EUS are more likely to contain metastases than are smaller nodes. Heinz and colleagues found that over 70 percent of lymph nodes > 10 mm contained disease.[55] Other criteria for determining lymph node metastases include shape and the inability to visualize the lymph node hilum. Aibe and colleagues noted that round lymph nodes contained metastases more frequently than ellipsoid lymph nodes of similar size.[54] Tio and Tytgat found that sharply demarcated lymph nodes with an inhomogeneous echo pattern that was either similar to or more hypoechoic than that of the primary lesion were more likely to contain metastases. In contrast, inflammatory lymph nodes were homogeneous, had indistinct boundaries, and were more hyperechoic than the primary lesions.[56]

The accuracy of EUS for predicting metastases is reduced in distant lymph nodes. Akahoshi and colleagues noted that EUS diagnosed 86 percent of perigastric lymph nodes; 25 percent of left gastric, common hepatic, splenic, or celiac artery lymph nodes; and only 14 percent of retropancreatic- and mesenteric-root lymph nodes.[46] Other studies confirmed that EUS predicts regional lymph node disease with 80 percent accuracy but predicts distant lymph node disease with less than 60 percent accuracy.[44–48,53,57] Recent technological advances have allowed EUS-guided fine-needle aspiration of suspicious nodes, thus improving the accuracy of the evaluation.

Laparoscopy and Laparoscopic Ultrasonography

The introduction of laparoscopy to the diagnostic armamentarium has had a dramatic effect on the staging of gastric cancer. Laparoscopy allows direct visualization of the primary tumor as well as assessment of the liver and peritoneal cavity. Figure 12–8 illustrates a locally advanced tumor with serosal involvement (T3). Subradiologic metastatic disease can be identified. Proponents of laparoscopy note that 20 to 40 percent of patients with clinically localized M0 disease will be up-staged by laparoscopy and have their management changed.[58–64] Laparoscopy is especially sensitive for detecting small peritoneal and hepatic implants that are not detected by CT.[58,59,62,65] Figures 12–9 and 12–10 are laparoscopic images that reveal small-volume metastatic disease not seen on the preoperative work-up (including helical CT). Since curative resection was not possible, these asymptomatic patients were able to avoid the morbidity of a laparotomy.

The laparoscopic experience is typified in a study from our institution by Burke and colleagues.[62] In this study of 111 patients with gastric cancer judged to be free of metastatic disease by preoperative CT, laparoscopy diagnosed metastatic disease in 32 patients, with an overall accuracy of 94 percent. The peritoneum and liver made up 97 per-

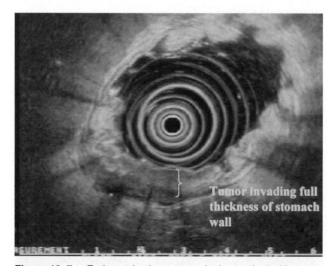

Figure 12–7. Endoscopic ultrasonography in a patient with a gastric adenocarcinoma. The tumor disrupts all layers of the stomach wall, indicating a T3 lesion.

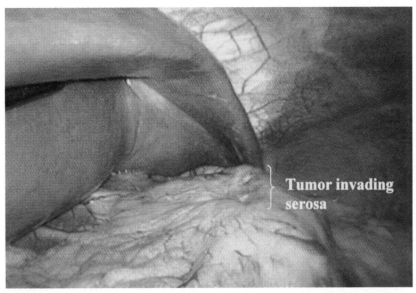

Figure 12–8. Laparoscopy in a patient with gastric adenocarcinoma reveals serosal invasion (a T3 lesion). This constitutes locally advanced disease, and this patient would be offered preoperative (neoadjuvant) chemotherapy.

cent of the metastatic disease that was detected by laparoscopy only (Figure 12–11). The asymptomatic patients diagnosed with M1 disease at laparoscopy avoided a laparotomy and were discharged, usually the day after surgery. In contrast, patients who had M1 disease noted at open laparotomy were hospitalized for an average of 7 days. Interestingly, patients diagnosed with M1 disease by laparoscopy did not require a subsequent open procedure for bleeding, perforation, or obstruction. Further, these patients had similar survivals to those of historical controls with M1 disease. These data question the role of prophylactic bypass or resection in asymptomatic patients with M1 disease.

Concern has been expressed regarding the possibility that laparoscopy could lead to tumor dissemi-

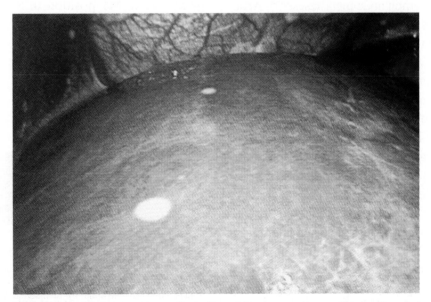

Figure 12–9. Laparoscopy in a patient with gastric adenocarcinoma without evidence of metastatic disease on preoperative helical computed tomography. Small-volume disease is seen in the liver. Since curative resection is not possible, this patient can be spared the morbidity of laparotomy.

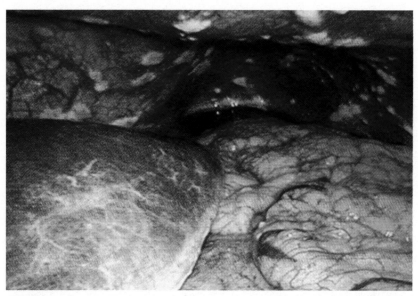

Figure 12–10. Laparoscopy in a patient (different from patient represented in Figure 12–9) with gastric adenocarcinoma without evidence of metastatic disease as seen by preoperative helical computed tomography. Small-volume disease is seen in the peritoneum. Since curative resection is not possible, the patient can be spared the morbidity of laparotomy.

nation and subsequent port site implantation. However, recent work suggests that the incidence of port site implantation is less than 1 percent after laparoscopy for abdominal malignancy.[66]

The addition of ultrasonography to laparoscopy (laparoscopic ultrasonography [LUS]) partially compensates for the lack of tactile sensation and may improve the surgeon's ability to determine tumor depth and to detect lymph node metastases.[67–69] Articulating LUS probes that can be placed through a 10-mm port have been developed (Figure 12–12). With LUS, the stomach wall appears as alternating hyper- and hypoechnoic layers (Figure 12–13). Invasion is seen as disruption of the normal architecture. Figure 12–14 shows a deep T2 lesion with interruption of the second hypoechoic layer of the stomach wall.

Evidence suggests that LUS complements laparoscopy. Smith and colleagues noted that 18 of 93 patients found to have resectable disease by standard preoperative imaging had additional disease identified by laparoscopy, which negated attempts at curative resection.[70] Laparoscopic ultrasonography provided evidence of unresectability in 7 additional patients. Overall, 27 percent of patients in this study avoided a laparotomy.

Common to most studies on laparoscopic staging for gastric cancer is the difficulty of diagnosing occult lymph node disease. In the study of 111 patients by Burke and colleagues, 6 patients at laparotomy were found to have M1 disease by virtue of distant nodal disease that was not documented by laparoscopy.[62] By improving the nodal assessment, LUS may reduce the incidence of false-negative laparoscopies. By using laparoscopy and LUS, Rau and colleagues noted enlarged lymph nodes in the M1 position in 8 of 40 patients with esophageal and gastric cancer.[71] Biopsy specimens

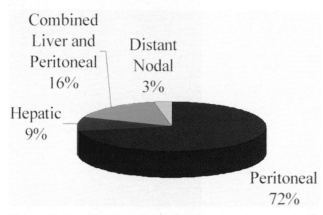

Figure 12–11. Pie chart depicting the location of metastatic disease seen in patients by laparoscopy but missed by routine preoperative imaging. The majority of disease is small-volume disease located in the liver and on the peritoneal surface. (Reproduced with permission from Burke EC, Karpeh MS, Conlon KC, Brennan MF. Laparoscopy in the management of gastric adenocarcinoma. Ann Surg 1997;225:262–7.)

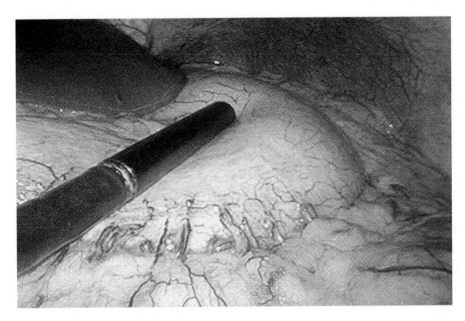

Figure 12–12. Laparoscopic ultrasonography, using a 10-mm probe.

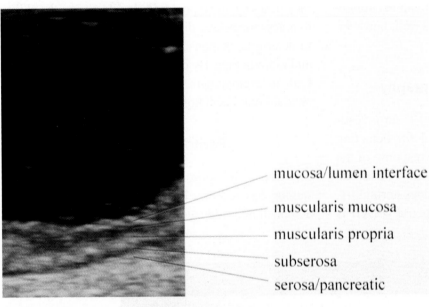

mucosa/lumen interface

muscularis mucosa

muscularis propria

subserosa

serosa/pancreatic

Figure 12–13. Laparoscopic ultrasonography depicts the normal stomach wall as alternating hyper- and hypoechoic layers. The probe is placed on the anterior gastric wall, and the posterior gastric wall is visualized. The stomach is filled with saline.

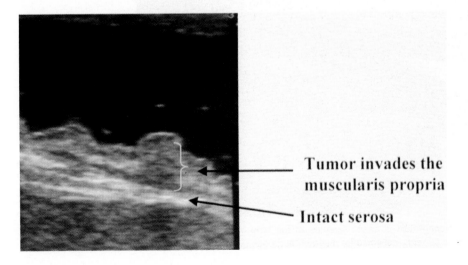

Tumor invades the muscularis propria

Intact serosa

Figure 12–14. Laparoscopic sonogram, depicting a posterior gastric adenocarcinoma with interruption of the second hypoechoic layer (muscularis propria) of the stomach wall. This image represents a deep T2 lesion.

of these lymph nodes showed metastases in 6 (75%) of these 8 patients.

Other techniques, including peritoneal-fluid sampling, can be performed at the time of laparoscopy (Figure 12–15). Patients with viable tumor cells in the peritoneal fluid have poor outcomes, and peritoneal cytology is expected to become a component of routine staging in the future (see below).

Magnetic Resonance Imaging

Magnetic resonance imaging (MRI) has gained popularity as an imaging modality for gastrointestinal and liver pathology. Currently the greatest benefit of MRI is its increased sensitivity for detecting liver metastases. Some reports suggest that MRI appears to have greater resolution than CT for this indication.[72–74] There is evidence that MRI can accurately stage tumor depth of gastric cancer as well; however, this remains investigational.[75]

Positron Emission Tomography

Positron emission tomography (PET) is an investigational imaging tool with potential for detecting metastatic disease and measuring the response of the primary tumor to chemotherapy. Malignant tissue consumes glucose more avidly than does normal tissue. Intravenous 18F-fluorodeoxyglucose (FDG) is

transported into tumor cells, where it emits positrons that are detected by a gamma camera (Figure 12–16). Beneficial results in esophageal cancer have suggested that PET may be useful in gastric cancer as well. In a study of 91 patients with esophageal cancer, PET detected 30 percent of metastases missed by CT.[76] Although more accurate than CT, PET was less sensitive than laparoscopy.[76]

Although there are few PET studies specifically involving gastric cancer, there are data indicating that gastric tumors are avid consumers of FDG and are detectable by PET.[77] The data on the ability of PET to diagnose lymph node metastases in patients with gastroesophageal cancer is somewhat mixed.[77–81] A number of studies indicate that PET has approximately a 90 percent accuracy in detecting lymph node metastases[79] whereas other studies have reported an accuracy of less than 50 percent.[81] In addition to the ability to assess metastatic disease, PET may have the ability to determine responses to neoadjuvant chemotherapy and radiotherapy. By comparing a post-treatment PET scan to pretreatment scans, one can determine if a residual mass contains metabolically active cells.[82]

Peritoneal Cytology

The impact of peritoneal cytology as an adjunct to staging has recently been investigated. Studies have demonstrated reduced survival when viable tumor

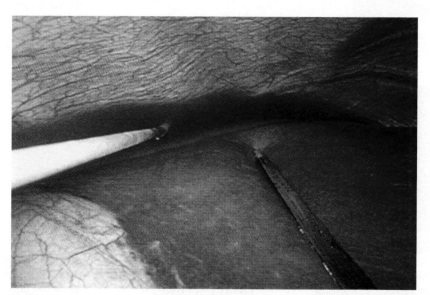

Figure 12–15. Peritoneal fluid is easily sampled at the time of laparoscopy. (At the authors' center, fluid is currently collected for research purposes.)

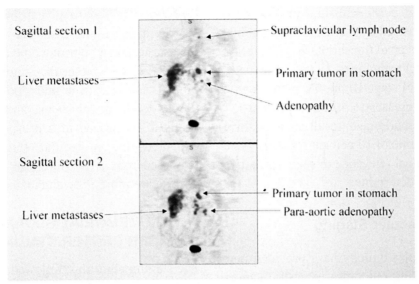

Figure 12–16. Two sagittal views produced by positron emission tomography (PET), showing metastatic disease involving the supraclavicular, periaortic, and perigastric lymph nodes and the liver.

cells are noted in the peritoneal lavage fluid taken at the time of gastric resection.[83–88] Figure 12–17 shows tumor cells in a cytology specimen stained by the Papanicolaou technique. The likelihood of detecting positive peritoneal cytology appears related to the stage of disease. Of 127 patients in a study in which peritoneal cytology was analyzed by the Papanicolaou method, no patients with T1 or T2 tumors, 10 percent of patients with T3 and T4 tumors, and 59 percent of patients with M1 disease had positive cytology.[84] Within the subgroup of completely resected patients with stage III gastric cancer, positive cytology predicts reduced survival. In fact, the outcome is similar to that of patients with M1 disease.[84] This has led many groups to suggest that cytology be included in the staging of gastric cancer.[84,87,88]

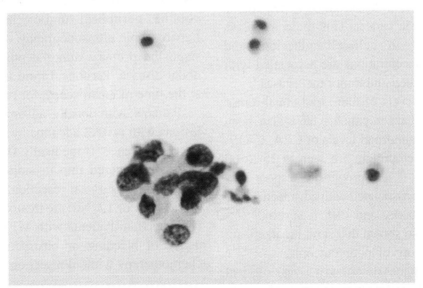

Figure 12–17. Malignant cells, stained by the Papanicolaou technique, in the peritoneal fluid of a gastric cancer. patient. Patients with positive peritoneal cytology have survival rates similar to those of patients with M1 disease. (Reproduced with permission from Burke EC, Karpeh MS, Conlon KC, Brennan MF. Laparoscopy in the management of gastric adenocarcinoma. Ann Surg 1997;225:262–7.

The sensitivity of peritoneal-fluid cytology can be dramatically increased by the use of immunohistochemistry and reverse transcriptase polymerase chain reaction (PCR) techniques. Using these methods, the proportion of stage III and IV patients with positive cytology increases to 46 to 64 percent.[85,86] However, these methods also result in a positive peritoneal cytology rate of 10 percent for stage I and II patients. The clinical relevance of such a sensitive method is yet to be determined.

Molecular Staging

Advances in molecular biology have provided new methods for predicting outcomes in gastric cancer patients. The expression of various molecular markers has been correlated with poor outcomes. The tumor-suppressor gene *p53* has been implicated in the sequence of gastric carcinogenesis,[89] and over-expression of *p53* is associated with reduced survival in patients with diffuse-type gastric cancer.[90] Similarly, adhesion molecule overexpression has been implicated in the development of early metastases. These molecules are believed to control the migration of tumor cells through the vasculature. Tumor expression of the cell adhesion receptor sialyl-Le(x) is associated with venous invasion and a poor outcome.[91] Similarly, the cell adhesion molecule CD44 is elevated in the serum of some patients with advanced gastric cancer. This molecule plays an important role in cell-cell adhesion, and increased serum concentrations are associated with increased tumor burden and tumor metastases.[92]

Elevated serum levels of more traditional tumor markers in gastric cancer patients have also been noted. Specifically, abnormal levels of CEA, CA19-9, CA72-4, and α-fetoprotein are seen in 15 to 60 percent of patients[17–23] and prognosticate poor outcomes since they are associated with advanced tumor depth, nodal metastases, and distant spread.[18–23,93] Some series have also shown that serum markers are independent predictors of poor outcome.[17–19,23,93,94] Tachibana and colleagues described a 5-year survival rate of 32 percent following the resection of gastric cancer in patients with an elevated preoperative CEA level, compared to 77 percent for patients with a normal preoperative CEA level.[19] Similarly, high serum levels of CA72-4 (a glycoprotein associated with gastric cancer) are associated with lymph node metastases and a poor outcome.[94]

The value of molecular staging and its ability to predict survival over and above factors such as tumor depth, nodal status, and distant metastases needs to be proven in a prospective manner. It is expected that molecular staging will have an increased role in the future as the mechanisms of disease are more fully elucidated.

THE MEMORIAL SLOAN-KETTERING CANCER CENTER STAGING ALGORITHM

The staging algorithm followed at Memorial Sloan-Kettering Cancer Center for gastric cancer patients is depicted in Figure 12–2. Diagnosis is usually accomplished with endoscopy. Endoscopic ultrasonography may be used to determine the depth of invasion and perigastric adenopathy for patients with early lesions and for those whose tumor is located at the gastroesophageal junction. For lesions involving the body and antrum of the stomach, EUS has been mostly replaced by LUS. In all cases, CT is performed to detect obvious metastases that would preclude a curative resection. Biopsies of metastatic disease to the liver are usually performed under the guidance of CT. For patients without evidence of M1 disease, laparoscopy is performed to rule out small-volume peritoneal and/or hepatic metastases. Laparoscopic ultrasonography is frequently used to stage the primary tumor depth and the extent of nodal disease. Peritoneal fluid is currently sampled at the time of laparoscopy, for research purposes.

Patients with locally advanced disease (T3/T4 lesions with N1/N2 adenopathy) are at high risk for local recurrence. If medically fit, these patients are preferably entered into neoadjuvant chemotherapy trials prior to surgical resection. Patients with early disease (T1 or T2, N0) are treated by immediate gastric resection. Patients with M1 disease and no evidence of bleeding or obstruction usually receive chemotherapy without resection.

SUMMARY

The diagnosis and staging of gastric cancer have evolved in recent years as improvements in diagnostic modalities have been coupled with the development of a multimodal approach to therapy. Further advances are expected in the future as our understanding of the molecular basis of the disease progresses.

REFERENCES

1. Landis SH, Murray T, Bolden S, Wingo PA. Cancer statistics, 1999. CA Cancer J Clin 1999;49:8–31, 1.

2. Brennan MF, Karpeh MS Jr. Surgery for gastric cancer: the American view. Semin Oncol 1996;23:352–9.

3. Karpeh MS Jr, Brennan MF. Gastric carcinoma. Ann Surg Oncol 1998;5:650–6.

4. Lawrence W Jr, Menck HR, Steele GD Jr, Winchester DP. The National Cancer Data Base report on gastric cancer. Cancer 1995;75:1734–44.

5. Wanebo HJ, Kennedy BJ, Chmiel J, et al. Cancer of the stomach. A patient care study by the American College of Surgeons. Ann Surg 1993;218:583–92.

6. Low VH, Levine MS, Rubesin SE, et al. Diagnosis of gastric carcinoma: sensitivity of double-contrast barium studies. AJR Am J Roentgenol 1994;162:329–34.

7. Gore RM, Levine MS, Ghahremani GG, Miller FH. Gastric cancer. Radiologic diagnosis. Radiol Clin North Am 1997;35:311–29.

8. Nava HR, Arredondo MA. Diagnosis of gastric cancer: endoscopy, imaging, and tumor markers. Surg Oncol Clin North Am 1993;2:371–92.

9. Graham DY, Schwartz JT, Cain GD, Gyorkey F. Prospective evaluation of biopsy number in the diagnosis of esophageal and gastric carcinoma. Gastroenterology 1982;82:228–31.

10. Hatfield AR, Slavin G, Segal AW, Levi AJ. Importance of the site of endoscopic gastric biopsy in ulcerating lesions of the stomach. Gut 1975;16:884–6.

11. Winawer SJ, Posner G, Lightdale CJ, et al. Endoscopic diagnosis of advanced gastric cancer. Factors influencing yield. Gastroenterology 1975;69:1183–7.

12. Witzel L, Halter F, Gretillat PA, et al. Evaluation of specific value of endoscopic biopsies and brush cytology for malignancies of the oesophagus and stomach. Gut 1976;17:375–7.

13. Oshima A, Hirata N, Ubukata T, et al. Evaluation of a mass screening program for stomach cancer with a case-control study design. Int J Cancer 1986;38:829–33.

14. Hallissey MT, Allum WH, Jewkes AJ, et al. Early detection of gastric cancer. BMJ 1990;301:513–5.

15. Parsonnet J, Hansen S, Rodriguez L, et al. *Helicobacter pylori* infection and gastric lymphoma. N Engl J Med 1994;330:1267–71.

16. Parsonnet J, Friedman GD, Orentreich N, Vogelman H. Risk for gastric cancer in people with CagA positive or CagA negative *Helicobacter pylori* infection. Gut 1997;40:297–301.

17. Tocchi A, Costa G, Lepre L, et al. The role of serum and gastric juice levels of carcinoembryonic antigen, CA19.9 and CA72.4 in patients with gastric cancer. J Cancer Res Clin Oncol 1998;124:450–5.

18. Kodera Y, Yamamura Y, Torii A, et al. The prognostic value of preoperative serum levels of CEA and CA19-9 in patients with gastric cancer. Am J Gastroenterol 1996;91:49–53.

19. Tachibana M, Takemoto Y, Nakashima Y, et al. Serum carcinoembryonic antigen as a prognostic factor in resectable gastric cancer. J Am Coll Surg 1998;187:64–8.

20. Marrelli D, Roviello F, De Stefano A, et al. Prognostic significance of CEA, CA 19-9 and CA 72-4 preoperative serum levels in gastric carcinoma. Oncology 1999;57:55–62.

21. Nakajima K, Ochiai T, Suzuki T, et al. Impact of preoperative serum carcinoembryonic antigen, CA 19-9 and alpha fetoprotein levels in gastric cancer patients. Tumour Biol 1998;19:464–9.

22. Kodama I, Koufuji K, Kawabata S, et al. The clinical efficacy of CA 72-4 as serum marker for gastric cancer in comparison with CA19-9 and CEA. Int Surg 1995;80:45–8.

23. Maehara Y, Kusumoto T, Takahashi I, et al. Predictive value of preoperative carcinoembryonic antigen levels for the prognosis of patients with well-differentiated gastric cancer. A multivariate analysis. Oncology 1994;51:234–7.

24. Roder JD, Bottcher K, Busch R, et al. Classification of regional lymph node metastasis from gastric carcinoma. German Gastric Cancer Study Group. Cancer 1998;82:621–31.

25. Miller FH, Kochman ML, Talamonti MS, et al. Gastric cancer. Radiologic staging. Radiol Clin North Am 1997;35:331–49.

26. Cho JS, Kim JK, Rho SM, et al. Preoperative assessment of gastric carcinoma: value of two-phase dynamic CT with mechanical IV injection of contrast material. AJR Am J Roentgenol 1994;163:69–75.

27. Hori S, Tsuda K, Murayama S, et al. CT of gastric carcinoma: preliminary results with a new scanning technique. Radiographics 1992;12:257–68.

28. Minami M, Kawauchi N, Itai Y, et al. Gastric tumors: radiologic-pathologic correlation and accuracy of T staging with dynamic CT. Radiology 1992;185:173–8.

29. Rossi M, Broglia L, Graziano P, et al. Local invasion of gastric cancer: CT findings and pathologic correlation using 5-mm incremental scanning, hypotonia, and water filling. AJR Am J Roentgenol 1999;172:383–8.

30. Dux M, Richter GM, Hansmann J, et al. Helical hydro-CT for diagnosis and staging of gastric carcinoma. J Comput Assist Tomogr 1999;23:913–22.

31. Ziegler K, Sanft C, Zimmer T, et al. Comparison of computed tomography, endosonography, and intraoperative assessment in TN staging of gastric carcinoma. Gut 1993;34:604–10.

32. Takao M, Fukuda T, Iwanaga S, et al. Gastric cancer: evaluation of triphasic spiral CT and radiologic-pathologic correlation. J Comput Assist Tomogr 1998;22:288–94.

33. Fukuya T, Honda H, Kaneko K, et al. Efficacy of helical CT in T-staging of gastric cancer. J Comput Assist Tomogr 1997;21:73–81.

34. Davies J, Chalmers AG, Sue-Ling HM, et al. Spiral computed tomography and operative staging of gastric carcinoma: a comparison with histopathological staging. Gut 1997;41:314–9.

35. Adachi Y, Sakino I, Matsumata T, et al. Preoperative assessment of advanced gastric carcinoma using computed tomography. Am J Gastroenterol 1997;92:872–5.

36. Greenberg J, Durkin M, Van Drunen M, Aranha GV. Computed tomography or endoscopic ultrasonography in preoperative staging of gastric and esophageal tumors. Surgery 1994;116:696–701.

37. Stell DA, Carter CR, Stewart I, Anderson JR. Prospective comparison of laparoscopy, ultrasonography and computed tomography in the staging of gastric cancer. Br J Surg 1996;83:1260–2.

38. Fukuya T, Honda H, Hayashi T, et al. Lymph-node metastases: efficacy for detection with helical CT in patients with gastric cancer. Radiology 1995;197:705–11.

39. Paramo JC, Gomez G. Dynamic CT in the preoperative evaluation of patients with gastric cancer: correlation with surgical findings and pathology. Ann Surg Oncol 1999;6:379–84.

40. Vallgren S, Hedenbro J, Gotberg S, Walther B. Preoperative computed tomography for evaluation of tumour growth in patients with gastric cancer. Acta Chir Scand 1985; 151:571–3.

41. Watt I, Stewart I, Anderson D, et al. Laparoscopy, ultrasound and computed tomography in cancer of the oesophagus and gastric cardia: a prospective comparison for detecting intra-abdominal metastases. Br J Surg 1989;76:1036–9.

42. Young N, Sing T, Wong KP, et al. Use of spiral and non-spiral computed tomography arterial portography in the detection of potentially malignant liver masses. J Gastroenterol Hepatol 1997;12:385–91.

43. Gunven P, Makuuchi M, Takayasu K, et al. Preoperative imaging of liver metastases. Comparison of angiography, CT scan, and ultrasonography. Ann Surg 1985;202:573–9.

44. Akahoshi K, Chijiwa Y, Hamada S, et al. Pretreatment staging of endoscopically early gastric cancer with a 15 MHz ultrasound catheter probe. Gastrointest Endosc 1998; 48:470–6.

45. Wang JY, Hsieh JS, Huang YS, et al. Endoscopic ultrasonography for preoperative locoregional staging and assessment of resectability in gastric cancer. Clin Imaging 1998;22:355–9.

46. Akahoshi K, Chijiiwa Y, Sasaki I, et al. Pre-operative TN staging of gastric cancer using a 15 MHz ultrasound miniprobe. Br J Radiol 1997;70:703–7.

47. Grimm H, Binmoeller KF, Hamper K, et al. Endosonography for preoperative locoregional staging of esophageal and gastric cancer. Endoscopy 1993;25:224–30.

48. Caletti G, Ferrari A, Brocchi E, Barbara L. Accuracy of endoscopic ultrasonography in the diagnosis and staging of gastric cancer and lymphoma. Surgery 1993;113:14–27.

49. Smith JW, Brennan MF, Botet JF, et al. Preoperative endoscopic ultrasound can predict the risk of recurrence after operation for gastric carcinoma. J Clin Oncol 1993;11:2380–5.

50. Yanai H, Tada M, Karita M, Okita K. Diagnostic utility of 20-megahertz linear endoscopic ultrasonography in early gastric cancer. Gastrointest Endosc 1996;44:29–33.

51. Saito N, Takeshita K, Habu H, Endo M. The use of endoscopic ultrasound in determining the depth of cancer invasion in patients with gastric cancer. Surg Endosc 1991; 5:14–9.

52. Lightdale CJ. Endoscopic ultrasonography in the diagnosis, staging and follow-up of esophageal and gastric cancer. Endoscopy 1992;24 Suppl 1:297–303.

53. Akahoshi K, Misawa T, Fujishima H, et al. Preoperative evaluation of gastric cancer by endoscopic ultrasound. Gut 1991;32:479–82.

54. Aibe T, Ito T, Yoshida T, et al. Endoscopic ultrasonography of lymph nodes surrounding the upper GI tract. Scand J Gastroenterol Suppl 1986;123:164–9.

55. Heintz A, Mildenberger P, Georg M, et al. Endoscopic ultrasonography in the diagnosis of regional lymph nodes in esophageal and gastric cancer—results of studies in vitro. Endoscopy 1993;25:231–5.

56. Tio TL, Tytgat GN. Endoscopic ultrasonography in analysing peri-intestinal lymph node abnormality. Preliminary results of studies in vitro and in vivo. Scand J Gastroenterol Suppl 1986;123:158–63.

57. Botet JF, Lightdale CJ, Zauber AG, et al. Preoperative staging of gastric cancer: comparison of endoscopic US and dynamic CT. Radiology 1991;181:426–32.

58. Feussner H, Omote K, Fink U, et al. Pretherapeutic laparoscopic staging in advanced gastric carcinoma. Endoscopy 1999;31:342–7.

59. Arnold JC, Neubauer HJ, Zopf T, et al. Improved tumor staging by diagnostic laparoscopy. Z Gastroenterol 1999; 37:483–8.

60. Hunerbein M, Rau B, Hohenberger P, Schlag PM. The role of staging laparoscopy for multimodal therapy of gastrointestinal cancer. Surg Endosc 1998;12:921–5.

61. Asencio F, Aguilo J, Salvador JL, et al. Video-laparoscopic staging of gastric cancer. A prospective multicenter comparison with noninvasive techniques. Surg Endosc 1997; 11:1153–8.

62. Burke EC, Karpeh MS, Conlon KC, Brennan MF. Laparoscopy in the management of gastric adenocarcinoma. Ann Surg 1997;225:262–7.

63. Possik RA, Franco EL, Pires DR, et al. Sensitivity, specificity, and predictive value of laparoscopy for the staging of gastric cancer and for the detection of liver metastases. Cancer 1986;58:1–6.

64. Jimenez RE, Warshaw AL, Rattner DW, et al. Impact of laparoscopic staging in the treatment of pancreatic cancer. Arch Surg 2000;135:409–14.

65. D'Ugo DM, Coppola R, Persiani R, et al. Immediately preoperative laparoscopic staging for gastric cancer. Surg Endosc 1996;10:996–9.

66. Pearlstone DB, Mansfield PF, Curley SA, et al. Laparoscopy in 533 patients with abdominal malignancy. Surgery 1999;125:67–72.

67. Conlon KC, Karpeh MS Jr. Laparoscopy and laparoscopic ultrasound in the staging of gastric cancer. Semin Oncol 1996;23:347–51.

68. Romijn MG, van Overhagen H, Spillenaar Bilgen EJ, et al. Laparoscopy and laparoscopic ultrasonography in staging of oesophageal and cardial carcinoma. Br J Surg 1998; 85:1010–2.

69. Goletti O, Buccianti P, Chiarugi M, et al. Laparoscopic sonography in screening metastases from gastrointestinal cancer: comparative accuracy with traditional procedures. Surg Laparosc Endosc 1995;5:176–82.

70. Smith A, John TG, Garden OJ, Brown SP. Role of laparoscopic ultrasonography in the management of patients with oesophagogastric cancer. Br J Surg 1999;86:1083–7.

71. Rau B, Hunerbein M, Reingruber B, et al. Laparoscopic lymph node assessment in pretherapeutic staging of gastric and esophageal cancer. Recent Results Cancer Res 1996;142:209–15.

72. Schultz JF, Bell JD, Goldstein RM, et al. Hepatic tumor imaging using iron oxide MRI: comparison with computed tomography, clinical impact, and cost analysis. Ann Surg Oncol 1999;6:691–8.

73. Semelka RC, Worawattanakul S, Kelekis NL, et al. Liver lesion detection, characterization, and effect on patient management: comparison of single-phase spiral CT and current MR techniques. J Magn Reson Imaging 1997;7:1040–7.

74. Zeman RK, Dritschilo A, Silverman PM, et al. Dynamic CT vs 0.5 T MR imaging in the detection of surgically proven hepatic metastases. J Comput Assist Tomogr 1989;13:637–44.

75. Matsushita M, Oi H, Murakami T, et al. Extraserosal invasion in advanced gastric cancer: evaluation with MR imaging. Radiology 1994;192:87–91.

76. Luketich JD, Friedman DM, Weigel TL, et al. Evaluation of distant metastases in esophageal cancer: 100 consecutive positron emission tomography scans. Ann Thorac Surg 1999;68:1133–6.

77. McAteer D, Wallis F, Couper G, et al. Evaluation of 18F-FDG positron emission tomography in gastric and oesophageal carcinoma. Br J Radiol 1999;72:525–9.

78. Flanagan FL, Dehdashti F, Siegel BA, et al. Staging of esophageal cancer with 18F-fluorodeoxyglucose positron emission tomography. AJR Am J Roentgenol 1997;168:417–24.

79. Kole AC, Plukker JT, Nieweg OE, Vaalburg W. Positron emission tomography for staging of oesophageal and gastroesophageal malignancy. Br J Cancer 1998;78:521–7.

80. Block MI, Patterson GA, Sundaresan RS, et al. Improvement in staging of esophageal cancer with the addition of positron emission tomography. Ann Thorac Surg 1997;64:770–6.

81. Rankin SC, Taylor H, Cook GJ, Mason R. Computed tomography and positron emission tomography in the pre-operative staging of oesophageal carcinoma. Clin Radiol 1998;53:659–65.

82. Couper GW, McAteer D, Wallis F, et al. Detection of response to chemotherapy using positron emission tomography in patients with oesophageal and gastric cancer. Br J Surg 1998;85:1403–6.

83. Bonenkamp JJ, Songun I, Hermans J, van de Velde CJ. Prognostic value of positive cytology findings from abdominal washings in patients with gastric cancer. Br J Surg 1996;83:672–4.

84. Burke EC, Karpeh MS Jr, Conlon KC, Brennan MF. Peritoneal lavage cytology in gastric cancer: an independent predictor of outcome. Ann Surg Oncol 1998;5:411–5.

85. Benevolo M, Mottolese M, Cosimelli M, et al. Diagnostic and prognostic value of peritoneal immunocytology in gastric cancer. J Clin Oncol 1998;16:3406–11.

86. Kodera Y, Nakanishi H, Yamamura Y, et al. Prognostic value and clinical implications of disseminated cancer cells in the peritoneal cavity detected by reverse transcriptase-polymerase chain reaction and cytology. Int J Cancer 1998;79:429–33.

87. Kodera Y, Yamamura Y, Shimizu Y, et al. Peritoneal washing cytology: prognostic value of positive findings in patients with gastric carcinoma undergoing a potentially curative resection. J Surg Oncol 1999;72:60–4.

88. Suzuki T, Ochiai T, Hayashi H, et al. Peritoneal lavage cytology findings as prognostic factor for gastric cancer. Semin Surg Oncol 1999;17:103–7.

89. Brito MJ, Williams GT, Thompson H, Filipe MI. Expression of p53 in early (T1) gastric carcinoma and precancerous adjacent mucosa. Gut 1994;35:1697–700.

90. Lee WJ, Shun CT, Hong RL, et al. Overexpression of p53 predicts shorter survival in diffuse type gastric cancer. Br J Surg 1998;85:1138–42.

91. Amado M, Carneiro F, Seixas M, et al. Dimeric sialyl-Le(x) expression in gastric carcinoma correlates with venous invasion and poor outcome. Gastroenterology 1998;114:462–70.

92. Guo YJ, Liu G, Wang X, et al. Potential use of soluble CD44 in serum as indicator of tumor burden and metastasis in patients with gastric or colon cancer. Cancer Res 1994;54:422–6.

93. Sakamoto J, Nakazato H, Teramukai S, et al. Association between preoperative plasma CEA levels and the prognosis of gastric cancer following curative resection. Tumor Marker Committee, Japanese Foundation for Multidisciplinary Treatment of Cancer, Tokyo, Japan. Surg Oncol 1996;5:133–9.

94. Spila A, Roselli M, Cosimelli M, et al. Clinical utility of CA 72-4 serum marker in the staging and immediate post-surgical management of gastric cancer patients. Anticancer Res 1996;16:2241–7.

13

Surgical Treatment of Localized Gastric Cancer

JOHN I. LEW, MD

MITCHELL C. POSNER, MD

Theodor Billroth performed the first successful gastric resection (a distal subtotal gastrectomy for stomach cancer) in 1881.[1] Billroth operated on a 43-year-old woman with gastric outlet obstruction caused by pyloric carcinoma. Despite tolerating the surgical procedure well and having a benign hospital course, the patient died of recurrent gastric cancer 14 months later. Nevertheless, the new surgical technique proved to be a great success for Billroth, whose clinic would later report 257 gastric resections for stomach cancer in 1894.[2] In 1889, Mikulicz began to espouse lymph node dissection in addition to gastrectomy and (if required) distal pancreatectomy for the treatment of gastric cancer.[3] In 1898, Charles B. Brigham performed the first successful gastric resection in the United States, a total gastrectomy, on a 66-year-old woman using a Murphy button in the reconstruction phase of the operation, to help create an esophago-duodenal anastomosis.[4] The contributions of these surgeons and others in the late nineteenth century provided the cardinal foundations for current surgical management of patients with gastric cancer.

Resection remains the only potentially curative treatment for localized gastric cancer. The basic surgical approach for stomach cancer that is amenable to potential cure has essentially remained the same since Billroth's time. In the early 1940s, Coller and colleagues recommended radical resection, including regional lymphadenectomy, for all gastric cancers since lymph node metastasis could be insidious and because identification of the correct resection plane is difficult.[5] However, other contemporaries were not convinced of Coller's assertions and found the high postoperative mortality rate associated with radical gastrectomy unacceptable.[6] Since that time, there has been an ongoing discourse as to which surgical procedure is associated with the most optimal outcome and the least postoperative morbidity and mortality. Efforts to enhance the surgical cure of patients have focused on defining the appropriate extent of lymphadenectomy. The principal areas addressed in this chapter include the extent of both gastric resection and lymph node dissection, the adequacy of proximal and distal margins, the role of adjacent-organ resection and splenectomy in localized disease, and the surgical treatment of recurrent gastric cancer.

ANATOMIC CONSIDERATIONS

The stomach serves as a reservoir for the mechanical and chemical digestion of ingested foodstuffs and is anatomically defined proximally by the gastroesophageal junction and distally by the retroperitoneal duodenum. The organ is also bounded on the right by the liver and on the left by the spleen. The stomach is divided into anatomic regions based on these external landmarks (Figure 13–1). The gastric cardia includes the region of the stomach just distal to the gastroesophageal junction and is relatively stable due to the gastrophrenic ligament. At the gastroesophageal junction, the cardiac notch demarcates the esophagus and the gastric fundus. The cardiac notch, along with the decussating and circular fibers of the lower esophagus, forms the lower

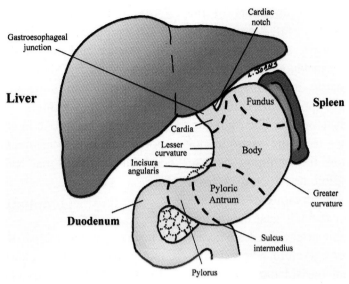

Figure 13–1. The anatomy of the stomach.

esophageal sphincter that prevents gastroesophageal reflux in normal conditions. The gastric fundus includes the part of the stomach above and left of the gastroesophageal junction. The gastric corpus or body makes up the region between the fundus and pyloric antrum and is anatomically defined by a line from the incisura angularis on the lesser curvature to a point that is one-fourth the distance from the pylorus along the greater curvature. The incisura angularis is a sharp indentation line that serves to separate the body and pyloric portion of the stomach; it is surgically used as the proximal line of tran-

section for antrectomy. The gastric pylorus includes the pyloric antrum and pyloric sphincter, consisting of a thickened ring of smooth muscle.

Blood Supply

The gastric blood supply is extensive and is derived primarily from the celiac trunk. The major vessels that supply the stomach include the right and left gastric arteries and the right and left gastroepiploic arteries (Figure 13–2). The right gastric artery, which usually branches off the common hepatic

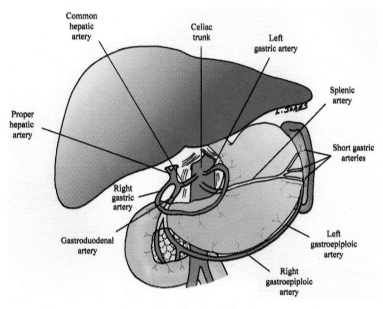

Figure 13–2. The arterial supply of the stomach.

artery, supplies the distal lesser curvature of the stomach and anastomoses with the left gastric artery. Less commonly, the right gastric artery may originate from the left hepatic, gastroduodenal, or proper hepatic artery. The left gastric artery, the smallest branch of the celiac trunk, supplies the cardia and upper lesser curvature of the stomach. The right gastroepiploic artery originates from the gastroduodenal artery that arises from the common hepatic artery. The right gastroepiploic artery courses from right to left along the greater curvature of the stomach and anastomoses with the left gastroepipoloic artery, a branch of the splenic artery, to create a vascular arch along the greater curvature. Short gastric arteries that originate from the splenic artery also supply the gastric fundus. The rich blood supply of the stomach allows preservation of gastric viability after ligation of most arteries, thus simplifying gastric reconstructive procedures.

The venous drainage of the stomach parallels the arterial supply and drains into the portal venous system (Figure 13–3). The left gastric vein or "coronary" vein passes from left to right along the gastric cardia, where it receives esophageal veins, and onward to the right, where it courses beyond the celiac trunk to drain into the portal vein. The small right gastric vein forms from tributaries of the pylorus and passes from left to right, ending directly in the portal vein. The right gastroepiploic vein drains the inferior portions of the stomach and crosses the uncinate process of the pancreas to end in the superior mesenteric vein. The left gastroepiploic vein completes the venous arch along the greater curvature and ends in the origin of the splenic vein. The short gastric veins drain the fundus and superior part of the greater curvature of the stomach, where they terminate in the splenic vein. Most of these veins become clinically significant in cases of portal vein hypertension and splenic vein thrombosis as both conditions may lead to variceal formation.

Lymphatic Supply

The four major routes of lymphatic drainage normally parallel the gastric blood supply (Figure 13–4). First, lymph vessels drain the lesser curvature of the stomach to the left gastric nodes that extend to the cardia. These left gastric nodes eventually drain into the celiac nodes. A second group of suprapyloric nodes drains the gastric pylorus of the lesser curvature, runs along the right gastric artery, and drains into the hepatic and celiac nodes. A third group of lymphatic vessels drains the proximal part of the greater curvature of the stomach. These pancreaticosplenic nodes also drain the spleen and pancreas before draining into the celiac nodes. Finally, lymphatic vessels drain to right gastroepiploic nodes from the greater curvature of the distal portion of the stomach into the infrapyloric nodes. Secondary drainage from all of these lymphatic groups eventually traverses nodes at the base of the celiac axis.

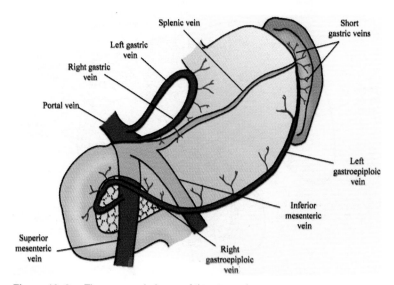

Figure 13–3. The venous drainage of the stomach.

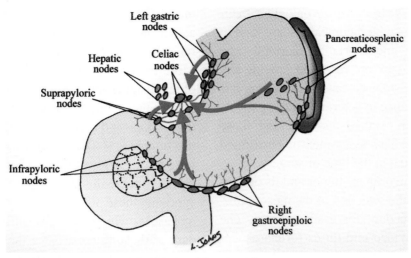

Figure 13–4. The lymphatic drainage of the stomach.

Of note, like the blood supply, the lymphatics of the stomach exhibit extensive intramural and extramural communications; in disease states, this allows for intramural spread beyond the site of origin and to distant nodal groups from the primary lymphatics.

Nerve Supply

The nerves of the stomach are both parasympathetic and sympathetic (Figure 13–5). The left (anterior) and right (posterior) vagal nerves of the parasympathetic system descend parallel with the esophagus to the gastroesophageal junction. At this anatomic site, the vagal nerves run along the lesser curvature of the stomach, sending nerve branches to accompany the blood supply of the lesser curvature. At the junction of the fundus and antrum of the stomach, the vagal nerves innervate the antrum. The sympathetic innervation of the stomach passes through the celiac ganglion, and the postganglionic fibers accompany the gastric blood supply.

Primary Tumor Location

The primary objectives of resection for gastric cancer are to provide the best chance for cure in patients

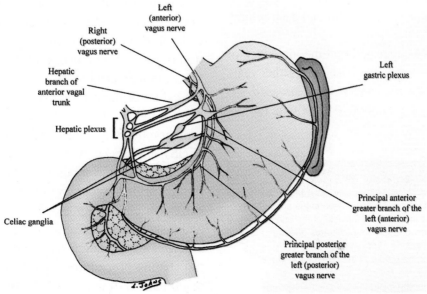

Figure 13–5. The nerve supply of the stomach.

with localized disease, to optimize palliative treatment in those patients with incurable disease, and to minimize morbidity and mortality. Currently, no therapeutic modalities except resection provide any possibility for cure of stomach cancer. Therefore, it is of paramount importance to determine those patients who are suitable for curative resection and those patients who are not. This assessment is performed both preoperatively and at the time of surgery.

The location of the primary tumor and its pattern of spread determine the selection of the most appropriate operative procedure for gastric cancer. The stomach has been divided into thirds for classification.[7] The proximal third consists of the gastroesophageal junction and extends to the fundus. Such tumors of the gastroesophageal junction have recently been classified into three types, based solely on topographic and anatomic criteria[8] (Table 13–1). The middle third of the stomach includes the body of the stomach and extends from the fundus to the incisura angularis of the lesser curvature. The distal third of the stomach consists of the pyloric antrum and originates from the incisura angularis to the pylorus. Although there is some controversy regarding which surgical procedure to apply, in general, proximal-third tumors that include the gastric cardia require a total gastrectomy, with resection of up to 10 cm of distal esophagus. Likewise, large tumors of the middle third and fundus of stomach are treated by total gastrectomy. Distal-third and small midcorpus tumors, however, are treated surgically with a radical (75 to 85%) subtotal gastrectomy (Figure 13–6).[7,9,10]

Past studies have suggested that the incidence of proximal gastric cancers has risen over the years while that of distal gastric cancers has decreased.[11,12] This shift from distal tumors to proximal tumors may reflect a relative increase or the stabilization of actual numbers of proximal tumors with a concurrent decrease in the incidence of distal tumors.[7] More important, because of the borderline location of the distal esophagus and proximal stomach, many discrepancies are found in the literature describing the etiology and classification of these proximal gastric tumors.[13–15] The varied surgical approaches and long-term survival rates after resection that are reported in the literature reflect the confusion in categorizing these proximal tumors as either esophageal or gastric, which may also influence the incidence data of these tumors. Nevertheless, such trends are of some significance as most distal gastric cancers are related to diet and may arise from dysplastic mucosa whereas proximal cancers are not related to diet.[16] Furthermore, the postoperative morbidity and mortality rates for patients with proximal gastric cancers are higher than those for patients with middle and distal gastric tumors. Of equal importance, the long-term prognosis in patients with proximal gastric tumors is also worse. Since the location of the primary tumor does have an influence on nodal metastasis and prognosis, the choice of a specific surgical procedure according to tumor location remains of paramount importance in the management of gastric cancer.

PREOPERATIVE EVALUATION

The diagnosis of gastric cancer is usually made by upper gastrointestinal (GI) endoscopy, with biopsy or barium studies. Although they provide visualization of the gastric mucosa, these diagnostic modalities cannot determine the depth of tumor invasion or the extent of metastasis that is important for preoperative tumor staging. In recent years, computed tomography (CT) and endoscopic ultrasonography (EUS) have been used primarily to stage gastric tumors since both modalities are able to determine (with varying accuracy) depth of wall invasion, extragastric tumor spread, lymph node involvement, and distant metastases (Figure 13–7).

After tissue diagnosis has been established, initial staging procedures involve a thorough physical examination, routine blood tests, and abdominal/ pelvis and chest CT. Computed tomography can

Table 13–1. CLASSIFICATION OF TUMORS OF THE GASTROESOPHAGEAL JUNCTION	
Type I	Adenocarcinoma of the distal esophagus arises from specialized intestinal metaplasia of the esophagus (Barrett's esophagus) and infiltrates gastroesophageal junction from above.
Type II	Carcinoma of the cardia at the gastroesophageal junction.
Type III	Gastric carcinoma infiltrates the gastroesophageal junction and distal esophagus from below.

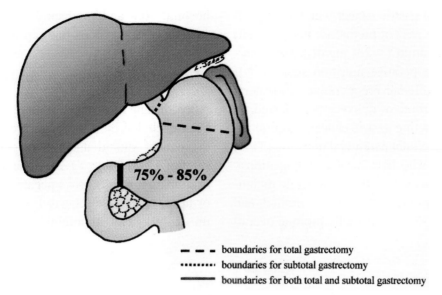

- - - boundaries for total gastrectomy
········· boundaries for subtotal gastrectomy
———— boundaries for both total and subtotal gastrectomy

Figure 13–6. Landmarks for gastric resection.

detect carcinomatosis with diffuse peritoneal seeding, malignant ascites, and pelvic metastasis. Although the stomach, perigastric nodes, and such distant sites as the liver and lung are visualized, up to 50% of patients will be found to have gross disease (missed by preoperative CT) at the time of laparotomy.[17–19] Endoscopic ultrasonography is more accurate than CT for determining lymph node involvement in the perigastric region. The advantages of EUS reside with its ability to visualize all layers of the gastric wall, perigastric lymph nodes, and surrounding tissues. Since CT is able to identify distant metastatic sites (eg, liver, lungs, and ovaries), CT and EUS are considered complementary tests. Studies with pathologic specimens have shown EUS to be very accurate in determining depth of invasion and lymph node involvement.[20,21] The overall accuracy for tumor staging ranges from 80 to 90%. The diagnostic accuracy of EUS in determining nodal status ranges from 70 to 90%. Endoscopic ultrasonography not only detects malignant lymph nodes by size but also by shape, homogeneity, and hypoechogenicity of the lymph node and by tumor proximity.[20,21] Recent technologic advances allow EUS-guided tissue sampling of lymph nodes. One limitation, however, is the ability of EUS to detect lymph nodes that are > 3 cm from the gastric wall. More recently, laparoscopic ultrasonography (LUS) has been a valuable modality for

identifying missed metastases to the liver and peritoneum and may prove more accurate in detecting lymph node metastasis and tumor stage.[22]

Although highly accurate, EUS will not necessarily change the overall surgical approach to gastric cancer. This diagnostic modality, however, may be useful in identifying patients who are candidates for preoperative chemotherapy and radiotherapy trials. We routinely use CT and endoscopy (with or without ultrasonography) as part of our preoperative staging work-up in patients with gastric cancer.

SURGICAL MANAGEMENT

Preoperative Preparation

After the decision for surgery has been made, the preoperative preparation should include optimization of cardiac and respiratory status. Patients should be typed and screened, in case blood transfusion during surgery is necessary. Patients with gastric cancer often have an increased pH and bacterial colonization of the stomach and therefore have a higher risk for wound infection. At the time of intubation, a single dose of a first-generation cephalosporin should be given to cover such common organisms as *Streptococcus viridans*, *Streptococcus fecalis*, *Escherichia coli*, *Clostridium* species, and *Bacteroides* species.[23]

For patients with gastric cancer who have significant weight loss (> 15% of predisease body weight) and low serum albumin (< 2.9 mg/dL), some surgeons advocate preoperative nutrition support.[24] If such patients can tolerate preoperative nasoenteral tube feedings, this route of delivery is preferred. In patients with obstructing gastric cancer, hospitalization for preoperative total parenteral nutrition (TPN) may benefit those who have severe malnutrition.[24] However, for patients with mild or moderate malnutrition, the role of preoperative TPN is limited, and this nutritional support may actually prolong overall hospital stay and predispose patients to infection such as central venous line sepsis.

Resection Techniques for Gastric Cancer

After distant metastasis or unresectable tumor has been excluded by a thorough preoperative work-up, the patient should undergo diagnostic laparoscopy (Figure 13–8; Table 13–2). Should the laparoscopic examination results prove negative, an upper midline or upper transverse (chevron) incision is made (Figure 13–9). The abdominal contents are initially

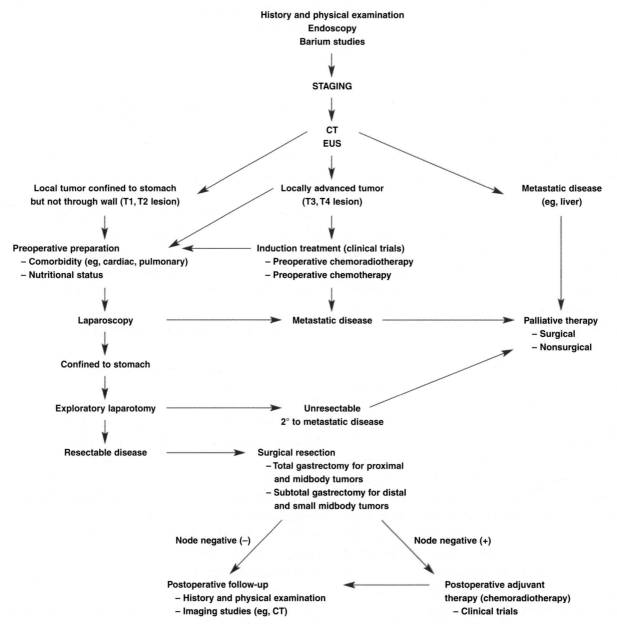

Figure 13–7. An algorithm for the management of gastric cancer. (CT = computed tomography; EUS = endoscopic ultrasonography.)

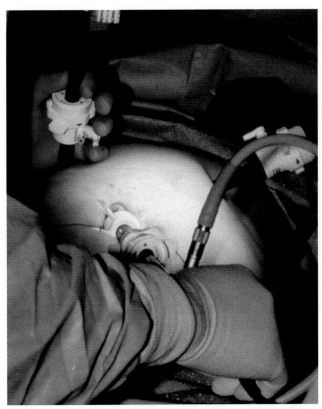

Figure 13–8. Diagnostic laparoscopy allows the evaluation of nodal, visceral, and peritoneal metastases prior to planned gastric resection.

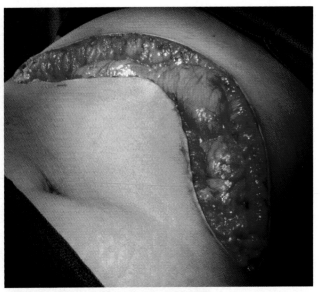

Figure 13–9. A bilateral subcostal or chevron incision provides optimal exposure for gastric resection. This incision permits wide exposure of the upper abdomen and allows the costal margin to be retracted superiorly.

explored for any evidence of metastatic disease. Inspection for the presence of ascites, peritoneal seeding, and "drop" metastasis in the pelvis should be performed to confirm the previous laparoscopic observations. In the upper abdomen, examination should be directed to the liver, greater omentum, and origin of the mesentery below the transverse colon and periaortic lymph nodes (Figure 13–10). The stomach itself should be inspected to determine the location and extent of the primary tumor (Figure 13–11). Careful palpation of the primary tumor is necessary to

determine whether there is direct invasion into adjacent structures such as the pancreas. If no liver metastasis or peritoneal seeding has occurred, gastrectomy should be performed with curative intent.

Total Gastrectomy

Retracting the greater omentum upward and gently withdrawing the transverse colon from the peritoneal cavity may allow the determination of tumor extension involving the underlying pancreas or regional major vessels by manual palpation. The transverse colon is freed from the omentum. The greater omentum is then retracted upward and the transverse colon caudad to allow for the dissection of the anterior leaf from the posterior leaf of the mesocolon with electrocautery. The plane between the anterior and posterior folds of the mesocolon is usually bloodless. As the omentum is mobilized, the venous branch between the right gastroepiploic and middle colic veins is identified and ligated. The lesser omentum is then dissected from the inferior edge of the liver and reflected downward. If present, a replaced left hepatic artery will be identified at this time and should be preserved.

Since metastasis may spread to the infrapyloric lymph nodes, this basin should be included in the

---

Table 13–2. FUNCTIONS OF DIAGNOSTIC LAPAROSCOPY FOR GASTRIC CANCER

Identifies tumor extension into contiguous organs (eg, liver, colon, pancreas, spleen)

Identifies bloodborne metastasis (eg, liver)

Identifies peritoneal dissemination (serosal penetration by tumor, ascites, carcinomatosis)

Identifies lymphatic spread involving local and distant lymph nodes

Enables lymph node sampling

Enables peritoneal lavage for identification of intra-abdominal free cancer cells (cytology)

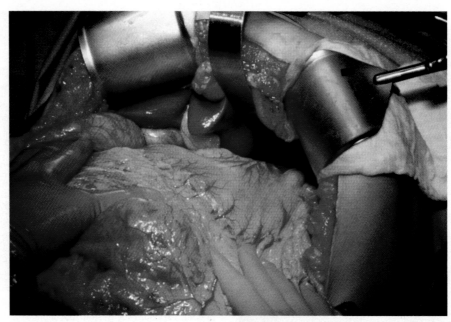

Figure 13–10.   The entire abdomen is carefully explored for gross metastasis.

total gastric resection. The right gastroepiploic artery is identified originating from the gastroduodenal artery, is doubly ligated, and is divided away from the duodenal wall with 2-0 silk sutures, to include adjacent lymph nodes. The right gastric vessels are also identified and doubly ligated away from the superior margin of the second portion of the duodenum with 2-0 silk sutures. For adequate margins, the mobilized duodenum is divided approximately 1 to 3 cm distal to the pyloric ring, using a GIA or TA stapling device (Figure 13–12).

The avascular triangular ligament that supports the left lateral segment of the liver is divided. The left lobe is gently mobilized upward with a moist pack and a manual retractor. The remaining gastrohepatic ligament is then divided close to the liver, which includes a branch of the inferior phrenic artery. The stomach is next retracted upward and to the left,

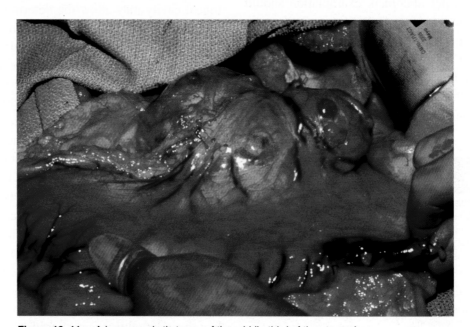

Figure 13–11.   A large exophytic tumor of the middle third of the stomach.

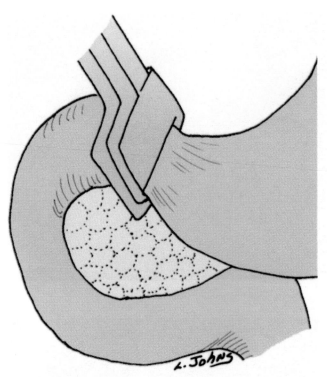

Figure 13–12. Transection of the duodenum with a TA stapling device.

which allows optimal exposure of the pancreas and easier en bloc dissection of the anterior pancreatic capsule, along with the lymph nodes parallel to the splenic artery (Figure 13–13). This maneuver enables the surgeon to be in a proper plane to perform an optimal lymph node dissection. The lymphatics in the hepatoduodenal ligament along the common hepatic artery and celiac axis are identified and removed, completely clearing the periaortic structures of all lymph nodes.

The left gastric vessels are then identified and isolated from adjacent tissues by blunt and sharp dissection (Figure 13–14) and are then doubly ligated and divided with 2-0 silk sutures. The ligation of the left gastric vessels located on the lesser curvature of the stomach further enhances the subsequent exposure of the gastroesophageal (GE) junction. Of importance, the inadvertent division of an aberrant or accessory left hepatic artery stemming from the left gastric artery may cause significant postoperative hepatic ischemia.[25] Early identification and careful surgical technique must be emphasized to avoid complications related to the division of the anatomic variants of the left hepatic artery.

The left gastroepiploic vessels are doubly ligated. The greater curvature of the stomach is then mobilized up to the esophagus (Figure 13–15). If tumor is adherent to the spleen, pancreas, liver, diaphragm, or mesocolon, the involved structures are removed en bloc. If the spleen is to remain, the gastrosplenic ligament is divided. Short gastric vessels are also ligated up to the GE junction with 3-0 silk sutures or surgical clips. Alternatively, the short gastric vessels may be divided with a harmonic scalpel or a similar coagulating device. The peritoneum over the esophagus is divided, and all bleeding points are ligated. The distal esophagus is then dissected free, and the vagal nerves are divided, which facilitates mobilization of the esophagus for 10 to 12 cm into the peritoneal cavity. Since the esophagus tends to retract upward when divided, two stay sutures are placed to provide downward traction.

After mobilization of the entire stomach and lower esophagus, the nasogastric tube is retracted; an automatic purse-string applier is placed approximately 6 to 10 cm above the GE junction, and the esophagus is then divided (Figures 13–16 and 13–17). The specimen, which consists of stomach, proximal duodenum, greater omentum, and regional lymph nodes, is sent to pathology to confirm the adequacy of the resected margins before reconstruction. Various reconstructive techniques have been used in an attempt to ensure better postoperative nutrition and fewer symptoms following total gastrectomy. A large jejunal loop with an enteroenterostomy has been described. Reflux esophagitis secondary to regurgitation may be alleviated by a Roux-en-Y procedure. Once the margins are cleared, reconstruction is performed either by stapled or hand-sewn anastomosis, depending on the preference of the operating surgeon. Although both reconstructive techniques are used, we prefer the stapling method since this approach simplifies the anastomosis and lessens the overall time for this procedure.

Stapled Anastomosis

After the removal of the specimen and after disease-free margins are confirmed histologically, a Roux-en-Y end-to-side esophagojejunostomy is performed. A 28 EEA anvil is placed into the lumen of the divided esophagus, and the purse-string suture is

Figure 13–13. The stomach is retracted upward and to the left for en bloc dissection of the anterior pancreatic capsule along with lymph nodes along the common hepatic and splenic artery.

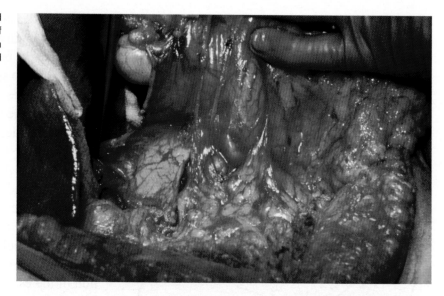

Figure 13–14. The forceps point out the celiac axis. The left gastric artery is doubly ligated and divided. Inadvertent division of an aberrant or accessory left hepatic artery originating from the left gastric artery may cause significant postoperative hepatic ischemia. The forceps point to the left gastric pedicle.

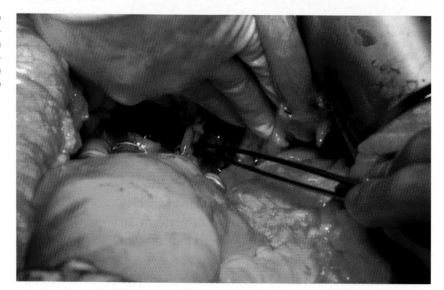

Figure 13–15. The greater curvature of the stomach is mobilized up to the esophagus, using a Ligasure® or a similar coagulating device to divide the short gastric vessels.

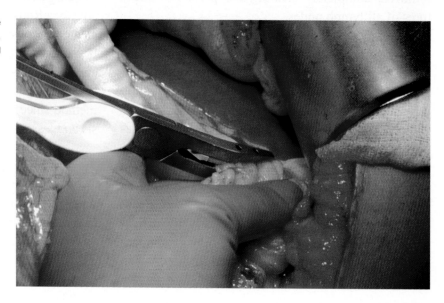

tied (Figures 13–18 and 13–19). Once this is accomplished, the jejunum is divided distal to the ligament of Treitz, with a GIA stapler. The jejunum is mobilized, and its mesenteric blood supply is examined to confirm that it is intact. The divided distal loop of jejunum is then brought up through an opening in the mesocolon just left of the middle colic vessels. This retrocolic approach enables the jejunal limb to reach the end of the esophagus in a tension-free manner. The jejunal staple line is removed, and an EEA instrument is placed into the jejunum. The trocar from the EEA is brought through the side of the jejunum, and the instrument is then attached to the anvil, closed, and fired (Figure 13–20). The EEA is opened, slightly rotated, and then removed. The

opened end of the jejunal limb is closed with a TA-30 stapler. The nasogastric tube is then passed beyond the anastomosis (Figure 13–21). To examine for air leaks, air is insufflated with the esophagojejunal anastomosis submerged under sterile saline.

A side-to-side jejunojejunostomy 40 cm from the esophagojejunostomy completes the Roux-en-Y reconstruction and re-establishes alimentary continuity beyond the ligament of Treitz (Figure 13–22). The side-to-side anastomosis is performed with a GIA stapler introduced into the antimesenteric sides of the jejunum. The enteroenterotomy is then closed with a TA-60 stapler. The jejunum is anchored to the margins of the mesocolon opening, which must be closed to avoid internal herniation, with interrupted

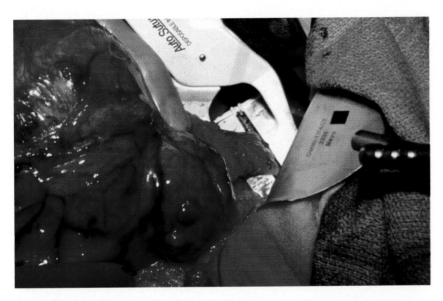

Figure 13–16. After the stomach and esophagus are mobilized, an automatic purse-string applier is placed about 6 to 10 cm above the gastroesophageal junction.

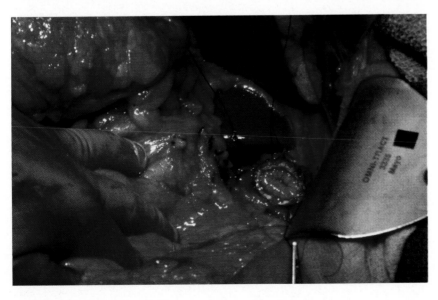

Figure 13–17. The esophagus is divided. Stay sutures are used to prevent the retraction of the remaining distal esophagus into the mediastinum and to ensure easy approximation with the jejunum.

Figure 13–18.   A 28 EEA anvil is inserted into the lumen of the divided esophagus.

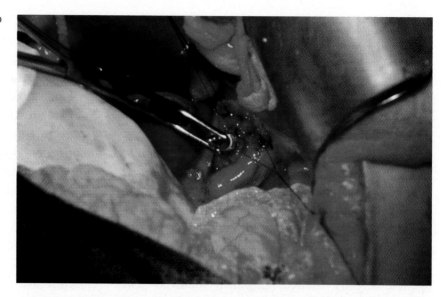

Figure 13–19.   The purse-string suture is tightened to hold the anvil of the circular stapler in place.

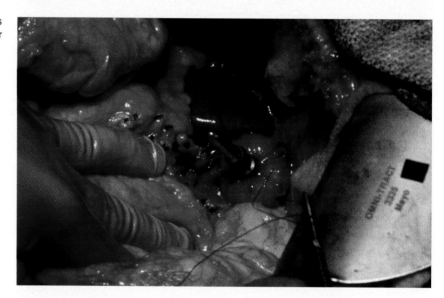

Figure 13–20.   The shaft of the EEA circular stapling device is introduced into the divided jejunal limb, and the trocar from the EEA is brought through the jejunal wall, attached to the anvil, and fired.

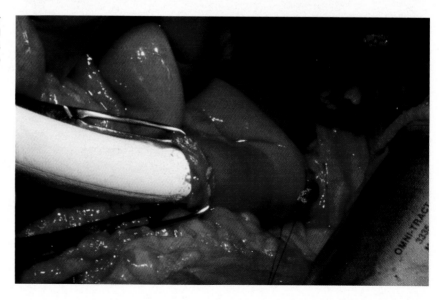

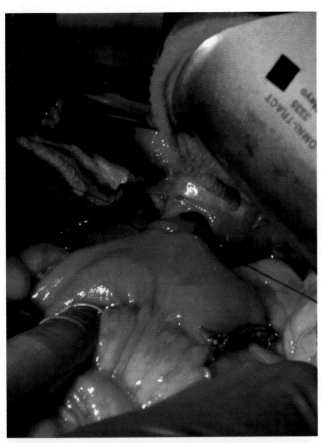

Figure 13–21. A completed end-to-side esophagojejunostomy. The opened end of the jejunal limb is closed with a TA-30 linear stapler.

3-0 silk sutures. At this time, a needle catheter feeding jejunostomy is placed just past the enteroenterostomy and is secured to the abdominal wall with 3-0 silk sutures.

Subtotal Gastrectomy

A subtotal gastrectomy, which includes regional lymphadenectomy, is the operation of choice for distal gastric cancers. This procedure is approached in a similar fashion as that previously described for total gastrectomy, except that only 75 to 85% of distal stomach is resected. About a 75% gastric resection can be performed when the line of division includes most of the lesser curvature, with the ligation of the left gastric and left gastroepiploic vessels. The stomach is divided with a TA-90 stapling device (Figure 13–23). A small stomach remnant supplied by the short gastric vessels provides some gastric reservoir to minimize postgastrectomy sequelae (Figure 13–24).

After negative margins are obtained, a Roux-en-Y gastrojejunostomy is our reconstructive method of choice. The distal limb of jejunum is brought up through the mesocolon in a retrocolic fashion, and an end-to-side gastrojejunostomy is made, using a running inner layer of 3-0 absorbable suture and an interrupted outer layer of 3-0 silk Lambert sutures (Figure 13–25). A 40-cm distal limb is measured, and a side-to-side jejunojejunostomy is made, using either a stapled or hand-sewn method as previously described. An alternate technique involves using a Billroth II loop gastrojejunostomy.

Postoperative Management

After surgery has been completed, postoperative care begins, with the ultimate goal of optimizing and maintaining the patient in a normal physiologic state. Postoperative pain is controlled with the use of judicious narcotics in the form of an epidural catheter left in place for a few days or a patient-controlled analgesia (PCA) system administering morphine or meperidine. The use of a nasogastric tube is controversial, and such use is based on surgeon preference. During the initial postoperative period, fluid and electrolyte balance is maintained intravenously. Early ambulation is encouraged, usually on the first postoperative day. With the resumption of bowel function, the patient's diet is gradually advanced. If the patient has

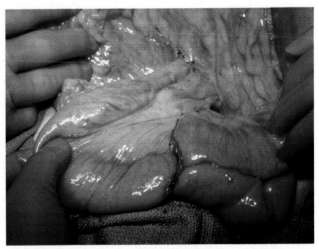

Figure 13–22. A side-to-side jejunojejunostomy 40 cm from the esophagojejunostomy completes the Roux-en-Y reconstruction. The side-to-side anastomosis shown was created with the GIA-60 linear stapling device, and the enteroenterotomy was closed with a TA-60 stapler.

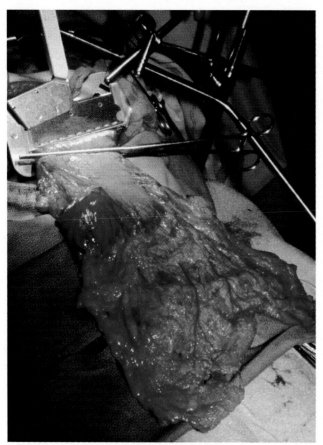

Figure 13–23. For subtotal gastrectomy, approximately 75 to 85% of distal stomach is resected with a TA-90 stapling device.

difficulty with the oral consumption of foodstuffs, a previously placed feeding jejunostomy tube may be used for postoperative nutritional support.

Guidelines for follow-up after resection for gastric cancer have not been standardized. Nevertheless, patients should be monitored closely for the first 2 years as most recurrences fall within this period. Patients are seen every 3 months and are questioned about dysphagia, changes in bowel habits, abdominal pain, and weight loss. The physical examination should focus on the appearance of any abdominal tenderness, masses, or ascites, and a rectal examination should be performed to check for occult blood and pelvic peritoneal recurrence (Blumer's shelf). Follow-up visits may be scheduled every 6 months for years 3 to 5 and yearly thereafter. No strict recommendations can be made for periodic chest radiography, CT, or routine blood tests. The development of symptoms, however, usually warrants imaging or endoscopic studies to rule out recurrence.

Other Surgery-Related Options: The Role of Laparoscopy

The usefulness of laparoscopy lies in its ability to detect nodal metastases, subclinical peritoneal carcinomatosis, and occult hepatic metastases. Failure to detect these diseased states may ultimately affect the resectability rate and outcome. Several studies show that laparoscopy may be more accurate in assessing nodal involvement and detecting hepatic metastases than compared to ultrasonography and CT and that peritoneal carcinomatosis can be conclusively excluded by laparoscopy. In one report, laparoscopy detected nodal involvement with a diagnostic accuracy of 72%, compared to 52% for ultrasonography and 57% for CT.[26] Laparoscopy detected hepatic metastases more accurately (96%) than ultrasonography (83%) and CT (85%). Furthermore, laparoscopy had an 83% sensitivity for the detection of peritoneal carcinomatosis.[27]

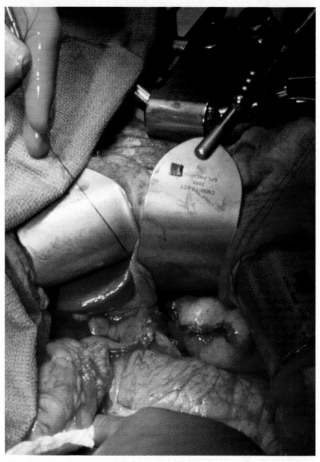

Figure 13–24. A small gastric remnant supplied by short gastric vessels acts as a reservoir to minimize postgastrectomy sequelae.

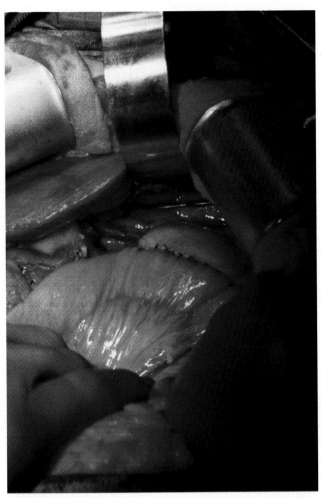

Figure 13–25. A completed gastrojejunostomy. The distal jejunal limb is brought up in a retrocolic fashion to help create a Roux-en-Y end-to-side gastrojejunostomy.

The value of laparoscopy in the management of gastric cancer is highlighted in two studies. In one report of preoperative CT and laparoscopy, subclinical peritoneal carcinomatosis and occult hepatic metastases were detected by laparoscopy in 28% of the patients with gastric cancer.[28] The median survival of these patients was 5 months, and only one patient required reoperation for palliation. In another study of patients in whom laparoscopic exploration was performed following a reported normal CT scan, subclinical metastatic disease was found in 37% of these patients, with an 84% sensitivity and a 100% specificity.[29] No patients who initially underwent only laparoscopy required reoperation for palliation.

Laparoscopy has also been shown to be a safe and useful method for examining occult disseminated gastric cancer through peritoneal-lavage cytology.[30,31] Since many patients with gastric cancer have undetectable disseminated disease, resection is not likely to alter their outcome. Therefore, it would be important to accurately identify these patients for exclusion from surgery and for placement into protocols exploring new or novel therapeutic regimens. Laparoscopically obtained peritoneal washings and the use of Giemsa and Papanicolaou stains to identify intraperitoneal free cancer cells (IFCCs) are of great value in detecting microscopic intra-abdominal spread and in identifying that subset of patients who are at high risk of peritoneal recurrence. Furthermore, positive laparoscopic peritoneal-lavage cytology may be a good predictor of poor outcomes in patients with advanced disease and may be used in treatment planning, especially for patients who are entering either neoadjuvant or adjuvant treatment protocols.

In a report of 127 patients with gastric cancer, the prevalence of IFCCs was 0% (0 in 45) in patients with T1/T2 M0 disease, 10% (3 in 31) in patients with T3/T4 M0 disease, and 59% in patients with M1 disease.[30] The three T3/T4 M0 patients with positive cytology had recurrences at a median follow-up of 8.5 months, and their survival was significantly decreased when compared to that of stage-matched controls with negative cytology who underwent resection for cure. There was also no difference in survival between the three stage III M0 patients and stage IV patients who did not undergo resection. The study suggested that patients with positive lavage cytology are equivalent to those with stage IV disease, even in the absence of macroscopic peritoneal disease or distant metastases, and that this technique identifies the subset of T3/T4 M0 patients who are unlikely to benefit from resection alone.

In a study of 49 patients with gastric cancer, laparoscopy with cytologic examination for staging revealed IFCCs in 41% of patients.[31] In 8 cases, laparoscopy revealed carcinomatosis and liver metastases precluding laparotomy. All patients who tested positive for IFCCs developed peritoneal recurrence. The absence of IFCCs was associated with improved overall survival. The report concluded that laparoscopic peritoneal-lavage cytology is valuable in identifying patients at high risk of peritoneal recurrence and thereby improves the selection of patients suitable for curative or palliative resection. Furthermore, the study demonstrated that a positive cytologic test is a significant prognostic factor for survival.

Laparoscopic techniques are useful for confirming the absence or presence of incurable disease. Laparoscopy allows easy access to intra-abdominal structures for biopsy and for determining local resectability, thereby avoiding unnecessary high-risk surgical procedures. Furthermore, laparoscopic peritoneal-lavage cytology may play an important role in staging, evaluating, and classifying patients with gastric cancer for appropriate treatment. This approach may be especially valuable in the diagnosis of occult abdominal M1 disease missed by standard ultrasonography or CT. For all of the above reasons, we routinely perform laparoscopy prior to attempting curative gastric resection.

SURGICAL ISSUES IN GASTRIC CANCER

Extended Lymph Node Dissection

The role of extended lymphadenectomy for gastric cancer is a controversial issue that continues to receive much attention. Radical lymph node dissection was embraced as an integral part of gastrectomy procedures, based on an initial report from Japan that demonstrated a survival benefit for patients with serosal or involved regional lymph nodes who underwent D2 lymphadenectomy.[32] The Japanese have made significant contributions to the classification of regional lymph nodes, which is essential to the understanding of extended lymph node resection. The Japanese staging of lymph node involvement is different from the American Joint Committee on Cancer (AJCC) system in that it describes four major nodal groups (N1 to N4) that comprise 16 separate locations of nodal tissue. Group 1 (N1) nodes are located closest to the primary tumor and within the perigastric tissue along the greater and lesser curvature of the stomach. Group 2 (N2) nodes are found along the major vessels from the celiac axis, including the common hepatic, splenic, and left gastric arteries. Group 3 (N3) nodes are located at the celiac axis, near the origin of the superior mesenteric artery, near the

hepatoduodenal ligament, and behind the pancreas. Group 4 (N4) nodes reside in the periaortic tissue. The N3 and N4 locations would be the equivalent of distant metastatic disease (M1) in the AJCC system. Importantly, the location of lymph nodes in relation to the primary tumor, rather than number of nodes, is used to define the stage of lymph node disease and is ultimately used to determine the extent of lymph node dissection.

In Japan, gastric resection with extended lymphadenectomy is classified into five types. A D0 resection includes a gastrectomy with the incomplete resection of N1 nodes whereas a D1 gastric resection includes the complete dissection of N1 nodes. A D2 resection includes the removal of both the N1 and N2 nodes. A D3 resection includes the dissection of N1 to N3 nodes. A D4 resection is the most extensive and includes the removal of all nodal groups. The Japanese Research Society for Gastric Cancer defines a curative resection as a resection that involves a gastric resection with lymph node dissection one level beyond that of pathologic lymph node involvement in a patient without peritoneal or hepatic metastasis.[33] In Japan, the meticulous surgical dissection and pathologic staging of specific nodal basins in relation to the primary tumor are based on the premise of an orderly progression in the spread of metastasis from primary tumor to regional lymph nodes and then to the next higher echelon of nodes. From this assumption, the Japanese believe that more extensive surgery involving the removal of progressively higher echelons of lymph nodes will result in improved survival rates per stage of disease.[34,35] Thus, for positive N1 nodes, a D2 dissection would be required for adequate resection.

According to one Japanese study, the 5-year survival rates for patients with nodal involvement at N0, N1, N2, N3, and N4 nodes are 81.5%, 49.7%, 24%, 5.9%, and 1.9%, respectively.[34] These findings suggest that a greater number of involved nodes indicates a higher incidence of positive nodes at multiple levels and therefore a lower 5-year survival rate. As extended lymph node resection for gastric cancer has become more universally accepted in Japan, the operative mortality for such radical dissections has declined while 5-year survival rates after curative resection have increased. In another nonrandomized study, Japanese patients who underwent D3 resection had a 5-year survival rate of 21.4%, compared to 10.0% for those patients who underwent D2 resection for N2 gastric cancer.[35] Other studies from Japan reported 5-year survival rates approaching 50% in node-positive patients after extended lymphadenectomy.[36]

These impressive survival outcomes from Japan have not been reliably reproduced in Western reports and have undoubtedly contributed to the controversy over whether or not extended lymphadenectomy confers a survival advantage. A more aggressive surgical approach involving a total gastrectomy with en bloc resection of adjacent organs with standard extended lymphadenectomy is believed by Japanese surgeons to be the main reason for such good stage-specific survival. Other factors that may explain such results include the younger age of Japanese patients, less comorbidity in this population, earlier detection due to mass screening programs, and stage migration (described below). Finally, there may exist the possibility that gastric cancers in Japan are inherently different from gastric cancers in other Western countries and that the Japanese have developed a less aggressive form of the intestinal type of disease.

In the last two decades, D2 resections have become more commonplace in Western countries. Nonrandomized studies from Germany, Norway, and the United States have reported postoperative morbidity rates of around 30%, mortality rates between 4 and 5%, and 5-year survival rates between 26.3 and 47% for D2 resections[37–39] (Table 13–3). This variability in outcome is probably due to the varied definitions of D2 resections.

On the basis of the aforementioned retrospective data, four randomized studies comparing D1 to D2 resections have been performed (Table 13–4). In a small study from South Africa, no survival differences were reported in patients who underwent either D1 or D2 resection for T1–3 N0–1 M0 gastric cancer.[40] Furthermore, the patients who underwent D2 resections had longer operative times, longer hospital stays, and higher complication rates. In a report from Hong Kong, no benefit in morbidity, mortality, or survival was demonstrated in patients undergoing more extended D3 resections when compared to patients undergoing D1 resections.[41]

In a prospective randomized trial from Great Britain, patients undergoing D1 resections were compared to patients undergoing D2 resection.[42] Postoperative complications were significantly higher in the D2 group than in the D1 group (46% vs. 28%, $p \leq .001$). Postoperative mortality rates were also significantly higher in the D2 group (13% vs. 6.5% in the D1 group, $p \leq .05$). There were no significant differences in 5-year survival rates between the D2 group and the D1 group (33% vs. 35%, respectively). Likewise, a phase III clinical trial from the Netherlands reported that patients who underwent more extensive D2 resections experienced more postoperative complications than those who underwent D1 resections (43% vs. 25%, respectively, $p \leq .001$) and had a significantly higher operative mortality (10% vs. 4% for the D1 patients, $p \leq .0005$).[43] The 5-year survival rates for patients undergoing D1 and D2 resections were 45% and 47%, respectively.

Some conclusions can be drawn from these randomized trials. Although there were substantial differences in the design and conduct of these studies, the postoperative morbidity and mortality were significantly higher in the D2 resection group than in the D1 resection group. Furthermore, in all studies,

	Table 13–3. NONRANDOMIZED STUDIES OF D1 AND D2 GASTRECTOMIES							
	D1 Gastrectomy				D2 Gastrectomy			
Study, Year (Country)	n	Morbidity (%)	Mortality (%)	5-Yr Survival (%)	n	Morbidity (%)	Mortality (%)	5-Yr Survival (%)
Siewert et al, 1993 (Germany)	558	29	5.2	51.2	1,096	30.6	5	46.6
Viste et al, 1994 (Norway)	78	37	13.0	30.0	105	30.0	4	47.0
Wanebo et al, 1996 (United States)	1,529	—	—	30.0	695	—	—	26.3

n = sample size.

Table 13–4. RANDOMIZED STUDIES OF D1 AND D2 GASTRECTOMIES								
	D1 Gastrectomy				D2 Gastrectomy			
Study, Year (Country)	n	Morbidity (%)	Mortality (%)	5-Yr Survival (%)	n	Morbidity (%)	Mortality (%)	5-Yr Survival (%)
Dent et al, 1988 (South Africa)	22	22	0.0	69	21	43.0	0.0	67
Robertson et al,* 1994 (Hong Kong)	25	0	0.0	45	30	58.6	3.3	35
Cuschieri et al, 1999 (Great Britain)	200	28	6.5	35	200	46.0	13.0	33
Bonenkamp et al, 1999 (The Netherlands)	380	25	4.0	45	331	43.0	10.0	47

n = sample size.
*Study involved extended D3 resections vs. D1 resections.

there was no 5-year survival advantage for D2 resections. Thus, the adopted practice of D2 resection for Western patients with N1 gastric cancers warrants reconsideration as this surgical approach is associated with higher postoperative morbidity and mortality rates and no apparent survival benefit.

Extent of Gastric Resection

For proximal gastric tumors, surgical management remains controversial in regard to the extent of gastric and esophageal resection and in regard to the optimal surgical approach. The options include performing a total gastrectomy through a transabdominal approach versus performing a proximal gastrectomy through an Ivor Lewis or transabdominal approach. In general, proximal tumors often have an advanced presentation and have a poorer prognosis than distal tumors. In one report, a survival advantage and a lower recurrence rate have been shown for patients with stage I and II disease of the proximal stomach who undergo a radical total gastrectomy with esophagojejunal anastomosis.[44] This procedure can be accomplished with minimal morbidity and a mortality of < 5%.[45] The advantages of total gastrectomy when compared to proximal gastrectomy include the increased probability of achieving negative histologic distal margins and the relative ease of complete perigastric lymph node removal. Furthermore, total gastrectomy with Roux-en-Y reconstruction for proximal gastric lesions also precludes the possibility of alkaline reflux esophagitis that is frequently associated with disabling symptoms after proximal subtotal gastrectomy. However, in a recent study of 391 patients with proximal gastric

cancers, the extent of resection did not affect the long-term outcome.[46] The report concluded that both total and proximal gastrectomy could equally be safely accomplished and that they had similar times for recurrence, similar recurrence rates, and similar 5-year survival rates.

Midbody lesions account for approximately 15 to 30% of all gastric cancers, and these tumors tend to remain asymptomatic until they are locally advanced. Although the decision to perform a radical total gastrectomy versus a subtotal gastrectomy (75 to 85%) remains controversial, most midstomach tumors are large and invade adjacent structures that may require a radical total gastrectomy or an extended total gastrectomy (en bloc splenectomy and distal pancreatectomy) to achieve negative margins. In a comparative study, there were no convincing data regarding the superiority of one procedure over another.[47] This finding may reflect the fact that the majority of patients in the study had stage III and IV disease and that no surgical procedure was therefore likely to have a favorable impact on survival. The lowest local recurrence rate (16%) was achieved in patients who underwent extended total gastrectomy. Overall, these data suggest that tumor biology, rather than the extent of gastrectomy, dictates the eventual outcome.

Approximately 35% of all remaining gastric cancers occur in the distal third of the stomach. These lesions are detected earlier than the more proximal lesions in the stomach because they have the tendency to cause symptoms of gastric outlet obstruction even when relatively small. For distal gastric cancers, radical subtotal gastrectomy is the surgical procedure of choice. This operation requires the resection of approximately 75% or more of the distal stomach, including most of the lesser curvature. At least 1 cm of the first portion of the duodenum and 5 to 7 cm of normal gastric tissue proximal to the tumor should be resected to ensure adequate margins. As with all gastric resections, removal of the omental bursa with regional lymph node dissection is routinely performed if the surgeon subscribes to the concept that D2 resection improves survival. For posterior tumors, extended distal subtotal gastrectomy with en bloc resection of the pancreatic tail and spleen may be necessary if the primary tumor is adherent or invades surrounding tissues. In comparative studies, patients undergoing distal resection have the lowest incidence of postoperative complications and mortality, compared to other patients undergoing other surgical procedures for gastric cancer. In a study of 55 patients with antral cancers, patients treated with a D1 subtotal gastrectomy had better overall survival and lower postoperative morbidity when compared to patients who underwent D3 total gastrectomy.[41] Although it had a low operative mortality rate, D3 total gastrectomy was also associated with increased postoperative intra-abdominal sepsis. The report concluded that such findings did not support the routine use of D3 total gastrectomy in distal-third cancers.

Adequacy of Proximal and Distal Margins

The importance of adequate margins of resection is apparent and was highlighted by a study that reported a 5-year survival rate of 28% for patients with positive proximal margins after gastrectomy.[48] Local recurrence was a cause of death in 23% of these patients. The patients had a 6-cm or larger gross margin of resection from the primary tumor. Further studies suggest that local recurrences usually are not due to disease in the mucosa but rather to infiltration of cancer in the surrounding lymphatic vessels and adjacent organs.

Distal margins are usually histologically negative when the duodenum is divided 2 to 3 cm or more distal to the gastric pylorus. Proximal resections, in contrast, require larger margins of resection from the gross primary tumor. Furthermore, re-excision to obtain negative margins is rarely indicated. For tumors of the GE junction, up to 10 cm of distal esophagus should be included within the resected specimen since these cancers tend to spread throughout the submucosa.

Splenectomy and Resection of Adjacent Organs

Routine splenectomy during resection for gastric cancer has not been shown to improve patient outcome. In a retrospective study of 392 patients undergoing potentially curative resection, splenectomy in association with extended resections caused significantly more complications than did those procedures without splenectomy.[49] Importantly, patients who underwent splenectomy had a higher percentage of infectious complications than patients who did not undergo the procedure. No survival benefit was attributed to splenectomy. The report concluded that splenectomy increased the morbidity of curative gastrectomy and should be reserved for tumors that invade the spleen or require splenectomy to facilitate gastrectomy. Another recent report attributed no survival benefit to splenectomy for any given stage of gastric cancer.[50]

Advanced gastric cancer with direct invasion into adjacent organs indicates a poor prognosis. Although there have been studies of extended en bloc resection that includes the spleen, distal pancreas, and transverse colon in patients with advanced gastric cancer, no data support an improved 5-year survival in those patients undergoing such an approach if adjacent organs are uninvolved with tumor. En bloc resection that does not remove all gross disease is not indicated for gastric cancer.

Surgical Treatment of Locally Recurrent Gastric Cancer

Despite complete resection of all gross tumor with negative margins, recurrence of gastric cancer is nevertheless common. Certain patterns of locoregional failure and distant metastasis are apparent. The disease spreads by local extension into contiguous structures, metastasizes to regional lymph nodes, seeds throughout the peritoneal cavity, and metastasizes to distant sites such as the liver and lungs. Locoregional recurrences occur at the site of anastomosis, within the bed of gastric resection, or in the adjacent lymph nodes, and occur in approximately 20 to 50% of patients after gastrectomy.[51–54] Approximately 90% of all recurrences appear within the first 2 years after the initial resection.[55] The patients who are at highest risk of locoregional failure are those with (1) locally advanced tumors penetrating through the gastric serosa, (2) lymph node involvement, and (3) invasion of adjacent organs. Histologic studies suggest that locoregional failure occurs in about 45% of patients who have primary lesions that extend through the stomach wall and in 19% of those without stomach-wall infiltration.[54]

There is some evidence to suggest that re-excision may be appropriate and potentially beneficial for a select group of patients with locoregional recurrence after initial surgical resection. In a retrospective study from Japan of 51 patients with recurrent gastric cancer following partial or subtotal gastrectomy, 25% of patients underwent re-excision for recurrent lesions; 92% of those patients underwent total resection of the gastric remnant, with en bloc removal of the distal pancreas, spleen, transverse colon, and liver segment.[56] The operative mortality rate was 7.6%, and the 1-year survival rate was 41.7%. The authors of the study concluded that aggressive surgical re-excision might be indicated for locally recurrent disease, which histologically proved to be stage I and II disease after the initial operation.

In another report, re-excision was possible in 53.5% of 75 patients who were explored for locally recurrent gastric cancer.[53] Total gastrectomy with reconstruction was performed in 55% of the patients who underwent re-excision, and gastrectomy combined with en bloc adjacent organ resection was performed in 45% of patients, with an overall mortality rate of 15%. Of those patients who underwent re-excision for recurrent gastric cancer, 31.2% received preoperative radiation whereas 28.2% underwent postoperative systemic chemotherapy. The 2-year survival rates for those patients who underwent re-excision were as follows: re-excision alone, 20%; preoperative radiation and re-excision, 31.3%; and re-excision with postoperative chemotherapy, 66.4%. The report concluded that re-excision benefits select patients with recurrent gastric cancer and that preoperative

radiation or postoperative chemotherapy may provide some additional benefit.

RESULTS OF SURGERY

As a consequence of the advanced disease stage at presentation, the overall 5-year survival rate in most Western countries ranges from 10 to 20% for all patients with gastric cancer and from 24 to 58% for patients who undergo curative resection. In contrast, the Japanese consistently report higher survival rates, which they attribute to increased detection and to the subsequent treatment of early gastric cancer with more extensive lymph node dissections.[57] Although earlier diagnosis, a higher incidence of intestinal-type tumors, and more extensive surgeries in Japan may account for such disparity, a major contributing factor may be the differences between Japan and most Western countries in regard to the surgical and pathologic staging of gastric cancer. The differing classifications of lymph node dissection used in the United States and in Japan suggest a stage migration bias that may confound the interpretation of comparative surgical results between the two countries.

Within the Japanese system of meticulous surgical dissection and staging of nodal basins in relation to the primary tumor, a so-called stage migration may arise. In stage migration, a subset of patients may be assigned to a more advanced disease stage.[58] This migration may lead to statistical improvements in stage survival, as depicted in Table 13–5. For example, a subset of staged patients from group A are assigned (or migrate to) more advanced stages according to group-B staging criteria, as shown in the middle column. The combined staged results of group B are shown on the right of the table. Twenty-four stage I patients from group A migrate to an advanced stage under group B. All except two patients migrate to stage III of group B. The 22 patients now considered to have stage III disease have a 5-year survival rate (59%) that is lower than the original survival rate in stage I (79%) but higher than the original survival rate in stage III (31%). Thus, the number of patients increases in more advanced stages, and the survival results within each stage improve under group B. The overall survival

Table 13–5. EXAMPLE OF STAGE MIGRATION ON 5-YEAR SURVIVAL RATE*								
Group A			Stage Migration			Group B		
Stage	No. of Patients	(5-Yr Survival)	Stage	No. of Patients	(5-Yr Survival)	Stage	No. of Patients	(5-Yr Survival)
I	41/52	(79%)	I	26/28	(93%)	I	26/28	(93%)
			II	2/2	(100%)			
			III	13/22	(59%)			
II	15/30	(50%)	II	13/21	(62%)	II	15/23	(65%)
			III	2/9	(22%)			
III	21/68	(31%)	III	21/68	(31%)	III	36/99	(36%)
Overall 5-yr survival rate	77/150	(52%)					77/150	(52%)

*Numbers are arbitrary and not from actual studies.

rate of those patients under group B, however, remains the same as that of group A (52%).

This apparent increase in stage-specific survival without an influence on overall survival or stage migration is caused by a reclassification of staging by lymph node dissection and may explain the difference in survival between Japanese and Western patients. The controversy regarding the role of extended lymph node dissection and the observed stage migration in the staging system used in the United States versus that used in Japan not only can be difficult to interpret but also raises concerns about the accuracy of staging and the appropriate selection of surgical treatment. Currently, no distinct advantage to staging gastric cancer according to the Japanese system has been shown in Western patients. Until proven otherwise, the tumor-node-metastasis (TNM) staging system advocated by the AJCC remains the standard in the United States.

To further add to this confusion, the terminology used to characterize the various types of surgical resections has changed. Resections that remove N1, N1 to N2, and N1 to N3 nodes were previously termed R1, R2, and R3 resections, respectively. Presently, they are respectively termed D1, D2, and D3 resections. The term R0 represents curative resection with no residual tumor whereas the term R1 indicates incomplete tumor resection.

To identify specific variables that might correlate with a poor prognosis and long-term survival following gastrectomy, Shiu and colleagues performed a retrospective prognostic study of 246 patients undergoing curative resection for gastric cancer.[59] Lesions of the gastric cardia and GE junction were

excluded. Of nine clinicopathologic variables, three were found to have independent prognostic significance by multivariate analysis. These variables were advanced TNM stage, metastatic involvement of four or more lymph nodes, and histologic evidence of poorly differentiated tumors. Of six treatment variables, only two variables—splenectomy and inadequate scope of lymphadenectomy—were independent predictors of outcome. Both variables proved to have a negative impact on survival.

In a study of 211 gastric cancer patients from the United States, 83% underwent laparotomy, and of these patients, 34% underwent gastrectomy with curative intent whereas 24% underwent palliative surgery. Although the overall survival rate for all 211 patients was 21%, those patients who underwent resection had a 5-year survival rate of 36%.[11] For those patients who underwent surgery with curative intent, the 5-year survival increased significantly to 58%. The survival rate of patients with distal tumors undergoing curative resection was twice that of patients with proximal tumors. Of all patients, 15% had linitis plastica, with a median survival of 12 months. The report recommended that resection be avoided in this patient group unless palliation of an obstructing or bleeding tumor was necessary. The report concluded that the appropriate selection of patients for resection with curative intent consistently improved outcomes, as shown by higher median and 5-year survival rates.

In a review of 1,710 cases of gastric cancer over a 35-year period, the 5-year survival rates after resection according to stage were as follows: stage 0 or I, 27%; stage II, 25%; and stages III and IV, 6%.[60] The report emphasized that regional lymph node spread did not always equate with aggressive tumor biology. Also, the report revealed that stage III and IV patients who underwent resection during a 20-year period made up 48% of all 5-year survivors in the study. In addition, antral tumors proved to be more common than proximal gastric tumors, and most 5-year survivors were those patients who were surgically treated for antral lesions. The long-term survival rate for patients with proximal lesions did, however, improve from 0% in the first 25 years to 14% during the last decade. The study also suggested that the morphology of the lesions related to 5-year survival, ulcerating tumors having the worst prognosis.

In a review of 5-year survival rates for gastric cancer in English-language publications from 1960 to 1990, results from Japan, Europe, and the United States were combined and analyzed separately.[36] The 5-year survival rate following all reported gastric resections increased from 20.7% before 1970 to 28.4% in 1990. During this period, the 5-year survival rate for patients undergoing curative or radical resection increased from 37.6 to 55.4%. When the Japanese experience was analyzed separately from the Western experience, the 5-year survival rate after curative resection was 60.5% in Japan and 39.4% in the Western countries. Other findings included a decreased incidence of exploratory laparotomies (due to improved staging methods prior to surgery) and decreased operative mortality during this period. The report concluded that the outcome for patients with gastric cancer improved due to earlier diagnosis, better preoperative staging, more extensive resections, and better perioperative care.

The experience with gastric cancer in the United States was reported in a comprehensive study of 18,365 patients that was conducted by the American College of Surgeons. As expected, survival after surgical treatment was stage dependent.[61] Patients with stage I and II disease had an overall 5-year survival rate of 50% and 29%, respectively, after resection. Patients with stage III and IV disease had survival rates of 13% and 3%, respectively. Approximately 66% of patients presented with either stage III or stage IV disease. Patients rarely underwent extensive lymphadenectomy. Tumor recurrence was shown to be 40% locoregional and 60% distant. Adjuvant radi-

ation, chemotherapy, or both yielded no survival benefit when compared to surgical resection alone. When the findings from this study were compared to experiences reported from 56 Japanese hospitals, a higher incidence of stage I gastric cancer was noted among patients from Japan (33.7%), compared to patients from the United States (17.1%). The overall survival rate of patients who underwent resection was 19% in the United States, compared to 56.3% in Japan. The stage-for-stage 5-year survival rate was also better in Japan. The reasons for such discrepancy may be due to the understaging of patients in the American series whereas in the Japanese series, a more aggressive surgical approach to lymph node dissection may have provided more accurate staging. Although the results of surgery for gastric cancer in the United States are less favorable than those reported by the Japanese and by centers in other Eastern countries, the report concluded that earlier diagnosis and appropriate surgical technique for controlling locoregional disease are essential for optimizing outcomes.

In a subsequent study conducted by the American College of Surgeons and the American Cancer Society, the demographics, grade, subsite, treatment, and rate of survival of Japanese Americans were investigated to explain the international differences in stage-stratified survival for gastric cancer patients.[62] The stage-stratified 5-year and 10-year survival rates based on the fifth edition of the AJCC staging system were as follows, respectively: stage 1A, 78% and 65%; stage IB, 58% and 42%; stage II, 34% and 26%; stage IIIA, 20% and 14%; stage IIIB, 8% and 3%; and stage IV, 7% and 5%. The report revealed that Japanese Americans had a superior stage-for-stage survival, which was attributed partly to this group's predilection for fewer proximal tumors, a lower male-female ratio, and fewer adjacent-organ resections. Furthermore, the fifth edition of the AJCC system, which stages lymph nodes according to number rather than location, proved to be a superior prognostic tool. Finally, the report asserted that the consideration of proximal tumors as being located at a separate disease site might improve the current TNM staging system and concluded that surgical undertreatment of patients with gastric cancer remains a problem in the United States.

EARLY GASTRIC CANCER

In 1962, the Japanese first characterized early gastric cancer as adenocarcinoma that was limited to the mucosa or submucosa, regardless of lymph node involvement. This histologic classification is distinguished by a high cure rate associated with patients who are surgically treated for this disease. Because of aggressive screening programs, a greater incidence of early gastric cancer has been reported in Japan (from 5 to 30% of all stomach cancers) whereas the incidence has increased only slightly (from 5 to 15%) in the United States during the past two decades. The diagnosis of early gastric cancer is made by endoscopic biopsy that demonstrates adenocarcinoma superficial to the muscularis propria. Therefore, by TNM classification, all T1 tumors with any N stage of disease are considered early gastric cancers.

In a Japanese study of 396 patients, the 10-year survival rate for patients with T1 tumors ranged from 82 to 97% when there were no involved nodes but decreased with nodal involvement, from 57 to 87%.[63] Approximately 10% of patients with T1 tumors present with nodal metastases. Multivariate analysis identified large tumor size (> 2 cm) and submucosal invasion as independent risk factors for lymph node involvement in patients with early gastric cancer. For patients with early gastric cancer and no involved nodes, extended lymph node resection has not proved to be beneficial. For early gastric cancer patients with large tumors, lymphatic involvement, or submucosal invasion, however, extended lymphadenectomy may be indicated due to the increased risk of nodal metastases.

In a retrospective study of 60 patients with early gastric cancer from the United States, the disease-free 5-year survival rate after gastrectomy was 76.4% and did not correlate with sex, tumor site, macroscopic tumor appearance, extent of gastric resection, or histologic type.[64] Lower survival rates, however, were associated with larger (> 1.5 cm) early gastric tumors that invaded the submucosa or involved regional lymph nodes. The authors of the study concluded that a high index of suspicion was necessary for earlier detection of early gastric cancers and that gastrectomy with extended D2 lymphadenectomy was necessary to achieve the highest rate of cure. In another study from the same institution, of 165 patients with early gastric cancer staged as T1, the 5-year survival rate after surgical resection was 91% in those patients with negative nodes, compared to 78% in those patients with positive nodes.[65] Although multivariate analysis showed that nodal disease and tumors > 4.5 cm in size were associated with decreased survival, only the presence of nodal disease predicted decreased survival. Moderately or well-differentiated tumors < 4.5 cm and limited to the mucosa had no incidence of nodal metastasis. The authors of the study concluded that early gastric cancer patients with T1 tumors in the United States have a prognosis that is as good as that of similar patients in Japan after surgical resection and that favorable pathologic tumors should be considered for limited resection without lymphadenectomy.

Current surgical treatment for early gastric cancer should therefore consist of subtotal gastrectomy with regional lymph node dissection. Patients with multifocal and proximal lesions should be treated with total gastrectomy. Although extended lymphadenectomy for more advanced lesions remains controversial, the majority of patients with early gastric cancers do well with limited lymphadenectomy, and extended dissections may not be indicated. A limited resection without lymphadenectomy may be considered in patients with small T1 tumors who have comorbid conditions that would put these patients at prohibitive risk if subjected to a more formal and conventional gastrectomy.

In Japan, endoscopic treatment for early gastric cancer has been evaluated in elderly or other poor-risk patients as well as in those patients who refuse gastric resection. In one report, endoscopic therapy in the form of laser ablation, multiple or strip biopsies, or chemical injections followed by careful monitoring resulted in a disease-free survival rate of close to 100%.[66] The best results are obtained when tumors are < 2 cm and less likely to be metastatic. Patients with small elevated tumors found to be limited to the gastric mucosa by EUS evaluation are the best candidates for endoscopic treatment.[67] Although short-term survival has been promising thus far in poor-risk patients and in those who refuse gastrectomy, more experience with this "minimally invasive" treatment modality is needed before endoscopic treatment can replace surgical resection as standard therapy for early gastric cancer.

CONCLUSION

Gastric cancer remains a deadly disease worldwide. Resection remains the only potentially curative treatment for localized stomach cancer. With the exception of early gastric cancer, overall 5-year survival rates for gastric cancer remain dismal (10 to 20% in most Western countries). Recent studies from the United States show that 5-year survival rates for patients undergoing resection with curative intent range from 20 to 58%, indicating occult microscopic metastatic spread in a large number of patients. Although studies show that extended D2 resections can be performed safely and may be indicated in cases of locoregional lymph node involvement, more extensive resections may not provide any further survival benefit. The Japanese have demonstrated the effectiveness of mass screening and meticulous staging in high-risk patients, with impressive results. If such favorable outcomes are to be duplicated in the West, greater efforts at earlier detection and prevention must be made. Further investigations into the nature of the disease are ongoing and may ultimately lead to better strategies for the diagnosis and treatment of gastric cancer in the future.

REFERENCES

1. Billroth T. Offenes schreiben an Herrn Dr. L. Wittelschofer. Wien Med Wochenschr 1881;31:162–5.
2. Haberkant H. Ueber die bis jetzl erzielten unmittelbaren und weiterer Erfolage der verschiedenen Operationen am Magen. Arch Klin Chir 1896;51:484.
3. Mikulicz J. Beitrage zur Technik der Operation des Magencarcinomas. Arch Klin Chir (Berlin) 1898;1:524–32.
4. Brigham CB. Case of removal of the entire stomach for carcinoma; successful esophagoduodenostomy; recovery. Boston Med Surg J 1898;138:415–9.
5. Coller FA, Kay EB, MacIntyre RS. Regional lymphatic metastases of carcinoma of the stomach. Arch Surg 1941;43:748–50.
6. Pack GT, McNeer GP. Total gastrectomy for cancer: a collective review of the literature and an original report on 20 cases. Int Abstracts Surg 1943;77:265–99.
7. Smith JW, Brennan MF. Surgical treatment of gastric cancer. Surg Clin North Am 1992;72:381–99.
8. Siewert JR, Feith M, Werner M, et al. Adenocarcinoma of the esophagogastric junction. Ann Surg 2000;232:353–61.
9. Cady B, Ramsden D, Chloe D. Treatment of gastric cancer. Surg Clin North Am 1976;56:599–605.
10. Dupont J, Lee J, Bunton G, et al. Adenocarcinoma of the stomach: review of 1,497 cases. Cancer 1978;41:941–7.
11. Cady B, Rossi R, Silverman ML, et al. Gastric adenocarcinoma: a disease in transition. Arch Surg 1989;124:303–8.
12. Meyers W, Damiano RJ, Postlewaite RW, et al. Adenocarcinoma of the stomach: changing patterns over the last 4 decades. Ann Surg 1987;205:1–8.
13. Walsh TN, Noonan N, Hollywood D, et al. A comparison of multimodal therapy and surgery for esophageal adenocarcinoma. N Engl J Med 1996;335:462–7.
14. Graham AJ, Finley RT, Clifton JC, et al. Surgical management of adenocarcinoma of the cardia. Am J Surg 1998;175:418–21.
15. Wijnhoven BP, Siersema PD, Hop WC, et al. Adenocarcinomas of the distal esophagus and gastric cardia are one clinical entity. Br J Surg 1999;86:529–35.
16. Correa P. Clinical implications of recent developments in gastric cancer pathology and epidemiology. Semin Oncol 1985;1:2–10.
17. Cook AO, Levine BA, Sirinek KR, Gaskil HV 3rd. Evaluation of gastric adenocarcinoma. Abdominal computed tomography does not replace celiotomy. Arch Surg 1986;121:603–6.
18. Miller FH, Kochman ML, Talamonti MS, et al. Gastric cancer. Radiologic staging. Radiol Clin North Am 1997;35:331–49.
19. Fukuya T, Honda H, Hayashi T, et al. Lymph node metastases: efficacy of detection with helical CT in patients with gastric cancer. Radiology 1995;197:705–11.
20. Botet JF, Lightdale CJ, Zauber AG, et al. Preoperative staging of gastric cancer: comparison of endoscopic US and dynamic CT. Radiology 1991;181:426–32.
21. Caletti G, Ferrari A, Brocchi E, Barbara L. Accuracy of endoscopic ultrasonography in the diagnosis and staging of gastric cancer and lymphoma. Surgery 1993;113:14–27.
22. Bartlett DL, Conlon KC, Gerdes H, Karpeh MS. Laparoscopic ultrasonography: the best pretreatment staging modality in gastric adenocarcinoma? Case report. Surgery 1995;118:562–6.
23. Gatehouse D, Dimock F, Burdon DW, et al. Prediction of wound sepsis following gastric operations. Br J Surg 1978;65:551–4.
24. Buzby GP, the VA TPN Cooperative Study Group. Perioperative total parenteral nutrition in surgical patients. N Engl J Med 1991;325:525.
25. Okano S, Sawai K, Taniguchi H, Takahashi T. Aberrant left hepatic artery arising from the left artery and liver function after radical gastrectomy for gastric cancer. World J Surg 1993;17:70–3.
26. Watt I, Stewart I, Anderson D, et al. Laparoscopy, ultrasound and computed tomography in cancer of the esophagus and gastric cardia: a prospective comparison for detecting intra-abdominal metastasis. Br J Surg 1989;76:1036–9.
27. Possik RA, Franco EL, Pires DR, et al. Sensitivity, specificity, and predictive value of laparoscopy for the staging of gastric cancer and for the detection of liver metastasis. Cancer 1986;58:1–6.
28. Lowy AM, Mansfield PF, Leach SD, Ajani J. Laparoscopic staging for gastric cancer. Surgery 1996;119:611–4.
29. Burke EC, Karpeh MS, Conlon KC, Brennan MF. Laparo-

scopy in the management of gastric adenocarcinoma. Ann Surg 1997;225:262–7.

30. Burke EC, Karpeh MS, Conlon KC, Brennan MF. Peritoneal lavage cytology in gastric cancer: an independent predictor of outcome. Ann Surg Oncol 1997;5:411–5.

31. Ribeiro U, Gama-Rodrigues JJ, Safatle-Ribeiro AV, et al. Prognostic significance of intraperitoneal free cancer cells obtained by laparoscopic peritoneal lavage in patients with gastric cancer. J Gastrointest Surg 1998;2:224–49.

32. Kodama Y, Sugimachi K, Soejima K, et al. Evaluation of extensive lymph node dissection for carcinoma of the stomach. World J Surg 1981;5:241–8.

33. Kajitani T. The general rules for the gastric cancer study in surgery and pathology. Part I. Clinical classification. Jpn J Surg 1981;11:127–39.

34. Maruyama K, Gunven P, Okabayashi K, et al. Lymph node metastases of gastric cancer. General pattern in 1931 patients. Ann Surg 1989;210:596–602.

35. Maruyama K, Okabayashi K, Kinoshita T. Progress in gastric cancer surgery in Japan and its limits of radicality. World J Surg 1987;11:418–25.

36. Akoh JA, Macintyre IMC. Improving survival in gastric cancer: review of 5-year survival rates in English language publications from 1970. Br J Surg 1992;79:293–9.

37. Siewert JR, Bottcher K, Roder JD, et al. Prognostic relevance of systemic lymph node dissection in gastric carcinoma. Br J Surg 1993;80:1015–8.

38. Viste A, Svanes K, Janessen CW Jr, et al. Prognostic importance of radical lymphadenectomy in curative resections for gastric cancer. Eur J Surg 1994;160:497–502.

39. Wanebo HJ, Kennedy BJ, Winchester DP, et al. Gastric carcinoma: does lymph node dissection alter survival? J Am Coll Surg 1996;183:616–24.

40. Dent DM, Madden MV, Price SK. Randomized comparison of R1 and R2 gastrectomy for gastric carcinoma. Br J Surg 1988;75:110–2.

41. Robertson CS, Chung SCS, Woods SDS, et al. A prospective randomized trial comparing R1 subtotal gastrectomy with R3 total gastrectomy for antral cancer. Ann Surg 1994;220:176–82.

42. Cuschieri A, Weeden S, Fielding J, et al. Patient survival after D1 and D2 resection for gastric cancer. Br J Cancer 1999; 79:1522–30.

43. Bonenkamp JJ, Hermans J, Sasako M, et al. Extended lymph-node dissection for gastric cancer. N Engl J Med 1999; 340:908–14.

44. Papachristou DN, Fortner JG. Adenocarcinoma of the gastric cardia: the choice of gastrectomy. Ann Surg 1979;192: 58–64.

45. Boddie AW, McBride CM, Balch CM. Gastric cancer. Am J Surg 1989;157:595–606.

46. Harrison LE, Karpeh MS, Brennan MF. Total gastrectomy is not necessary for proximal gastric cancer. Surgery 1998; 123:127–30.

47. Shiu MH, Papachristou DN, Kosloff C, et al. Selection of operative procedure for adenocarcinoma of midstomach. Ann Surg 1980;192:730–7.

48. Bozzetti F, Bonafanti G, Bufalino R, et al. Adequacy of mar-gins of resection in gastrectomy for cancer. Ann Surg 1984;148:645–8.

49. Brady MS, Rogatko A, Dent LL, Shiu MH. Effect of splenectomy on morbidity and survival following curative gastrectomy for carcinoma. Ann Surg 1991;216:359–64.

50. Wanebo HJ, Kennedy BJ, Winchester DP, et al. Role of splenectomy in gastric cancer surgery: adverse effect of elective splenectomy on long-term survival. J Am Coll Surg 1997;185:177–84.

51. Gunderson LL, Sosin H. Adenocarcinoma of the stomach: areas of failure in a re-operation series clinicopathologic correlation and implications for adjuvant therapy. Int J Radiat Oncol Biol Phys 1982;8:1–11.

52. Blomjous JG, Hop WC, Langenhorst BL, et al. Adenocarcinoma of the gastric cardia. Recurrence and survival after resection. Cancer 1992;70:569–74.

53. Shchepotin I, Evans SRT, Shabahang M, et al. Radical treatment of locally recurrent gastric cancer. Am Surg 1995; 6:371–6.

54. Landry J, Tepper JE, Wood WC, et al. Patterns of failure following curative resection of gastric carcinoma. Int J Radiat Oncol Biol Phys 1990;19:1357–62.

55. Papachristou DN, Fortner JG. Local recurrence of gastric adenocarcinoma after gastrectomy. J Surg Oncol 1981;18: 47–50.

56. Sunagawa M, Takeshita K, Nakajima A, et al. [Reoperation of recurrent gastric cancer—a comparative study of a resected and nonresected group.] Gan No Rinsho 1984; 30:1899–903.

57. Noguchi Y, Imada T, Matsumoto A, et al. Radical surgery for gastric surgery. Cancer 1989;64:2053–62.

58. Feinstein AR, Sosin DM, Wells CK. The Will Rogers phenomenon. Stage migration and new diagnostic techniques as a source of misleading statistics for survival in cancer. N Engl J Med 1985;312:1604–8.

59. Shiu MH, Perrotti M, Brennan MF. Adenocarcinoma of the stomach: a multivariate analysis of clinical, pathologic, and treatment factors. Hepatogastroenterology 1989;36:7–12.

60. Breaux JR, Bringaze W, Chappuis C, et al. Adenocarcinoma of the stomach: a review of 35 years and 1,710 cases. World J Surg 1990;14:580–6.

61. Wanebo HJ, Kennedy BJ, Chmiel J, et al. Cancer of the stomach. Ann Surg 1993;218:583–92.

62. Hundahl SA, Phillips JL, Menck HR. The national cancer database report on poor survival of U.S. gastric carcinoma patients treated with gastrectomy. Cancer 2000;88:921–32.

63. Maehara Y, Orita H, Okuyama T, et al. Predictors of lymph node metastases in early gastric cancer. Br J Surg 1992; 79:245–7.

64. Lawrence M, Shiu MH. Early gastric cancer. Twenty-eight year experience. Ann Surg 1991;213:327–34.

65. Hochwald SN, Brennan MF, Klimstra DS, et al. Is lymphadenectomy necessary for early gastric cancer? Ann Surg Oncol 1999;6:664–70.

66. Hioki K, Nakane Y, Yamamoto M. Surgical strategy for early gastric cancer. Br J Surg 1990;77:1330–4.

67. Farley DR. Donohue JH. Early gastric cancer. Surg Clin North Am 1992;72:401–21.

14

Adjuvant Therapy
for Gastric Cancer

DANIEL G. HALLER, MD

In 2001, Approximately 21,700 Americans will be diagnosed with gastric cancer, and gastric cancer will cause over 12,800 deaths.[1] Worldwide, gastric cancer is the third most common cancer, with 798,000 new cases in 1999.[2] The prognosis for gastric cancer depends on the disease stage at diagnosis; cure rates exceed 70 percent after surgery alone for early-stage disease (T1 N0 or shallow-penetrating T2 N0 M0 tumors). Postoperatively, patients with locally advanced cancers (T3 N0 M0) have a 50 percent or greater chance of dying within 5 years, and those with lymph node metastases fare much worse. In the United States, 80 to 90 percent of patients fall into these high-risk groups, and only 40 percent of patients are eligible to undergo potentially curative surgery. Even for those patients who undergo a complete resection, the rate of recurrence is very high. Conversely, in other countries, such as Japan, the presentation (and even the biology) of gastric cancer may be different, so that it becomes difficult to compare the results of surgery or postoperative treatment programs. As methods for potentially increasing the rate of cure after surgery for gastric cancer, multidisciplinary approaches using postoperative adjuvant and preoperative neoadjuvant therapies are receiving increasing attention, particularly in light of evidence of benefit from such therapies in cases of other common tumors of the gastrointestinal tract, such as colon and rectal cancer. Many of these approaches have been investigated for many years, but no obvious survival benefit has been shown in any large-scale well-controlled trial until recently.

ADJUVANT CHEMOTHERAPY

Postoperative chemotherapy alone for gastric cancer has been extensively evaluated, with generally equivocal results. A number of prospective randomized trials have been performed by different groups, but few studies have demonstrated any statistically significant benefit. It is difficult to perform a post hoc analysis of why these trials failed, but it may be that some of the same problems that were present in the early trials of colon cancer could also be found in these trials of postoperative treatment of gastric cancer. Many of these trials used relatively inactive chemotherapy regimens or were underpowered to detect small but clinically relevant survival benefits. In the Gastrointestinal Tumor Study Group (GITSG) study, 142 patients were randomized to receive adjuvant chemotherapy of semustine (methyl CCNU) and 5-fluorouracil (5-FU) or to be followed with no further treatment after curative-intent resection.[3] At a median follow-up of 4 years, a statistically significant survival advantage appeared in favor of the chemotherapy arm. However, an identical study performed by the Eastern Cooperative Oncology Group (ECOG) during the same time period and using the same dose schedule of the identical drugs did not show benefit.[4] Mitomycin-C has been studied in a series of trials in Europe and Japan. Although a small Spanish trial (in which 33 patients received mitomycin after surgery and 37 had surgery alone) showed a survival benefit for mitomycin treatment (at 10 years of follow-up, 31 of the 37 patients in the control arm and 16 of the 33 patients in the treatment arm were dead because of relapse of disease, [$p < .01$]),[5] this has not been confirmed by larger multicenter studies that have used mitomycin either as a single agent or in combination.[6,7]

Several anthracycline-containing regimens used as adjuvant treatment of gastric cancer have also been reported. No significant difference in disease-free survival or overall survival has been reported, although there have been trends in favor of adjuvant chemotherapy. The International Collaborative Cancer Group conducted a randomized study in 315 gastric cancer patients after curative resection.[8] Patients were randomized to receive either a combination of 5-FU, doxorubicin, and mitomycin (FAM) or no treatment. The final analysis included 181 patients. There was no difference noted in disease-free or overall survival ($p = .21$) with a median follow-up of 68 months, although a retrospective subset analysis suggested that the patients with more advanced disease (T3 or T4) may have benefited from treatment. Indeed, few adjuvant trials for gastric cancer have entered enough patients within discrete disease stages to allow for more than a hypothesis-generating analysis of which patients within a trial may have benefited or not. A different study of doxorubicin randomized 125 patients who had undergone potential curative resection to treatment with 5-FU plus doxorubicin or to observation alone. The two groups showed almost identical 5-year survival rates (32% in the treatment arm and 33% in the control arm).[9] In a small study combining epirubicin with 5-FU/leucovorin as adjuvant treatment for patients with node-positive gastric cancer,[10] 48 patients were randomized to the chemotherapy arm, and 55 patients were randomized to the observation arm. The median survival rate was 20.4 months for patients in the chemotherapy arm but only 13.6 months for the patients having only surgery ($p = .01$). However, this study had a small sample size, and larger trials would be required to confirm the benefit observed. An Italian Trials in Medical Oncology (ITMO) study suggested a small benefit from postoperative adjuvant chemotherapy with etoposide, doxorubicin, and cisplatin followed by 5-FU and leucovorin in the subset of gastric cancer patients with widespread node involvement. For those patients with 7 or more involved nodes, 5-year overall survival rates were 42 percent in the treatment arm and 22 percent in the observation arm.[11]

Several meta-analyses of adjuvant chemotherapy for gastric cancer have been undertaken. A meta-analysis of randomized trials (published since 1980) of adjuvant 5-FU–based chemotherapy following curative resection for localized gastric cancer did not demonstrate a survival benefit, with an odds ratio of 0.88 (95% confidence interval [CI], 0.78 to 1.08).[12] This meta-analysis has been criticized for lacking sufficient power to detect a clinically relevant difference in survival.[13] A second meta-analysis (including 13 randomized controlled trials of adjuvant chemotherapy versus observation following curative resection for gastric cancer in non-Asian patients) has also been performed.[14] These results suggest that adjuvant chemotherapy may produce a small survival benefit of borderline statistical significance in patients with curatively resected gastric cancer (Figure 14–1). The odds ratio for death in the treated group was 0.80 (95% CI, 0.66 to 0.97), corresponding to a relative risk of 0.94 (95% CI, 0.89 to 1.00). A larger magnitude of the effect appeared when the analysis was restricted to trials in which at least two-thirds of patients had node-positive disease (odds ratio of 0.74 [95% CI, 0.59 to 0.95]). A small survival benefit of adjuvant chemotherapy after curative resection for gastric cancer has been demonstrated from a recently published third meta-analysis, which included 20 randomized trials (3 trials of a single agent, 7 trials of 5-FU with an anthracycline, and 10 trials of 5-FU combinations without an anthracycline).[15] The study collected information on 3,658 patients and 2,180 deaths, using death from any cause as the end point. The result showed that chemotherapy reduced the risk of death by 18 percent (a hazard ratio of 0.82 [95% CI, 0.75 to 0.89, $p < .001$]), which translates to an absolute survival advantage of 2 to 4 percent, depending on the stage of the disease. The use of chemotherapy alone in a routine fashion cannot be supported by the results of single trials or from these meta-analyses. The meta-analyses do, however, suggest that chemotherapy could play a role in adjuvant treatment. This seems quite reasonable, given the activity of chemotherapy in gastric cancer and given the benefits of adjuvant chemotherapy in other solid

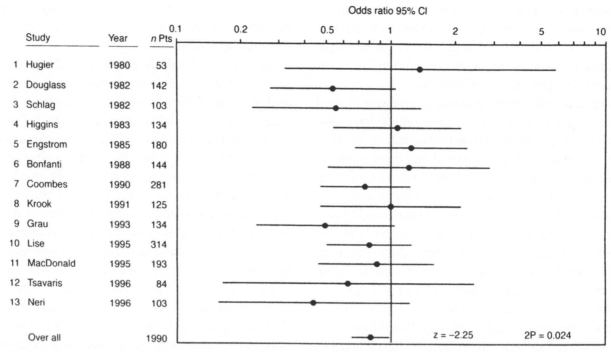

Figure 14–1.   Forrest plot of a meta-analysis of randomized trials comparing adjuvant chemotherapy with observation after curative resection of gastric cancer. (z = degree of freedom; 2P = two-sided p value; nPts = number of patients.) (Reproduced with permission from Earle CC, Maroun JA. Adjuvant chemotherapy after curative resection for gastric cancer in non-Asian patients: revisiting a meta-analysis of randomized trials. Eur J Cancer 1999;35:1059–64.)

tumors. Appropriately designed and statistically powered studies will be required to accomplish this.

ADJUVANT RADIATION THERAPY

Based on the high likelihood of local and regional recurrence after surgery for gastric cancer, there may be a role for adjuvant radiation. However, the position of the stomach limits the radiation dose that can be safely delivered, owing to the location of the spinal cord, kidneys, small bowel, and liver. After partial gastrectomy, the residual stomach is also a radiation-sensitive organ; thus, adjuvant radiation may result in significant ulceration and bleeding. Acute side effects including nausea, fatigue, and weight loss may occur when the upper abdomen is irradiated, which may make postoperative treatment difficult in a recovering patient.

Most reports of adjuvant radiation as a single modality have been of intraoperative radiation used alone or in combination with external beam radiation. A phase II study reported by the Radiation Therapy Oncology Group combined intraoperative radiation (12.5 to 16.5 Gy) and postoperative 45-Gy

external beam radiation.[16] Twenty-seven patients received intraoperative radiation, and 23 of those also received external beam radiation. Eighty-three percent of the patients had serosal involvement, and 70 percent had lymph node metastases. The actuarial 2-year survival was 47 percent, and there was local recurrence of disease in 15 percent of patients. Three small phase III trials using intraoperative radiation and/or external beam radiation postoperatively have also been reported. A survival advantage of a single dose of intraoperative radiation (20 to 25 Gy) after resection for patients with stages II, III, and IV disease (gross residual disease without metastases) was reported by Japanese researchers.[17] Unfortunately, these patients were randomized without regard to stratification criteria. A small randomized trial conducted by the National Cancer Institute compared external beam radiation (45 Gy) alone to intraoperative radiation plus external beam radiation following gastrectomy.[18] No survival difference was demonstrated, but the group that received intraoperative radiation plus external beam radiation had a lower local recurrence rate. A three-arm randomized trial from Britain compared gastrectomy alone to gastrectomy followed by 5-FU, doxorubicin, and methotrexate or postoperative radiation (45 Gy in 25 fractions).[20] There was no survival benefit for either adjuvant chemotherapy or the radiation. The second prospective randomized trial by the British Stomach Cancer Group also failed to demonstrate a survival benefit for postoperative adjuvant radiation; however, there was an apparent decrease in the rate of locoregional failure, from 27 to 10 percent.[20]

ADJUVANT CHEMORADIATION THERAPY

In a series of early trials at the Mayo Clinic, there was evidence of the superiority of 5-FU plus external beam radiation over radiation alone in a small randomized controlled trial involving patients with unresectable gastric cancer.[21] Based on these encouraging results, clinical investigators have considered the use of such therapy (which has been applied in patients with pancreatic, esophageal, and rectal tumors) in patients with resectable disease as well. Several single-institution phase II studies have suggested an improved survival for patients given postoperative adjuvant chemoradiation (Table 14–1).[22–25] A study done at the Massachusetts General Hospital reported a 4-year survival rate of 43 percent for 14 patients with poorly differentiated disease (80% of

them with lymph node metastases) who received adjuvant chemoradiation, a rate that was better than that expected in patients who underwent surgery only (38% survival for patients with negative lymph nodes, 15% survival for patients with positive lymph nodes).[22] Similar results were reported from another study with 25 patients who had locally advanced gastric cancer and who received postresection 5-FU–based chemoradiation.[23]

A few phase III studies have been performed to evaluate the benefit of adjuvant chemoradiation therapy for locally advanced gastric cancer.[26,27] Dent and colleagues conducted an early study comparing surgery alone in 31 patients to adjuvant chemoradiation with 20 Gy of external beam radiation and 5-FU in 35 patients.[26] There was no significant difference noted between the control and the treatment arms. However, the Mayo Clinic conducted a prospective randomized trial comparing gastrectomy alone with gastrectomy followed by adjuvant external beam radiation (37.5 Gy in 24 fractions) plus 5-FU (15 mg/kg bolus on days 1 through 3).[27] The patients, including those with scirrhous carcinomas, regional lymph node metastases, or adjacent organ involvement, were all considered to have poor prognoses. The 5-year survival rate in the adjuvant chemoradiation group was 23 percent, versus 4 percent in the surgery-only group ($p = .05$). Fifty-five percent of those patients who were treated by surgery alone had locoregional relapse as the first clinical recurrence, compared to 39 percent of those who had with adjuvant chemoradiation. However, the results of this trial are confounded by the fact that the study was done with a technique known as prerandomization. Ultimately, 10 patients who were randomized to adjuvant treatment refused chemoradiation, and these patients did as well as those patients who received adjuvant treatment.

In an attempt to clarify whether combined-modality chemoradiotherapy following curative-intent resection may benefit patients with locally advanced gastric cancer, a phase III intergroup study (INT-0116) was conducted in the United States.[28] For the first time, both disease-free survival (DFS) and overall survival (OS) in high-risk resected locally advanced adenocarcinoma of the stomach and gastroesophageal (GE) junction were demonstrated by this well-designed prospective phase III

Study (Reference No.)	No. of Patients	Median Survival (mo)	5-Year Survival (%)
Table 14–1. PHASE II TRIALS OF ADJUVANT CHEMORADIATION			
Gunderson et al (23)			
Surgery alone	110	NR	38 (node –); 15 (node +)
Surgery → 5-FU + XRT	14	24	43[*]
Gez et al (24)			
Surgery → 5-FU + XRT	25	33	40
Regine et al (25)			
Surgery alone	70	12	13
Surgery → chemo + XRT	20	19	21
Whittington et al (26)			
Surgery alone	40	16	31
Surgery → XRT	17	15	50
Surgery → chemo + XRT	20	21	55

chemo = chemotherapy; NR = not recorded; 5-FU = 5-fluorouracil; XRT = radiation therapy.
*4-year survival rate.

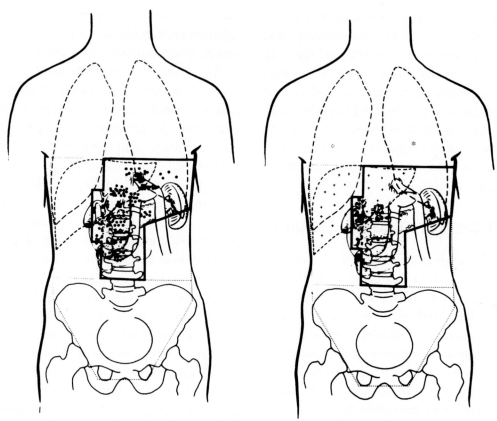

Figure 14–2.   Radiation field for gastric cancer in an adjuvant setting. The areas enclosed by the proposed radiation fields encompass the majority of locoregional failure sites. (Reproduced with permission from Gunderson LL, Sosin H. Adenocarcinoma of the stomach: areas of failure in a re-operation series [second or symptomatic look] clinicopathologic correlation and implications for adjuvant therapy. Int J Radiol Biol Phys 1982;8:1–11.)

trial. In INT-0116, patients with complete resections (ie, R0 resections), negative margins, and no evidence of residual disease were randomized to receive surgery alone or surgery plus postoperative chemotherapy with 5-FU and leucovorin and concurrent radiation therapy (Figure 14–2). The type of lymphadenectomy was not mandated by the study protocol although D2 resection was recommended. From the analysis, it was observed that only 54 patients (9.9%) underwent formal D2 dissections, 199 patients (36%) underwent D1 dissections (removal of all N1 nodes), and the rest of the patients (54%) underwent D0 dissections (ie, less than complete dissection of the N1 nodal stations). This has prompted the criticism that more complete surgery should have been performed and that the results of the study would not be applicable if more D2 dissections had been done. Randomization was performed between 20 and 40 days after surgery, with stratification based on tumor stage (T1 to T2 vs T3 vs T4) and nodal sta-

tus (none vs 1 to 3 vs 4 or more positive). The treatment consisted of one cycle of 5-FU (425 mg/m²) and leucovorin (20 mg/m²) in a 5-times-daily regimen (the Mayo Clinic regimen), followed by 45 Gy (180 cGy/d) of radiation 28 days later, given with 5-FU (400 mg/m²) and leucovorin (20 mg/m²) on days 1 through 4 and on the last 3 days of radiation. One month after completion of radiation therapy, two cycles of 5-FU (425 mg/m²) and leucovorin (20 mg/m²) daily for 5 days were given at monthly intervals. Doses of 5-FU were reduced in patients experiencing grade 3 and grade 4 toxicity. Modified schedules of 5-FU/leucovorin were given with radiation therapy. Based on the knowledge and experience from previous studies in gastrointestinal tumors, specific attention was given to the designation and monitoring of radiation, to allow for optimal quality control. The therapy was designed in a "sandwich" fashion to allow for the delayed start of radiation and to allow for a prospective external review of radiation

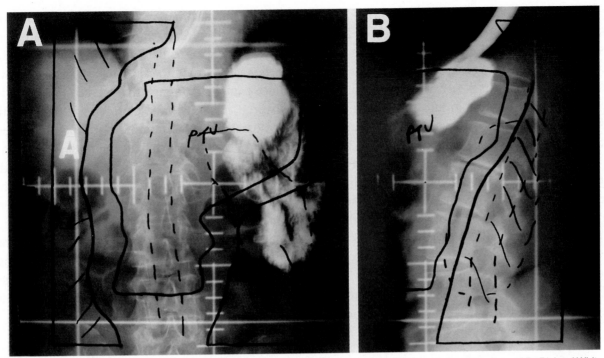

Figure 14–3. Radiation port for treatment of gastric cancer. *A,* Anteroposterior view. *B,* lateral view. (Courtesy of Dr Richard Whittington, Professor of Medicine, Radiation Oncology, University of Pennsylvania.)

ports before treatment commenced. Radiotherapy consisted of 45 Gy in 25 fractions, 5 days per week, to the original tumor bed, regional nodes, and proximal and distal resection margins plus 2 cm. The designed size and coverage area for radiation were based on the results of early studies of the locoregional patterns of recurrence of gastric cancer (Figure 14–3).[29] The original tumor bed was defined on the basis of preoperative computed tomographic imaging, barium studies, and surgical clips. The Japanese Research Society for the Study of Gastric Cancer (JRSGC) definition of the extent of the regional lymph node involvement was used.[30] Perigastric, celiac, local para-aortic, splenic, hepatoduodenal, portahepatic, and pancreaticoduodenal lymph nodes were included in the radiation fields (Figure 14–4). Patients with GE-junction tumors had the additional inclusion of paracardial and paraesophageal nodes in radiation fields, but pancreaticodudenal radiation was not required. Splenic nodes were excluded in patients with antral lesions if doing so was necessary to spare volumes of the left kidney. Dose limiting of radiation to structures was defined as follows: for the liver, < 60 percent of hepatic volume exposed to > 30 Gy; for the kidneys, the equivalent of at least two-thirds of one kidney spared from the radiotherapy field; for the heart, < 30 percent of the cardiac silhouette exposed to > 40 Gy.

At the initial radiotherapy quality control review, prior to treatment implementation, 35 percent of treatment plans were found to contain major or minor deviations due either to critical-organ toxicity or to failure to treat protocol-defined target volumes. The overwhelming majority of these errors were corrected prior to the initiation of radiotherapy. The final radiotherapy quality assurance review (following the delivery of radiation) for those with complete documentation revealed 6.5 percent major deviations. The importance of nutrition was emphasized in the study, and careful attention was paid to the patient's nutritional status. Most of the patients had appropriate nutritional support before and during treatment. Between August 1991 and July 1998, 603 patients were accrued, and 556 patients were eligible for the study. The surgery-alone observation arm included 275 patients; 281 patients were in the combined-modality arm. For all eligible patients, the median follow-up was 5 years. The median survival was 36 months for patients in the adjuvant-chemoradiation arm versus 26 months for patients in the surgery-only arm (a hazard ratio of 1.35) (p = .005; 95% CI, 1.09 to 1.66) (Figure 14–5). The 3-year OS rates were 50 percent for the treatment group and 40 percent for the observation group. The 3-year DFS rates were 48 percent for the treatment group and 31 percent for the observation group. The median DFS rates were 30 months for treated patients and 19 months for surgery-only patients, with a hazard ratio of 1.52 (p < .001; 95% CI, 1.23 to 1.86) (Figure 14–6). The toxicities of the chemoradiation appeared acceptable, with hematologic and gastrointestinal toxicities being the predominant adverse events. Grade 3 and grade 4 toxicity occurred in 41 percent and 32 percent of cases, respectively, and three patients (1%) died due to toxicities.

This study was the first large well-controlled study demonstrating a significant survival advan-tage to adjuvant therapy for gastric cancer. Com-bined-modality treatment should therefore be con-sidered the new standard of care in gastric cancer when gastric resection has been performed with curative intent. Although this therapy may be safely delivered, it is important to emphasize that radiation oncologists must be familiar with the proper tech-niques of delivering upper-abdominal radiation in postgastrectomy patients, and care must be paid to the maintenance of adequate nutrition during ther-apy. In this study, there was no compelling evidence that more extensive surgery (ie, D2 dissection) obviated the need for radiation and chemotherapy postoperatively. However, some investigators have questioned whether the more aggressive D2 dissec-tion could eliminate the need for radiation therapy in future trials.

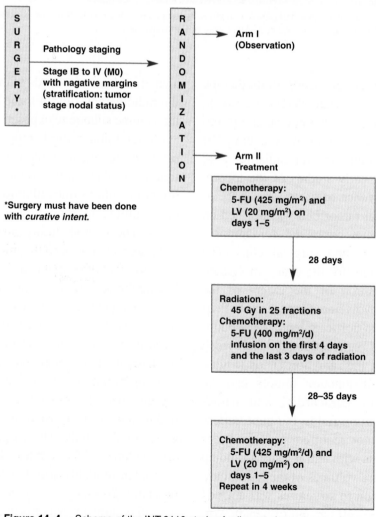

Figure 14–4. Schema of the INT-0116 study of adjuvant chemotherapy for gas-tric cancer. (5-FU = 5-fluorouracil; LV = leucovorin.)

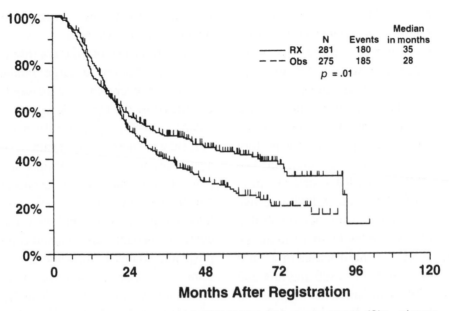

Figure 14–5. Overall survival rates in the INT-0116 study, by treatment arm. (Obs = observation arm; RX = radiation arm; N = population size). (Data from Dr. John S. Macdonald.)

NEOADJUVANT CHEMORADIATION AND CHEMOTHERAPY

It has been shown that neoadjuvant chemoradiation therapy can down-stage gastric cancer and the pathologic complete responses can be achieved, but no obvious long-term survival benefit has yet been proven in a randomized trial.[31–33] Down-staging of the tumor may benefit a subgroup of patients with favorable tumor characteristics, but this has been difficult to prove clinically. Obvious down-staging benefits have been shown in several phase II studies. In one study, three cycles of docetaxel (75 mg/m^2 on day 1) and cisplatin (75 mg/m^2 on day 1) were given as induction chemotherapy, with the support of prophylactic granulocyte colony–stimulating factor (G-

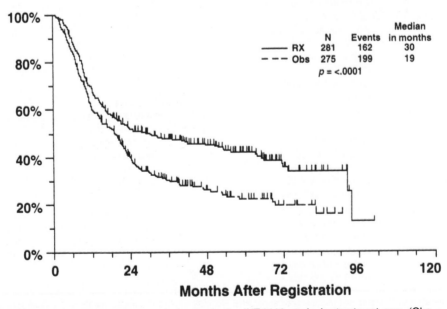

Figure 14–6. Relapse-free survival rates in the INT-0116 study, by treatment arm. (Obs = observation arm; RX = radiation arm; N = population size.) (Data from Dr. John S. Macdonald.)

CSF).[34] Radiation therapy (200 cGy/d, to a total of 50 Gy) with concurrent weekly docetaxel (20 mg/m^2) was given 3 to 4 weeks before surgery. Thirty-two patients underwent surgical resection. Of these, 14 had pathologic complete responses and 10 had only microscopic residual disease. In another study, induction therapy of irinotecan (CPT-11) and cisplatin (75 mg/m^2 and 25 mg/m^2, respectively, four times weekly every 6 weeks, delivered in two courses) was given, followed by R0 gastric resection in 10 patients.[35] Out of 10 patients, 8 had objective partial responses to the neoadjuvant therapy. With a median follow-up of 6.8 months (5 to 12 months), all 10 patients were free of the disease. In a third study, continuous-infusion 5-FU (300 mg/m^2) and 45 Gy of external beam radiation were given to patients with gastric cancer, followed by a D2 gastrectomy with 10 Gy of intraoperative radiation.[36] Of 34 patients who underwent resection, 5 had pathologic complete responses while 18 had partial responses with evidence of down-staging. It is therefore clear that preoperative chemoradiation can down-stage patients, but no data as to whether such

treatment affects the ultimate curability of such patients are yet available.

To further explore the contribution of perioperative chemotherapy, a large randomized study of neoadjuvant chemotherapy for esophageal cancer was conducted by the United Kingdom Medical Research Council (MRC) Upper GI Tract Cancer Group and has shown encouraging results. These results may also apply to patients with gastric cancer, since 67 percent of the patients had adenocarcinomas and 64 percent had lower-third esophageal tumors.[37] Eight hundred and two patients were randomized to two cycles of neoadjuvant chemotherapy before surgery (cisplatin, 80 mg/m^2 for 4 hours; 5-FU, 1 g/m^2 by continuous infusion for 4 days) or to surgery alone. Resectability was significantly higher in the treatment arm (78% vs 70% [$p < .001$]), as was the overall survival ($p = .003$). The European Organization for the Research and Treatment of Cancer (EORTC) initiated a phase III randomized multicenter study to compare surgery alone to preoperative chemotherapy with cisplatin, leucovorin, and 5-FU followed by surgery in patients with locally advanced gastric carcinoma

Table 14–2. PHASE III NEOADJUVANT CHEMOTHERAPY TRIALS					
Trial	No. of Patients	Neoadjuvant Treatment Arm	Control Arm	Postsurgery Treatment	Other Tests
EORTC 40954	360	Cisplatin IV over 1 h on days 1, 15, 29 Leucovorin IV over 2 h, followed by 5-FU IV over 24 h on days 1, 8, 15, 22, 29, 36 Repeat the treatment in 2 wk	—	See "Other Tests"	QOL is assessed before randomization, every 3 mo for 1 yr, and at 2 yr
FRE-FNCLCC9012	250	5-FU CI IV on days 1–5 Cisplatin IV on days 1, 2, for 2 cycles 3 cycles (for patients with response and without serious toxicity)	—	3–4 courses of same chemotherapy to patients who responded to neoadjuvant chemotherapy	R2 resection with at least 8 nodal groups recommended
MRCST02	500	5-FU CI IV for 3 wk Cisplatin IV over 4 h (4 h after 5-FU initiated) on day 1 Epirubicin IV on day 1 (ECF) for 3 cycles	—	3 additional ECF cycles for patients in neoadjuvant arm	QOL is assessed at baseline, at completion of study therapy, then every 6 mo for 2 y

EORTC = European Organization for Research and Treatment of Cancer; FRE-FNCLCC = French-Federation Nationale des Centres de Lutte Contre le Cancer; MRC = Medical Research Council; CI = continuous infusion; 5-FU = 5-fluorouracil; QOL = quality of life; IV = intravenous; ECF = epirubicin/cisplatin [CDDP]/5-FU; wk = weeks.

(Table 14–2). A similar phase III study (surgery alone vs neoadjuvant fluorouracil/cisplatin plus surgery for the lower third of esophagus or cardia adenocarcinoma) is now being performed by the French-Federation Nationale des Centres de Lutte Contre le Cancer (FRE-FNCLCC). The MRC is currently conducting a phase III randomized study of perioperative chemotherapy with epirubicin/cisplatin/5-FU (ECF) versus surgery alone for resectable gastric adenocarcinoma.

OTHER TREATMENTS IN THE ADJUVANT SETTING

Intraperitoneal Chemotherapy and Intraperitoneal Hyperthermic Chemoperfusion

The rationale of intraperitoneal chemotherapy is that locoregional failure occurs in 40 to 65 percent of patients who relapse after curative gastric resections.[29,38] Reports from autopsy and second-look laparotomy have revealed that up to 50 percent of patients have peritoneal carcinomatosis as a site of failure. Significantly higher drug concentrations within the peritoneal cavity can be achieved by intraperitoneal delivery than by intravenous or oral administration. Results of intraperitoneal chemotherapy in other cancers, such as ovarian cancer, support its use in gastric cancer. Intraperitoneal chemotherapy may be delivered intraoperatively or after surgery; the most commonly used procedure involves intraperitoneal treatment (with or without hyperthermia) following surgery. Mitomycin-C, 5-FU, floxuridine (FUDR), and cisplatin have all been used, but no difference in overall survival is apparent among these agents.[39,40]

Most of the studies of intraperitoneal hyperthermic chemoperfusion (IHCP) have been conducted by Japanese investigators. For those patients with peritoneal disease or a high risk of developing carcinomatosis, IHCP has been administered during exploratory laparotomy.[41,42] The efficacy of prophylactic or therapeutic IHCP with mitomycin-C (with or without cisplatin) administered immediately after resection for gastric cancer has been evaluated in several multiarm studies, mainly in Japan.[43–45] Suggestions of survival benefit have been reported from these relatively small trials.[46] The feasibility of IHCP is currently being evaluated at several centers in the United States and Europe.

Immunochemotherapy

Immunochemotherapy has also been used as adjuvant treatment following the resection of gastric cancer; most trials of such treatment have been conducted in Japan and Korea. Japanese investigators conducted studies of the administration of protein-bound polysaccharide (PSK) in the adjuvant setting, either alone or combined with 5-FU and/or mitomycin-C after gastrectomy.[47] One study randomized postresection gastric cancer patients to weekly chemotherapy with mitomycin and 5-FU or to PSK plus the same chemotherapy. The 5-year DFS rate was 70.7 percent in the PSK-plus-chemotherapy group versus 59.4 percent in the standard-treatment group ($p = .047$). The 5-year survival rates were 73 percent and 60 percent, respectively ($p = .044$).[48] Korean investigators reported a trial that compared FAM to intradermally administered OK-432 (a *Streptococcus progenes* preparation) plus the standard FAM regimen in patients with gastric carcinoma who underwent curative resection.[49] Fifty patients received chemotherapy only, and 49 patients had chemotherapy with OK-432 as an immunostimulant. A significant improvement in survival with chemotherapy plus immunotherapy over chemotherapy alone was reported (respective 5-year survival rates of 62 percent and 52 percent [$p = .04$]). The prognostic advantage of preoperative intratumoral injection of OK-432 for patients with gastric cancer has also been suggested by a Japanese study.[50] These data suggest that it is possible that immunotherapy or immunochemotherapy may benefit the outcome for those gastric cancer patients who have had potentially curative gastrectomy. However, these trials were small and were without sufficient statistical power to convincingly demonstrate a clinical benefit.

CONCLUSION

The use of adjuvant treatment in gastric cancer is dictated by the high rate of recurrence in optimally resected patients. The risk of recurrence is even higher in patients with serosal extension, positive lymph nodes, or positive surgical margins. The result of the large and well-controlled intergroup INT-0116 study demonstrated a survival advantage for chemoradiation therapy with acceptable toxicity; in the United States, this therapy is the standard adjuvant treatment today for gastric cancer, following curative intent-resection. From the conduct of the study, it must be stressed that radiation oncologists must be well trained in the proper techniques of delivering upper-abdominal radiation in postgastrectomy patients, and attention must also be paid to the maintenance of adequate nutrition during therapy. Whether such treatment is appropriate in other countries, where surgical treatments and tumor biology may be different, is open to question. Of particular interest is the question of whether a large properly controlled program of adjuvant chemotherapy would be as effective as the chemoradiation administered in the INT-0116 study, particularly when a D2 dissection is performed. Neoadjuvant chemotherapy or chemoradiation is under active study to ascertain whether an increase in the number of patients undergoing potentially curative operations will translate into a survival benefit. More information from large well-controlled studies is necessary to evaluate intraperitoneal chemotherapy (including IHCP), immunochemotherapy, and other biologic treatments. More studies are also needed to assess molecular prognostic risk factors for gastric cancer (eg, loss of heterozygosity of chromosome 5q, p53, ras, E-cadherin, microsatellite instability, HER-2/neu, epidermal growth factor receptor [EGFR], and cyclooxygenase-2 [COX-2]) and to assess target-oriented treatments for these molecular alterations.

ACKNOWLEDGMENT

The author would like to thank Dr. Richard Whittington, Dr. John S. Macdonald, Dr. Leonard Gunderson, and Dr. Craig Earle for their support.

REFERENCES

1. Greenlee RT, Hill-Harmon MB, Murray T, et al. Cancer statistics, 2001. CA Cancer J Clin 2001;51:15–36.
2. Parkin D, Pisani P, Ferlay J. Global cancer statistics. CA Cancer J Clin 1999;49:33–64.
3. Gastrointestinal Tumor Study Group. Controlled trial of adjuvant chemotherapy following curative resection for gastric cancer. Cancer 1982;49:1116-22.
4. Engstrom P, Lavin P, Douglass H. Postoperative adjuvant 5-fluorouracil plus methyl CCNU therapy for gastric cancer. Cancer 1985;55:1868–73.
5. Estape J, Grau JJ, Alcobends F, et al. Mitomycin C as an adjuvant treatment to resected gastric cancer. A 10-year follow-up. Ann Surg 1991;213:219–21.
6. Carrato A, Diaz-Rubio E, Medrano J, et al. Phase III trial of surgery versus adjuvant chemotherapy with mitomycin C and tegafur plus uracil, starting within the first week after surgery, for gastric adenocarcinoma. Proc Am Soc Clin Oncol 1995;14:A198.
7. Allum WH, Hallissey MT, Kelly KA. Adjuvant chemotherapy in operable gastric cancer: 5-year follow-up of first British Stomach Cancer Group trial. Lancet 1989;1:571–4.
8. Coombes RC, Schein PS, Chilvers CE, et al. A randomized trial comparing adjuvant fluorouracil, doxorubicin, and mitomycin with no treatment in operable gastric cancer. International Collaborative Cancer Group. J Clin Oncol 1990;8:1362–9.
9. Krook JE, O'Connell MJ, Wieand HS, et al. A prospective, randomized evaluation of intensive-course 5-fluorouracil plus doxorubicin as surgical adjuvant chemotherapy for resected gastric cancer. Cancer 1991;67:2454–8.
10. Neri B, de Leonardis V, Romano S, et al. Adjuvant chemotherapy after gastric resection in node-positive cancer patients: a multicenter randomized study. Br J Cancer 1996;73:549–52.
11. Bartolomeo MD, Bajetta E, Bordogna G, et al. Improved adjuvant therapy outcome in resected gastric cancer patients (Pts) according to node involvement. 5-year results of randomized study by the Italian Trials in Medical Oncology (ITMO) Group. Proc Am Soc Clin Oncol 2000;19:A934.
12. Hermans J, Bonenkamp JJ, Boon MC, et al. Adjuvant therapy after curative resection for gastric cancer: meta-analysis of randomized trials. J Clin Oncol 1993;11:1441–7.
13. Pignon JP, Ducreux M, Rougier P. Meta-analysis of adjuvant chemotherapy in gastric cancer: a critical reappraisal. J Clin Oncol 1994;12:877–8.
14. Earle CC, Maroun JA. Adjuvant chemotherapy after curative resection for gastric cancer in non-Asian patients: revisiting a meta-analysis of randomized trials. Eur J Cancer 1999;35:1059–64.
15. Mari E, Floriani I, Tinazzi A, et al. Efficacy of adjuvant chemotherapy after curative resection for gastric cancer: a meta-analysis of published randomized trials. A study of the GISCAD. Ann Oncol 2000;11:837–43.
16. Avizonis VN, Buzydlowski J, Lanciano R, et al. Treatment of adenocarcinoma of the stomach with resection, intraoperative radiotherapy, and adjuvant external beam radiation: a phase II study from Radiation Therapy Oncology Group 85-01. Ann Surg Oncol 1995;2:295–302.
17. Abe M, Takahashi M. Intraoperative radiotherapy: the Japanese experience. Int J Radiat Oncol Biol Phys 1981;7:863–8.
18. Sindelar WF, Kinsella TJ, Tepper JE, et al. Randomized trial of intraoperative radiation in carcinoma of the stomach. Am J Surg 1993;165:178–87.

19. Allum WH, Hallissey MT, Ward LC, et al. A controlled, prospective, randomized trial of adjuvant chemotherapy or radiotherapy in respectable gastric cancer: interim report: British Stomach Cancer Group. Br J Cancer 1989; 60:739–44.

20. Hallissey MT, Dunn JA, Ward LC, et al. The second British Stomach Cancer Group trial of adjuvant radiotherapy or chemotherapy in resectable gastric cancer: five-year follow-up. Lancet 1994;343:1309–12.

21. Moertel CG, Childs DS Jr, Reitemeier RJ, et al. Combined 5-FU and supervoltage radiation therapy of locally unresectable gastrointestinal cancer. Lancet 1969;2:865–7.

22. Gunderson LL, Hoskins RB, Cohen AC. Combined modality treatment of gastric cancer. Int J Radiat Oncol Biol Phys 1983;9:965–75.

23. Gez E, Sulkes A, Yablonsky-Peretz T, et al. Combined 5-fluorouracil (5-FU) and radiation therapy following resection of locally advanced gastric carcinoma of the stomach. J Surg Oncol 1986;31:139–42.

24. Regine WF, Mohiuddin M. Impact of adjuvant therapy on locally advanced adenocarcinoma of the stomach. Int J Radiat Oncol Biol Phys 1992;24:921–7.

25. Whittington R, Coia LR, Haller DG, et al. Adenocarcinoma of the esophagus and esophagogastric junction: the effects of single and combined modalities on the survival and patterns of failure following treatment. Int J Radiat Oncol Biol Phys 1990;19:593–603.

26. Dent DM, Werner ID, Novis B, et al. Prospective randomized trial of combined oncological therapy for gastric carcinoma. Cancer 1979;44:385–91.

27. Moertel CG, Childs DS, O'Fallon JR, et al. Combined 5-fluorouracil and radiation therapy as a surgical adjuvant for poor prognosis gastric carcinoma. J Clin Oncol 1984;2: 1249–54.

28. Macdonald JS, Smalley SR, Benedetti J, et al. chemoradiotherapy after surgery compared with surgery alone for adenocarcinoma of the stomach or gastroesophageal junction. N Engl J Med 2001;345:725–30.

29. Gunderson LL, Sosin H. Adenocarcinoma of the stomach: areas of failure in a re-operation series (second or symptomatic look). Clinicopathologic correlation and implications for adjuvant therapy. Int J Radiat Biol Phys 1982; 8:1–11.

30. Nishi M, Omori Y, Miwa K, editors. Japanese classification of gastric carcinoma. 1st English ed. Japanese Research Society for Gastric Cancer. Tokyo: Kanehara and Co. Ltd.; 1995.

31. Kelsen DP. Adjuvant and neoadjuvant therapy for gastric cancer. Semin Oncol 1996;23:379–489.

32. Lowy AM, Mansfield PF, Leach SD, et al. Response to neoadjuvant chemotherapy best predicts survival after curative resection of gastric cancer. Ann Surg 1999;229:303–8.

33. Stein HJ, Sendler A, Fink U, et al. Multidisciplinary approach to esophageal and gastric cancer. Surg Clin North Am 2000;80:659–82.

34. Mauer AM, Haraf DC, Ferguson MK, et al. Docetaxel-based combined modality therapy for locally advanced carcinoma of the esophagus and gastric carcinoma. Proc Am Soc Clin Oncol 2000;19:A954.

35. Potmesil M, Newman E, Yee H, et al. Neoadjuvant therapy of gastric adenocarcinoma by CPT-11 (camptosar) and cisplatin: preliminary surgical and histopathologic finding. Proc Am Clin Oncol 2000;19:A1209.

36. Mansfield PF, Lowy AM, Feig BW, et al. Preoperative chemoradiation for potentially resectable gastric cancer. Proc Am Clin Oncol 2000;19:A955.

37. Clark P, MRC Clinic Trials Unit. Surgical resection with or without pre-operative chemotherapy in oesophageal cancer: an updated analysis of a randomized controlled trial conducted by the UK Medical Research Council upper GI tract cancer group. Proc Am Clin Oncol 2001;20:A502.

38. Landry J, Tepper J, Wood W, et al. Analysis of survival and local control following surgery for gastric cancer. Int J Radiat Oncol Biol Phys 1990;191:1357–62.

39. Yu W, Whang I, Suh I, et al. Prospective randomized trial of early postoperative intraperitoneal chemotherapy as an adjuvant to respectable gastric cancer. Ann Surg 1998; 228:347–54.

40. Sautner T, Hofbauer F, Dipisch D, et al. Adjuvant intraperitoneal cisplatin chemotherapy dose not improve long-term survival after surgery for advanced gastric cancer. J Clin Oncol 1994;12:970–4.

41. Dedrick RL. Theoretical and experimental bases of intraperitoneal chemotherapy. Semin Oncol 1985;12 Suppl 4:1–6.

42. Los G, Smals OA, van Vugt MJ, et al. A rationale for carboplatin treatment and abdominal hyperthemia in cancers restricted to the peritoneal cavity. Cancer Res 1992;52: 1252–8.

43. Fujimura T, Yonemura Y, Fushida S, et al. Continuous hyperthermic peritoneal perfusion for the treatment of peritoneal dissemination in gastric cancer and subsequent second-look operation. Cancer 1990;65:65–71.

44. Koga S, Hamazoe R, Maeta M, et al. Prophylactic peritoneal perfusion with mitomycin C. Cancer 1988;61:232–7.

45. Hamazoe R, Maeta M, Kaibara N. Intraperitoneal thermochemotherapy for prevention of peritoneal recurrence of gastric cancer. Cancer 1994;73:2048–52.

46. Fujimoto S, Takahashi M, Mutou T, et al. Successful intraperitoneal hyperhermic chemoperfusion for the prevention of postoperative peritoneal recurrence in patients with advanced gastric carcinoma. Cancer 1999;85:529–34.

47. Iguchi C, Nio Y Takeda H, et al. Plant polysaccharide PSK: cytostatic effects on growth and invasion; modulating effect on the expression of HLA and adhesion molecules on human gastric and colonic tumor cell surface. Anticancer Res 2001;21(2A):1007–13.

48. Nakazato H, Koike A, Saji S, et al. Efficacy of immunochemotherapy as adjuvant treatment after curative resection of gastric cancer. Lancet 1994;343:1122–6.

49. Kim SY, Park HC, Yoon C, et al. OK-432 and 5-fluorouracil, doxorubicin, and mitomycin C (FAM-P) versus FAM chemotherapy in patients with curatively resected gastric carcinoma: a randomized phase III trial. Cancer 1998;83: 2054–9.

50. Gochi A, Orita K, Fuchimoto S, et al. The prognostic advantage of preoperative intratumoral injection of OK-432 for gastric cancer patients. Br J Cancer 2001;84:443–51.

15

Nonsurgical Palliative Therapy of Advanced Gastric Cancer

TOMISLAV DRAGOVICH, MD, PHD
HEDY LEE KINDLER, MD

It is projected that more than two-thirds of the 21,700 patients diagnosed with gastric cancer in the United States in the year 2001 will have unresectable disease.[1] Even for those patients with resectable disease, the expected median survival is only 24 months, and the 5-year survival rate does not exceed 30 percent.[2] The high incidence of local and distant recurrences implies that even when localized, gastric cancer behaves as a systemic disease.[3,4] For patients with metastatic disease, treatment options are limited to palliative noncurative therapies.

The goals of palliative therapy are to control cancer-related symptoms and prolong survival without compromising quality of life. This can be achieved with chemotherapy, radiation therapy, palliative surgical interventions, or supportive medical care. Several small randomized trials have demonstrated a modest survival advantage for patients with metastatic gastric cancer who receive palliative chemotherapy. In spite of the innumerable single agents and combinations that have been tested, the impact of chemotherapy on patient survival has been disappointing. The median survival of patients with metastatic disease remains between 6 and 9 months. This does not differ significantly from the 1968 report by Moertel that described a cohort of untreated patients with advanced gastric cancer.[5]

The search for more effective therapies that will make a difference in the natural history of gastric cancer continues. Recent advances in molecular biology and experimental pharmacology provide hope that more active and less toxic therapies will soon become available. This chapter reviews the history and the current status of palliative nonsurgical therapy for metastatic gastric cancer. The palliation of advanced gastric cancer via invasive methods is reviewed in the following chapter.

CLINICAL CHARACTERISTICS OF ADVANCED DISEASE

Both local invasion and metastatic spread to distant sites are responsible for the clinical manifestations of advanced gastric cancer. The most commonly encountered symptoms are weight loss, epigastric pain, nausea, and vomiting. Anorexia and weight loss are unfavorable prognostic signs.[6] Patients frequently present with symptoms caused by metastases. Physical signs such as a palpable abdominal mass, a distended stomach with a succussion splash, and hepatomegaly indicate advanced disease. Other late manifestations may result from gastric outlet obstruction, from bleeding, or from invasion of surrounding organs such as the liver, pancreas, bile ducts, transverse colon, and celiac plexus.

Gastric cancer metastasizes initially to regional lymph nodes and then spreads to more distant locations, including periumbilical ("Sister Mary Joseph node"), left supraclavicular (Virchow's node), and left axillary ("Irish's node") sites. Peritoneal carcinomatosis is common; it may involve the pouch of Douglas, in which case a mass can be felt on rectal examination (Blumer's shelf). Metastasis to the ovary (Krukenberg's tumor) is another typical finding in patients with peritoneal dissemination. Other metastatic sites include the liver, lung, bone, and (less commonly) the adrenal glands, brain, and kidney (Table 15–1).[7]

Paraneoplastic manifestations commonly associated with gastric cancer include hypertrophic pulmonary osteoarthropathy, cancer cachexia, dermatomyositis, acanthosis nigricans, and thromboembolism (Trousseau's syndrome).[8–11]

CLINICAL EVALUATION OF PATIENTS WITH ADVANCED GASTRIC CANCER

The initial work-up of the patient with suspected metastatic disease should include an upper endoscopy for evaluation of the primary tumor. This is appropriate even for patients who are not surgical candidates since it can help to identify and treat local complications such as obstruction or bleeding from the primary lesion. A computed tomography (CT) of the abdomen, chest radiography, complete blood count, and chemistries including a hepatic panel will suffice as the initial work-up for most patients with advanced disease. Additional clinical evaluations are dictated by the patient's symptoms. Computed tomography of the brain or radionuclide bone scanning should not be routinely done in the absence of symptoms. Computed tomography is the most effective imaging modality for assessing the interval response to chemotherapy (Figure 15–1). Endoscopic ultrasonography (EUS) has a sensitivity superior to that of CT for the initial staging of gastric tumors.[12,13] The role of EUS in the evaluation of treatment response in more advanced disease is less well established.[14]

The role of tumor markers in evaluating cancer progression or response to therapy is limited. Carci-

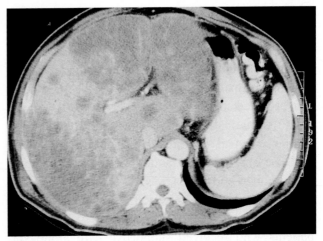

Figure 15–1. Computed tomography of the abdomen: gastric adenocarcinoma metastatic to the liver.

noembryonic antigen (CEA), CA19-9, CA125, and CA50 are elevated in a small proportion of patients with gastric cancer and have not been evaluated as indicators of treatment response.[15] Newer markers such as fibrinopeptide A, tissue polypeptide antigen, gastrointestinal cancer–associated antigen, and cobalamin-binding protein may prove more useful than CEA and CA19-9.[16]

For patients on chemotherapy, the toxicities of some of the drugs commonly used to treat gastric cancer may require additional laboratory monitoring. This includes assessments of hematopoietic, renal, hepatic, and cardiac functions.

CHEMOTHERAPY VERSUS SUPPORTIVE CARE

Although gastric cancer is a chemoresponsive malignancy, responses are of brief duration, and the impact of chemotherapy on patient survival is minimal. Four randomized trials have evaluated the impact of chemotherapy on survival and quality of life (QOL), compared to the best supportive care (BSC) (Table 15–2). The interpretation of this information is problematic since a total of only 174 patients have been randomized in the four trials.

Murad and colleagues compared the survival of patients treated with combined 5-fluorouracil, doxorubicin, and methotrexate (FAMTX) to that of a control group of patients who received only BSC.[17] Due to an observed survival difference in favor of the

| Table 15–1. COMMON SITES OF METASTASIS IN PATIENTS WITH METASTATIC GASTRIC CANCER ||
Site	% Involved
Liver	54
Peritoneum	24
Lung	22
Pancreas	29
Adrenal gland	15
Bone	11

Adapted from Dupont JB Jr, Lee Jr, Burton GR, et al. Adenocarcinoma of the stomach: review of 1,497 cases. Cancer 1978;41:941–7.

treatment group, the randomization was terminated after only 22 patients were enrolled; subsequent patients received chemotherapy. The median survival of the 30 patients who received chemotherapy was 9 months, compared with 3 months for the 10 patients who received supportive care only ($p < .001$).

A statistically significant improvement in median survival favoring the chemotherapy group was also observed in a randomized study conducted by Pyrhonen and colleagues.[18] Patients who received 5-fluorouracil, epirubicin, and methotrexate (FEMTX) achieved a median survival of 12 months; patients who received supportive care alone survived a median of only 3 months ($p < .001$). Similarly, in a 37-patient German study, the median survival of patients in the supportive care group was only 4 months whereas patients treated with etoposide, leucovorin, and fluorouracil (ELF) achieved a median survival of 7.5 months ($p < .05$).[19]

The largest trial, with 61 patients, was conducted by Glimelius and colleagues.[20] Patients were randomized either to immediate chemotherapy including BSC or to BSC alone. Those patients randomized to BSC could subsequently receive chemotherapy if supportive measures did not provide adequate palliation. Patients received ELF chemotherapy unless they were over 60 years of age or had a Karnofsky performance status of 70 percent or less, in which case they received 5-fluorouracil (5-FU) plus leucovorin. In addition to assessing patient survival, this trial assessed QOL, using a validated European Organization for Research and Treatment of Cancer (EORTC) Quality of Life Questionnaire–Core 30 (QLQ-C30) instrument. Forty-five percent of patients in the chemotherapy group reported an improved QOL for at least 4 months, compared with only 20 percent of patients in the supportive care group who reported an improved QOL. In the treatment group, there was a trend toward an increased median survival (8 months versus 5 months) that did not reach statistical significance ($p = .12$).

The analysis of these trials has been hampered by the small number of accrued patients and by differences in the chemotherapy regimens. Nevertheless, these four studies appear to support the use of palliative chemotherapy to improve QOL and lengthen survival in patients with advanced gastric cancer.

CHEMOTHERAPY

The role of systemic chemotherapy in patients with gastric cancer was first evaluated in the 1960s.[21] Among the first drugs tested were 5-FU, the nitrosoureas, mitomycin C, and doxorubicin (Table 15–3).[22,23] Response evaluation in these early clinical trials was limited by the lack of sensitive imaging tests such as CT or magnetic resonance imaging (MRI). Therefore, one needs to account for the effect of stage migration when comparing the outcomes of the early trials to those of more recent ones.

Table 15–2. TRIALS OF CHEMOTHERAPY VERSUS BEST SUPPORTIVE CARE IN GASTRIC CANCER PATIENTS

Regimen	No. of Patients	Median Survival (mo)	p-Value	Reference
FAMTX	30	9	< .001	Murad et al, 1993
vs BSC	10	3		
FEMTX	17	12	< .001	Pyrhonen et al, 1995
vs BSC	19	3		
ELF	18	7.5	< .05	Scheithauer et al, 1995
vs BSC	19	4		
ELF or LF	31	8	< .12	Glimelius et al, 1997
vs BSC	30	5		

FAMTX = 5-fluorouracil, doxorubicin, methotrexate; BSC = best supportive care; FEMTX = 5-fluorouracil, epirubicin, methotrexate; ELF = etoposide, leucovorin, 5-fluorouracil; LF = leucovorin, 5-fluorouracil.

Table 15–3. SINGLE-AGENT CHEMOTHERAPY FOR GASTRIC CANCER

Drug	Number of Patients	Response Rate (%)	Reference
Older agents			
5-Fluorouracil	392	21	Comis and Carter, 1974
Ftorafur	73	10	Blokhina et al, 1972
Mitomycin-C	211	30	Comis et al, 1974
Doxorubicin	141	17	Moertel et al, 1979
Epirubicin	50	16	Cersosimo et al, 1986
Cisplatin	139	19	Perry et al, 1986
Hydroxyurea	31	19	Comis and Carter, 1974
Newer agents			
CPT-11	60	23	Futatsuki et al, 1994
Paclitaxel	30	17	Ajani et al, 1998
Oral etoposide	26	17	Ajani et al, 1992
Carboplatin	41	5	Preusser et al, 1990
Docetaxel	33	24	Sulkes et al, 1994
UFT/leucovorin	26	15	Ravaud et al, 1999
S-1	51	49	Sakata et al, 1998
Trimetrexate	33	21	Raman et al, 1999
Gemcitabine	18	0	Christman et al, 1994

CPT-11 = irinotecan.

Single-Agent Chemotherapy

5-Fluorouracil

The activity of 5-FU against gastric cancer has been a focus of preclinical and clinical investigations for the past three decades (Figure 15–2). A variety of doses and schedules were investigated in the early studies. Comis and Carter analyzed data on 450 patients with gastric cancer who were treated with various schedules of 5-FU that included bolus, weekly, and continuous intravenous administration. They reported an overall objective response rate of 22 percent.[22] The major side effects of 5-FU are myelosuppression, diarrhea, and mucositis.

Biomodulation of 5-Fluorouracil

In the absence of other effective chemotherapeutic agents, other investigators attempted to enhance the activity of 5-FU with biologic modulators such as leucovorin (folinic acid), methotrexate, interferon-α, and N-phosphonacetyl-L-aspartic acid (PALA).[24] Leucovorin potentiates the stability of the ternary complex between 5-FU and thymidylate synthase (TS), further enhancing TS inhibition by 5-FU (see Figure 15–2). Methotrexate inhibits tetrahydrofolate reductase, thus decreasing the cellular pool of folate and increasing the incorporation of the 5-FU metabolite fluorodeoxyuridine monophosphate (FdUMP) into ribonucleic acid (RNA) and deoxyribonucleic acid (DNA).

Machover and colleagues treated 27 gastric cancer patients with 5-FU (340 to 400 mg/m²/d) and high-dose leucovorin (200 mg/m²/d) for 5 days every 3 weeks.[25] Twenty-six of the 27 patients with gastric cancer had undergone no previous chemotherapy. The overall response rate was 48 percent; median survival was 7 months. Using a different dose and schedule of 5-FU (600 mg/m² IV bolus weekly for 6 weeks, followed by a 2-week rest) and leucovorin (500 mg/m² IV weekly), Arbuck and colleagues reported a modest 12 percent response rate and a 5.5-month median survival.[26] Almost half of the patients enrolled in this trial had been previously treated with chemotherapy containing 5-FU. The combination of 5-FU and leucovorin remains one of the standard treatment options for this disease, especially for patients deemed unsuitable for more toxic regimens.

The concept of 5-FU biomodulation by leucovorin and methotrexate has been exploited in some commonly used combination regimens for gastric

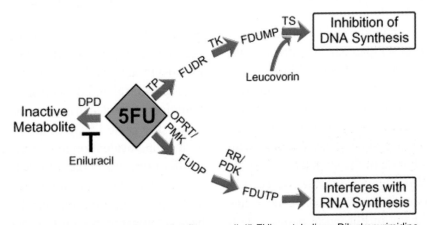

Figure 15–2. Major pathways of 5-fluorouracil (5-FU) metabolism. Dihydropyrimidine dehydrogenase (DPD) catalyzes the rate-limiting step in 5-FU inactivation. Eniluracil and other DPD inhibitors interfere with this step. In order to exert cytotoxic activity, 5-FU requires enzymatic conversion to active nucleotides. Two major activation pathways are (a) conversion to fluorodeoxyuridine monophosphate (FdUMP), which forms a stable ternary complex with thymidylate synthase (TS) and causes sustained inhibition of deoxyribonucleic acid (DNA) synthesis; and (b) conversion to fluorodeoxyuridine triphosphate (FdUTP), which interferes with ribonucleic acid (RNA) synthesis. Leucovorin stabilizes the complex between the FdUMP and TS. (OPRT = orotate phosphorybosyl transferase; PMK = pyrimidine monophosphate kinase; RR = ribonucleotide reductase; TK = thymidine kinase; TP = thymidine phosphorylase; FUDR = 5-fluoro-2'-deoxyuridine; FUDP = fluoro-2'-deoxyuridine-5'-diphosphate; PDK = pyrimidine diphosphate kinase.)

cancer, such as FAMTX.[2]

Although PALA and interferon-α have been effective in vitro modulators, they failed to enhance the activity of 5-FU in clinical trials.[27–29]

More recently, the combination of 5-FU, hydroxyurea, and interferon-α was evaluated in a phase II trial in patients with refractory gastrointestinal malignancies, including 31 patients with gastric cancer.[30] Hydroxyurea inhibits ribonucleotide reductase and depletes intracellular deoxyuridine monophosphate (dUMP). Interferon-α is thought to modulate the cellular effects of both 5-FU and hydroxyurea.[31,32] The overall response rate in the 30 assessable gastric cancer patients was 37 percent, including 7 percent complete responses. The regimen was myelotoxic: grade 3 or 4 granulocytopenia developed in 49 percent of patients, and thrombocytopenia developed in 22 percent of patients.

Other Single Agents

Mitomycin-C is an antitumor antibiotic that acts as a DNA alkylator.[33] As a single agent, mitomycin-C has been reported to produce responses in 30 percent of patients with stomach cancer.[22] The clinical use of mitomycin-C is limited by its cumulative and often delayed myelotoxicity (up to 8 weeks after treatment).

Doxorubicin, a commonly used anthracycline, produced responses in 17 percent of patients with gastric cancer.[21] Common side effects of doxorubicin are myelosuppression, mucositis, and a cumulative risk of cardiotoxicity. Mitoxantrone, another anthracycline, produced no objective responses when given weekly at a dose of 5 mg/m^2 to 15 patients with advanced adenocarcinoma of the stomach.[34]

Epirubicin, a doxorubicin derivative recently approved in the United States for breast cancer, has been studied extensively in Europe in patients with gastric cancer. As a single agent, it has demonstrated modest activity, with an overall response rate of 17 percent.[35] In an International Collaborative Cancer Group trial (ICCG), 70 patients were randomized to either epirubicin (100 to 140 mg/m^2 every 3 weeks) or 5-FU (500 to 700 mg/m^2 on days 1 to 5 every 3 weeks).[36] Response rates were disappointing: 8 percent for epirubicin and 6 percent for 5-FU. Epiru-

bicin is less cardiotoxic than doxorubicin and thus has been substituted for doxorubicin in several combination chemotherapy regimens.[37]

Platinum compounds have shown modest activity in gastric cancer. Cisplatin has been the most extensively investigated derivative. Lacave and colleagues administered 100 mg/m^2 of cisplatin every 3 weeks to 34 patients who were refractory to previous chemotherapy. The overall response rate was 18 percent, including three complete responses.[38] Common side effects seen with cisplatin are nausea and vomiting, nephrotoxicity, and neurotoxicity.[39–41] Carboplatin, a less toxic platinum derivative, has no significant activity when used as a single agent.[42] Twenty-four patients were treated with 130 to 160 mg/m^2 of carboplatin on days 1, 3, and 5 every 4 weeks. The overall response rate was only 9 percent.

Etoposide, a type II topoisomerase inhibitor, has shown clinical activity when administered intravenously in untreated patients, with a response rate of about 20 percent.[43] More recently, an oral formulation of etoposide was tested in patients with previously untreated gastric cancer.[44] This therapy produced a modest 17 percent response rate in 26 evaluable patients and was well tolerated.

Newer Single Agents

Several new classes of chemotherapeutic drugs have been tested in patients with advanced gastric cancer. Promising activity has been observed with the taxanes (paclitaxel and docetaxel), type I topoisomerase inhibitors (irinotecan), and the oral fluoropyrimidines (see Table 15–3). Some of these drugs are now undergoing evaluation in combination regimens.

Taxanes. Paclitaxel (Taxol) and docetaxel (Taxotere) exert their antitumor activity by binding to and stabilizing microtubular assembly. Both agents have demonstrated significant antitumor activity in breast, lung, and ovarian malignancies.[45] Paclitaxel is active in patients with esophageal adenocarcinoma, both as a single agent and in combination with 5-FU.[46] Based on this evidence, taxanes have been investigated for patients with advanced gastric adenocarcinoma.

In a phase II study, Ajani and colleagues investigated two schedules of paclitaxel, 200 mg/m^2

infused either over 3 hours or over 24 hours.[47] They reported an objective response rate of 17 percent in chemotherapy-naive patients who received the 3-hour infusion and a 23 percent response rate for patients receiving the 24-hour infusion. The median duration of response was 6.5 months. Other trials of paclitaxel have reported varying response rates. Ohtsu and colleagues treated 15 patients with 210 mg/m² of paclitaxel infused over 3 hours;[48] they reported a 20 percent overall response rate. In a study of a 24-hour paclitaxel infusion (250 mg/m²), Einzig and colleagues reported only a 5 percent response rate in 22 assessable patients.[49]

Docetaxel has also demonstrated clinical activity against gastric cancer. The European Organization for Research and Treatment of Cancer (EORTC) evaluated docetaxel (100 mg/m², every 3 weeks) in 37 patients with untreated gastric cancer;[50] the partial response rate was 24 percent. Investigators from Japan reported a 24 percent overall response rate in 59 patients treated with 60 mg/m² of docetaxel every 3 to 4 weeks.[51] The most common grade three-to-four toxicities in both trials were neutropenia and thrombocytopenia. Vanhoefer and colleagues reported a 20 percent response rate when docetaxel (100 mg/m², every 3 weeks) was given as second-line therapy to patients who progressed on 5-FU/cisplatin.[52]

Topoisomerase I Inhibitors. Irinotecan (CPT-11) and topotecan (Hycamptin) belong to a family of natural products known as the camptothecins.

Camptothecins exert their antitumor activity by binding to the enzyme topoisomerase I and causing single-strand breaks in DNA (Figure 15–3). Early clinical trials of CPT-11 (mostly from Japan) in patients with advanced gastric cancer reported response rates ranging from 18 to 43 percent.[53] Irinotecan is currently approved in Japan for the treatment of gastric cancer.

In a European trial of CPT-11 (350 mg/m², every 3 weeks), there were 3 complete responses and 1 partial response among 18 evaluable patients (the overall response rate was 17.6 %).[54] The North Central Cancer Treatment Group (NCCTG) reported excessive toxicity in their study when CPT-11 (320 mg/m², every 3 weeks) was delivered to patients with advanced cancer of the stomach or gastroesophageal junction.[55] Six of nine patients enrolled in this trial were hospitalized for severe treatment-related diarrhea.

Another type I topoisomerase inhibitor, topotecan, was assessed in a phase II study of 13 patients with gastric cancer. The drug was administered intravenously at a dose of 1.5 mg/m²/d for 5 consecutive days; cycles were repeated every 21 days.[56] There were no objective responses. Myelosuppression was the principal toxicity.

Oral Fluoropyrimidines and Other Newer Agents. Oral administration of 5-FU is hampered by its erratic bioavailability due to substantial inter- and intrapatient variability in 5-FU metabolism. Dihydropyrimidine dehydrogenase (DPD) is the rate-lim-

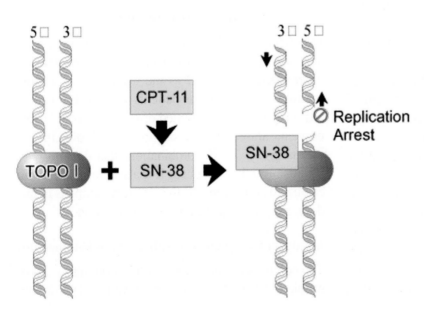

Figure 15–3. Irinotecan (CPT-11) and its active derivative SN-38 are topoisomerase I (TOPO-I) poisons. TOPO-I plays a role in deoxyribonucleic acid (DNA) replication, recombination, and repair. Topoisomerase I poisons such as CPT-11 and SN-38 create a stable "cleavable complex" with TOPO-1 and DNA strands, leading to irreversible DNA breakage, replication arrest, G_2 cycle arrest, and apoptosis.

iting enzyme involved in 5-FU catabolism; its inhibition greatly enhances the bioavailability of orally administered fluoropyrimidines (see Figure 15–2). Inhibitors of DPD such as uracil, eniluracil, and gimestat (5-chloro-2, 4-dihydroxypyridine [CDHP]), are currently being investigated.[57,58] The potential advantages of the oral fluoropyrimidines are the maintenance of sustained drug levels, convenient administration, and potentially lower cost.

The drug known as uracil:tegafur (UFT) is a combination of the DPD inhibitor uracil and the 5-FU prodrug tegafur in a 4:1 molar ratio.[59] This drug has been widely used in Japan as a front-line therapy for patients with gastric cancer. Pooled data from multiple Japanese institutions reveal an overall response rate of 27 percent.[60] The major toxic effects of UFT are anorexia, nausea, vomiting, and diarrhea. Pharmacologic studies have shown that the addition of low-dose leucovorin to UFT enhances the rate of TS inhibition.[58] Kim and colleagues reported a 29 percent overall response rate, including one complete response, in 16 patients with gastric cancer who received oral UFT plus leucovorin.[61] The main toxic effects were diarrhea and mucositis. In another phase II trial, Ravaud and colleagues reported an overall response rate of 15 percent in 26 evaluable patients.[62] Further clinical evaluation of UFT plus leucovorin is ongoing in the United States and Europe.

The drug known as S-1 is a combination of the 5-FU prodrug tegafur, gimestat (CDHP), and otastat potassium (Oxo).[63] Gimestat is an inhibitor of DPD, and Oxo is thought to alleviate the gastrointestinal side effects of 5-FU. In a study that included 51 patients with gastric cancer, Sakata and colleagues reported an overall response rate of 49 percent (95% confidence interval [CI], 35.9 to 62.3%).[57] The median survival was 8.5 months. Twenty percent of the patients developed grade 3 or 4 toxicity, principally as myelosuppression and diarrhea.

Two other oral agents that may have potential for the treatment of gastric cancer but that have not yet been evaluated for this disease are eniluracil and capecitabine. Eniluracil is a potent and irreversible inhibitor of DPD.[64] In combination with 5-FU, it was well tolerated in phase I trials, and it is currently being evaluated for patients with gastrointestinal malignancies.[65] Capecitabine (Xeloda) is a 5-FU prodrug that preferentially accumulates in tumor tissues;[66] the results of capecitabine therapy for patients with metastatic colo-rectal cancer are encouraging.[67] This is the only oral fluoropyrimidine currently approved in the United States.

Oxaliplatin is diaminocyclohexane (DACH) platinum with a different toxicity and activity profile from cisplatin.[68] Given the activity of cisplatin in gastric cancer, investigations of oxaliplatin in this disease are ongoing.[69]

Gemcitabine, a nucleoside analogue active in patients with pancreatic cancer, has been investigated in chemotherapy-naive patients with metastatic gastric cancer. There were no objective responses noted in 18 patients treated with weekly gemcitabine.[70]

Trimetrexate (TMX) is a nonclassic folate antagonist. Ramanathan and colleagues treated 33 patients who had unresectable or metastatic gastric cancer.[71] The overall response rate was 21 percent, and the median survival was 5.9 months. Trimetrexate should be further evaluated in combination with 5-FU and leucovorin since it is thought to enhance the activity of 5-FU.

Multitargeted antifolate (MTA) is novel antifolate that inhibits several enzymes involved in folate metabolism and DNA synthesis. The targeted enzymes are TS, dihydrofolate reductase, and glycinamide ribonucleotide formyltransferase.[72,73] Preliminary results from early clinical trials of MTA suggest that it has activity in gastric cancer (P. Paoletti, personal communication, August 2000).

Multidrug Regimens

Experience with the biochemical modulation of 5-FU and the success of combination chemotherapy in other malignancies led to the evaluation of various multidrug regimens for patients with gastric cancer. Early regimens incorporated drugs such as 5-FU, mitomycin, ara-C, the nitrosoureas, and doxorubicin (Adriamycin).[21,22,74] Combinations that demonstrated promising activity in phase II trials were subsequently evaluated and compared to reference regimens in randomized phase III studies (Tables 15–4 and 15–5).

5-Fluorouracil plus Doxorubicin plus Mitomycin-C

The combination of 5-fluorouracil (600 mg/m^2), doxorubicin (30 mg/m^2), and mitomycin-C (10 mg/m^2)

Table 15–4. SELECTED PHASE II TRIALS OF MULTIDRUG REGIMENS FOR GASTRIC CANCER

Chemotherapy Regimen	Response Rate (%)	Median Survival (mo)	Reference
FAM	42	5.5	MacDonald et al, 1980
FAMe	47	6	O'Connell, 1985
FU/cisplatin	43	7	Ohtsu et al, 1994
EAP	64	9	Preusser et al, 1989
FAMTX	59	6	Klein et al, 1989
ELF	48	10	Wilke et al, 1990
ECF	56	9	Zaniboni et al, 1995
PELF	62	11	Cascinu et al, 1997
TAX/FU	65	12	Murad et al, 1999
CPT/CDDP	48	10	Boku et al, 1999

FAM = 5-fluorouracil, doxorubicin, mitomycin-C; FAMe = 5-fluorouracil, doxorubicin, methyl lomustine (CCNU); FU = 5-fluorouracil; EAP = etoposide, doxorubicin, cisplatin; FAMTX = 5-fluorouracil, doxorubicin, methotrexate; ELF = etoposide, leucovorin, 5-fluorouracil; ECF = epirubicin, cisplatin, 5-fluorouracil; PELF = cisplatin, epirubicin, 5-fluorouracil, 6-stereoisomer of leucovorin, filgrastim, glutathione; TAX/FU = paclitaxel and 5-fluorouracil; CPT/CDDP = irinotecan (CPT-11) and cisplatin.

(FAM) given on an 8-week schedule was first introduced in the 1970s.[75] Of 62 patients enrolled in the initial trial of FAM, 26 achieved a partial response, for an overall response rate of 42 percent. The median survival for all patients was 5.5 months (12.5 months in responders and 3.5 months in nonresponders). The regimen was well tolerated and there were no toxic deaths associated with the therapy. The major toxic events were myelosuppression, nausea, and vomiting.

In the 1980s, FAM became the reference treatment for gastric cancer. However, subsequent clinical studies reported variable response rates, without evidence of a survival benefit.[76,77] The NCCTG compared FAM to 5-FU/doxorubicin and to 5-FU in a three-arm phase III trial that enrolled patients with gastric and pancreatic cancer. In gastric cancer patients with measurable disease, the objective response rates to 5-FU, 5-FU/doxorubicin, and FAM were 18 percent, 27 percent, and 38 percent, respectively. Despite the apparently higher response rate with FAM, the median survival in all three arms was identical (7 months).[78] The FAM regimen also produced more anorexia, nausea, vomiting, and cumulative bone marrow suppression than the other regimens.

Other combinations developed on the basis of FAM included 5-FU plus doxorubicin (Adriamycin) plus methyl lomustine (CCNU) (FAMe) and 5-FU plus mitomycin-C plus cytosine arabinoside (FMC).[79]

The addition of leucovorin to FAM (FAM-CF) failed to further improve the response rate or the survival.[80] In spite of the moderate response rates observed in some trials, the impact of FAM and FAM variants on patient survival has been disappointing.[81,82]

5-Fluorouracil plus Doxorubicin plus Methotrexate

Based on preclinical observations, the addition of methotrexate (MTX) to 5-FU–based chemotherapy would be expected to result in enhanced clinical activity. This concept was exploited with the next-generation regimen, FAMTX, a combination of 5-fluorouracil, doxorubicin, and methotrexate.[76] A moderately high dose of MTX ($1,500$ mg/m^2) is administered on day 1 and is followed by 5-FU ($1,500$ mg/m^2) 1 hour later. Leucovorin rescue begins 24 hours after MTX and doxorubicin (30 mg/m^2) is given on day 15. Cycles are repeated every 28 days. The initial phase II trial of FAMTX reported a

Table 15–5. SELECTED PHASE III TRIALS OF MULTIDRUG REGIMENS FOR GASTRIC CANCER

Regimen	No. Patients Randomized	Response (%)	Median Survival (mo)	Reference
Dox vs	110	21	3	O'Connell, 1985
FAMe vs		47	6	
FMC		14	3	
FU vs	144	18	7	Cullinan et al, 1985
FU/dox vs		27	7	
FAM		38	7	
FAMTX vs	213	41	10	Wils et al, 1991
FAM		9	7	
FP vs	295	51	9	Kim et al, 1993
FAM vs		25	7	
FU		26	7	
FAMTX vs	60	33	7	Kelsen et al, 1992
EAP		20	6	
FAMTX vs	283	25	7	Wilke et al, 1995
FP vs		30	9	
ELF		17	7	
FAM vs	137	15	6	Cocconi et al, 1994
PELF		43	8	
FAMTX vs	274	21	9	Waters et al, 1999
ECF		46	6	

Dox = doxorubicin; FAM = 5-fluorouracil, doxorubicin, mitomycin-C; FAMe = 5-fluorouracil, doxorubicin, methyl lomustine (CCNU); FMC = 5-fluorouracil, mitomycin C, cytosine arabinoside; FU = 5-fluorouracil; FP = 5-fluorouracil, cisplatin; EAP = etoposide, doxorubicin, cisplatin; FAMTX = 5-fluorouracil, doxorubicin, methotrexate; ELF = etoposide, leucovorin, 5-fluorouracil; PELF = cisplatin, epirubicin, 5-fluorouracil, 6-S-leucovorin, filgrastim, glutathione; ECF = epirubicin, cisplatin, 5-fluorouracil.

response rate of 58 percent, including 12 percent complete responders and 3 percent treatment-related deaths out of 100 patients enrolled.[83] In a confirmatory phase II study by the EORTC, the response rate was 33 percent, including 13 percent complete responses.[84] Grade 4 leukopenia was noted in 14 percent of the patients, severe mucositis in 11 percent, and neurotoxicity in 3 percent.

In a follow-up phase III study, FAMTX was compared to FAM.[85] The response rates were 41 percent for FAMTX and 9 percent for FAM. The 1- and 2-year survival rates were 41 percent and 9 percent for FAMTX and 22 percent and 0 percent for FAM, respectively ($p = .004$). The toxic death rate was 4 percent for FAMTX and 3 percent for FAM. Thus, FAMTX became one of the most commonly used combination chemotherapy regimens for patients with advanced gastric cancer in the early 1990s.

Cisplatin-Based Combinations

Cisplatin-based regimens such as etoposide, doxorubicin, and cisplatin (EAP) and 5-FU, doxorubicin, and cisplatin (FAP) were also developed in the late 1980s.

In a phase II trial of EAP reported by Preusser and colleagues, 67 patients received etoposide (120 mg/m^2) on days 4, 5, and 6; doxorubicin (20 mg/m^2) on days 1 and 7, and cisplatin (40 mg/m^2) on days 2 and 8.[86] Cycles were repeated every 21 to 28 days. The overall response rate was 64 percent, including 21 percent complete responses. The median duration of response was 7 months, and the median survival reached 9 months.

However, a high toxicity rate and several treatment-related deaths were reported in subsequent phase II trials of EAP. A phase II study from the Dana Farber Cancer Institute demonstrated a 33 percent response rate including 8 percent complete responses.[87] Toxicity was excessive; 11 percent of patients died of treatment-related toxicity, and hospitalization for neutropenic fever was required over 22 percent of patients in all administered cycles. The Eastern Cooperative Oncology Group (ECOG) evaluated EAP in 31 patients with advanced disease.[88] Partial responses were observed in 23 percent of patients; there were no complete responses. There were 4 treatment-related deaths from neutropenia and sepsis.

The EAP regimen was compared to FAMTX in a phase III trial conducted by investigators from the Memorial Sloan-Kettering Cancer Center.[89] Of the patients on the FAMTX arm, 33 percent responded, including 10 percent complete responses. Among those treated with EAP, 20 percent had a partial response, and there were no complete responders. Four patients (13%) died of therapy-related causes on the EAP arm as opposed to no therapy-related deaths on the FAMTX arm ($p = .04$). The overall survivals were not significantly different (7 months for the FAMTX arm versus 6 months for the EAP arm).

Variants of the EAP regimen, such as 5-FU, doxorubicin, and cisplatin (FAP) and epirubicin, etoposide, and cisplatin (FEP) do not appear to offer any additional advantage to other combination chemotherapy regimens.[90,91] Due to its unacceptably high toxicity and unconfirmed efficacy, EAP and its variants have been largely abandoned in clinical practice.[92]

5-Fluorouracil plus Cisplatin

The combination of 5-FU and cisplatin has been tested in several phase II trials. Ohtsu and colleagues treated 55 chemotherapy-naive patients with continuous-infusion 5-FU (800 mg/m^2 on days 1 to 5) and cisplatin (20 mg/m^2 on days 1 to 5). Objective responses were noted in 43 percent of the 40 patients with measurable disease; the median survival was 7 months.[93] The regimen was well tolerated, and grade 3 or 4 myelosuppression occurred in less than 20 percent of patients. Other investigators have also reported response rates of 40 to 50 percent and good tolerability.[94,95] A low-dose continuous infusion of 5-FU ($200 \text{ mg/m}^2/\text{d}$) with cisplatin was somewhat better tolerated but less active (the overall response rate was 10%), suggesting the importance of full-dose 5-FU for the activity of this regimen.[96]

5-Fluorouracil plus cisplatin (FP) was compared to FAMTX and ELF in a phase III trial conducted by the EORTC. The response rates for FAMTX, FP, and ELF were 25 percent, 30 percent and 17 percent, respectively. There was no significant difference in survivals among the three arms (survivals ranged from 7 to 9 months).[97]

The combination of 5-FU and cisplatin remains a reasonable option for off-protocol therapy of metastatic gastric cancer (Table 15–6). There is no convincing evidence that other multidrug combinations are superior.

Etoposide plus Leucovorin plus 5-Fluorouracil

The marginal performance status of many elderly patients with gastric cancer created interest in combination chemotherapy regimens that might be less toxic. The addition of etoposide to 5-FU and leucovorin (ELF) produces response rates and survivals similar to those seen with FAMTX.[98] In a phase II trial, 32 patients older than 65 years of age or with underlying cardiac disease were treated with ELF. The overall response rate was 48 percent, including 12 percent complete responses. Median survival reached 10.5 months. The major toxic effects of ELF are leukopenia and diarrhea. There were no toxic deaths. A phase II study of ELF, conducted in patients unsuitable for aggressive chemotherapy, reported a 32 percent overall response rate and 7 percent complete responses.[99] Thus, ELF appears to be a less toxic alternative for elderly patients or for patients who cannot tolerate the toxicities of doxorubicin or cisplatin. Interestingly, investigators from M.D. Anderson Cancer Center reported a much lower response rate in their phase II trial of ELF plus granulocyte-macrophage colony–stimulating factor (GM-CSF): a partial response rate of only 14 percent was reported for 29 assessable patients.[100]

The addition of epirubicin to ELF (ELF-E) may also form a potentially effective and well-tolerated regimen for patients with advanced gastric cancer

according to Colluci and colleagues.[101] Of 51 assessable patients, 49 percent responded, including 8 percent who achieved a complete response (95% CI, 35 to 63%). The median survival in this study was 8 months.

Epirubicin-Based Combinations

In a phase I/II study, the combination of epirubicin (starting at 50 mg/m^2 on day 1), 5-FU, and leucovorin (425 mg/m^2 and 20 mg/m^2, respectively, on days 1 to 5) was administered every 4 weeks to 37 patients with advanced gastric cancer.[102] The regimen produced objective responses in 38 percent of treated patients and was well tolerated.

A combination of epirubicin (50 mg/m^2, every 3 weeks), cisplatin (60 mg/m^2, every 3 weeks), and 5-FU (200 mg/m^2/d, continuous) (ECF) was tested in 53 patients with locally advanced (n = 7) and metastatic gastric cancer (n = 46).[103] The overall response rate was 56 percent including 8 complete responses (95% CI, 43 to 69%), and the median survival reached 9 months. There were no toxic deaths, and only 3 patients required hospitalization for neutropenic fever.

The ECF combination was compared to FAMTX in a randomized multicenter phase III trial that involved 274 patients with advanced esophageal or gastric adenocarcinoma.[104] The ECF regimen was superior to FAMTX in terms of both response rate (46% versus 21%, p = .0003) and survival (median of 8.7 months versus 6.1 months, p = .0005). The 2-year survival rate was 14 percent for the ECF group and 5 percent for the FAMTX group (p = .03). In Europe, ECF is considered one of the standard frontline regimens for advanced gastric cancer. With the recent Food and Drug Administration (FDA) approval of epirubicin (Ellence) in the United States for breast cancer, it is expected that this active regimen may undergo further evaluation in the United States.

Cisplatin, epirubicin, 5-FU, and leucovorin (PELF) (repeated every 3 weeks) are another active epirubicin-based combination. In a randomized trial comparing PELF to FAM, PELF was more active (a response rate of 43%, versus 15% for FAM) but also more toxic; 2 toxic deaths were reported among 85 treated patients.[105] The median survivals were not

Table 15–6. COMMONLY USED COMBINATION CHEMOTHERAPY REGIMENS FOR GASTRIC CANCER			
Regimen	Chemotherapy Drugs	Dose*	Schedule
FP	5-FU	1,000 mg/m^2	Days 1–5, CIV
	Cisplatin	100 mg/m^2	Day 2
FAMTX	Methotrexate	1,500 mg/m^2	Day 1
	5-FU	1,500 mg/m^2	Day 1
	Doxorubicin	30 mg/m^2	Day 15
ELF	Etoposide	120 mg/m^2	Days 1–3
	Leucovorin	300 mg/m^2	Days 1–3
	5-FU	500 mg/m^2	Days 1–3

*Repeated every 4 weeks.
CIV = continuous intravenous infusion; ELF = etoposide, leucovorin, 5-fluorouracil; FAMTX = 5-fluorouracil, doxorubicin, methotrexate; FP = 5-fluorouracil, cisplatin; 5-FU = 5-fluorouracil.

significantly different: 8.1 months for PELF and 5.6 months for FAM ($p = .24$).

A more recent trial of intense "modified PELF" (with glutathione and filgrastim) given weekly to 105 patients reported an overall response rate of 62 percent, including 17 percent complete responses (95% CI, 53 to 71%). The median survival was 11 months, with 1- and 2-year survival rates of 42 percent and 5 percent, respectively.[106] Grade 3 and 4 toxicities (manifest principally as myelosuppression and mucositis) were reported in 38 percent of the patients.

Taxane-Based Combinations

The known activity of single-agent taxanes in gastric cancer prompted the evaluation of their activity when they are combined with other agents.

Murad and colleagues investigated the combination of paclitaxel (175 mg/m^2 over 3 hours on day 1) and 5-FU (1,500 mg/m^2 over 3 hours on day 2) in 31 patients with advanced gastric cancer. Of 29 evaluated patients, 19 had objective responses (the overall response rate was 65% [95% CI, 48 to 83%]); these included 7 complete responses.[107] The overall median survival was 12 months.

The combination of docetaxel and cisplatin was assessed in a phase I/II study that included chemotherapy-naive patients with advanced gastric cancer.[108] Of 45 evaluable patients, 2 patients achieved a complete response and 22 patients had a partial response (the overall response rate was 53%; [95% CI, 38 to 68%]). The median survival was 8.6 months. Sixty-eight percent of patients experienced grade 3 or 4 neutropenia, including 9 episodes (19%) of febrile neutropenia.

Irinotecan plus Cisplatin

The combination of irinotecan (CPT-11) (60 to 80 mg/m^2 on days 1 and 15) and cisplatin (80 mg/m^2 on day 1) was evaluated in a phase I/II trial in 24 patients, most of whom had been treated previously. The maximum tolerated dose of CPT-11 was established at 80 mg/m^2. Neutropenia was the dose-limiting toxicity.[109] A follow-up phase II trial reported an overall response rate of 48 percent (95% CI, 33 to 63%) in 44 evaluable patients.[110] The overall median patient survival on this study was 10.2 months.

Ajani and colleagues treated 35 patients with gastric and gastroesophageal (GE)-junction carcinomas with CPT-11 and cisplatin and reported a 51 percent overall-response rate, including 3 complete responses.[111]

In summary, although many combination regimens have been evaluated in clinical trials, there is no uniformly accepted standard therapy for advanced or metastatic gastric cancer (see Table 15–6). Many of these regimens achieve moderate response rates, some of them at the expense of increased toxicity. However, even the most intense regimens cannot produce complete responses in more than 10 to 15 percent of patients nor can they extend median survival beyond 1 year. Therefore, the search for new approaches for the systemic therapy of gastric cancer is continuing. Combinations of newer drugs such as irinotecan, the taxanes, and the oral fluoropyrimidines will be evaluated in a new generation of multidrug regimens. Considering that available treatments have not yet demonstrated a significant impact on survival, patients should be offered the option to participate in well-designed clinical trials whenever possible. In the absence of that option, 5-FU plus cisplatin or multidrug regimens such as ECF or ELF should be considered for patients with good performance status.

Miscellaneous Agents

The role of noncytotoxic therapies in the treatment of gastric cancer has been less completely explored. Anecdotal reports of remission of gastric cancer in patients taking H$_2$ blockers and the proposed inhibition of suppressor T cells by H$_2$ blockers led to a prospective randomized evaluation of cimetidine in patients with gastric cancer.[112] The study's authors found no significant differences in 5-year survival between the patients who received cimetidine and those who took placebo.

In vitro investigations have shown that peptide hormones such as gastrin and cholecystokinin have a mitogenic effect on some gastric carcinoma cells. Proglumide, a synthetic gastrin/cholecystokinin receptor antagonist, was tested in 110 patients with all stages of gastric cancer.[113] The median survival in patients in the antagonist group was 13 months, versus 11 months in the placebo group, a difference that was not statistically significant.

Immunostimulants such as bacterial polysaccharides have also been assessed, mostly in the adjuvant setting. Bacille Calmette-Guérin (BCG) has been investigated in patients with gastric cancer.[114] There was a trend for a modest benefit from BCG in patients with operable gastric cancer. No benefit was reported in the group of patients with unresectable disease.

THE ROLE OF RADIATION THERAPY IN ADVANCED DISEASE

Although the reported results from the Gastrointestinal Tumor Study Group (GITSG) trials suggest a role for chemoradiation in treating locally advanced gastric cancer,[115,116] radiation therapy has a limited role for patients with metastatic disease. This is primarily due to the technical difficulties of delivering a sufficient therapeutic dose of radiation to the upper abdomen.

However, there is still a definite role for radiation therapy in controlling pain, bleeding, and/or obstructive symptoms. It also has a role in the palliation of symptoms caused by metastatic involvement of the central nervous system (CNS) or skeleton.

SUPPORTIVE MEDICAL CARE

Supportive care complements other treatment modalities. The goal is to help patients tolerate aggressive therapy and to control both disease and therapy-related symptoms. In advanced stages of the disease, when other treatment modalities have failed, supportive care often becomes the primary mode of care.

The focus of supportive care is on improving and maintaining quality of life (QOL). This is very important for patients with metastatic gastric cancer since few patients achieve durable objective responses with currently available therapies. Patients with advanced or metastatic gastric cancer frequently suffer from pain, malnutrition, cachexia, and fatigue.

Cancer pain can result from tumor infiltration of visceral organs, stretching of Glisson's capsule (liver), bone involvement, or direct infiltration of nerves. To adequately control the pain, it is important to determine its cause and to quantitate its severity. There are several reliable and validated instruments for pain measurement, such as the Wisconsin Brief Pain Questionnaire, the McGill Pain Questionnaire, and the Memorial Pain Assessment Card.[117–119] The management of cancer pain incorporates pharmacologic control, anesthetic and neurosurgical interventions, and cognitive-behavioral interventions. A stepwise approach to pharmacologic analgesia, outlined by the Cancer Relief Program of the World Health Organization (WHO), results in pain control for more than 70 percent of cancer patients.[120] This concept is based on the combined and incremental use of non-opioids, opioid drugs, and adjuvant agents. Difficult and complicated cases of pain management may be referred to a specialized pain service if available.

Celiac plexus blockade with ethanol injection may provide effective and lasting pain control in some patients with cancer of the stomach.[121] When pain is caused by infiltration of the viscera or bone, a localized course of radiation therapy may be effective.

Anorexia and weight loss are commonly encountered problems in patients with gastric cancer. The causes are multifactorial and include anatomic and functional defects, cancer cachexia, side effects from chemotherapy and radiation, and depression. Maintenance of an adequate caloric intake is important, especially in the setting of active therapy. Megestrol acetate (Megace) has been shown to help improve appetite and increase body weight in more than two-thirds of cancer patients.[122] The optimal dose appears to be 800 mg/d.[123] Therapy with megestrol acetate is associated with an increased risk for thromboembolism (9% in patients on megestrol acetate [Megace] versus 2% in a control group of patients).[124] Corticosteroids such as dexamethasone are also effective as appetite stimulants but are associated with more severe toxicity.[125] The role of total parenteral nutrition (TPN) for patients with advanced disease is limited. In several randomized trials, the addition of TPN has failed to demonstrate a beneficial impact on treatment response or patient survival.[126]

The nutritional support of patients with stomach cancer is often limited by obstruction from the primary tumor. In selected cases, adequate enteral feeding can be established by the placement of a feeding (gastrostomy or jejunostomy) tube. Some patients with total obstruction may benefit from the placement of a draining gastric tube and a feeding J tube. Unfortunately, many patients with ascites and significant peritoneal carcinomatosis cannot undergo the placement of a feeding tube, because of the associated increased risk of intra-abdominal infection.

As it is for patients with other solid tumors, fatigue is a major QOL issue for patients with stomach cancer. Many causes are involved, including anemia, malnutrition, metabolic dysfunction, depression, and sleep disorders. Anemia can be caused by bleeding or it can be caused by insufficient erythropoiesis due to advanced cancer or from chemotherapy. Management includes red blood cell transfusions and erythropoietin (Epogen, Procrit) therapy. Erythropoietin therapy has been shown to decrease the need for blood transfusions in patients with solid tumors and in patients with chemotherapy-induced anemia.[127,128]

Malignant ascites is another complication seen with gastric cancer, and it often heralds a terminal stage.[129] In general, loop diuretics and potassium-sparing agents are not effective in malignant ascites in the absence of portal hypertension. Therapeutic paracentesis provides immediate relief, but fluid quickly reaccumulates. Repeated taps increase the risk of infection or injury to the viscera. Other palliative measures include external drains or peritoneovenous shunts. Unfortunately, none of these approaches have been shown to make a difference in patient survival or quality of life.[130]

Despite advances in diagnosis and treatment, most patients with advanced gastric cancer will die of their disease. The role of the oncologist is not only to recommend and conduct active treatments but also to recognize the moment when these treatments are no longer helpful and may even be harmful. In these situations, efforts should focus on supportive and symptomatic care. This is often facilitated by hospice services that specialize in providing supportive care to terminally ill cancer patients.

THE FUTURE: TARGET-BASED APPROACHES

Recent advances in cancer biology and genomics have greatly improved our understanding of carcinogenesis and tumor progression. This information is now being used to develop new and more selective anticancer therapies. With the help of combinatorial chemistry and rational drug design, a number of target-based anticancer therapeutics have been developed. Some of these agents are now in the preclinical or early clinical phase of development and could possibly become effective therapies for gastric cancer.

Receptors belonging to the receptor tyrosine kinase (RTK) family act as oncogenes by raising the threshold for apoptosis in the cancer cell (Figure 15–4). Epidermal growth factor receptor (EGFR), HER-2/*neu*, and vascular endothelial growth factor (VEGF) receptors are among the members of this family.[131,132] When overexpressed in well-differenti-

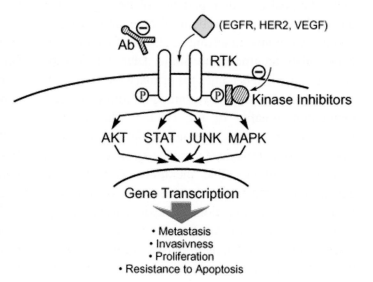

Figure 15–4. Receptor tyrosine kinases (RTKs) are transmembrane glycoproteins serving as membrane receptors for epidermal growth factors (EGF and HER-2), vascular endothelial growth factor (VEGF), and many other factors involved in cancer cell signaling. The binding of a ligand to an RTK results in receptor dimerization and phosphorylation of its intracellular domain. This leads to downstream activation of other kinases such as Mapk, Junk, Stat, and Akt. Ultimately, signals are transduced to the nucleus, resulting in a new gene transcription. Deregulation of some of the RTK pathways in the cancer cell is linked to cell proliferation, invasion, metastasis, and resistance to apoptosis (programmed cell death). Receptor tyrosine kinases have recently emerged as promising targets for anticancer drug development. Some of the concepts under investigation include receptor-directed monoclonal antibodies and small molecule inhibitors of the intracellular kinase domain (*arrows*). (EGFR = epidermal growth factor receptor.)

ated gastric tumors, ERB-B2 (HER-2/*neu*) is associated with a poor prognosis.[133] Inhibitors of some of the RTKs, such as trastuzumab (Herceptin) and *bcr/abl* kinase inhibitors, have already demonstrated clinical activity in some malignancies.[134,135] Trastuzumab (Herceptin) therapy is currently being investigated in patients with upper-gastrointestinal malignancies.

Another class of target-based agents that may possibly play a role in the treatment of gastric cancer is the antiangiogenesis drugs. Increased expression of VEGF and its receptor KDR correlates with an increased rate of neovascularization associated with metastatic gastric cancer.[132] Agents such as endostatin and inhibitors of fibroblast growth factor (FGF), platelet-derived growth factor (PDGF), and VEGF are undergoing early clinical investigation.[136]

Matrix metalloproteinase (MMP) inhibitors have been tested in preclinical and clinical studies. Marimastat, a competitive and reversible broad-spectrum inhibitor of MMPs, was compared to placebo in 369 patients with inoperable gastric cancer who had received no more than one prior chemotherapy regimen. Although progression-free survival was improved in the marimastat group, no significant difference in overall survival was observed.[137]

Tumor antigens that are expressed by gastric cancer (such as CEA and other membrane glycoproteins) are immunogenic and are capable of inducing a cellular or humoral immune response. Currently, several tumor vaccines against CEA and other antigens are undergoing early clinical investigation in patients with gastrointestinal neoplasms (including gastric cancer).[138]

Validation of the molecular predictors of cancer chemoresistance and chemosensitivity in clinical trials may allow selective patient-targeted therapy and may ultimately improve response rates. The expression of enzymes involved in purine metabolism (such as TS and thymidine phosphorylase) is often altered in gastric cancer cells. This variability in enzyme expression has been shown to affect the therapeutic response to fluoropyrimidines.[139,140] Overexpression of the excision-repair-cross-complementing (ERCC) gene may affect the response to cisplatin-based therapy in patients with gastric cancer.[141]

SUMMARY

In spite of advances in diagnosis and treatment, the prognosis for the majority of patients with advanced gastric cancer remains poor. Many of the known chemotherapeutic drugs show some clinical activity against this disease, but unfortunately, this does not translate into prolonged patient survival. Many regimens welcomed as new "gold standards" after phase II trials failed to prove their efficacy in larger randomized trials. Unlike in the case of many other malignancies, there is still no consensus for a standard chemotherapy regimen for metastatic gastric cancer. Nevertheless, results from clinical trials of some of the new drugs such as the taxanes, topoisomerase inhibitors, and oral fluoropyrimidines are encouraging. When these agents are combined together, it is hoped it will yield a regimen with a higher rate of complete and durable remissions.

Cancer of the stomach is a disabling disease, causing a great deal of discomfort and suffering. Supportive care measures focusing on the control of pain, nutrition, and fatigue can significantly improve the quality of life in this group of patients.

Finally, a recent explosion of knowledge in the fields of cancer biology, immunology, and experimental pharmacology has resulted in the development of a number of novel therapeutics. Some of these target-based anticancer agents are already entering clinical investigation. These trials may demonstrate whether these new approaches, alone or in combination with conventional chemotherapy, can alter the natural history of advanced gastric cancer.

REFERENCES

1. Greenlee RT, Murray T, Bolden S, et al. Cancer statistics, 2000. CA Cancer J Clin 2000;50:7–33.
2. Ajani JA. Chemotherapy for gastric carcinoma: new and old options. Oncology (Huntingt) 1998;12:44–7.
3. Gunderson LL, Sosin H. Adenocarcinoma of the stomach: areas of failure in a re-operation series (second or symptomatic look) clinicopathologic correlation and implications for adjuvant therapy. Int J Radiat Oncol Biol Phys 1982;8:1–11.
4. Weed TE, Nuessle W, Ochsner A. Carcinoma of the stomach. Why are we falling to improve survival? Ann Surg 1981;193:407–13.
5. Moertel CG. The natural history of advanced gastric cancer. Surg Gynecol Obstet 1968;126:1071–4.
6. Dewys WD, Begg C, Lavin PT, et al. Prognostic effect of

weight loss prior to chemotherapy in cancer patients. Eastern Cooperative Oncology Group. Am J Med 1980; 69:491–7.

7. Dupont JB Jr, Lee JR, Burton GR, et al. Adenocarcinoma of the stomach: review of 1,497 cases. Cancer 1978;41:941–7.

8. Long BW, Thigpen JT, Morrison FS. Paraneoplastic manifestations in gastric carcinoma. J Miss State Med Assoc 1975;16:337–9.

9. Coenen C, Wedmann B, Bauer KH, et al. Dermatomyositis as a paraneoplastic syndrome. A case report. Fortschr Med 1989;107:720–2.

10. Yeh JS, Munn SE, Plunkett TA, et al. Coexistence of acanthosis nigricans and the sign of Leser-Trelat in a patient with gastric adenocarcinoma: a case report and literature review. J Am Acad Dermatol 2000;42:357–62.

11. Cafagna D, Ponte E. Pulmonary embolism of paraneoplastic origin. Minerva Med 1997;88:523–30.

12. Ajani JA, Mansfield PF, Lynch PM, et al. Enhanced staging and all chemotherapy preoperatively in patients with potentially resectable gastric carcinoma. J Clin Oncol 1999;17:2403–11.

13. Dittler HJ, Siewert JR. Role of endoscopic ultrasonography in gastric carcinoma. Endoscopy 1993;25:162–6.

14. Bergman JJ, Fockens P. Endoscopic ultrasonography in patients with gastro-esophageal cancer. Eur J Ultrasound 1999;10:127–38.

15. Pectasides D, Mylonakis A, Kostopoulou M, et al. CEA, CA 19-9, and CA-50 in monitoring gastric carcinoma. Am J Clin Oncol 1997;20:348–53.

16. Wakatsuki Y, Inada M, Kudo H, et al. Immunological characterization and clinical implication of cobalamin binding protein in human gastric cancer. Cancer Res 1989;49: 3122–8.

17. Murad AM, Santiago FF, Petroianu A, et al. Modified therapy with 5-fluorouracil, doxorubicin, and methotrexate in advanced gastric cancer. Cancer 1993;72:37–41.

18. Pyrhonen S, Kuitunen T, Nyandoto P, et al. Randomised comparison of fluorouracil, epidoxorubicin and methotrexate (FEMTX) plus supportive care with supportive care alone in patients with non-resectable gastric cancer. Br J Cancer 1995;71:587–91.

19. Scheithauer WKG, Zeh B. Palliative chemotherapy versus supportive care in patients with metastatic gastric cancer: a randomized trial. Proceedings of the Second International Conference on Biology, Prevention and Treatment of GI Malignancy; 1995; Koln, Germany. p. 68.

20. Glimelius B, Ekstrom K, Hoffman K, et al. Randomized comparison between chemotherapy plus best supportive care with best supportive care in advanced gastric cancer. Ann Oncol 1997;8:163–8.

21. Moertel CG, Lavin PT. Phase II-III chemotherapy studies in advanced gastric cancer. Eastern Cooperative Oncology Group. Cancer Treat Rep 1979;63:1863–9.

22. Comis RL, Carter SK. A review of chemotherapy in gastric cancer. Cancer 1974;34:1576–86.

23. Cocconi G, DeLisi V, Di Blasio B. Randomized comparison of 5-FU alone or combined with mitomycin and cytarabine (MFC) in the treatment of advanced gastric cancer. Cancer Treat Rep 1982;66:1263–6.

24. Schilsky RL. Biochemical and clinical pharmacology of 5-fluorouracil. Oncology (Huntingt) 1998;12:13–8.

25. Machover D, Goldschmidt E, Chollet P, et al. Treatment of advanced colorectal and gastric adenocarcinomas with 5-fluorouracil and high-dose folinic acid. J Clin Oncol 1986;4:685–96.

26. Arbuck SG, Douglass HO Jr, Trave F, et al. A phase II trial of 5-fluorouracil and high-dose intravenous leucovorin in gastric carcinoma. J Clin Oncol 1987;5:1150–6.

27. Windschitl HE, O'Connell MJ, Wieand HS, et al. A clinical trial of biochemical modulation of 5-fluorouracil with N-phosphonoacetyl-L-aspartate and thymidine in advanced gastric and anaplastic colorectal cancer. Cancer 1990;66:853–6.

28. Wadler S, Gleissner B, Hilgenfeld RU, et al. Phase II trial of N-(phosphonacetyl)-L-aspartate (PALA), 5-fluorouracil and recombinant interferon-alpha-2b in patients with advanced gastric carcinoma. Eur J Cancer 1996;32A:1254–6.

29. Jager E, Bernhard H, Klein O, et al. Combination 5-fluorouracil (FU), folinic acid (FA), and alpha-interferon 2B in advanced gastric cancer: results of a phase II trial. Ann Oncol 1995;6:153–6.

30. Wadler S, Damle S, Haynes H, et al. Phase II/pharmacodynamic trial of dose-intensive, weekly parenteral hydroxyurea and fluorouracil administered with interferon alfa-2a in patients with refractory malignancies of the gastrointestinal tract. J Clin Oncol 1999;17:1771–8.

31. Wadler S, Horowitz R, Mao X, et al. Effect of interferon on 5-fluorouracil-induced perturbations in pools of deoxynucleotide triphosphates and DNA strand breaks. Cancer Chemother Pharmacol 1996;38:529–35.

32. Wadler S, Horowitz R, Rao J, et al. Interferon augments the cytotoxicity of hydroxyurea without enhancing its activity against the M2 subunit of ribonucleotide reductase: effects in wild-type and resistant human colon cancer cells. Cancer Chemother Pharmacol 1996;38:522–8.

33. Cummings J, Spanswick VJ, Smyth JF. Re-evaluation of the molecular pharmacology of mitomycin C. Eur J Cancer 1995;31A:1928–33.

34. DeSimone PA, Gams R, Birch R. Phase II evaluation of mitoxantrone in advanced carcinoma of the stomach: a Southeastern Cancer Study Group Trial. Cancer Treat Rep 1986;70:1043–4.

35. Scarffe JH, Kenny JB, Johnson RJ, et al. Phase II trial of epirubicin in gastric cancer. Cancer Treat Rep 1985;69:1275–7.

36. Coombes RC, Chilvers CE, Amadori D, et al. Randomised trial of epirubicin versus fluorouracil in advanced gastric cancer. An International Collaborative Cancer Group (ICCG) study. Ann Oncol 1994;5:33–6.

37. Wils JA. Epirubicin in advanced gastrointestinal (GI) cancer. Onkologie 1986;9 Suppl 1:21–3.

38. Lacave AJ, Wils J, Diaz-Rubio E, et al. cis-Platinum as second-line chemotherapy in advanced gastric adenocarcinoma. A phase II study of the EORTC Gastrointestinal Tract Cancer Cooperative Group. Eur J Cancer Clin Oncol 1985;21:1321–4.

39. Perry MC, Green MR, Mick R, et al. Cisplatin in patients with gastric cancer: a Cancer and Leukemia Group B phase II study. Cancer Treat Rep 1986;70:415–6.

40. Wilke H, Preusser P, Fink U, et al. New developments in the treatment of gastric carcinoma. Semin Oncol 1990;17: 61–70.

41. Kim R, Murakami S, Ohi Y, et al. A phase II trial of low dose

administration of 5-fluorouracil and cisplatin in patients with advanced and recurrent gastric cancer. Int J Oncol 1999;15:921–6.

42. Preusser P, Wilke H, Achterrath W, et al. Phase II study of carboplatin in untreated inoperable advanced stomach cancer. Eur J Cancer 1990;26:1108–9.

43. Macdonald JS, Havlin KA. Etoposide in gastric cancer. Semin Oncol 1992;19:59–62.

44. Ajani JA, Dumas P. Evaluation of oral etoposide in patients with metastatic gastric carcinoma: a preliminary report. Semin Oncol 1992;19:45–7.

45. Rowinsky EK. Paclitaxel pharmacology and other tumor types. Semin Oncol 1997;24:S19-1–12.

46. Ajani JA, Ilson DH, Daugherty K, et al. Activity of taxol in patients with squamous cell carcinoma and adenocarcinoma of the esophagus. J Natl Cancer Inst 1994;86:1086–91.

47. Ajani JA, Fairweather J, Dumas P, et al. Phase II study of Taxol in patients with advanced gastric carcinoma. Cancer J Sci Am 1998;4:269–74.

48. Ohtsu A, Boku N, Tamura F, et al. An early phase II study of a 3-hour infusion of paclitaxel for advanced gastric cancer. Am J Clin Oncol 1998;21:416–9.

49. Einzig AI, Lipsitz S, Wiernik PH, et al. Phase II trial of taxol in patients with adenocarcinoma of the upper gastrointestinal tract (UGIT). The Eastern Cooperative Oncology Group (ECOG) results. Invest New Drugs 1995;13:223–7.

50. Sulkes A, Smyth J, Sessa C, et al. Docetaxel (Taxotere) in advanced gastric cancer: results of a phase II clinical trial. EORTC Early Clinical Trials Group. Br J Cancer 1994; 70:380–3.

51. Taguchi T, Sakata Y, Kanamaru R, et al. Late phase II clinical study of RP56976 (docetaxel) in patients with advanced/recurrent gastric cancer: a Japanese Cooperative Study Group trial (group A). Gan To Kagaku Ryoho 1998;25:1915–24.

52. Vanhoefer U, Wilke H, Harstrick A, et al. Phase II study of docetaxel as second line chemotherapy in metastatic gastric cancer. Proc Am Soc Clin Oncol 1999;18:303a.

53. Bleiberg H. CPT-11 in gastrointestinal cancer. Eur J Cancer 1999;35:371–9.

54. Kohne CH, Thuss-Patience P, Catane R, et al. Final results of a phase II trial of CPT-11 in patients with advanced gastric cancer. Proc Am Soc Clin Oncol 1999;18:258a.

55. Egner JR, Goldberg RM, Sargent DJ, et al. CPT-11 at 320 mg/m2 caused excessive toxicity in patients with advanced adenocarcinoma of the stomach or gastroesophageal junction: A NCCTG trial. Proc Am Soc Clin Oncol 1999;18:282a.

56. Saltz LB, Schwartz GK, Ilson DH, et al. A phase II study of topotecan administered five times daily in patients with advanced gastric cancer. Am J Clin Oncol 1997;20:621–5.

57. Sakata Y, Ohtsu A, Horikoshi N, et al. Late phase II study of novel oral fluoropyrimidine anticancer drug S-1 (1 M tegafur-0.4 M gimestat-1 M otastat potassium) in advanced gastric cancer patients. Eur J Cancer 1998;34:1715–20.

58. Ichikura T, Tomimatsu S, Okusa Y, et al. Thymidylate synthase inhibition by an oral regimen consisting of tegafur-uracil (UFT) and low-dose leucovorin for patients with gastric cancer. Cancer Chemother Pharmacol 1996;38:401–5.

59. Hoff PM, Lassere Y, Pazdur R. Tegafur/uracil + calcium foli-

nate in colorectal cancer: double modulation of fluorouracil. Drugs 1999;58:77–83.

60. Ota K, Taguchi T, Kimura K. Report on nationwide pooled data and cohort investigation in UFT phase II study. Cancer Chemother Pharmacol 1988;22:333–8.

61. Kim YH, Cheong SK, Lee JD, et al. Phase II trial of oral UFT and leucovorin in advanced gastric carcinoma. Am J Clin Oncol 1996;19:212–6.

62. Ravaud A, Borner M, Schellens JH, et al. UFT and oral calcium folinate as first-line chemotherapy for metastatic gastric cancer. Oncology (Huntingt) 1999;13:61–3.

63. Shirasaka T, Nakano K, Takechi T, et al. Antitumor activity of 1 M tegafur-0.4 M 5-chloro-2,4-dihydroxypyridine- 1 M potassium oxonate (S-1) against human colon carcinoma orthotopically implanted into nude rats. Cancer Res 1996;56:2602–6.

64. Porter DJ, Chestnut WG, Merrill BM, et al. Mechanism-based inactivation of dihydropyrimidine dehydrogenase by 5-ethynyluracil. J Biol Chem 1992;267:5236–42.

65. Schilsky RL, Hohneker J, Ratain MJ, et al. Phase I clinical and pharmacologic study of eniluracil plus fluorouracil in patients with advanced cancer. J Clin Oncol 1998;16: 1450–7.

66. Verweij J. Rational design of new tumoractivated cytotoxic agents. Oncology 1999;57 Suppl 1:9–15.

67. Van Cutsem E, Findlay M, Osterwalder B, et al. Capecitabine, an oral fluoropyrimidine carbamate with substantial activity in advanced colorectal cancer: results of a randomized phase II study. J Clin Oncol 2000;18:1337–45.

68. Cvitkovic E, Bekradda M. Oxaliplatin: a new therapeutic option in colorectal cancer. Semin Oncol 1999;26:647–62.

69. Eriguchi M, Osada I, Fujii Y, et al. Pilot study for preoperative administration of l-OHP to patients with advanced scirrhous type gastric cancer. Biomed Pharmacother 1997;51:217–20.

70. Christman K, Kelsen D, Saltz L, et al. Phase II trial of gemcitabine in patients with advanced gastric cancer. Cancer 1994;73:5–7.

71. Ramanathan RK, Lipsitz S, Asbury RF, et al. Phase II trial of trimetrexate for patients with advanced gastric carcinoma: an Eastern Cooperative Oncology Group study (E1287). Cancer 1999;86:572–6.

72. John W, Picus J, Blanke CD, et al. Activity of multitargeted antifolate (pemetrexed disodium, LY231514) in patients with advanced colorectal carcinoma: results from a phase II study. Cancer 2000;88:1807–13.

73. Adjei AA, Erlichman C, Sloan JA, et al. Phase I and pharmacologic study of sequences of gemcitabine and the multitargeted antifolate agent in patients with advanced solid tumors. J Clin Oncol 2000;18:1748–1757.

74. Rake MO, Mallinson CN, Cocking JB, et al. Chemotherapy in advanced gastric cancer: a controlled, prospective, randomised multi-centre study. Gut 1979;20:797–801.

75. MacDonald JS, Schein PS, Woolley PV, et al. 5-Fluorouracil, doxorubicin, and mitomycin (FAM) combination chemotherapy for advanced gastric cancer. Ann Intern Med 1980;93:533–6.

76. Klein HO, Wils J, Bleiberg H, et al. An EORTC gastrointestinal (GI) group randomized evaluation of the toxicity of sequential high dose methotrexate and 5-fluorouracil

combined with adriamycin (FAMTX) vs 5-fluorouracil, adriamycin and mitomycin (FAM) in advanced gastric cancer. Med Oncol Tumor Pharmacother 1989;6:171–4.

77. Wils J, Bleiberg H. Current status of chemotherapy for gastric cancer. Eur J Cancer Clin Oncol 1989;25:3–8.

78. Cullinan SA, Moertel CG, Fleming TR, et al. A comparison of three chemotherapeutic regimens in the treatment of advanced pancreatic and gastric carcinoma. Fluorouracil vs fluorouracil and doxorubicin vs fluorouracil, doxorubicin, and mitomycin. JAMA 1985;253:2061–7.

79. O'Connell MJ. Current status of chemotherapy for advanced pancreatic and gastric cancer. J Clin Oncol 1985;3:1032–9.

80. Arbuck SG, Silk Y, Douglass HO Jr, et al. A phase II trial of 5-fluorouracil, doxorubicin, mitomycin C, and leucovorin in advanced gastric carcinoma. Cancer 1990;65:2442–5.

81. Lacave A, Wils J, Bleiberg H, et al. An EORTC Gastrointestinal Group phase III evaluation of combinations of methyl-CCNU, 5-fluorouracil, and adriamycin in advanced gastric cancer. J Clin Oncol 1987;5:1387–93.

82. Levi JA, Fox RM, Tattersall MH, et al. Analysis of a prospectively randomized comparison of doxorubicin versus 5-fluorouracil, doxorubicin, and BCNU in advanced gastric cancer: implications for future studies. J Clin Oncol 1986;4:1348–55.

83. Klein HO. Long-term results with FAMTX (5-fluorouracil, adriamycin, methotrexate) in advanced gastric cancer. Anticancer Res 1989;9:1025–6.

84. Wils J, Bleiberg H, Dalesio O, et al. An EORTC Gastrointestinal Group evaluation of the combination of sequential methotrexate and 5-fluorouracil, combined with adriamycin in advanced measurable gastric cancer. J Clin Oncol 1986;4:1799–803.

85. Wils JA, Klein HO, Wagener DJ, et al. Sequential high-dose methotrexate and fluorouracil combined with doxorubicin—a step ahead in the treatment of advanced gastric cancer: a trial of the European Organization for Research and Treatment of Cancer Gastrointestinal Tract Cooperative Group. J Clin Oncol 1991;9:827–31.

86. Preusser P, Wilke H, Achterrath W, et al. Phase II study with the combination etoposide, doxorubicin, and cisplatin in advanced measurable gastric cancer. J Clin Oncol 1989;7:1310–7.

87. Lerner A, Gonin R, Steele GD Jr, et al. Etoposide, doxorubicin, and cisplatin chemotherapy for advanced gastric adenocarcinoma: results of a phase II trial. J Clin Oncol 1992;10:536–40.

88. Clark JL, Kucuk O, Neuberg DS, et al. Phase II trial of etoposide, doxorubicin, and cisplatin combination in advanced measurable gastric cancer. An Eastern Cooperative Oncology Group study. Am J Clin Oncol 1995;18:318–24.

89. Kelsen D, Atiq OT, Saltz L, et al. FAMTX versus etoposide, doxorubicin, and cisplatin: a random assignment trial in gastric cancer. J Clin Oncol 1992;10:541–8.

90. Cazap EL, Gisselbrecht C, Smith FP, et al. Phase II trials of 5-FU, doxorubicin, and cisplatin in advanced, measurable adenocarcinoma of the lung and stomach. Cancer Treat Rep 1986;70:781–3.

91. Bajetta E, Di Bartolomeo M, Carnaghi C, et al. FEP regimen (epidoxorubicin, etoposide and cisplatin) in advanced gastric cancer, with or without low-dose GM-CSF: an Italian Trial in Medical Oncology (ITMO) study. Br J Cancer 1998;77:1149–54.

92. O'Connell MJ. Etoposide, doxorubicin, and cisplatin chemotherapy for advanced gastric cancer: an old lesson revisited. J Clin Oncol 1992;10:515–6.

93. Ohtsu A, Shimada Y, Yoshida S, et al. Phase II study of protracted infusional 5-fluorouracil combined with cisplatinum for advanced gastric cancer: report from the Japan Clinical Oncology Group (JCOG). Eur J Cancer 1994;14:2091–3.

94. Rougier P, Ducreux M, Mahjoubi M, et al. Efficacy of combined 5-fluorouracil and cisplatinum in advanced gastric carcinomas. A phase II trial with prognostic factor analysis. Eur J Cancer 1994;9:1263–9.

95. Chung YS, Yamashita Y, Inoue T, et al. Continuous infusion of 5-fluorouracil and low dose cisplatin infusion for the treatment of advanced and recurrent gastric adenocarcinoma. Cancer 1997;80:1–7.

96. Williamson SK, Tangen CM, Maddox AM, et al. Phase II evaluation of low-dose continuous 5-fluorouracil and weekly cisplatin in advanced adenocarcinoma of the stomach. A Southwest Oncology Group study. Am J Clin Oncol 1995;18:484–7.

97. Wilke H, Wils J, Rougier P, et al. Preliminary analysis of a randomized phase III trial of FAMTX versus ELF versus cisplatin/FU in advanced gastric cancer: a trial of the EORTC gastrointestinal tract cancer cooperative group and the AIO. Proc Am Soc Clin Oncol 1995;14:206.

98. Wilke H, Preusser P, Fink U, et al. High dose folinic acid/etoposide/5-fluorouracil in advanced gastric cancer—a phase II study in elderly patients or patients with cardiac risk. Invest New Drugs 1990;8:65–70.

99. di Bartolomeo M, Bajetta E, de Braud F, et al. Phase II study of the etoposide, leucovorin and fluorouracil combination for patients with advanced gastric cancer unsuitable for aggressive chemotherapy. Oncology 1995;52:41–4.

100. Partyka S, Dumas P, Ajani J. Combination chemotherapy with granulocyte-macrophage-colony stimulating factor in patients with locoregional and metastatic gastric adenocarcinoma. Cancer 1999;85:2336–9.

101. Colucci G, Giuliani F, Gebbia V, et al. Epirubicin, folinic acid, fluorouracil, and etoposide in the treatment of advanced gastric cancer: phase II study of the Southern Italy Oncology Group (GOIM). Am J Clin Oncol 1999;22:262–6.

102. Kornek G, Schulz F, Depisch D, et al. A phase I-II study of epirubicin, 5-fluorouracil, and leucovorin in advanced adenocarcinoma of the stomach. Cancer 1993;71:2177–80.

103. Zaniboni A, Barni S, Labianca R, et al. Epirubicin, cisplatin, and continuous infusion 5-fluorouracil is an active and safe regimen for patients with advanced gastric cancer. An Italian Group for the Study of Digestive Tract Cancer (GISCAD) report. Cancer 1995;76:1694–9.

104. Waters JS, Norman A, Cunningham D, et al. Long-term survival after epirubicin, cisplatin and fluorouracil for gastric cancer: results of a randomized trial. Br J Cancer 1999; 80:269–72.

105. Cocconi G, Bella M, Zironi S, et al. Fluorouracil, doxorubicin, and mitomycin combination versus PELF chemotherapy in advanced gastric cancer: a prospective randomized trial of the Italian Oncology Group for Clinical Research. J Clin Oncol 1994;12:2687–93.

106. Cascinu S, Labianca R, Alessandroni P, et al. Intensive weekly chemotherapy for advanced gastric cancer using fluorouracil, cisplatin, epi-doxorubicin, 6S-leucovorin, glutathione, and filgrastim: a report from the Italian Group for the Study of Digestive Tract Cancer. J Clin Oncol 1997;15:3313–9.

107. Murad AM, Petroianu A, Guimaraes RC, et al. Phase II trial of the combination of paclitaxel and 5-fluorouracil in the treatment of advanced gastric cancer: a novel, safe, and effective regimen. Am J Clin Oncol 1999;22:580–6.

108. Roth AD, Maibach R, Fazio N, et al. Taxotere-cisplatin in advanced gastric carcinoma: an active drug combination. Proc Am Soc Clin Oncol 1998;17:283a.

109. Shirao K, Shimada Y, Kondo H, et al. Phase I-II study of irinotecan hydrochloride combined with cisplatin in patients with advanced gastric cancer. J Clin Oncol 1997; 15:921–7.

110. Boku N, Ohtsu A, Shimada Y, et al. Phase II study of a combination of irinotecan and cisplatin against metastatic gastric cancer. J Clin Oncol 1999;17:319–23.

111. Ajani JA, Fairweather J, Pisters PW, et al. Phase II study of CPT-11 plus cisplatin in patients with advanced gastric and GE junction carcinomas. Proc Am Soc Clin Oncol 1999;18:241a.

112. Langman MJ, Dunn JA, Whiting JL, et al. Prospective, double-blind, placebo-controlled randomized trial of cimetidine in gastric cancer. British Stomach Cancer Group. Br J Cancer 1999;81:1356–62.

113. Harrison JD, Jones JA, Morris DL. The effect of the gastrin receptor antagonist proglumide on survival in gastric carcinoma. Cancer 1990;66:1449–52.

114. Popiela T, Zembala M, Kulig J, et al. Postoperative immunochemotherapy (BCG + 5-FU) in advanced gastric cancer. Anticancer Res 1988;8:1423–7.

115. A comparison of combination chemotherapy and combined modality therapy for locally advanced gastric carcinoma. Gastrointestinal Tumor Study Group. Cancer 1982;49:1771–7.

116. The concept of locally advanced gastric cancer. Effect of treatment on outcome. The Gastrointestinal Tumor Study Group. Cancer 1990;66:2324–30.

117. Daut RL, Cleeland CS, Flanery RC. Development of the Wisconsin Brief Pain Questionnaire to assess pain in cancer and other diseases. Pain 1983;17:197–210.

118. Graham C, Bond SS, Gerkovich MM, et al. Use of the McGill pain questionnaire in the assessment of cancer pain: replicability and consistency. Pain 1980;8:377–87.

119. Fishman B, Pasternak S, Wallenstein SL, et al. The Memorial Pain Assessment Card. A valid instrument for the evaluation of cancer pain. Cancer 1987;60:1151–8.

120. Ventafridda V, Tamburini M, Caraceni A, et al. A validation study of the WHO method for cancer pain relief. Cancer 1987;59:850–6.

121. Rosen SM. Procedural control of cancer pain. Semin Oncol 1994;21:740–7.

122. Loprinzi CL. Management of cancer anorexia/cachexia. Support Care Cancer 1995;3:120–2.

123. Loprinzi CL, Bernath AM, Schaid DJ, et al. Phase III evaluation of 4 doses of megestrol acetate as therapy for patients with cancer anorexia and/or cachexia. Oncology 1994;51 Suppl 1:2–7.

124. Rowland KM Jr, Loprinzi CL, Shaw EG, et al. Randomized double-blind placebo-controlled trial of cisplatin and etoposide plus megestrol acetate/placebo in extensive-stage small-cell lung cancer: a North Central Cancer Treatment Group study. J Clin Oncol 1996;14:135–41.

125. Loprinzi CL, Kugler JW, Sloan JA, et al. Randomized comparison of megestrol acetate versus dexamethasone versus fluoxymesterone for the treatment of cancer anorexia/cachexia. J Clin Oncol 1999;17:3299–306.

126. Chlebowski RT. Critical evaluation of the role of nutritional support with chemotherapy. Cancer 1985;55:268–72.

127. Nowrousian MR. Recombinant human erythropoietin in the treatment of cancer-related or chemotherapy-induced anaemia in patients with solid tumours. Med Oncol 1998;15 Suppl 1:S19–28.

128. Oberhoff C, Neri B, Amadori D, et al. Recombinant human erythropoietin in the treatment of chemotherapy-induced anemia and prevention of transfusion requirement associated with solid tumors: a randomized, controlled study. Ann Oncol 1998;9:255–60.

129. Sonnenfeld T, Tyden G. Peritoneovenous shunts for malignant ascites. Acta Chir Scand 1986;152:117–21.

130. Gough IR, Balderson GA. Malignant ascites. A comparison of peritoneovenous shunting and nonoperative management. Cancer 1993;71:2377–82.

131. Tsugawa K, Yonemura Y, Hirono Y, et al. Amplification of the c-met, c-erbB-2 and epidermal growth factor receptor gene in human gastric cancers: correlation to clinical features. Oncology 1998;55:475–81.

132. Takahashi Y, Cleary KR, Mai M, et al. Significance of vessel count and vascular endothelial growth factor and its receptor (KDR) in intestinal-type gastric cancer. Clin Cancer Res 1996;2:1679–84.

133. Brien TP, Depowski PL, Sheehan CE, et al. Prognostic factors in gastric cancer. Mod Pathol 1998;11:870–7.

134. Perez EA. HER-2 as a prognostic, predictive, and therapeutic target in breast cancer. Cancer Control 1999;6:233–240.

135. Druker BJ, Lydon NB. Lessons learned from the development of an abl tyrosine kinase inhibitor for chronic myelogenous leukemia. J Clin Invest 2000;105:3–7.

136. Kerbel RS. Tumor angiogenesis: past, present and the near future. Carcinogenesis 2000;21:505–15.

137. Nelson AR, Fingleton B, Rothenberg ML, et al. Matrix metalloproteinases: biologic activity and clinical implications. J Clin Oncol 2000;18:1135–49.

138. Laheru DA, Jaffee EM. Potential role of tumor vaccines in GI malignancies. Oncology (Huntingt) 2000;14:245–56, 259–60.

139. Lenz HJ, Leichman CG, Danenberg KD, et al. Thymidylate synthase mRNA level in adenocarcinoma of the stomach: a predictor for primary tumor response and overall survival. J Clin Oncol 1996;14:176–82.

140. Johnston PG, Lenz HJ, Leichman CG, et al. Thymidylate synthase gene and protein expression correlate and are associated with response to 5-fluorouracil in human colorectal and gastric tumors. Cancer Res 1995;55:1407–12.

141. Metzger R, Leichman CG, Danenberg KD, et al. ERCC1 mRNA levels complement thymidylate synthase mRNA levels in predicting response and survival for gastric cancer patients receiving combination cisplatin and fluorouracil chemotherapy. J Clin Oncol 1998;16:309–16.

16

Invasive Techniques for Palliation of Advanced Gastric Cancer

EDDIE K. ABDALLA, MD

MADHUKAR KAW, MD

PETER W.T. PISTERS, MD, FACS

Because of the low cure rate for gastric cancer and the advanced stage at which most patients present with gastric cancer, appropriate palliative techniques are essential. A large proportion (30 to 80%) of patients with gastric adenocarcinoma present with stage IV disease,[1] and an additional proportion (28 to 37%) initially believed to have localized disease are found to have metastatic disease after state-of-the-art staging.[2,3] Further, the 5-year survival rate for patients with stage IV disease approaches 0 percent.[4] Hence, the majority of newly diagnosed gastric cancers are incurable.

Gastric adenocarcinoma spreads locally, via lymphatic and hematogenous routes. Thus, invasion of adjacent organs, nodal metastases, and distant metastases are common. Invasion through the gastric serosa can occur early and leads to the increased risk of peritoneal spread, invasion of local structures, and lymphatic metastasis (in up to 75% of patients).[5] Spread through the intramural gastric lymphatics to the esophagus and the duodenum occurs in 30 to 65 percent of patients.[6] Analysis of patterns of failure after potentially curative therapy reveals that occult distant metastases are almost universal. The relatively poor overall prognosis of gastric cancer makes palliation a central theme in gastric cancer management.

Optimal palliation relieves or abates symptoms while causing minimal morbidity, and it improves the patient's quality of life. Prolonged survival is generally not a goal of palliative intervention, but palliation may relieve debilitating and potentially life-threatening problems such as gastrointestinal bleeding and gastric-outlet obstruction. Surgical palliation of advanced gastric cancer may include resection or bypass, alone or in combination with endoscopic, percutaneous, or radiational interventions. This chapter reviews surgical, endoscopic, and other modes of palliative therapy for gastric cancer.

SURGICAL PALLIATION

Resection

Accurate pretreatment staging (which includes laparoscopy) has lowered the rate of nontherapeutic laparotomies for gastric cancer. Treatment planning is greatly facilitated when the extent of disease and the presence of metastases are defined before planned laparotomy. Therapy for most patients with visceral metastatic disease or peritoneal carcinomatosis is nonsurgical because of the short median survival—about 6 months—and the lack of a defined benefit for palliative gastrectomy in this setting.[7,8] Patients with positive peritoneal lavage cytology have a prognosis comparable to that of patients with macroscopic visceral or peritoneal disease.[9] At the University of Texas M.D. Anderson Cancer Center, therapy is carefully individualized for patients whose only evidence of distant disease is positive peritoneal lavage cytology. At the Center, we favor neoadjuvant chemotherapy, with or without chemoradiotherapy. Patients are then restaged, and further treatment planning is based on symptoms, response to therapy, and performance status. Following repeat laparoscopic or open restaging, carefully selected patients in this high-risk group may be offered resection.

Gastrectomy for gastric cancer can be classified postoperatively (after pathologic evaluation of surgical margins) by the presence or absence of residual disease (R status). The ideal goal of complete gross and microscopic removal of tumor (R0 resection) may not always be achieved, resulting in microscopic (R1) or macroscopic (R2) residual disease. State-of-the-art staging combined with standardized resection techniques has minimized the incidence of noncurative (R1 and R2) resections.

The extent to which noncurative resection provides palliation depends on several factors, including pretreatment performance status, nutritional status, preoperative symptoms, volume of disease, and the morbidity of the palliative procedure (Table 16–1). The operative mortality rate (primarily related to anastomotic leak) for palliative resections is higher than that for curative resections in most series, probably because patients who undergo R1 or R2 resections generally have worse preoperative performance and nutritional statuses than do patients with localized disease.[10] Thus, avoidance of deliberate palliative resection is recommended, except for carefully selected patients.

The Mayo Clinic has historically promoted resection, even total gastrectomy, as the best palliation in advanced technically resectable gastric cancer.[11] In a review of 53 consecutive patients treated by palliative total gastrectomy, the median survival was 19 months. Twenty-four percent of patients survived beyond 2 years, with a quality of life considered good in 59 percent, satisfactory in 28 percent, and poor in 13 percent of these surviving patients. The operative mortality rate was 8 percent. Butler and colleagues reported similar results in a series of 27 patients who underwent palliative total gastrectomy.[12] Ellis and colleagues reported favorable results in a series of 167 esophagogastrectomies, with an in-hospital mortality rate of 1.3 percent, a major complication rate of 15 percent, and a 5-year survival rate of 22 percent.[13] However, this report included patients with tumors at earlier stages (stages I, II, and III); hence, these more favorable-appearing results likely reflect the inclusion of patients with better prognoses.

Particular controversy surrounds palliative surgery for advanced proximal gastric cancer since palliative resection requires total gastrectomy or esophagogastrectomy, which carries higher overall morbidity and mortality rates than does palliative distal gastrectomy. Such tumors can be large, may be associated with bulky adenopathy, and may involve adjacent structures, including the esophagus, liver, diaphragm, spleen, and celiac axis (Figures 16–1 and 16–2). A few centers that treat large numbers of patients with advanced proximal gastric cancers have reported performing palliative resections with acceptable morbidity and mortality rates.[14–16] However, this approach is probably not advisable for the majority of patients with advanced proximal gastric cancer, given the high risk of such procedures and the established relationship between the number of patients treated and the outcomes of patients undergoing major cancer surgery.[17] Less morbid approaches, such as endoscopic recanalization or the use of stents, may improve the quality (and possibly the quantity) of life in this population.[18]

Meijer and colleagues evaluated the usefulness of surgical palliation by examining outcomes after laparotomy in 204 patients with gastric cancer believed to be resectable on the basis of preoperative studies (see Table 16–1).[19] Of these patients, 121 (59%) underwent R0 resection. Tumors in the remaining patients (41%) were unresectable for cure; 26 (13% of all) of these patients underwent palliative (R1 or R2) resection, 25 (12%) underwent gastroenterostomy, and 32 (16%) underwent nontherapeutic laparotomy. Results for those who underwent gastroenterostomy were poor. Those who underwent palliative resection achieved a mean survival of 9.5 months, but only one-half of these patients experienced good palliation (defined as relief of preoperative symptoms, absence of new symptoms, acceptable body weight, and solid-food intake); 27 percent experienced moderate palliation, and 15 percent experienced poor palliation. Of 14 patients who underwent palliative total gastrectomy, 2 died after developing an anastomotic leak. Overall, only 13 percent of the gastric cancer patients who underwent surgery were candidates for palliative resection on the basis of operative findings, and 28 percent underwent a surgical procedure that provided neither meaningful relief of symptoms nor

Table 16–1. REPORTED SERIES OF PALLIATIVE SURGICAL PROCEDURES FOR ADVANCED GASTRIC ADENOCARCINOMA

First Author (Patient Date Range)	Ref. No.	No. of Patients Total	No. of Patients Operated	No. of Patients Resected	Palliative Therapy (No. of Patients)	Morbidity (%)	Mortality* (%)	Comments on Patients Surviving > 30 Days†
ReMine (NR)	20	206	206	69	EG (17) TG (6) ST (46) GJ (98) Stent (16)	NR	6 0 6.5 3 13	EG: 35% experienced good palliation, 47% fair, 12% failed TG: palliation considered fair-poor in all ST: 30% good, 13% fair, 50% failed/poor GJ: 19% benefited, 46% equivalent, 32% failed Stent: 25% good, 44% fair, 19% poor
Ekbom (1957–78)	14	144	144	124	ST (40) T/P/E (15) GJ (20)	22 33 20	15 27 25	88% of all PRs experienced good palliation for average of 14.6 months. 80% of GJs: good palliation for mean 5.9 months.
Boddie (1941–81) (1941–69) (1970–81)	15	198	198	196	T/P/E T/P/E T/P/E	37 (leak) 16 (abscess) 9 (fistula)	17.8 11.1 22.2	For all PRs 1941–81: 0% experienced good palliation, 85.7% fair, 14.3% poor
Boddie (1941–81) (1941–69) (1970–81)	15	21	21	NA	NT or GJ NT or GJ	5 (leak) 0 (abscess) 5 (fistula)	23.8 33.3 11.1	For all NT or GJ patients, 1941–81: 0% experienced good palliation, 60% fair, 40% poor
Meijer (1965–81)	19	256	204	147	TG (14) ST (12) GJ (25) NT (32)	NR	14.3 0 0 0	For all PRs: 50% experienced good palliation, 27% moderate, 15% poor. GJ: 100% poor palliation NT: quality of palliation not reported
Welvaart (1970–82)	48	54	54	54	TG (17) Prox ST (37)	NR	29 24	Of those discharged from hospital, nearly all prox STs tolerated regular diet until death, and those with TG had a fair result overall.
Lo (1986–88)	21	51	51	NA	GJ (51)	55	22	78% of all could take food PO by postoperative day 18, but 63% required re-admission to hospital, and 10% required reoperation.
Monson (1980–89)	11	53	53	53	TG (53)	NR	8	Of 47 evaluable after hospital discharge, 59% experienced good palliation, 28% satisfactory, 13% poor. 17% required further surgery before death.
Geoghegan (1982–86)	10	114	77	54	PR (32) GJ (12) NT (9)	22 NR NR	12.5 25 44	PR: 82% were symptom-free for 6 months. GJ: 56% experienced satisfactory palliation. NT: None experienced satisfactory palliation.

*30-day or in-hospital mortality.
†Though the number of total patients and number operated are provided, morbidity, mortality, and comments are restricted to patients who underwent palliative procedures. Noncurative (palliative) resections include both R1 and R2 resections.
NR = not reported; EG = esophagogastrectomy; TG = total gastrectomy; ST = subtotal gastrectomy; GJ = gastrojejunostomy; T/P/E = total, proximal, or esophagogastrectomy; PR = palliative resection; NA = not applicable; NT = nontherapeutic laparotomy; Prox ST = proximal subtotal gastrectomy; PO = per os (orally).

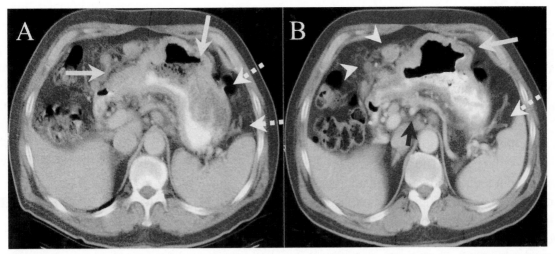

Figure 16–1. Computed tomography scans show a large mass involving the body and antrum of the stomach (*long arrows*), with enlarged left gastric lymph nodes and nodes along the right gastroepiploic artery (*arrowheads in B*), consistent with metastatic disease. The infiltrative change surrounding the perigastric fat along the greater curvature (*dashed arrows*) suggests extragastric extension of tumor as well as celiac and splenic arterial involvement (*black arrow in B*).

extension of life. These results from a major referral center with experienced gastric surgeons emphasize the considerable risk for morbidity and death and the relatively poor "return on investment" for many patients who undergo palliative major resection.

Local recurrence in the absence of distant disease is exceedingly rare, and the surgical management of patients with such recurrence is highly individualized. As for patients with positive peritoneal cytology (and no demonstrable visceral metastases), those with isolated local recurrence should be considered for neoadjuvant chemotherapy with or without radiotherapy. Patients are then restaged, and further treat-

ment planning is based on symptoms, response to therapy, and performance status. Following open restaging, carefully selected patients in this high-risk group may be offered resection.

Gastroenteric Bypass

Before the advent of endoscopic techniques, operative bypass with gastroenteric anastomosis was used in nearly three-fourths of patients with unresectable distal gastric cancer and gastric-outlet obstruction.[20] Two reports have focused on the efficacy of this approach. Lo and colleagues reported that 88 percent

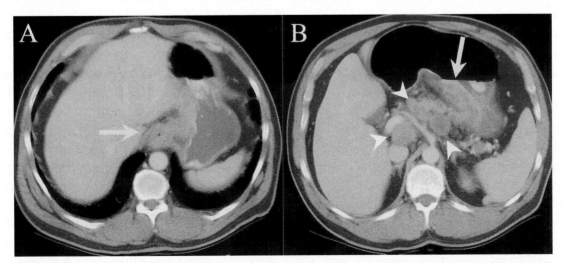

Figure 16–2. Computed tomography scans show a large mass involving the esophagogastric junction (*long arrows*), with enlarged lymph nodes along the celiac axis and its visceral branches (*arrowheads in B*).

of 51 patients who underwent palliative gastroen-terostomy could tolerate a soft diet by postoperative day 8 and that 60 percent could "cope with progression of disease" at home.[21] Nonetheless, this left 40 percent with poor results; furthermore, the operative mortality and morbidity rates were 22 percent and 55 percent, respectively. A recent Japanese review of 52 patients who underwent gastrojejunostomy for unresectable cancer of the antrum revealed poor palliation and a median duration of effective palliation of only 2.8 months (range of 0 to 13 months) in this population with a median survival of 5.0 months.[22] Furthermore, survival and quality of life were not significantly improved by the procedure. Thus, there is little in the literature to support laparotomy with gastroenteric bypass as an approach for palliation in patients with advanced disease and luminal obstruction. With the significant progress in minimally invasive surgery over the past decade, some investigators have evaluated therapeutic laparoscopy as a potentially low-morbidity means of surgical palliation. Advances in laparoscopic techniques now permit the creation of a gastrojejunostomy at the time of laparoscopy, relieving gastric-outlet obstruction without the morbidity of a larger surgical incision.[23] Increasing experience with this technique may make possible a greater improvement in symptoms and in quality of life, with less morbidity than that associated with gastroenterostomy performed at open laparotomy. Clinical trials with uniform staging criteria for entry and quality-of-life end points are needed to help define the role of laparoscopic approaches to the palliation of gastrointestinal symptoms.

Standard bypass techniques for the palliation of gastric-outlet obstruction, such as simple gastrostomy (Figure 16–3, A), side-to-side gastroenterostomy (see Figure 16–3, B), or Roux-en-Y gastrojejunostomy (see Figure 16–3, C), are usually possible. Techniques of palliative reconstruction that are more creative and extensive have been proposed for minimizing the problems of postprandial dumping and small reservoir after a patient has undergone palliative total gastrectomy with the standard Roux-en-Y esophagojejunostomy. These include (a) transdiaphragmatic Roux-en-Y esophagojejunostomy to bypass distal esophageal or gastroesophageal-junction tumors[24] and (b) esophageal mucosectomy with colon interposition.[25]

Operative Intubation

Operative intubation of esophageal and gastroesophageal-junction tumors has largely been abandoned. Advances in technology and materials have shifted the focus to endoscopically placed stents. Endoscopic stent placement can be performed on an outpatient basis, with low morbidity.[26,27] Endoscopic techniques for palliation are discussed below.

NONSURGICAL INVASIVE PALLIATIVE INTERVENTIONS

Dilatation and Laser Ablation

The considerable morbidity of surgical bypass has prompted advances in endoscopic techniques for palliating dysphagia. Dilatation, tumor ablation with laser or argon coagulation, various endoluminal stenting techniques, and radiation have been investigated as means of re-establishing oral feeding with less morbidity than that seen with laparotomy. Dilatation is a simple means of re-establishing a conduit for the passage of intestinal contents; however, doing so can be technically impossible because of complete or near-complete luminal obstruction.

The neodymium:yttrium-aluminum-garnet laser can be used to ablate tumor and re-establish the intestinal lumen. This approach is effective in the palliation of cardia lesions that are nearly completely obstructive or that are problematic because of bleeding; initial palliation is achieved in 90 percent of patients, and durable palliation is achieved in about 70 percent. However, about one-third of patients may require further treatment.[28–31]

Endoscopic argon electrocoagulation may provide palliation similar to that achieved with laser recanalization, at lower cost and with similar morbidity. In one report of 83 patients, 58 percent of patients were able to tolerate a normal diet after one argon electrocoagulation treatment, 26 percent of patients required multiple treatments but were ultimately able to eat, and 16 percent of patients failed to tolerate a regular diet regardless of endoscopic treatment.[32] Perforation complicated treatment in 8 percent, but only one of these patients required operative management.

These reports emphasize that although ablative therapy is effective in re-establishing oral intake, repeat therapy is necessary in most patients. Radiotherapy has been studied as a means of extending the duration of effect after ablative therapy. External beam radiotherapy (30 Gy in 10 fractions) after laser recanalization extends the treatment interval to 9 weeks (from 4 to 5 weeks without radiotherapy).[33]

Endolumenal Stents

Celestin esophageal stents have been replaced by the newer expandable metal stents because of the high mortality (up to 27%) and relatively poor long-term palliation associated with Celestin stents.[34] Tumor can grow through the interstices of expandable stents, but newer coated expandable metallic stents

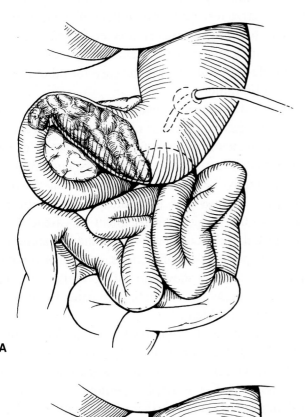

A

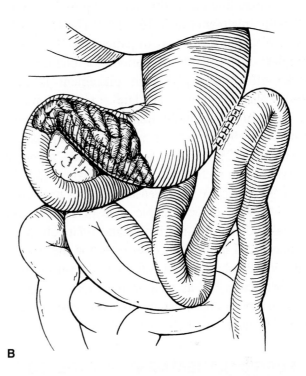

B

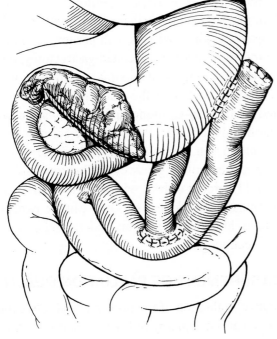

C

Figure 16–3. *A,* Open or percutaneous gastrostomy. This may be the only option for palliation in patients with intractable vomiting and advanced disease. *B,* Gastroenterostomy; *C,* Roux-en-Y gastrojejunostomy. For palliation of gastric-outlet obstruction, patients with acceptable performance status may be candidates for gastroenterostomy or Roux-en-Y gastrojejunostomy.

may minimize this problem.[35] Fewer complications, shorter hospital stays, and similar rates of recurrent dysphagia are reported for the coated expandable stents, compared to noncoated stents[35] (Table 16–2).

For patients with gastric-outlet obstruction from locally advanced distal gastric lesions, expandable metal stents have been shown to be effective for the palliation of intractable nausea and vomiting, and patients may tolerate a soft diet for up to 3 months following treatment (Table 16–3).[36,37] The stent cannot be placed in a minority of patients (< 10%), and complete inability of the patient to tolerate oral intake after successful stent placement is rare (9%).[38] The overall (early and late) complication rate (ie, rate of perforation, migration, dislodgment, obstruction by tumor, or severe esophagitis) is acceptable (22%);[39] few patients require a major intervention to rectify these problems when they do occur. Two recent comprehensive reviews reiterated the advantages of endoscopic stent placement and emphasized the low morbidity and relatively high technical and clinical success rates for the use of endoscopic techniques for palliation of gastrointestinal obstruction,[26,27] as well as the shorter hospital stays and lower cost when compared to open procedures[27] (Figures 16–4, 16–5, and 16–6).

SURGICAL TREATMENT OF PATIENTS WITH DISTANT METASTASES

The surgical treatment of patients with metastatic gastric cancer is rarely indicated because of the significant morbidity of major surgery in the context of the short median survival of these patients. However, resectional and nonresectional therapies have been used selectively. Successful resection of metastases, with extended survival, has been achieved in rare instances (typically in the case of a solitary metastasis for which negative margins of > 1 cm are achieved).[40] Rarely, malignant small-bowel obstruction that is not amenable to endoscopic or percutaneous treatment requires laparotomy in a patient with an acceptable performance status. For many such patients, a side-to-side enteroenterostomy to a convenient loop of bowel is performed to address focal obstruction with minimum dissection (Figure 16–7).

Percutaneous chemoembolization under local anesthesia may be a means of managing metastatic disease limited to the liver and has the advantages of requiring minimal or no hospital stay and avoiding systemic chemotherapy and its attendant toxicities.[41] However, this therapy has not been applied extensively for patients with gastric cancer. Other nonresectional therapies, such as radiofrequency ablation and cryoablation, remain investigational. The selective resection or treatment of symptomatic bone or brain metastases is directed by the patient's clinical indications, performance status, and anticipated life expectancy, as is the case for other metastatic solid tumors.

Surgical treatment of malignant ascites related to a patient's gastric cancer is rarely indicated because life expectancy is so short for these patients. Severe abdominal discomfort and respiratory compromise are generally best treated by traditional means, including diuresis and paracentesis. Very little in regard to the surgical management of gastric cancer–related ascites can be found in the literature. In spite of periodic malfunctions, peritoneovenous shunts have been shown to be of limited use in selected patients for facilitating outpatient management of this problem.[42]

Novel aggressive approaches to patients with extensive disease limited to the peritoneal cavity (without visceral metastatic disease) are under investigation. For example, peritoneal debulking with intraperitoneal hyperthermic chemotherapy has been used for some patients with peritoneal disease. The procedure involves extended gastrectomy, complete peritonectomy with maximal cytoreduction (of all visible tumor), and the manual distribution of heated mitomycin-C, alone or in combination with cisplatin and etoposide. Postoperative complications are common, but the 5-year survival rate of patients in whom a complete gross cytoreduction has been done is 11 percent or less, with a median survival of 12 months. This modest survival can be expected only in highly selected patients undergoing protocol-based treatment.[43,44]

MEASUREMENT OF PALLIATION QUALITY

Objective evaluation of the impact of palliative therapies on patients' quality of life is important. Several

Table 16-2. ENDOSCOPIC TREATMENT OF MALIGNANT DISTAL ESOPHAGEAL OR GASTROESOPHAGEAL STENOSIS OR OCCLUSION

First Author* (Patient Date Range)	Ref. No.	Tumor Location (No. of Tumors)	Treatment (No. of Patients)	Treatments Initial	Treatments Interval	Treatments Total	Morbidity (%)	Mortality† (%)	Comments
Barr (NR)	47	All GEJ tumors (14/40 SCCA)	Laser only (20) Laser + stent (20) (Nd:YAG)	NR NR	1 mo 1 mo	4.6 2.9	10.0 40.0	0 0	25% recurrent dysphagia, complications trivial 45% recurrent dysphagia, all treated successfully with repeat endoscopy Equal QL improvement in both groups
Barr (NR)	49	Malignant dysphagia (40)	Nd:YAG laser (40)‡	>1	1 mo	NR	3.0 (major)	0	Significant improvement in dysphagia and QL by several QL instruments
Loizou (1987–89)	18	Distal esophagus and cardia (73)	Nd:YAG laser (43) Stent (30)	NR	4–5 wk	NR	NR	NR	QL improved until death in all pts followed (23) QL improved until death in all pts followed (15)
Spinelli (1978–92)	39	Distal esophagus (43), cardia (33)	Endoscopic stent (77)	1	10 repeat endoscopy for replace/ reposition		22.0	0	56% tolerated food, 35% liquids only, 8% unimproved. Complications: 3 perforations, 4 migrations, 6 late dislodgments, 2 obstructions, 1 severe esophagitis.
Carter (1985–88)	30	Esophagus and cardia (141)	Nd:YAG laser (141)	NR	NR	NR	11.3	4	92% tolerated semisolid or regular diet, 4% liquids only, 4% unable to recanalize. Complications: perforation, TEF, aspiration
Freitas (1987–92)	31	Cervical (18), mid (41), distal/cardia (45)	Nd:YAG laser (104)	3	1 mo	NR	6.0	1	75% good, 16% fair, 9% failed palliation. 49% required alternative treatment before death. Complications: 3 TEF, 3 perforations.
Hurley (1990–96)	29	Esophagus and cardia (67)	Nd:YAG laser (67)	2	25 d	4	9.0	0	90% initial palliation, 76% sustained after 3 mo, 71% within 1 mo of death. 29% required second-line palliation. Complications included perforation, bleeding.
Ell (Review)	26	Esophagus and cardia	Self-expanding metal stent	—	—	Review	—	—	Summarizes reports: early complication rate 0–24% (stent migration, delamination, incomplete expansion); late complication rate 25–40% (tumor ingrowth, stent migration, obstruction)
Heindorff (1993–95)	32	Upper (19), mid (18), distal/GEJ (46)	Argon electro coagulation (83)	1 (58%) > 1 (26%)	3–4 wk	NR	8.0	1	64% maintained patency until death, 36% required further treatment (stent). 16% failed to achieve regular diet.
Norberto (1992–97)	28	Distal esophagus (40), cardia (67)	Nd:YAG laser (107)	2	2 mo	6.3	0.0	0	82% excellent or good palliation

*There are no studies reporting outcomes for gastric cancer patients only.
†Procedure related
‡In all other studies, some patients may have received some other therapy (chemotherapy, photodynamic therapy, radiation therapy, surgery, stent). This is the only study including patients whose only treatment was laser recanalization.
NR = not reported; GEJ = gastroesophageal junction; SCCA = squamous cell carcinoma; Nd:YAG = neodymium:yttrium-aluminum-garnet; QL = quality of life; pts = patients; TEF = tracheoesophageal fistula.

instruments for measuring the quality of palliation have been studied, and many of them give consistent results. The instruments evaluate objective factors (dysphagia scores) and subjective factors (the patient's feelings of emotional and social well-being). Recent studies show concordance among rating scales such as the Quality of Life Index, the Linear Analogue Self-Assessment, the Gastrointestinal Quality-of-Life Index, and Karnofsky Performance Status.[45,46]

A prospective study of patients with T4 or M1 disease, 43 of whom underwent laser ablation alone for near-obstructing esophageal or gastroesophageal-junction tumors and 30 of whom underwent laser ablation plus endoscopic intubation for the same types of tumors, highlights the importance of objective evaluations of quality of life parameters in the assessment of palliative techniques. In this series, Loizou and colleagues showed that both therapies improve quality of life significantly but that a significant deterioration of quality of life precedes the patient's death regardless of treatment.[18] In a similar study of 46 patients, Barr and colleagues showed that although the complication rate for intubation after laser ablation was four times that of ablation alone, fewer repeat procedures were necessary with laser ablation, and improvement in quality of life was the same with both procedures.[47] Given the primary goals of palliation, the objective evaluation of the quality of palliation should be an important focus of future clinical research.

RECOMMENDATIONS AND CONCLUSION

Following optimal staging, patients found to have peritoneal disease, hepatic metastases, extensive nodal metastases, or ascites and patients with problems that include bleeding or proximal or distal gastric obstruction are best palliated by endoscopic means. The results of endoscopic palliation are generally superior to those of surgical bypass in these patients, and the overall morbidity is considerably less—an important factor for patients with a relatively short life expectancy. Laser recanalization or simple dilatation can reestablish oral intake, with or without the placement of a stent in the proximal stomach. Repeat endoscopy may be required at peri-

Table 16–3. ENDOSCOPIC TREATMENT OF MALIGNANT GASTRIC OUTLET OBSTRUCTION OR DUODENAL STENOSIS OR OCCLUSION

First Author* (Patient Date Range)	Ref. No.	Stent Location (No.)	Treatment	Morbidity (%)	Mortality† (%)	Comments on Patient Results
Feretis (1993–94)	36	Gastric outlet (12)	Self-expanding metal stent	0	0	All able to eat semisolid food 4 days after insertion and until discharge; none required more than 1 endoscopy.
Pinto (1991–95)	37	Gastric outlet and duodenum (6)	Self-expanding metal stent	0	0	All tolerated soft diet 4 days after procedure; 1 failed at 4 weeks, refused therapy; 2 others successfully re-stented for recurrent obstruction.
Yates (1994–96)	38	Gastric outlet and duodenum (11)	Self-expanding metal stent	0	0	91% success (single failure due to distal small-bowel obstruction); 4/11 developed recurrent obstruction (of whom 2 required repeat stenting); 1 required 2 repeat procedures.
Jung (1998–99)	50	Gastric outlet and duodenum (19)	Covered metal stent	25	0	All but 1 tolerated oral diet after stent or re-stent (5 stents migrated and were re-stented); 1 developed jaundice after migration.
Yim (1996–99)	27	Gastric outlet and duodenum (28); anastomosis (3)	Self-expanding metal stent	0	0	42% were stented as outpatients; 94% of stents were deployed successfully, with positive clinical outcomes in 81%; 2 (6%) technical failures were related to stent malposition and inability to cross a stenotic stricture with the guide wire.

*There are no studies reporting outcomes for gastric cancer patients only.
†Procedure related.

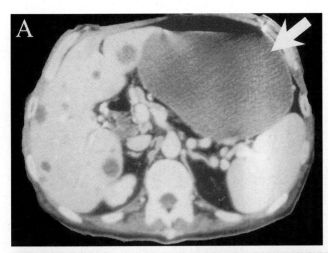

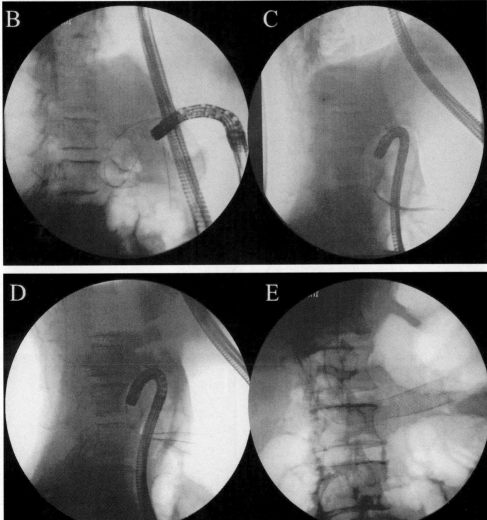

Figure 16–4. Endoscopic palliation was performed in this patient with multiple liver metastases and gastric distention from gastric-outlet obstruction, as demonstrated on computed tomography (*A*). Under fluoroscopic guidance, an endoscopic wire was passed through the stenotic gastric outlet (*B* [lateral oblique view]). The stent was positioned over the wire (*C* [lateral oblique view]) and subsequently deployed (*D* [lateral oblique view]). In this patient, a second stent was deployed distally for persistent narrowing in the distal duodenum (*E* [anteroposterior view]).

odic intervals. Patients who undergo stent placement for gastric-outlet obstruction are often able to eat solid or semisolid food and may not require any further intervention.

Selecting patients for palliative resection is complex. Clearly, R2 resection is to be avoided whenever possible since the outcome of such procedures is uniformly poor. In patients with an excellent perfor-

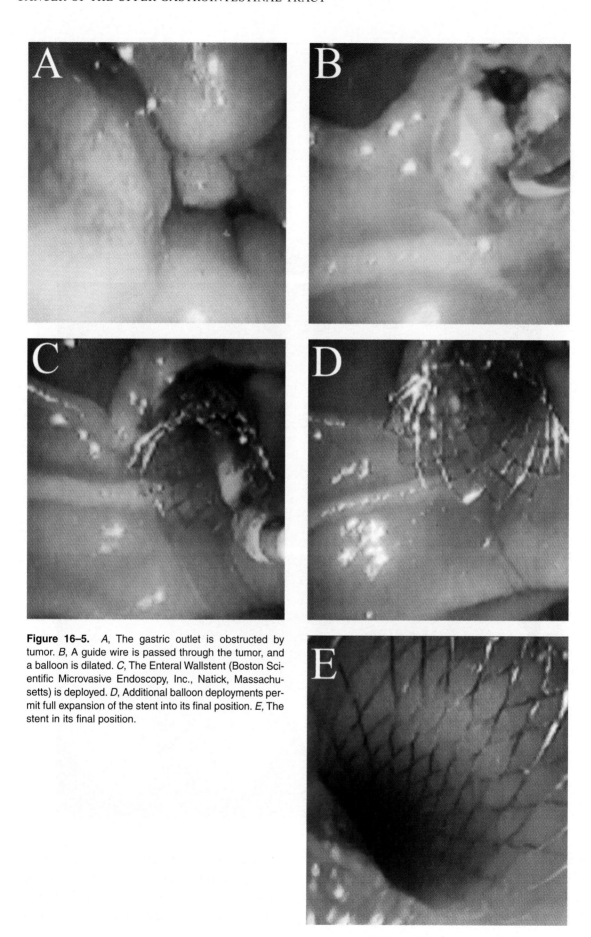

Figure 16–5. *A*, The gastric outlet is obstructed by tumor. *B*, A guide wire is passed through the tumor, and a balloon is dilated. *C*, The Enteral Wallstent (Boston Scientific Microvasive Endoscopy, Inc., Natick, Massachusetts) is deployed. *D*, Additional balloon deployments permit full expansion of the stent into its final position. *E,* The stent in its final position.

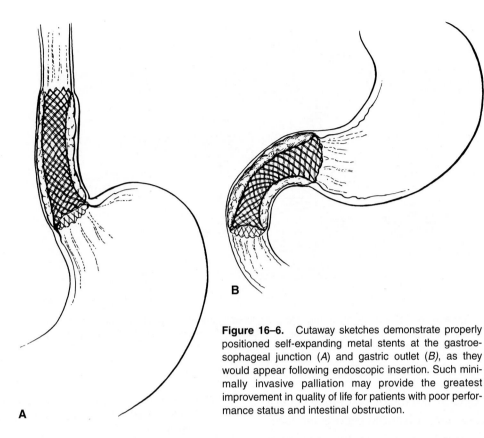

Figure 16–6. Cutaway sketches demonstrate properly positioned self-expanding metal stents at the gastroesophageal junction (*A*) and gastric outlet (*B*), as they would appear following endoscopic insertion. Such minimally invasive palliation may provide the greatest improvement in quality of life for patients with poor performance status and intestinal obstruction.

mance status, experienced surgeons can perform palliative R1 distal gastrectomy with minimal morbidity and acceptable mortality rates. Palliative total gastrectomy and esophagogastrectomy should be approached with greater caution as the morbidity from these procedures is significantly greater and as there is little evidence that quality of life is improved by these procedures.

The treatment of advanced gastric cancer continues to evolve. The cure rate remains low, but surgery may be considered in the palliative treatment of selected patients with advanced disease. Nontherapeutic laparotomy must be avoided whenever possible. The algorithm used at the University of Texas M.D. Anderson Cancer Center carefully applies these principles on a case-by-case basis after consideration by a multidisciplinary team consisting of surgical oncologists, gastroenterologists, and medical and radiation oncologists (Figure 16–8).

Specific indications for palliative resection, surgical bypass (open or laparoscopic), or endoscopic palliation remain undefined. However, assessment of morbidity, mortality, and quality of life has shown that carefully selected patients (particularly those

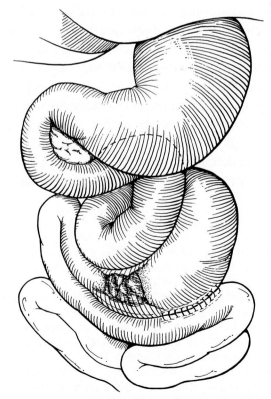

Figure 16–7. Side-to-side enteroenterostomy. In rare cases when the patient's performance status is acceptable and the only clinical problem is intestinal obstruction from metastasis, side-to-side enteroenterostomy may palliate small-bowel obstruction.

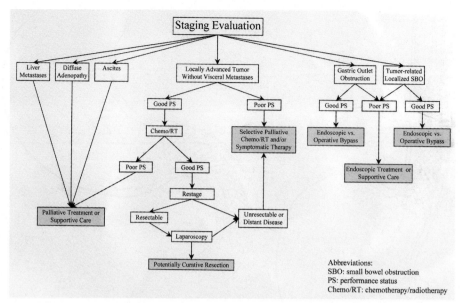

Figure 16–8. The University of Texas M.D. Anderson Cancer Center algorithm (2001) for palliative management of advanced gastric cancer. (Chemo/RT = chemotherapy/radiotherapy; PS = performance status; SBO = small-bowel obstruction.)

without macroscopic metastatic disease) may benefit from palliative resection. Advanced endoscopic techniques, including laser or argon beam tumor ablation and the endoscopic placement of metallic stents, provide better palliation of dysphagia than does surgical bypass, with less morbidity. Other techniques using multimodality therapy (radiation, surgery, and endoscopy) are likely to lead to continued improvements in quality of life and to less morbidity with palliative therapy. However, earlier diagnosis and advances in curative therapy will ultimately be required to definitively reduce the impact of advanced disease for patients with gastric adenocarcinoma.

REFERENCES

1. Wanebo HJ, Kennedy BJ, Chmiel J, et al. Cancer of the stomach. A patient care study by the American College of Surgeons. Ann Surg 1993;218:583–92.

2. Lowy AM, Mansfield PF, Leach SD, Ajani J. Laparoscopic staging for gastric cancer. Surgery 1996;119:611–4.

3. Burke EC, Karpeh MS, Conlon KC, Brennan MF. Laparoscopy in the management of gastric adenocarcinoma. Ann Surg 1997;225:262–7.

4. Fujii K, Isozaki H, Okajima K, et al. Clinical evaluation of lymph node metastasis in gastric cancer defined by the fifth edition of the TNM classification in comparison with the Japanese system. Br J Surg 1999;86:685–9.

5. Kennedy BJ. T N M classification for stomach cancer. Cancer 1970;26:971–83.

6. Zinniger M. Extent of gastric cancer in the intramural lymphatics and its relation to gastrectomy. Am Surg 1954; 20:920.

7. Dupont JB Jr, Lee JR, Burton GR, Cohn I Jr. Adenocarcinoma of the stomach: review of 1,497 cases. Cancer 1978;41:941–7.

8. Gastrointestinal Tumor Study Group. A comparison of combination chemotherapy and combined modality therapy for locally advanced gastric carcinoma. Cancer 2000; 49:1771–7.

9. Burke EC, Karpeh MS Jr, Conlon KC, Brennan MF. Peritoneal lavage cytology in gastric cancer: an independent predictor of outcome. Ann Surg Oncol 1998;5:411–5.

10. Geoghegan JG, Keane TE, Rosenberg IL, et al. Gastric cancer: the case for a more selective policy in surgical management. J R Coll Surg Edinb 1993;38:208–12.

11. Monson JR, Donohue JH, McIlrath DC, et al. Total gastrectomy for advanced cancer. A worthwhile palliative procedure. Cancer 1991;68:1863–8.

12. Butler JA, Dubrow TJ, Trezona T, et al. Total gastrectomy in the treatment of advanced gastric cancer. Am J Surg 1989; 158:602–4.

13. Ellis FH Jr, Gibb SP, Watkins E Jr. Esophagogastrectomy. A safe, widely applicable, and expeditious form of palliation for patients with carcinoma of the esophagus and cardia. Ann Surg 1983;198:531–40.

14. Ekbom GA, Gleysteen JJ. Gastric malignancy: resection for palliation. Surgery 1980;88:476–81.

15. Boddie AW Jr, McMurtrey MJ, Giacco GG, McBride CM. Palliative total gastrectomy and esophagogastrectomy. A reevaluation. Cancer 1983;51:1195–200.

16. Saario I, Schroder T, Tolppanen EM, Lempinen M. Total gastrectomy with esophagojejunostomy. Analysis of 100 consecutive patients. Am J Surg 1986;151:244–6.

17. Begg CB, Cramer LD, Hoskins WJ, Brennan MF. Impact of hospital volume on operative mortality for major cancer surgery. JAMA 1998;280:1747–51.

18. Loizou LA, Rampton D, Atkinson M, et al. A prospective assessment of quality of life after endoscopic intubation and laser therapy for malignant dysphagia. Cancer 1992; 70:386–91.

19. Meijer S, De Bakker OJ, Hoitsma HF. Palliative resection in gastric cancer. J Surg Oncol 1983;23:77–80.

20. ReMine WH. Palliative operations for incurable gastric cancer. World J Surg 1979;3:721–9.

21. Lo NN, Kee SG, Nambiar R. Palliative gastrojejunostomy for advanced carcinoma of the stomach. Ann Acad Med Singapore 1991;20:356–8.

22. Kikuchi S, Tsutsumi O, Kobayashi N, et al. Does gastrojejunostomy for unresectable cancer of the gastric antrum offer satisfactory palliation? Hepatogastroenterology 1999;46:584–7.

23. Kum CK, Yap CH, Goh PM. Palliation of advanced gastric cancer by laparoscopic gastrojejunostomy. Singapore Med J 1995;36:228–9.

24. Orel JJ, Vidmar SS, Hrabar BA. Intrathoracic gastric and jejunal bypass for palliation of nonresectable esophageal carcinoma. Int Surg 1982;67:147–51.

25. Saidi F, Keshoofy M, Abbassi-Dezfuli A, et al. A new approach to the palliation of advanced proximal gastric cancer. J Am Coll Surg 1999;189:259–68.

26. Ell C, May A. Self-expanding metal stents for palliation of stenosing tumors of the esophagus and cardia: a critical review. Endoscopy 1997;29:392–8.

27. Yim HB, Jacobson BC, Saltzman JR, et al. Clinical outcome of the use of enteral stents for palliation of patients with malignant upper GI obstruction. Gastrointest Endosc 2001;53:329–32.

28. Norberto L, Ranzato R, Marino S, et al. Endoscopic palliation of esophageal and cardial cancer: neodymium-yttrium aluminum garnet laser therapy. Dis Esophagus 1999;12:294–6.

29. Hurley JF, Cade RJ. Laser photocoagulation in the treatment of malignant dysphagia. Aust N Z J Surg 1997;67:800–3.

30. Carter R, Smith JS, Anderson JR. Palliation of malignant dysphagia using the Nd:YAG laser. World J Surg 1993; 17:608–13.

31. Freitas D, Gouveia H, Sofia C, et al. Endoscopic Nd-YAG laser therapy as palliative treatment for esophageal and cardial cancer. Hepatogastroenterology 1995;42:633–7.

32. Heindorff H, Wojdemann M, Bisgaard T, Svendsen LB. Endoscopic palliation of inoperable cancer of the oesophagus or cardia by argon electrocoagulation. Scand J Gastroenterol 1998;33:21–3.

33. Sargeant IR, Tobias JS, Blackman G, et al. Radiotherapy enhances laser palliation of malignant dysphagia: a randomized study. Gut 1997;40:362–9.

34. Qvist N, Ryttov N, Larsen KE. Inoperable oesophageal and cardia cancer. Benefits from Celestin intubation. Scand J Thorac Cardiovasc Surg 1987;21:61–3.

35. Siersema PD, Hop WC, Dees J, et al. Coated self-expanding metal stents versus latex prostheses for esophagogastric cancer with special reference to prior radiation and chemotherapy: a controlled, prospective study. Gastrointest Endosc 1998;47:113–20.

36. Feretis C, Benakis P, Dimopoulos C, et al. Palliation of malignant gastric outlet obstruction with self-expanding metal stents. Endoscopy 1996;28:225–8.

37. Pinto IT. Malignant gastric and duodenal stenosis: palliation by peroral implantation of a self-expanding metallic stent. Cardiovasc Intervent Radiol 1997;20:431–4.

38. Yates MR III, Morgan DE, Baron TH. Palliation of malignant gastric and small intestinal strictures with self-expandable metal stents. Endoscopy 1998;30:266–72.

39. Spinelli P, Cerrai FG, Ciuffi M, et al. Endoscopic stent placement for cancer of the lower esophagus and gastric cardia. Gastrointest Endosc 1994;40:455–7.

40. Miyazaki M, Itoh H, Nakagawa K, et al. Hepatic resection of liver metastases from gastric carcinoma. Am J Gastroenterol 1997;92:490–3.

41. Fiorentini G, Poddie DB, Giorgi UD, et al. Global approach to hepatic metastases from colorectal cancer: indication and outcome of intra-arterial chemotherapy and other hepatic-directed treatments. Med Oncol 2000;17:163–73.

42. Gough IR, Balderson GA. Malignant ascites. A comparison of peritoneovenous shunting and nonoperative management. Cancer 1993;71:2377–82.

43. Loggie BW, Fleming RA, McQuellon RP, et al. Cytoreductive surgery with intraperitoneal hyperthermic chemotherapy for disseminated peritoneal cancer of gastrointestinal origin. Am Surg 2000;66:561–8.

44. Sugarbaker PH, Yonemura Y. Clinical pathway for the management of resectable gastric cancer with peritoneal seeding: best palliation with a ray of hope for cure. Oncology 2000;58:96–107.

45. Svedlund J, Sullivan M, Liedman B, et al. Quality of life after gastrectomy for gastric carcinoma: controlled study of reconstructive procedures. World J Surg 1997;21:422–33.

46. Jentschura D, Winkler M, Strohmeier N, et al. Quality-of-life after curative surgery for gastric cancer: a comparison between total gastrectomy and subtotal gastric resection. Hepatogastroenterology 1997;44:1137–42.

47. Barr H, Krasner N, Raouf A, Walker RJ. Prospective randomised trial of laser therapy only and laser therapy followed by endoscopic intubation for the palliation of malignant dysphagia. Gut 1990;31:252–8.

48. Welvaart K, de Jong PL, Palliation of patients with carcinoma of the lower esophagus and cardia: the question of quality of life. J Surg Oncol 1986;32:197–9.

49. Barr H, Krasner N. Prospective quality-of-life analysis after palliative photoablation for the treatment of malignant dysphagia. Cancer 1991;68:1660–4.

50. Jung GS, Song HY, Kang SG, et al. Malignant gastroduodenal obstructions: treatment by means of a covered expandable metallic stent—initial experience. Radiology 2000; 216:758–63.

17

Gastric Lymphoma

RICHARD B. ARENAS, MD

Primary gastric lymphoma accounts for less than 5 percent of all gastric cancers.[1,2] The incidence and pathophysiology of gastric lymphomas differ clinically from the more common adenocarcinomas of the stomach. Unlike adenocarcinoma, primary gastric lymphoma generally responds to current treatment modalities, which include surgery, chemotherapy, and radiotherapy. Gastric lymphoma presents in the sixth decade of life, rarely occurring under the age of 40 years.[1,3] Men and women are equally affected. Whereas gastric cancer has been on the decline in the United States, gastric lymphoma has steadily increased.[4] According to data from the Surveillance, Epidemiology and End Results (SEER) program and some isolated reports, there has been a nearly twofold increase in the incidence of primary gastric lymphoma within the last two decades.[4,5] The age-adjusted incidence has especially risen in the population over 60 years of age.[4] This rise in incidence has gained considerable attention due to the increasing awareness of *Helicobacter pylori* and mucosa-associated lymphoid tissue lymphomas.

Patients with primary gastric lymphoma demonstrate an increased risk for other malignancies.[6] This association with other cancers coincidentally occurs with lymphomas (both Hodgkin's and non-Hodgkin's) that affect the peripheral lymph node tissue. The incidence of associated cancers in reported series of patients with primary gastric lymphoma can be as high as 20 to 25 percent.[7,8] Whereas many of these patients present with other lymphoid neoplasms, synchronous or metachronous gastric adenocarcinoma develops with relative frequency. One particular series from Japan estimated the incidence of synchronous gastric adenocarcinoma and lym-

phoma at 3.7 percent.[9] Although it is speculative that *Helicobacter pylori* may play a common role in these patients through malignant degeneration along epithelial and/or lymphoid lines, *H. pylori* has been documented in patients with synchronous and metachronous primary gastric lymphoma and adenocarcinoma.[9]

PATHOPHYSIOLOGY

The stomach is normally devoid of lymphoid tissue despite the stomach being the most common site for extranodal lymphoma.[1,10] Primary non-Hodgkins's lymphoma of the gastrointestinal tract is present from 41 to 73 percent of the time within the stomach.[10,11] In a population-based analysis of 580 patients from the Netherlands with non-Hodgkin's lymphoma, 209 (36%) patients presented with primary extranodal disease.[12] Within that group with extranodal lymphoma, 96 patients exhibited disease within the gastrointestinal tract; 56 percent of these patients had disease limited to the stomach. Gastric lymphoma can also occur in many cases of disseminated nodal lymphoma.[13] In an autopsy report from Roswell Park Cancer Center, occult gastrointestinal involvement was present in 46 percent of patients with non-Hodgkin's lymphoma.[14]

Ever since Isaacson and colleagues first described mucosa-associated lymphoid tissue (MALT) lymphomas within the gastrointestinal tract, primary gastric lymphoma has been considered a separate entity from non-Hodgkin's lymphoma of the peripheral nodal tissue.[15,16] The significance of MALT is based on the appearance of extranodal lymphoid tissue within the stomach in response to certain inflammatory conditions. *Helicobacter pylori* infection, transplant-related immunosuppression, celiac disease, inflammatory bowel disease, and human immunodeficiency virus (HIV) infection have all been considered risk factors for gastrointestinal lymphoma.[17]

Gastric MALT lymphomas represent a spectrum of disease that ranges from low-grade to high-grade disease. They are clinically distinct from the benign lymphoid infiltrates that are usually observed with chronic gastritis. Nevertheless, benign lymphoid tissue is present in up to 75 percent of cases of gastric lymphoma.[18,19] Several reported series that examined the morphologic changes in the gastric mucosa adjacent to MALT lymphomas demonstrated the presence of reactive lymphoid follicles, with mucosal atrophy and intestinal metaplasia within the neighboring gastric epithelium.[20,21] This reactive inflammatory response presenting with lymphoid hyperplasia is also known as pseudolymphoma and was once considered a premalignant condition for gastric lymphoma.[22] But the term "pseudolymphoma" is now considered inappropriate on the basis of the increasing immunohistochemical information that suggests that pseudolymphoma is actually a low-grade variant of MALT lymphomas.[1] Furthermore, deoxyribonucleic acid (DNA) hybridization techniques have demonstrated immunoglobulin heavy-chain gene re-arrangement in histologically benign reactive perigastric lymph nodes, confirming the hypothesis that MALT is one component of gastric lymphoma and is probably more widespread than was previously expected.[23]

Despite technical advances in histology and immunohistochemistry, low-grade gastric lymphomas with features of MALT still can be difficult to distinguish from benign inflammatory conditions such as gastritis. The hallmark of gastric lymphoma is the presence of a clonal population of B cells. To detect such clonality, molecular-biology techniques such as polymerase chain reaction have been used to identify monoclonal immunoglobulins from lymphoma cells.[24] Immunohistochemical staining for certain cellular markers such as CD10, CD75, and CD43 can distinguish gastritis from MALT-type lymphomas although such markers are used more frequently in differentiating high-grade from low-grade lymphomas.[25]

The distinction of low-grade MALT lymphoma from gastritis is becoming increasingly important because early treatment could prevent the progression toward a high-grade malignancy. Such transformation (previously postulated never to occur) is now believed to be mediated through increasing genetic instability and specific gene mutations. Inactivation of the p53 tumor-suppressor gene, expression of the replication error repair (RER) phenotype, and mutation of the *c-myc* proto-oncogene have been demonstrated to occur with the development of high-grade lymphomas.[26] Cytogenetics has also detected specific chromosomal abnormalities in primary gastric lymphoma. Trisomy of chromosome 3 has been associated with low-grade lymphomas whereas trisomy of chromosomes 12 and 18 has been demonstrated in high-grade lymphomas.[27]

The concept of gastric MALT lymphoma has gained considerable interest, especially in regard to its association with *H. pylori*–related infections.[28] Whereas the simultaneous presence of *H. pylori* and gastric cancer has been repeatedly demonstrated in epidemiologic studies, the causal relationship of *H. pylori* with primary gastric lymphoma remained only speculative until Parsonnet and colleagues demonstrated a sixfold increase in the incidence of non-Hodgkin's gastric lymphoma with previous *H. pylori* infection.[29,30] Numerous studies have subsequently confirmed the presence of *H. pylori* colonization in 59 to 98 percent of patients with primary gastric lymphoma.[31,32]

The specific immunologic responses that occur with *H. pylori* infection and lead to the development of gastric lymphoma have been extensively investigated. It is now believed that certain strains of *H. pylori* produce specific autoantigens that initiate T-cell activation and neutrophil chemotaxis that are necessary for an appropriate inflammatory response.[33,34] Local humoral and T-cell responses induce the production of pro-inflammatory cytokines, which in turn stimulate the proliferation of B cells.[35] The genetic instability of these autoreactive B cells, which are not directly associated with the *H. pylori* infection, leads to the development of a monoclonal lymphoproliferative lesion. This monoclonal population of B cells is first responsive to *H. pylori*–activated T cells; later, it becomes autonomous, resulting in further T-cell proliferation, thus leading to malignant transformation.[28,36] This concept of genetically predisposed B cells that can develop into a gastric lymphoma through an external inflammatory stimulus such as *H. pylori* has gained increasing acceptance and has led to the current controversy over the treatment of low-grade MALT lymphomas (discussed later in this chapter).

DIAGNOSIS

The diagnosis of primary gastric lymphoma requires histologic confirmation of lymphoma without any evidence of peripheral lymphadenopathy or hepatosplenomegaly.[13] Secondary gastric lymphoma indicates the involvement of the stomach by a diffuse lymphoma that has developed elsewhere. Tertiary gastric lymphoma, which is quite rare, is a recurrence within the stomach after the treatment of a lymphoma of the peripheral nodal basin. The work-up for any lymphoma involving the stomach should include a computed tomography (CT) scan, which may prove useful in demonstrating extragastrointestinal disease within either the chest or abdomen. Whereas lymphoscintigraphy may not add any additional information, examination of the peripheral blood smear and bone marrow is necessary.

There is considerable overlap in the clinical presentation of gastric lymphoma as compared to adenocarcinoma. Gastric lymphoma can present with nonspecific upper-gastrointestinal symptoms such as abdominal pain, anorexia, nausea (with or without vomiting), and weight loss.[2,13,37] Less common symptoms include fatigue, diarrhea, and constipation.[38] In one particular series evaluating early gastric lymphoma, pain was the most frequent complaint (71%), followed by weight loss (34%) and vomiting (23%).[2] In some instances, an abdominal mass can be appreciated.[39] It is difficult to ascertain the prevalence of bleeding and perforation at the time of diagnosis, based on the limited number of reported series. Furthermore, the larger studies from tertiary referral centers are few and suffer from inherent biases that overestimate the incidence of these symptoms. Gastric lymphoma presents more commonly with bleeding (7 to 33% of cases) rather than perforation (6 to 18% of cases).[2,39–42] Obstruction is rare and tends to occur when there is involvement of the distal stomach or small bowel.[13]

Since the presentation of gastric lymphoma is relatively nonspecific, the time between the onset of symptoms and diagnosis can be significantly prolonged. In one particular series, 46 percent of patients described symptoms that exceeded 6 months, and 23 percent were symptomatic more than 12 months prior to diagnosis.[2] But with the increasing use of endoscopy and CT (Figure 17–1), there has been a trend toward early diagnosis. Before the advent of endoscopy, the diagnosis of gastric lymphoma relied mainly on upper-gastrointestinal radiologic series or exploratory surgery. Radiologic findings can range widely, from the rounded confluent submucosal nodules of a superficial spreading lesion to the exophytic (polypoid) or ulcerating-type lesions. Unfortunately, these radiologic findings do not exclude gastric adenocarcinoma from the differential diagnosis of primary gastric lymphoma.[43] Large gastric folds that are characteristic of thickened rugae are the most difficult to interpret because other nonmalignant conditions, such as gastric varices and even gastritis, may also demonstrate these radiologic signs.[44]

In early studies, gastric lymphoma was diagnosed preoperatively in less than 50 percent of cases. Cytologic examination of gastric brushings can diagnose lymphoma in 28 to 56 percent of cases.[45] Fine-needle aspiration, even for large bulky tumors, has its limitations, leading to its replacement by more sophisticated methods of tissue procurement.[46] Due to improvements in endoscopic tissue sampling, more recent series have shown a greater accuracy in diagnosis with that method, without the need for formal surgery.[2,47] Endoscopy, alone or combined with barium radiography, approaches the highest diagnostic sensitivity.[38] A relatively large series of patients with gastric non-Hodgkin's lymphoma who underwent gastroendoscopy had their tumors classified as either exophytic or infiltrative (Figure 17–2).[48] Large exophytic lesions generally yield a higher success rate of diagnosis by endoscopic biopsy. The infiltrative lesions prove more difficult to diagnose, thereby requiring more invasive biopsy techniques such as endoscopic mucosal strip resection.[49] Whereas primary non-Hodgkin's lymphoma can involve any portion of the stomach, tumor location within the gastric fundus is particularly characteristic of secondary lymphoma.[37]

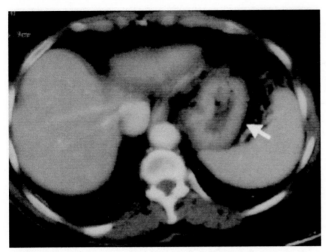

Figure 17–1. Computed tomography of a patient with primary gastric lymphoma. Note the diffuse thickening of the stomach (*arrow*).

Endoscopic ultrasonography (EUS) has recently been used to evaluate intraluminal changes that may be associated with certain gastric lymphomas. These subtle changes detected by EUS can assist in differentiating MALT lymphoma from other gastric conditions. One particular study proved EUS to be especially useful in the detection of lymphoma within enlarged gastric folds by demonstrating associated wall thickening that could not be appreciated with conventional endoscopy.[50] The identification of wall invasion by EUS is also helpful for targeting deep submucosal biopsies, especially in cases of lymphoma in which regeneration of the mucosa and fibrosis of the adjacent submucosa prohibit adequate sampling through conventional means.[49] Furthermore, the assessment of the depth of wall infiltration can predict regional lymph node involvement, which is important in planning chemotherapy in the neoadjuvant setting.[47]

STAGING

Primary gastric lymphomas are most commonly of B-cell origin (98% of cases in the Western countries).[1,4] T-cell lymphomas of the stomach are extremely rare. B-cell lymphomas can be divided into low-grade and high-grade tumors.[1] Low-grade lymphomas demonstrate centrocyte-like cells within reactive lymphoid follicles that infiltrate the stomach wall with some degree of distortion that recapitulates the structure of Peyer's patches rather than

peripheral lymph nodes. The lymphoepithelial lesion, which is pathognomonic for MALT lymphomas, presents with centrocyte-like cells that invade the glands of the gastric mucosa. High-grade lymphomas are characterized by cells that invade the mucosal glands with greater architectural destruction, leading to complete obliteration of glands within certain areas. Close examination of high-grade lymphomas may demonstrate areas of low-grade disease, further dividing high-grade lym-

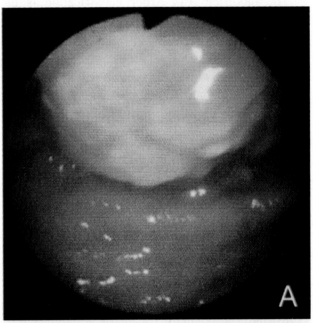

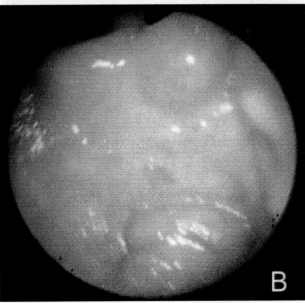

Figure 17–2. Gastroendoscopy primary gastric lymphoma. Note the submucosal mass-like effect in Image *A.* Diffuse thickening and irregularities of the mucosal folds are seen in image *B.*

phomas into mixed subgroups. In 1994, a revised European-American classification of lymphoid neoplasms was proposed by the International Lymphoma Study Group[51] (Table 17–1). The reclassification of lymphomas of the gastrointestinal tract was included by this workshop.[52] A consensus was made toward a unified criterion to histologically classify both B-cell and T-cell gastrointestinal lymphomas, in the realization that accurate grading was becoming more important as neo-adjuvant chemotherapy regimens were being introduced.

The modified Ann Arbor classification is the most widely accepted description of clinicopathologic staging criteria for primary gastric non-Hodgkin's lymphoma. It is based on the extent of disease (1) locally within the stomach (IE), (2) regionally within intra-abdominal lymph nodes (IIE), and (3) distally either below the diaphragm, such as in the liver or spleen (IIIE), or above the diaphragm or within the bone marrow (IVE)[53] (Table 17–2). Several reported series studying primary gastric lymphomas demonstrate a relatively wide distribution of stages at the time of diagnosis, in contrast to intestinal lymphomas, which tend to present with more advanced disease (Table 17–3).[3,18,41,54,55] More recent modifications of the Ann Arbor staging criteria have resembled the tumor-node-metastasis (TNM) staging system.[56] This revised classification adds depth of invasion (designated by T stage), which has been shown to be an important prognostic variable (Tables 17–4 and 17–5). However, both staging systems lack histologic classification and grading, which is an independent predictor of outcome for gastric lymphomas.

Table 17–2. CURRENT MODIFIED ANN ARBOR STAGING SYSTEM OF GASTROINTESTINAL NON-HODGKIN'S LYMPHOMA

Classification	Description
IE*	Confined to gastrointestinal tract
II1E	Spread to regional lymph nodes
II2E	Nodal involvement beyond regional lymph nodes (para-aortic, iliac, etc.)
IIIE	Spread to other intra-abdominal organs (liver, spleen)
IVE	Spread beyond abdomen (bone marrow, chest)

*E designates extralymphatic involvement.

TREATMENT OF *HELICOBACTER PYLORI*–ASSOCIATED (LOW-GRADE) MUCOSA-ASSOCIATED LYMPHOID TISSUE LYMPHOMA

Despite the clear association of *H. pylori* infection with gastric mucosa-associated lymphoid tissue (MALT) lymphoma, there remains some controversy as to the role of *H. pylori* antibiotic therapy in the treatment of primary gastric lymphoma. Ever since Wotherspoon and colleagues first described the regression of primary low-grade B-cell lymphoma after eradication of *H. pylori* infection, there has been an increasing number of studies showing similar response rates (ranging from 60 to 92%) with antimicrobial therapy alone.[57,58] One particular series, by Bayerdorffer and coleagues, described a 70 percent complete remission in 33 patients with low-grade MALT lymphoma. Nonresponders (12%) went on to more aggressive treatment, including surgery and chemotherapy.[59]

Table 17–1. REVISED PATHOLOGIC CLASSIFICATION OF GASTROINTESTINAL LYMPHOMAS

B-cell lymphoma
  Mucosa-associated lymphoid tissue (MALT)
    Low grade
    High grade (with or without a low-grade component)
    Immunoproliferative small intestinal
  Low grade (mixed high grade)
  Mantle cell
  Burkitt-like
  Other (similar to peripheral lymph node equivalents)
T-cell lymphoma
  Enteropathic-associated
  Other (non-enteropathic)

Table 17–3. DISTRIBUTION OF STAGES OF PRIMARY GASTRIC LYMPHOMA*

Study (Reference)	Stages (%)			
	IE	IIE	IE + IIE	IIIE/IVE
Radaszkiewicz et al (3)	51	49	—	—
Cogliatti et al (18)	61	39	—	—
Gobbi et al (41)	21	7	—	72
List et al (54)	—	—	54	46
Liang et al (55)	—	—	55	45

*Using the modified Ann Arbor classification criteria.

Table 17–4. TUMOR-NODE-METASTASIS STAGING FOR PRIMARY GASTRIC LYMPHOMA

T Stage (Tumor Invasion)	N Stage	M Stage
1: Lamina propria or submucosa 2: Muscularis propria 3: Subserosa 4: Serosa 5: Adjacent structures	0: Negative nodes 1: Perigastric (≤ 3 cm from tumor) 2: Perigastric (> 3 cm from tumor) 3: Distant abdominal nodes (including hepatoduodenal and para-aortic) 4: Extra-abdominal nodes	0: No metastasis 1: Distant (extranodal)

T = primary tumor; N = regional node; M = metastasis.

The presence of *H. pylori* can be determined by several non-endoscopic methods, such as the urea breath test (UBT), blood anti–*H. pylori* antibody detection, and a stool antigen assay that has been recently approved for clinical use. Because no therapy is 100 percent effective, several treatment regimens are available[60,61] (Table 17–6). The mainstay of therapy against *H. pylori* is the administration of at least two antimicrobial agents for 7 days (although more recent recommendations in the United States extend treatment durations to 10 to 14 days). Maintaining an increased pH in the stomach with antisecretory agents increases the effectiveness of antibiotic therapy. Post-treatment monitoring for resistant *H. pylori* colonization is essential (again, no regimen is 100% effective). In such instances, blood antibody testing is useless due to the delayed persistence of anti–*H. pylori* antibodies after successful treatment.

Antimicrobial therapy for low-grade gastric MALT lymphoma poses a special problem regarding the duration of therapy and subsequent surveillance. With most cases of MALT lymphoma, diagnosis is determined endoscopically. If histologic presence of *H. pylori* is absent, it is highly recommended that *H. pylori* colonization be ruled out by any of the previously described detection methods, especially if antibiotic therapy for MALT lymphoma is being

considered. The duration of therapy in most cases should extend beyond the recommended 2-week duration for *H. pylori* infections. In a recent prospective uncontrolled study, patients with stage I or stage II (N1) gastric MALT lymphoma were treated with two of three antibiotic regimens (see Table 17–6) for 21 days; these were repeated at 8 weeks.[61] Complete remission was defined by the absence of lymphoma on histopathologic evaluation on endoscopic biopsy. Fifty percent of treated patients achieved a complete remission; another 29 percent demonstrated a partial remission, as determined by a reduction of endoscopic tumor stage or tumor size. Of note, therapy failed in six patients who had no documented *H. pylori* colonization prior to treatment, emphasizing the need to demonstrate *H. pylori* infection in such instances.

The incomplete remission of certain cases of gastric lymphoma in response to antibiotic regimens against *H. pylori* has led to the understanding of the variability of MALT lymphomas that can present with concomitant *H. pylori* colonization. With a greater emphasis on the accurate grading of gastrointestinal lymphomas, many low-grade primary gastric lymphomas presumed to be related to *H. pylori* infection

Table 17–5. CRITERIA FOR TUMOR-NODE-METASTASIS STAGE DESIGNATION

Stage	Criteria*
I	T1, N0 or N1, M0
II	T1, N2, M0
	T2 or T3, N1–N3, M0
III	T4 or T5, any N, M0
	Any T, N4, M0
IV	Any T, any N, M1

*Expressed in subclassifications outlined in Table 17–4.

Table 17–6. RECOMMENDED TREATMENT REGIMENS* FOR *HELICOBACTER PYLORI* INFECTION

Antimicrobial therapy
  Amoxicillin 750 mg tid and clarithromycin 500 mg tid
  Tetracycline 500 mg qid and clarithromycin 500 mg tid
  Tetracycline 500 mg qid and metronidazole 500 mg tid
Antisecretory therapy
  Proton pump inhibitor (eg, lansoprazole or omeprazole)
  Selective H2-inhibitor (eg, ranitidine or cimetidine) and
    bismuth subsalicylate

qid = four times daily; tid = three times daily.
*One or two antimicrobial therapies administered sequentially in conjunction with an antisecretory regimen.

will demonstrate areas of mixed-grade differentiation, suggesting a possible predictor for relapse. A subsequent follow-up by Bayerdorffer and colleagues showed that patients who either relapsed or failed antimicrobial therapy most likely had prior evidence of high-grade lymphoma, as demonstrated on pathologic evaluation of surgically resected specimens.[62] Other series have similarly reported high-grade lymphomas in a large proportion (80%) of patients who did not respond to antimicrobial therapy.[63] This observation emphasizes the role of the pathologist in accurately defining the histology and grade of the lymphoma from endoscopic biopsy specimens since stomach preservation is highly feasible in this group of patients if they are properly treated.

A greater concern is whether patients with gastric MALT lymphoma who undergo treatment for *H. pylori* infection are actually cured of their lymphoma or are just in remission. Bayerdorffer and colleagues showed complete histologic regression of lymphoma cells, which was confirmed by a sensitive polymerase chain reaction analysis. However, Thiede and colleagues, in a series of 84 patients, showed a similar complete clinical response rate but with the persistence of immunoglobulin heavy-chain gene re-arrangement suggestive of residual lymphoma cells.[59,64] The clinical implications of such genetic changes that persist after a complete pathologic response can be determined only through long-term follow-up studies.

Guidelines are being developed to include antibiotic therapy for the efficacious eradication of *H. pylori* infection as the first-line treatment of low-grade gastric MALT lymphoma once the presence of *H. pylori* has been established[65] (Figure 17–3). A partial response or a nonresponse may require a more aggressive treatment, with surgery and/or chemotherapy, although the latter is reserved for when more extensive or high-grade disease is documented. However, controversy remains as to whether antimicrobial therapy has a role with systemic chemotherapy or radiotherapy in cases of mixed- or high-grade lymphomas, especially if stomach preservation is being considered. Although *H. pylori* colonization is detected in the majority of low-grade gastric MALT lymphomas, it is also present in a significant number of higher-grade lymphomas. Two particular series from Japan and the

Netherlands demonstrated the presence of *H. pylori* in 55 percent and 76 percent, respectively, of patients with high-grade primary gastric lymphoma.[66,67] In the Japanese series, 48 percent of cases with invasive lymphoma beyond the submucosa were strongly associated with persistent *H. pylori* colonization. Studies using a mouse model for human gastric MALT lymphoma determined that *Helicobacter*-infected animals have a greater likelihood of developing high-grade lymphoma if they are not treated for the infection.[68] It remains to be seen whether or not the presence of *H. pylori* in more advanced lymphomas adversely affects the prognosis of the disease either during treatment or in the long term.

SURGICAL MANAGEMENT OF GASTRIC LYMPHOMA

The role of surgery in the management of primary gastric lymphoma has changed significantly.

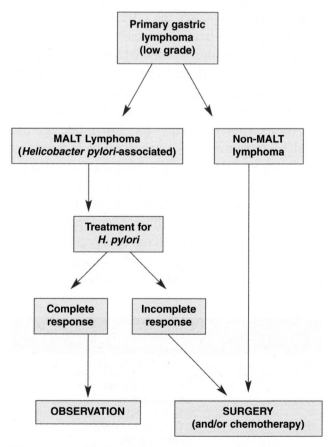

Figure 17–3.   Algorithm for the management of low-grade gastric lymphoma of the mucosa-associated lymphoid tissue (MALT) (associated with *Helicobacter pylori*) and non-MALT subtypes.

Advances in imaging techniques and endoscopy have reduced the need for formal laparotomy to definitively diagnose and stage the disease. Furthermore, with improvement in antineoplastic regimens (especially in the treatment of non-Hodgkin's lymphomas), there has been a greater emphasis on multimodality therapy and, more recently, a shift toward neo-adjuvant chemotherapy and stomach preservation. However, the role of surgery will continue to be debated and will remain controversial due to the relative rarity of this disease and the consquent lack of any large prospective experience that could provide answers in regard to appropriate therapy.[13]

In the past, surgical resection of a primary gastric lymphoma was necessary to prevent complications such as bleeding or perforation either during therapy or in the course of the disease, but the actual risk of such life-threatening complications is lower than previously expected. Recent studies evaluating the nonsurgical treatment of gastric lymphoma with chemotherapy alone or combined with radiotherapy have demonstrated that perforation is rare (most series described no cases of perforation).[69–71] Bleeding is more prevalent; however, the risk is usually less than the mortality associated with surgery.[72]

The standard treatment for gastric cancer has been radical gastrectomy, but recent staging and nonsurgical treatment modalities for primary gastric lymphoma have markedly changed this surgical approach. Nevertheless, numerous studies have demonstrated that resectability of the tumor affords a much better prognosis, especially if resection is performed through a radical approach.[2,42,56,73–78] Zinzani and colleagues emphasized that only through radical resection can complete surgical staging be achieved by the identification of three important pathologic features: (1) depth of invasion, (2) regional nodal involvement, and (3) margin status.[42] To understand how surgery can address such surgical issues as margin status and wide lymphadenectomy, however, it is important to review the pathophysiology of this disease.

Although criticized for their uniformly radical surgical approach, studies from Japan provide information about the role of extended lymphadenectomy for treatment of gastric lymphoma. Kodera and colleagues examined 60 patients with stage IE and IIE disease who underwent extended (D2) lymphadenectomy in conjunction with a partial or total gastrectomy.[73] They suggested that removal of the lymph node basin may be beneficial due to the relatively high incidence of nodal involvement (42% in their series) and the lack of peritoneal dissemination, unlike in the case of gastric adenocarcinoma. Stage IE patients had a 5-year survival rate of > 95 percent; the stage IIE patients demonstrated only a slight decrease in survival (85%) with surgery alone. Extension to regional lymph nodes had very little impact on survival, implying that limited nodal involvement in gastric lymphoma is amenable to surgery alone. The authors do discuss potential bias within the stage IIE patients, realizing that similarly staged patients with either bulky disease or extensive lymphatic involvement would not have undergone surgery.

Sano and colleagues applied the same technique of extended lymphadenectomy for stage IE and IIE primary gastric lymphoma. In their series, nodal metastases were confirmed in 25 patients (50%).[79] These patients went on to receive adjuvant chemotherapy. Splenectomy was performed in 36 patients (36%) although no parenchymal involvement was ever demonstrated. The stomach was divided equally into proximal, middle, and distal thirds to determine tumor location and multiplicity (Figure 17–4). At least two-thirds of the stomach was involved in 76 percent of patients; 62 had involvement of either the entire or the proximal two-thirds of the stomach, thereby requiring a total gastrectomy. Histologic examination accounted for the presence of multiple foci in 18 patients (36%). Of note, 1 patient had skip involvement of the proximal and distal third of the stomach. Zinzani and colleagues demonstrated a 9-year survival rate of 93 percent with radical gastrectomy for stage IE and IIE lymphoma.[42] In their series, postoperative radiotherapy was administered if there were extension to the serosa, regional lymph node involvement, or positive margins of resection. Both of these reports do emphasize the potential advantage of surgery and the disadvantages of the Ann Arbor classification (which does not include tumor-wall invasion) for properly staging the disease. These results have led many to suggest that surgery alone should be sufficient in cases of stage IE gastric lymphoma.[75]

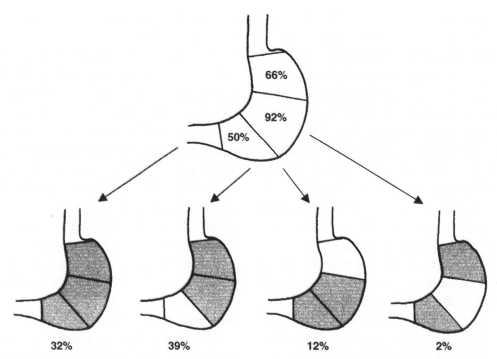

Figure 17–4. Distribution of pathologic involvement of primary gastric lymphoma. The relative frequency of lymphoma within the upper, middle, and lower thirds of the stomach from a series of 50 patients is depicted in the upper diagram. The lower diagrams demonstrate the distribution of involvement in each of the surgical specimens.

Only a few large (ie, more than 100 patients) reported series compare surgery alone to multimodality therapy including adjuvant chemotherapy and/or radiotherapy.[18,76,80] It must be cautioned that these studies are not randomized, and the results are therefore subject to significant bias. In many instances, 5-year survival rates range from 84 to 88 percent for patients with limited disease (stage IE and early IIE) who are treated with surgery alone. In most series, the addition of chemotherapy did not improve survival although there was a bias to treat patients with lymph node involvement with systemic therapy. A cumulative review of the published literature from 1974 to 1995, which included studies of more than 3,000 patients, demonstrated a high level of consensus for surgery alone for treating stage IE lymphoma.[74] For more advanced disease (ie, stage IIE and greater), there was still an emphasis on surgery (86% of authors expressed this view), but about half of the published series used multimodality therapy that included a combination of surgery, chemotherapy, and radiotherapy.

The management of primary gastric lymphoma when the disease is localized (stage IE or IIE) is resection of the entire stomach or a portion of the stomach. Any attempt at resection should include clear margins although there is some conflicting information as to whether microscopically involved margins compromise therapy, especially when adjuvant radiation or chemotherapy is being considered. The extent of lymphadenectomy (R0/R1 vs R2) remains controversial although the removal of selected lymphatic regions in cases of localized disease does allow for accurate staging and offers a potential for a cure with surgery alone (Figure 17–5). With a greater emphasis on multimodality therapy, patients with lymph node involvement or high-grade disease are receiving chemotherapy with greater frequency.

NONSURGICAL MANAGEMENT OF GASTRIC LYMPHOMA

Chemotherapy for gastrointestinal lymphoma is administered as a multidrug regimen. Whereas many of the protocols are still based on the cyclophosphamide, doxorubicin (Adriamycin) vincristine (Oncovin), and prednisone (CHOP) regimen, there

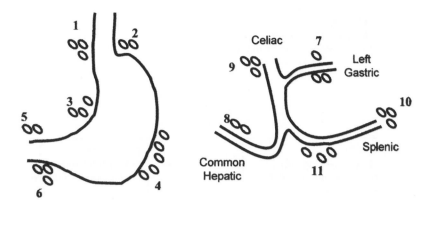

Lymph Node Regions:

1. Right Cardia
2. Left Cardia
3. Lesser Curvature
4. Greater Curvature
5. Suprapyloric
6. Infrapyloric
7. Left Gastric
8. Common Hepatic
9. Celiac
10. Splenic Hilum
11. Splenic Artery
12. Hepatoduodenal Ligament
13. Posterior Pancreas
14. Mesenteric Root
110. Paraespophageal (not shown)
111. Diaphragmatic (not shown)

R0/R1

R2

Figure 17–5. Lymphatic drainage of the stomach. The extent of lymph node dissection (R0/R1 vs R2) includes the removal of the designated lymph node regions that are in continuity to the segment of the stomach undergoing resection.

has been significant modification with the introduction of newer drugs.[69,81,82] The subsequent improvement in response rates with these regimens led (in part) to the development of neo-adjuvant protocols for primary gastric lymphoma, as a means of stomach preservation. Response rates in several series were extremely high (> 95%), especially in cases of stage IE and IIE disease (in these, stomach preservation was achieved in close to 100% of cases).[69–71,83] Again, the incidence of life-threatening complications (such as bleeding and perforation) from the primary tumor was extremely low.

A multi-institutional study from Germany is currently under way, comparing the operative and conservative management of primary gastric lymphoma[84,85] (Figure 17–6). Patients in the surgery group receive total abdominal radiation after complete resection of a low-grade tumor, with a boost to involved areas of any incomplete resection. High-grade lymphomas receive a combination of chemotherapy and radiotherapy after resection. In the conservatively managed group, patients receive a combination of chemotherapy and radiation. The decision to treat operatively or conservatively is not randomized but is based on the managing physician. Preliminary reports at 3 and 5 years of follow-up demonstrate comparable outcomes for patients with stage IE and IIE disease, with or without surgery (5-year survivals of 88% and 86%, respectively).[84,85] Although the results from this large prospective study of 280 patients are compelling, the experience with neo-adjuvant chemotherapy and stomach preservation for patients with primary gastric lymphoma needs further evaluation.

PROGNOSIS AND SUMMARY

The clinicopathologic stage of primary gastric lymphoma is an important predictor of tumor response to therapy, subsequent relapse, and overall survival.

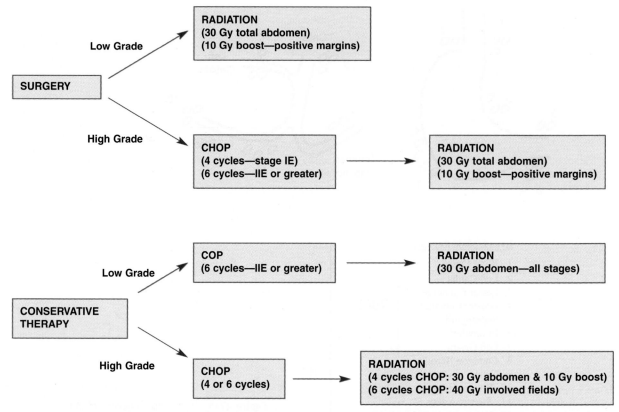

Figure 17–6. Treatment protocols for both operative and conservative management of stage IE and IIE primary gastric lymphoma. (CHOP = cyclophosphamide, doxorubicin, vincristine, and prednisone; COP = cyclophosphamide, vincristine, and prednisone.)

A meta-analysis of studies reported over a 20-year period (1974 to 1995) has demonstrated a steady improvement in survival rates from 37 percent to 87 percent, mainly due to changes in early diagnosis, proper staging, and treatment selection.[73] The spread of gastric lymphoma to intra-abdominal lymph nodes distant from the stomach or to other intra-abdominal organs has been considered a poor prognostic sign. In the review by Brands and colleagues, overall survival rates by the Ann Arbor classification were 77 percent for stage IE, 70 percent for stage II1E, 37 percent for stage II2E, 31 percent for stage IIIE, and 27 percent for stage IV.[74] Shimodaira and colleagues, in support of the TNM staging system, demonstrated that tumor invasion within the stomach wall was an independent prognostic indicator for primary gastric lymphoma.[56] Overall 5-year survival rates ranged from 82 to 100 percent for tumors extending up to the muscularis layer. Lymphomas that invade the serosa or adjacent structures had a significantly worse prognosis (53% and 33% 5-year survival rates, respectively).

Whereas most survival data for gastric lymphoma are reported on the basis of the pathologic stage of disease, the histologic subtype and (more important) the grade of the lymphoma can have a significant impact on the outcome[18,47,67] (Figure 17–7). Five-year survival rates for low-grade stage IE disease can be as high as 95 percent, thereby supporting treatment with surgery alone in this subgroup of patients.[47,72,74] For low-grade stage IIE disease (82% 5-year survival rate), surgical resection with clear margins alone offers excellent results, especially if the disease is limited to the perigastric nodal basin (stage II1E).[47,72,74] The use of adjuvant chemotherapy and/or radiotherapy in this setting remains somewhat controversial. High-grade lymphomas (stages IE and IIE) have 5-year survival rates that range from 39 to 74 percent, emphasizing the need for chemotherapy either as part of a multimodality treatment regimen or in a neo-adjuvant setting.[47,72] The grade of the lymphoma has not been shown to significantly alter the relatively poor survival rates of patients with advanced lymphomas (stage IIIE or IVE), suggesting

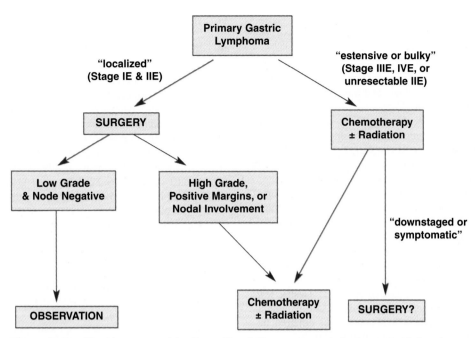

Figure 17–7. Algorithm summarizing the multimodality management of primary gastric lymphoma.

that these patients should not undergo surgery except to address symptoms of their local disease.

REFERENCES

1. Brenes F, Correa P. Pathology of gastric cancer. Surg Oncol Clin N Am 1993;2:347–70.

2. Schwarz RJ, Conners JM, Schmidt N. Diagnosis and management of stage IE and IIE gastric lymphomas. Am J Surg 1993;165:561–5.

3. Radaszkiewicz T, Dragosics B, Bauer P. Gastrointestinal malignant lymphomas of the mucosa-associated lymphoid tissue: factors relevant to prognosis. Gastroenterology 1992;102:1628–38.

4. Severson RK, Davis S. Increasing incidence of primary gastric lymphoma. Cancer 1990;66:1283–7.

5. Hayes J, Dunn E. Has the incidence of primary gastric lymphoma increased? Cancer 1989;63:2073–6.

6. Montalban C, Castrillo JM, Lopez-Abente G, et al. Other cancers in patients with gastric MALT lymphoma. Leuk Lymphoma 1999;33:161–8.

7. Fung CY, Grossbard ML, Linggood RM, et al. Mucosa-associated lymphoid tissue lymphoma of the stomach: long term outcome after local treatment. Cancer 1999;85:9–17.

8. Zucca E, Pinotti G, Roggero E, et al. High incidence of other neoplasms in patients with low-grade gastric MALT lymphoma. Ann Oncol 1995;6:726–8.

9. Nakamura S, Aoyagi K, Iwanaga S, et al. Synchronous and metachronous primary gastric lymphoma and adenocarcinoma: a clinicopathological study of 12 patients. Cancer 1997;79:1077–85.

10. Lewin KJ, Ranchod M, Dorfman RF. Lymphomas of the gastrointestinal tract: a study of 117 cases presenting with gastrointestinal disease. Cancer 1978;42:693–707.

11. Weingrad DN, Decosse JJ, Sherlock P, et al. Primary gastrointestinal lymphoma: a 30-year review. Cancer 1982; 49:1258–65.

12. Otter R, Bieger R, Kluin PM, et al. Primary gastrointestinal non-Hodgkin's lymphoma in a population-based registry. Br J Cancer 1989;60:745–50.

13. Bozzetti F, Audisio RA, Giardini R, Gennari L. Role of surgery in patients with primary non-Hodgkin's lymphoma of the stomach: an old problem revisited. Br J Surg 1993;80:1101–6.

14. Herrmann R, Panahon AM, Barcos MP, et al. Gastrointestinal involvement in non-Hodgkin's lymphoma. Cancer 1980;46:215–22.

15. Isaacson P, Wright DH. Malignant lymphoma of mucosa-associated lymphoid tissue: a distinctive type of B-cell lymphoma. Cancer 1983;52:1410–6.

16. Isaacson P, Wright DH. Extranodal malignant lymphoma arising from mucosa-associated lymphoid tissue. Cancer 1984;53:2515–24.

17. Crump M, Gospodarowicz M, Shepherd FA. Lymphoma of the gastrointestinal tract. Semin Oncol 1999;26:324–37.

18. Cogliatti SB, Schmid U, Schumacher U, et al. Primary B-cell gastric lymphoma: a clinicopathological study of 145 patients. Gastroenterology 1991;101:1159–70.

19. Moore I, Wright DH. Primary gastric lymphoma—a tumour of mucosa-associated lymphoid tissue. A histological and immunohistochemical study of 36 cases. Histopathology 1984;8:1025–39.

20. Herrera-Goepfert R, Arista-Nasr J, Alba-Campomanes A. Pathologic features of the gastric mucosa adjacent to primary MALT-lymphomas. J Clin Gastroenterol 1999;29: 266–9.

21. Driessen A, Ectors N, Creemers J, et al. Intestinal metaplasia in gastric malignancy: a comparison between carcinoma and lymphoma. Eur J Gastroenterol Hepatol 1998;10:595–600.

22. Sweeney JF, Muus C, McKeown PP, Rosemurgy AS. Gastric pseudolymphoma. Not necessarily a benign lesion. Dig Dis Sci 1992;37:939–45.

23. Sanchez L, Algara P, Villuendas R, et al. B-cell clonal detection in gastric low-grade lymphomas and regional lymph nodes: an immunohistologic and molecular study. Am J Gastroenterol 1993;88:413–9.

24. Weston AP, Banerjee SK, Horvat RT, et al. Specificity of polymerase chain reaction monoclonality for diagnosis of gastric mucosa-associated lymphoid tissue (MALT) lymphoma: direct comparison to Southern blot gene rearrangement. Dig Dis Sci 1998;43:290–9.

25. Arends JE, Bot FJ, Gisbertz IA, Schouten HC. Expression of CD10, CD75 and CD43 in MALT lymphoma and their usefulness in discriminating MALT lymphoma from follicular lymphoma and chronic gastritis. Histopathology 1999;35:209–15.

26. Isaacson PG. Gastric MALT lymphoma: from concept to cure. Ann Oncol 1999;10:637–45.

27. Hoeve MA, Gisbertz IA, Schouten HC, et al. Gastric low-grade MALT lymphoma, high-grade MALT lymphoma and diffuse large B cell lymphoma show different frequencies of trisomy. Leukemia 1999;13:799–807.

28. Nightingale TE, Gruber J. *Helicobacter* and human cancer. J Natl Cancer Inst 1994;86:1505–9.

29. The EUROGAST Study Group. An international association between *Helicobacter pylori* infection and gastric cancer. Lancet 1993;341:1359–62.

30. Parsonnet J, Hansen S, Rodriguez L, et al. *Helicobacter pylori* infection and gastric lymphoma. N Engl J Med 1994;330:1267–71.

31. Eidt S, Stolte M, Fischer R. *Helicobacter pylori* gastritis and primary gastric non-Hodgkin's lymphomas. J Clin Pathol 1994;47:436–9.

32. Miettinen A, Karttunen TJ, Alavaikko M. Lymphocytic gastritis and *Helicobacter pylori* infection in gastric lymphoma. Gut 1995;37:471–6.

33. Hussell T, Isaacson PG, Crabtree JE, Spencer J. The response of cells from low-grade B-cell gastric lymphomas of mucosa-associated lymphoid tissue to *Helicobacter pylori*. Lancet 1993;342:571–4.

34. Driessen A, Tierens A, Ectors N, et al. Primary diffuse large B cell lymphoma of the stomach: analysis of somatic mutations in the rearranged immunoglobulin heavy chain variable genes indicates antigen selection. Leukemia 1999;13:1085–92.

35. Crabtree JE, Wyatt JI, Trejdosiewicz LK, et al. Interleukin-8 expression in *Helicobacter pylori* infected, normal, and neoplastic gastroduodenal mucosa. J Clin Pathol 1994;47:61–6.

36. Crabtree JE, Spencer J. Immunologic aspects of *Helicobacter pylori* infection and malignant transformation of B cells. Semin Gastrointest Dis 1996;7:30–40.

37. Kolve M, Fischbach W, Greiner A, Wilms K. Differences in endoscopic and clinicopathological features of primary and secondary gastric non-Hodgkin's lymphoma. German Gastrointestinal Lymphoma Study Group. Gastrointest Endosc 1999;49:307–15.

38. Hansen PB, Vogt KC, Skov RL, et al. Primary gastrointestinal non-Hodgkin's lymphoma in adults: a population-based clinical and histopathologic study. J Intern Med 1998;244:71–8.

39. Hockey MS, Powell J, Crocker J, Fielding JW. Primary gastric lymphoma. Br J Surg 1987;74:483–7.

40. Shutze WP, Halpern NB. Gastric lymphoma. Surg Gynecol Obstet 1991;172:33–8.

41. Gobbi PG, Dionigi P, Barbieri F, et al. The role of surgery in the multimodal treatment of primary gastric non-Hodgkin's lymphomas. A report of 76 cases and review of the literature. Cancer 1990;65:2528–36.

42. Zinzani PL, Frezza G, Bendandi M, et al. Primary gastric lymphoma: a clinical and therapeutic evaluation of 82 patients. Leuk Lymphoma 1995;19:461–6.

43. Yoo CC, Levine MS, Furth EE, et al. Gastric mucosa-associated lymphoid tissue lymphoma: radiographic findings in six patients. Radiology 1998;208:239–43.

44. Kim YH, Lim HK, Han JK, et al. Low-grade gastric mucosa-associated lymphoid tissue lymphoma: correlation of radiographic and pathologic findings. Radiology 1999;212:241–8.

45. Sherman ME, Anderson C, Herman LM, et al. Utility of gastric brushing in the diagnosis of malignant lymphoma. Acta Cytol 1994;38:169–74.

46. Wakely PE Jr. Fine needle aspiration cytopathology of malignant lymphoma. Clin Lab Med 1998;18:541–59.

47. Taal BG, Boot H, van Heerde P, et al. Primary non-Hodgkin lymphoma of the stomach: endoscopic pattern and prognosis in low versus high-grade malignancy in relation to the MALT concept. Gut 1996;39:556–61.

48. Seifert E, Schulte F, Weismuller J, et al. Endoscopic and bioptic diagnosis of malignant non-Hodgkin's lymphoma of the stomach. Endoscopy 1993;25:497–501.

49. Suekane H, Iida M, Kuwano Y, et al. Diagnosis of primary early gastric lymphoma. Usefulness of endoscopic mucosal resection for histologic evaluation. Cancer 1993;71:1207–13.

50. Chen TK, Wu CH, Lee CL, et al. Endoscopic ultrasonography in the differential diagnosis of giant gastric folds. J Formos Med Assoc 1999;98:261–4.

51. Harris NL, Jaffe ES, Stein H, et al. A revised European-American classification of lymphoid neoplasms: a proposal from the International Lymphoma Study Group. Blood 1994;84:1361–92.

52. Rohatiner A, d'Amore F, Coiffier B, et al. Report on a workshop convened to discuss the pathological and staging classifications of gastrointestinal tract lymphoma. Ann Oncol 1994;5:397–400.

53. Carbone PP, Kaplan HS, Musshoff K, et al. Report of the Committee on Hodgkin's Disease Staging Classification. Cancer Res 1971;31:1860–1.

54. List AF, Greer JP, Ciusar JC, et al. Non-Hodgkin's lymphoma of the gastrointestinal tract: an analysis of clinical and pathologic features affecting outcome. J Clin Oncol 1988;6:1125–33.

55. Liang R, Todd D, Chan TK, et al. Gastrointestinal lymphoma in Chinese: a retrospective analysis. Hematol Oncol 1987;5:115–26.

56. Shimodaira M, Tsukamoto Y, Niwa Y, et al. A proposed staging system for primary gastric lymphoma. Cancer 1994;73:2709–15.

57. Wotherspoon AC, Doglioni C, Diss TC, et al. Regression of primary low-grade B-cell gastric lymphoma of mucosa-

associated lymphoid tissue type after eradication of *Helicobacter pylori*. Lancet 1993;342:575–7.

58. Wotherspoon AC. Gastric lymphoma of mucosa-associated lymphoid tissue and *Helicobacter pylori*. Annu Rev Med 1998;49:289–99.

59. Bayerdorffer E, Neubauer A, Rudolph B, et al. Regression of primary gastric lymphoma of mucosa-associated lymphoid tissue type after cure of *Helicobacter pylori* infection. Lancet 1995;345:1591–4.

60. Peterson WL, Fendrick AM, Cave DR, et al. *Helicobacter pylori*-related disease: guidelines for testing and treatment. Arch Intern Med 2000;160:1285–91.

61. Steinbach G, Ford R, Glober G, et al. Antibiotic treatment of gastric lymphoma of mucosa-associated lymphoid tissue. An uncontrolled study. Ann Intern Med 1999;131:88–95.

62. Bayerdorffer E, Neubauer A, Morgner A, et al. Regression of primary gastric low-grade MALT lymphoma after cure of *Helicobacter pylori* infection—German MALT lymphoma trial. Gastroenterology 1996;110:A490.

63. Neubauer A, Thiede C, Morgner A, et al. Cure of *Helicobacter pylori* infection and duration of remission of low-grade gastric mucosa-associated lymphoid tissue lymphoma. J Natl Cancer Inst 1997;89:1350–5.

64. Thiede C, Morgner A, Alpen B, et al. What role does the eradication of *Helicobacter pylori* play in gastric MALT and gastric MALT lymphoma? Gastroenterology 1997; 113:S61–4.

65. NCCN preliminary non-Hodgkin's lymphoma practice guidelines. Oncology 1997;11:281–46.

66. Nakamura S, Yao T, Aoyagi K, et al. *Helicobacter pylori* and primary gastric lymphoma. A histopathologic and immunohistochemical analysis of 237 patients. Cancer 1997;79:3–11.

67. de Jong D, Boot H, van Heerde P, et al. Histological grading in gastric lymphoma: pretreatment criteria and clinical relevance. Gastroenterology 1997;112:1466–74.

68. Enno A, O'Rourke J, Braye S, et al. Antigen-dependent progression of mucosa-associated lymphoid tissue (MALT)-type lymphoma in the stomach. Effects of antimicrobial therapy on gastric MALT lymphoma in mice. Am J Pathol 1998;152:1625–32.

69. Haim N, Leviov M, Ben-Arieh Y, et al. Intermediate and high-grade gastric non-Hodgkin's lymphoma: a prospective study of non-surgical treatment with primary chemotherapy, with or without radiotherapy. Leuk Lymphoma 1995;17:321–6.

70. Tondini C, Balzarotti M, Santoro A, et al. Initial chemotherapy for primary resectable large-cell lymphoma of the stomach. Ann Oncol 1997;8:497–9.

71. Ferreri AJ, Cordio S, Ponzoni M, Villa E. Non-surgical treatment with primary chemotherapy, with or without radiation therapy, of stage I-II high-grade gastric lymphoma. Leuk Lymphoma 1999;33:531–41.

72. Stephens J, Smith J. Treatment of primary gastric lymphoma and gastric mucosa-associated lymphoid tissue lymphoma. J Am Coll Surg 1998;187:312–20.

73. Kodera Y, Yamamura Y, Nakamura S, et al. The role of radical gastrectomy with systematic lymphadenectomy for the diagnosis and treatment of primary gastric lymphoma. Ann Surg 1998;227:45–50.

74. Brands F, Monig SP, Raab M. Treatment and prognosis of gastric lymphoma. Eur J Surg 1997;163:803–13.

75. Makela J, Karttunen T, Kiviniemi H, Laitinen S. Clinicopathological features of primary gastric lymphoma. J Surg Oncol 1999;70:78–82.

76. Salvagno L, Soraru M, Busetto M, et al. Gastric non-Hodgkin's lymphoma: analysis of 252 patients from a multicenter study. Tumori 1999;85:113–21.

77. Azab MB, Henry-Amar M, Rougier P, et al. Prognostic factors in primary gastrointestinal non-Hodgkin's lymphoma. A multivariate analysis, report of 106 cases and review of the literature. Cancer 1989;64:1208–17.

78. Radaszkiewicz T, Dragosics B, Bauer P. Gastrointestinal malignant lymphomas of the mucosa-associated lymphoid tissue: factors relevant to prognosis. Gastroenterology 1992;102:1628–38.

79. Sano T, Sasako M, Kinoshita T, et al. Total gastrectomy for primary gastric lymphoma at stage IE and IIE: a prospective study of fifty cases. Surgery 1997;121:501–5.

80. Brincker H, D'Amore F. A retrospective analysis of treatment outcome in 106 cases of localized gastric non-Hodgkin lymphomas. Danish Lymphoma Study Group, LYFO. Leuk Lymphoma 1995;18:281–8.

81. Smith MR. Non-Hodgkin's lymphoma. Curr Probl Cancer 1996;20:6–77.

82. Unterhalt M, Herrmann R, Tiemann M, et al. Prednimustine, mitoxantrone (PmM) vs cyclophosphamide, vincristine, prednisone (COP) for the treatment of advanced low-grade non-Hodgkin's lymphoma. Leukemia 1996;10:836–43.

83. Rabbi C, Aitini E, Cavazzini G, et al. Stomach preservation in low- and high-grade primary gastric lymphomas: preliminary results. Haematologica 1996;81:15–9.

84. Koch P, Grothaus-Pinke B, Hiddemann W, et al. Primary lymphoma of the stomach: three-year results of a prospective multicenter study. Ann Oncol 1997;8:85–8.

85. Willich NA, Reinartz G, Horst EJ, et al. Operative and conservative management of primary gastric lymphoma: interim results of a German multicenter study. Int J Radiol Oncol 2000;46:895–901.

18

Epidemiology of Small-Bowel Tumors

ROGER D. HURST, MD, FRCS (ED), FACS

Malignant tumors of the small intestine are rare. In fact, one of the more puzzling aspects of small-bowel tumors is the surprisingly low frequency with which they occur. Although the small intestine constitutes three-fourths of the length and approximately 90 percent of the surface area of the gastrointestinal (GI) tract, it is the site of less than 5 percent of GI malignancies.[1,2] In the United States, approximately 140,000 colo-rectal cancers and 22,000 gastric cancers occur annually whereas only 4,500 to 5,000 small-bowel cancers are seen each year.

Due to the rarity of these tumors, detailed knowledge of the epidemiology of small-bowel cancer is limited. Small-bowel cancer has been the subject of only a small number of population-based descriptive epidemiologic studies.[3–10] Detailed information and subpopulation analysis within these population-based studies are also limited. Hospital case studies, most requiring several decades to accumulate data, generally contain more detail than is available from cancer registries, and these studies (however flawed) have been the prime source of descriptive data regarding these rare cancers.

INCIDENCE

Four histologic tumors make up 90 percent of all small-bowel malignancies: adenocarcinoma, carcinoids, lymphoma, and sarcoma.[6] The relative frequencies of the differing histologies vary from reported studies. In general, however, adenocarcinoma and carcinoids have similar relative frequencies, and each constitute from 30 to 40 percent of all small-bowel malignancies. Small-bowel sarcomas and lymphomas are somewhat less common, each representing 10 to 20 percent of the total[3,5–7] (Figure 18–1).

The differing histologic forms of small-bowel cancer tend to occur in particular locations along the length of the small intestine. Adenocarcinomas most frequently occur in the duodenum, particularly in the vicinity of the ampulla. Sixty-two percent of the small-bowel adenocarcinomas reported in the Los Angeles County tumor registry were located within the duodenum,[7] and other studies also indicate a predominance for adenocarcinoma in the duodenum.[11] Carcinoids and lymphomas are typically more distal in the small bowel, being predominantly ileal or jejunal. Sarcomas appear to be evenly distributed throughout the small bowel.

The Surveillance, Epidemiology and End Results (SEER) data (1973 to 1991) indicate an overall annual rate of 9.9 cases per million population for all the histologic subtypes of small-bowel malignancies.[8,12] Combined statistics from the cancer registries of western Canada show a similar rate of 11 cases per million population.[5] This is approximately one-thirtieth of the incidence of colo-rectal carcinomas within the same population groups. Most population-based studies have indicated a slightly higher risk among men than among women, with the male-female ratio being approximately 1.2:1.[12] This higher incidence among males is consistent throughout all four of the more common histologic subtypes. The risk for small-bowel malignancies increases with age, with most occurring in individu-

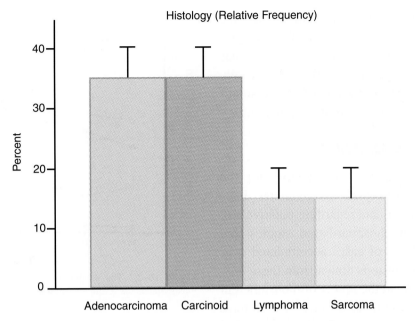

Figure 18–1.   Relative frequency of small-bowel tumors, by histology.

als who are 60 to 70 years of age. Over 90 percent of small-bowel malignancies occur in patients older than 40 years of age. In the industrialized countries, correlation with age occurs in all histologic subgroups although the mean age for the diagnosis of lymphoma and sarcoma is somewhat less than for carcinoids and adenocarcinoma. In the developing world, however, small-bowel lymphomas seem to occur more frequently in young adults.[13]

Few data exist describing the relative rates of small-bowel malignancies among people of differing races living within the same geographic location. Analysis of the SEER data by Chow and colleagues indicates that white individuals have a slightly increased risk for small-bowel malignancies when all histologic subtypes are taken into account.[4] The SEER data indicate an increased risk among African Americans for adenocarcinomas when compared to whites. The University of Southern California Cancer Surveillance Program also noted an increased age-adjusted risk for small-bowel adenocarcinoma among African Americans.[7] Small-bowel lymphomas, on the other hand, are somewhat less common among African Americans.

Population-based studies within the United States indicate a trend over time for an increasing incidence of small-bowel malignancies[4,6,8] (Figure 18–2). This increase in incidence has been for ade-

nocarcinomas and carcinoids but is most pronounced for lymphomas, which have risen from approximately 0.1 per million in 1973 to 3 per million in 1990[4] (Figure 18–3). This increase in small-bowel lymphomas parallels an increase in cases of gastric lymphoma over the same time period. This observation has led some to suggest a common etiology for small-bowel and gastric lymphomas. Immunosuppressive states, such as those that occur in acquired immunodeficiency syndrome (AIDS) and transplant patients, are an established risk factor for lymphomas in general; yet, it is not known

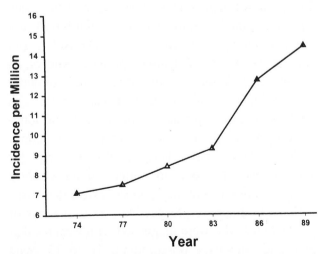

Figure 18–2.   The incidence of small intestinal malignancies in the United States, as a function of time.

whether such immunosuppressive states contribute specifically to the increased incidence in lymphomas of the small bowel. *Helicobacter pylori* has been associated with gastric lymphomas, but any relationship between *Helicobacter pylori* and small-bowel lymphomas is entirely based on conjecture.

RISK FACTORS

A wide variety of potential risk factors for the development of small-bowel malignancies have been investigated. Most data regarding putative risk factors originate from hospital-based studies that review a small number of cases accumulated over many years. The conclusions drawn from these hospital-based studies are at the mercy of their inherent deficiencies. A small number of such studies have used case-control comparisons in an attempt to find an association with certain dietary, social, and health factors. Along with increasing age and male sex, Crohn's disease and familial adenomatous polyposis (FAP) are clearly recognized as risk factors for small-bowel cancer. Many other factors have been studied, but their impact on the risk of small-bowel cancer is less certain (Table 18–1).

Crohn's Disease

The data clearly support Crohn's disease as a risk factor for small-intestinal adenocarcinoma. The expected incidence for these two rare conditions occurring in the same individual is approximately one in one billion;[14] yet, over 100 cases of Crohn's disease–associated small-bowel cancer have been reported in the literature since the initial report of a small-bowel Crohn malignancy by Ginsberg and colleagues in 1956.[15] Unlike sporadic cancers, in whose case adenocarcinomas occur predominantly in the proximal small bowel, adenocarcinomas with Crohn's disease typically occur in areas of long-standing active disease (most commonly, the ileum).

Many studies have shown a substantial risk for small-intestinal adenocarcinoma among Crohn's disease patients, but the precise calculated risks vary. In Denmark, a prospective cohort analysis of 373 patients who were diagnosed with Crohn's disease and who were observed for 10 to 15 years found 2 cases of small-bowel cancer, both in the

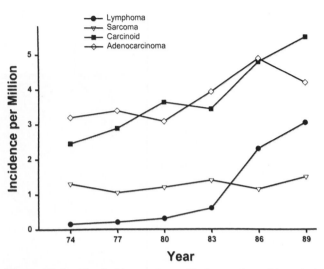

Figure 18–3. The incidence of specific forms of small-intestinal malignancies, as a function of time.

ileum, compared to an expected 0.04 cases.[16] Thus, in this study, the relative risk of small-bowel cancer in patients with Crohn's disease was 50 times that of the general population. A similar report from Stockholm found a lower but substantial relative risk of 15.6.[17] In a hospital-based study of patients with inflammatory bowel disease, Greenstein and colleagues estimated the incidence of small-bowel cancer to be increased 86-fold in patients with Crohn's disease.[18] In a case-control study by Chan and colleagues, 4 of 19 cases of small-bowel adenocarcinoma arose in the ileum, and 3 of these were associated with a history of Crohn's disease.[19] Although Crohn's disease patients are at risk for adenocarcinoma of the small bowel, their risk for other histologic subtypes of small-bowel malignancies is not increased.[19]

Table 18–1. RISK FACTORS FOR SMALL-BOWEL CANCER
Established factors
Age
Male sex
Crohn's disease
Familial adenomatous polyposis
Hereditary nonpolyposis colo-rectal cancer syndrome
Theoretic factors
High-fat/high-protein diet
Smoking
Alcohol
Peutz-Jeghers syndrome
Radiation injury
Celiac disease

There are three factors known to affect the risk for small-bowel adenocarcinoma in Crohn's disease patients. The first is duration of disease; the longer the history of active disease, the greater the risk. In fact, long-standing disease seems to be necessary; the appearance of small-bowel carcinoma in patients who have had Crohn's disease for less than 10 years is virtually unreported. The second established risk factor is male sex. Small-bowel cancer occurs with a male-to-female preponderance of 3:1 among Crohn's disease patients.[20–22] The final risk factor is the presence of diverted or excluded segments of small intestine. Although no longer recommended, intestinal bypass with the exclusion of diseased segments of small intestine was commonly performed for cases of active Crohn's disease. This practice resulted in a high incidence of adenocarcinoma developing in the diseased segment of intestine that was excluded from the normal intestinal stream. For this reason, this type of surgical approach to the management of Crohn's disease has been abandoned.

In addition to the archaic practice of intestinal bypass, other treatments for Crohn's disease have been studied for their potential to promote small-bowel cancer. Lashner and colleagues found a slight increase of risk for adenocarcinoma among Crohn's disease patients treated with 6-mercaptopurine.[22] This risk was not seen in patients treated with prednisone or sulfasalazine. Lashner and colleagues also found that patients with jejunal Crohn's disease seemed to be at higher risk when compared to patients with ileal Crohn's disease. Some surgeons have expressed concern regarding the use of strictureplasties to treat small-bowel Crohn's disease.[23] It has been suggested that this new technique may result in the retention of diseased segments for long durations and thus result in an increase in small-bowel cancer. To date, this theoretic concern has not demonstrated such a risk, and only two cases of adenocarcinoma in strictureplasty patients have been reported.[24]

Familial Adenomatous Polyposis and other Familial Cancer Syndromes

Patients with FAP are at high risk for small-bowel adenomas and adenocarcinomas, particularly of the duodenum. In fact, duodenal and periampullary adenocarcinomas are the most common extracolonic malignancies in FAP patients and represent the second most frequent cause of death among these patients.[25] Approximately 3 percent of FAP patients will develop small-bowel cancers, almost all of which will occur within the duodenum.[26] Among 1,391 patients in the Johns Hopkins FAP registry, 11 cases of duodenal and ampullary carcinoma occurred.[26] From this registry, the relative risk for duodenal adenocarcinoma among patients with FAP was calculated to be an extraordinary 330.8. Interestingly, however, FAP patients do not appear to have an increased risk for either gastric or nonduodenal small-bowel cancer.

In addition to patients with hereditary FAP, individuals with hereditary nonpolyposis colo-rectal cancer (HNPCC) also appear to be at higher risk for small-bowel cancer. Two studies have specifically addressed the issue of HNPCC and small-bowel cancer.[27,28] These studies indicate an estimated lifetime risk of 1 percent for small-bowel cancer among HNPCC patients. This is less than the risk associated with FAP but significantly higher than the risk in the general population.

Small-bowel tumors have been associated with other malignancies, aside from hereditary and non-hereditary colo-rectal cancers. Even sporadic colo-rectal cancer may be associated with an increased risk for small-intestinal cancer. From SEER data gathered between 1973 and 1988, Neuget and Santos investigated the association between the 2,581 cases of small-bowel cancer from the database and other second malignancies.[29] This study found relative risks for colo-rectal cancer following development of small-bowel adenocarcinoma of 5.0 in males and 3.7 in females. The risk of developing small-bowel adenocarcinoma following colo-rectal cancer was also increased, with risks of 7.1 in males and 9.0 in females.

From the Manitoba and British Columbia registries, 54 of 128 patients with small-bowel cancers also suffered from second malignancies.[30] This translates into a greater than eightfold increase in the incidence of second malignancies with small-bowel cancer. Thirty-eight of these associated tumors were diagnosed prior to the small-bowel cancer, eight were synchronous with it, and six were diagnosed after the small-bowel cancer. The most common sites for second malignancies were the large bowel, the prostate, the female genitalia, and the lung. In a separate report after a mean follow-up of 6 years, Frost and colleagues found that among 61 patients treated at the Kaiser-Permanente Los Angeles Medical Center for small-bowel cancer, 7 patients developed another primary cancer.[31] These new primary cancers included 3 breast cancers and 1 each of rectal cancer, renal cell cancer, lymphoma, and melanoma. In a study of 49 patients with adenocarcinoma of the small intestine recorded in the Hawaii tumor registry from 1960 to 1989, 11 patients had other cancers.[32] Six males had large-bowel cancer (one of these six also had prostate and stomach cancer; another had cancer of the ureter). Three other males had melanoma, stomach, and ureteral cancer; one male had each of the three cancers. Only two females had second malignancies (one case of colon cancer and one case of breast cancer).

Patients with Peutz-Jeghers syndrome, a rare familial disorder, have mucocutaneous pigmentation and multiple hamartomatous polyps of the GI tract. The risk for the development of invasive adenocarcinoma within these hamartomatous polyps or de novo within the small bowel has been the subject of controversy. Many reports of carcinoma within a Peutz-Jeghers polyp may have been misinterpretations resulting from the incorporation of muscle in the stroma of the polyp, giving the false impression of invasion.[33,34] Using strict criteria for establishing the diagnosis of malignancy in Peutz-Jeghers patients, Dozois and colleagues reviewed the published reports of 321 cases of Peutz-Jeghers syndrome and found 4 cases of established small-intestinal malignancy (3 of the duodenum and 1 of the ileum) and an incidence of 1.2 percent, suggesting an increased risk for small-bowel cancers in these patients.[35]

Radiation Therapy

Exposure to radiation therapy results in significant long-term injury to the small intestine. Radiation may also increase the risk for small-bowel malignancies within the segments exposed. In a cohort study, Kleinerman and colleagues compared 49,828 women with cervical cancer treated with radiation

therapy to 16,713 women with cervical cancer treated without radiation therapy. The relative risk for small-bowel cancer following radiation therapy was 1.8, and this risk remained high for up to 30 years following treatment.[36]

Celiac Disease

Celiac disease has been associated with an increased risk for the development of cancer, including small bowel adenocarcinoma and lymphoma. In a British National Collaborative Study, 235 patients with both celiac disease and malignancy were studied.[37] The most common tumor in these patients was small-bowel lymphoma, of which there were 67 cases. Nineteen patients had small-bowel adenocarcinoma, yet the expected incidence of this form of small-bowel cancer was only 0.23. The increased risk for small-bowel lymphoma and adenocarcinoma was not dependent on the clinical or histologic response to a gluten-free diet.

Diet

A limited number of studies have attempted to correlate the risk for small-bowel cancer with dietary habits. World Health Organization (WHO) data suggest a risk association with per capita intake of animal fat and protein.[38] Regions where traditional diets are high in animal fat and protein were noted to have higher rates of small-bowel cancer. Using cases and controls to compare patients suffering from small-bowel adenocarcinomas, Chow and colleagues reported a statistically significant risk with higher intakes of meat and smoked foods.[39] Other studies have suggested that sugar-sweetened nonalcoholic beverages may also pose a risk for the development of small-bowel tumors.[40] While these studies suggest an association between certain dietary habits and the risk of small-bowel cancer, no causal relationship between any specific food and small-bowel cancer has been established.

Smoking

Data regarding the risk of cigarette smoking to the development of small-bowel tumors are not conclusive. Chen and colleagues found an increased risk for small-bowel adenocarcinoma for smokers.[19] Among their patients, the age- and sex-adjusted odds ratios for cigarette smokers were 4.6 for adenocarcinoma and 4.2 for carcinoid of the small bowel. Wu and colleagues also reported an increased risk, albeit nonsignificant, of adenocarcinoma for male smokers but not for female smokers.[40] On the other hand, in two separate studies, Negri and colleagues[41] and Chow and colleagues[39] were unable to discern any tobacco-associated risk for small-bowel tumors.

Alcohol

Only a limited number of studies have investigated the risk of small-bowel cancer and the use of alcohol. The available data suggest that alcohol consumption increases the likelihood for small-bowel adenocarcinoma and possibly for small-bowel carcinoid tumors. Wu and colleagues reported a threefold increased risk for small-bowel adenocarcinomas among heavy drinkers (ie, > 80 g of alcohol a day).[40] Chen and colleagues reported an alcohol-related risk for both small-bowel adenocarcinomas and small-bowel carcinoids, with an adjusted odds ratio for alcohol consumption of 4.0 for adenocarcinomas and 3.1 for carcinoids.[19]

SUMMARY

Cancers of the small bowel are rare. Current data indicate an increasing incidence of these uncommon tumors, particularly small-bowel lymphomas. The risk for small-bowel cancer increases with age, and males are at slightly higher risk than females. Individuals suffering from FAP or long-standing Crohn's disease are at much higher risk for small-bowel adenocarcinoma, compared to the general population.

REFERENCES

1. Martin RG. Malignant tumors of the small intestine. Surg Clin North Am 1986;66:779–85.
2. Hirsch JE, Ahrens EH, Blankenhorn DH. Measurement of the human intestinal length vivo and some causes of variation. Gastroenterology 1956;31:274–84.
3. DiSario JA, Burt RW, McWhorter HVWP. Small bowel cancer: epidemiological and clinical characteristics from a population-based registry. Am J Gastroenterol 1994;89:699–701.
4. Chow JS, Chen CC, Ahsan H, Neugut AI. A population-based study of the incidence of malignant small bowel tumors: SEER, 1973–1990. Int J Epidemiol 1996;25:722–5.
5. Gabos S, Berkel J, Band P, et al. Small bowel cancer in western Canada. Int J Epidemiol 1993;22:198–206.
6. Weiss NS, Yang CP. Incidence of histologic types of cancer of the small intestine. J Natl Cancer Inst 1987;78:653–6.
7. Ross RK, Hartnett NM, Bernstein L, Henderson BE. Epidemiology of adenocarcinoma of the small intestine: is bile a small bowel carcinogen? Br J Cancer 1991;63:143–5.
8. Severson RK, Schenk M, Gurney JG, et al. Increasing incidence of adenocarcinomas and carcinoid tumors of the small intestine in adults. Cancer Epidemiol Biomarkers Prev 1996;5:81–4.
9. Howe JR, Karnell LH, Menck HR, Scott-Conner C. Adenocarcinoma of the small bowel: review of the national cancer data base, 1985–1995. Cancer 1999;86:2693–706.
10. Stang A, Stegmaier C, Eisinger B, et al. Descriptive epidemiology of small intestinal malignancies: the German Cancer Registry experience. Br J Cancer 1999;80:1440–4.
11. Neugut AI, Marvin MR, Rella VA, Chabot JA. An overview of adenocarcinoma of the small intestine. Oncology 1997;11:529–36.
12. Neugut AI, Jacobson JS, Suh S, et al. The epidemiology of cancer of the small bowel. Cancer Epidemiol Biomarkers Prev 1998;7:243–51.
13. Khojasteh A, Haghighi P. Immunoproliferative small intestinal disease: portrait of a potentially preventable cancer from the Third World. Am J Med 1990;89:483–90.
14. Ryan JC. Premalignant conditions of the small intestine. Semin Gastrointest Dis 1996;2:88–93.
15. Ginsburg L, Schneider KM, Dreizin DH, Levinson C. Carcinoma of the jejunum occurring in a case of regional enteritis. Surgery 1956;39:347–51.
16. Munkohlm P, Langholz E, Davidsen M, Binder V. Intestinal cancer risk and mortality in patients with Crohn's disease. Gastroenterology 1993;105:1716–23.
17. Persson PG, Darlen P, Bernell O, et al. Crohn's disease and cancer: a population-based cohort study. Gastroenterology 1994;107:1675–9.
18. Greenstein AJ, Sachar DB, Smith H, et al. A comparison of cancer risk in Crohn's disease and ulcerative colitis. Cancer 1981;48:2742–5.
19. Chen CC, Neugut AI, Rotterdam H. Risk factors for adenocarcinoma and malignant carcinoids of the small intestine: preliminary findings. Cancer Epidemiol Biomarkers Prev 1994;3:205–7.
20. Riberio MB, Greenstein AJ, Heimann T, et al. Adenocarcinoma of the small intestine in Crohn's disease. Surg Gynecol Obstet 1991;173:343–9.
21. Michelassi F, Testa G, Pomidor WJ, et al. Adenocarcinoma complicating Crohn's disease. Dis Colon Rectum 1993;36:654–61.
22. Lashner BA. Risk factors for small bowel cancer in Crohn's disease. Dig Dis Sci 1992;37:1179–84.
23. Fleshman JW. Invited editorial. Dis Colon Rectum 1997;40:238–9.
24. Marchetti F, Fazio VW, Ozuner G. Adenocarcinoma arising from a strictureplasty site in Crohn's disease: report of a case. Dis Colon Rectum 1996;39:1315–21.

25. Galle TS, Juel K, Bulow S. Causes of death in familial adenomatous polyposis. Scand J Gastroenterol 1999;34:808–12.

26. Offerhaus GJA, Giardiello FM, Krush AJ, et al. The risk of upper gastrointestinal cancer in familial adenomatous polyposis. Gastroenterology 1992;102:1980–2.

27. Aarnio M, Mecklin JP, Aaltonen LA, et al. Life-time risk of different cancers in hereditary non-polyposis colorectal cancer (HNPCC) syndrome. Int J Cancer 1995;64:430–3.

28. Watson P, Lynch HT. Extracolonic cancer in hereditary non-polyposis colorectal cancer. Cancer 1993;71:677–85.

29. Neugut AI, Santos J. The association between cancers of the small and large bowel. Cancer Epidemiol Biomarkers Prev 1993;2:551–3.

30. Ripley D, Weinerman BH. Increased incidence of second malignancies associated with small bowel adenocarcinoma. Can J Gastroenterol 1996;11:65–8.

31. Frost DB, Mercado PD, Tyrell JS. Small bowel cancer: a 30-year review. Ann Surg Oncol 1994;1:290–5.

32. Stemmermann GN, Goodman MT, Nomura AMY. Adenocarcinoma of the proximal small intestine. Cancer 1992;70:2766–71.

33. Reid JD. Intestinal carcinoma in the Peutz-Jeghers syndrome. JAMA 1974;229:833–4.

34. Perzin KH, Bridge MF. Adenomatous and carcinomatous changes in hamartomatous polyps of the small intestine (Peutz-Jeghers syndrome): report of a case and review of the literature. Cancer 1982;49:971–83.

35. Dozois RR, Judd ES, Dahlin DC, Bartholomew LG. The Peutz-Jeghers syndrome: is there a predisposition to the development of intestinal malignancy? Arch Surg 1969;98:509–16.

36. Kleinerman RA, Boice JD, Storm HH, et al. Second primary cancer after treatment for cervical cancer: an international cancer registries study. Cancer 1995;76:442–52.

37. Swinson CM, Slavin G, Coles EC, Booth CC. Coeliac disease and malignancy. Lancet 1983;1:111–5.

38. Lowenfels AB, Sonni A. Distribution of small bowel tumors. Cancer Lett 1977;3:83–6.

39. Chow WH, Linet MS, McLaughlin JK, et al. Risk factors for small intestine cancer. Cancer Causes Control 1993;4:163–9.

40. Wu AH, Yu MC, Mack TM. Smoking, alcohol use, dietary factors and risk for small bowel adenocarcinoma. Int J Cancer 1997;70:512–7.

41. Negri E, Bosetti C, LaVecchia C, et al. Risk factors for adenocarcinoma of the small intestine. Int J Cancer 1999;82:171–4.

19

Pathology of Small-Bowel Tumors

SHU-YUAN XIAO, MD

JOHN HART, MD

Like other segments of the gastrointestinal tract, masses or nodules in the small intestine include tumors and tumorlike (usually inflammatory) lesions and non-neoplastic (hamartomatous) polyps. Despite the length of the small intestine, malignant tumors are significantly less common there than in any other gastrointestinal site. Malignant tumors are most common in the duodenum and distal terminal ileum; they are actually quite rare in the jejunum and proximal ileum. Benign tumors and tumorlike lesions are more evenly distributed throughout the small bowel but are more often discovered as incidental findings in the distal terminal ileum and proximal duodenum, where they can be identified by endoscopy.

NON-NEOPLASTIC POLYPS AND MASSES

There are a large number of lesions in the category of non-neoplastic polyps and masses; some are typically incidental findings, and others can cause symptoms such as bleeding or obstruction. Lesions derived from mucosa include juvenile, Peutz-Jeghers, Cowden, and Cronkhite-Canada polyps. Nodular or mass lesions not derived from the mucosal epithelium include Brunner's gland hyperplasia, lymphoid polyp of the ileum, inflammatory fibroid polyp, duodenal adenomyosis, inflammatory myofibroblastic tumor of the terminal ileum, pancreatic heterotopia, and gastric heterotopia.[1-5] Many of these lesions are quite rare, and only selected lesions are discussed here.

Brunner's Gland Hyperplasia

Brunner's gland hyperplasia is characterized by smooth-surfaced sessile polyps or nodules found in the first or second portion of the duodenum (Figure 19–1). They may be single or may occur in clusters. Although sometimes called Brunner's gland adenomas, they are not dysplastic; thus, hyperplasia is a more appropriate term. Microscopically, they consist of large clusters of Brunner's glands within the submucosa, often with extension into the mucosa as

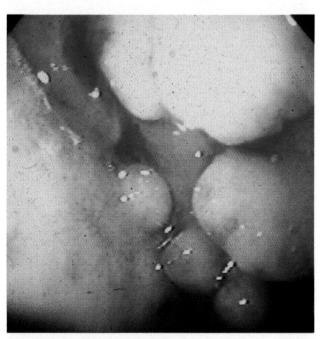

Figure 19–1. Brunner's gland hyperplasia. Several polyps are noted in the duodenal bulb.

well (Figure 19–2). Brunner's gland hyperplasia cannot be diagnosed accurately by endoscopic biopsy since normal Brunner's glands may extend into the lamina propria and occupy the submucosa sampled by a biopsy forceps.[3,5,6]

Peutz-Jeghers Syndrome

The small bowel is the most common site for Peutz-Jeghers polyps, which are true hamartomatous polyps. Typical presenting symptoms include gastrointestinal hemorrhage, obstruction, and intussusception. It is an autosomal dominant disease and is associated with mucocutaneous pigmentation. Since a sporadic form of this disease is not known, the presence of even a single polyp is diagnostic of the syndrome. Often, only one or two polyps are present. They may be sessile or pedunculated (Figure 19–3). Microscopically, Peutz-Jeghers polyps con-

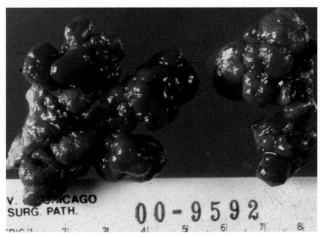

Figure 19–3. Peutz-Jeghers polyps. A multilobulated polypoid lesion.

sist of an increased number of glands, with a core of branching smooth-muscle fibers derived from the muscularis mucosa. The epithelial component of the Peutz-Jeghers polyp in the small bowel resembles normal small-bowel epithelium in that it contains both absorptive columnar cells and scattered goblet cells. While there is an increased risk of small-bowel and colonic adenocarcinoma in patients with this disease, the tumors do not appear to arise from the polyps themselves.[5,7]

Juvenile Polyps

Also known as retention polyps, juvenile polyps can occur in both children and adults. In the colon, they can occur either sporadically or as part of juvenile polyposis syndrome. Small-bowel polyps, on the other hand, occur only in patients with the autosomal dominant genetic defect and are usually multiple in that setting. They range from < 0.1 cm to 5.0 cm (usually 1 to 2 cm) in diameter and are typically pedunculated. Grossly, the polyps appear gray-pink, with a mushroom-like configuration. Small white patches can be seen endoscopically on the surface due to cystic dilatation of the crypt epithelium, which is one of the characteristic microscopic features (Figure 19–4). The cysts are surrounded by a prominent edematous stroma containing numerous inflammatory cells, including lymphocytes, plasma cells, eosinophils, and neutrophils. The neutrophils are usually seen surrounding the extravasated mucin from ruptured cysts. Prominent neovascularization and hemorrhage are

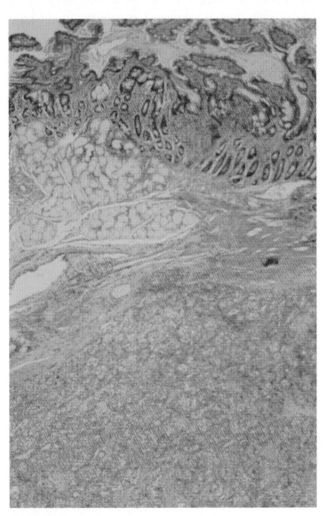

Figure 19–2. Brunner's gland hyperplasia.

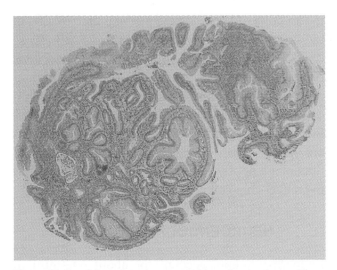

Figure 19–4. A juvenile polyp resected from the duodenum. There are multiple irregular dilated glands within abundant lamina propria that contain marked inflammatory cell infiltration.

also common. Dysplastic foci can develop in juvenile polyps in the setting of the polyposis syndrome, but this is much more common in colonic and gastric polyps than in small-bowel polyps.[2,5]

Cronkhite-Canada Syndrome

Cronkhite-Canada syndrome is a nonhereditary polyposis syndrome with associated protein-losing enteropathy, alopecia, nail atrophy, and hyperpigmentation of the skin. The polyps can occur within the stomach, small bowel, colon, and rectum. Microscopically, they are identical to juvenile polyps, with tortuous crypts that are cystically dilated. The lamina propria exhibits edema and inflammation. Characteristically, these microscopic changes are also seen in the intervening nonpolypoid mucosa.[5]

Lymphoid and Inflammatory Fibroid Polyps

Although they mostly occur in the rectum, lymphoid polyps can also be seen in the ileum. They range from a few millimeters to 3 cm in size. About 80 percent of them are solitary. Microscopically, they consist of aggregates of lymphoid follicles with prominent germinal centers involving the mucosa and submucosa.[2,5]

Although inflammatory fibroid polyps can occur throughout the gastrointestinal tract, the small bowel

is the most common site. These lesions are usually solitary, range from sessile (early) to pedunculated (later), and often cause mucosal ulceration. They arise from the submucosa and consist of loose to hyalinized connective tissue, with infiltration by plasma cells and eosinophils. The preponderance of evidence indicates that these lesions are inflammatory rather than neoplastic in nature, but they can recur if they are not completely excised.[5,8]

BENIGN EPITHELIAL TUMORS (ADENOMAS)

Adenomas are not commonly seen in the small bowel. These lesions may exhibit tubular, tubulovillous, or villous architecture and are usually sessile (Figure 19–5). They occur either sporadically or (most commonly) in patients with familial adenomatous polyposis (FAP) or Gardner's syndrome.[1–5] Over 90 percent of patients with FAP develop small-bowel adenomas (primarily at the ampulla of Vater), but only 5 percent will develop adenocarcinoma. Biopsies of an endoscopically normal-appearing ampulla will reveal microscopic foci of adenomatous change in up to 50 percent of adult patients with

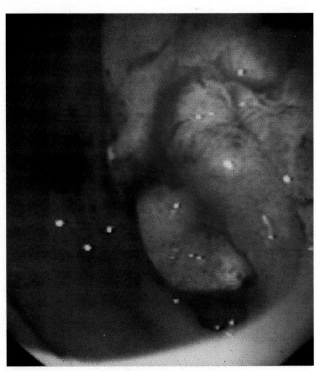

Figure 19–5. Duodenal adenoma. An endoscopic view of a large polypoid lesion in the duodenum.

FAP. Microscopically, small-bowel adenomas are nearly identical to adenomas that occur in the colon (Figure 19–6). They are lined by dysplastic columnar epithelial cells (ie, cells with enlarged, elongated [cigar-shaped], hyperchromatic, and stratified nuclei) that undergo frequent mitosis. The crypts show architectural irregularities such as branching, crowding, and cribriform formations. As is true also for colonic adenomas, complete excision is necessary to preclude the possibility of malignant degeneration. Complete excision can be problematic for large adenomas centered on the ampulla of Vater; despite the absence of invasive tumor, a pancreatoduodenectomy may be necessary if local excision is not feasible. However, it is not uncommon for a focus of invasive tumor (that was not sampled by the preceding endoscopic biopsy) to be discovered in the resection specimen.[1–5]

MALIGNANT EPITHELIAL TUMORS (ADENOCARCINOMAS)

Adenocarcinomas are rare in the small bowel (as opposed to the stomach and colon). However, they account for about 40 percent of small-bowel malignant tumors.[2,3] The most common sites of origin are the ampulla of Vater and the periampullary region of the duodenum (most in the setting of FAP). These tumors usually present as flat, stenosing, ulcerative, or polypoid lesions and are often associated with or arise from adenomas (Figure 19–7). Microscopically, most of the tumors are well to moderately differentiated (Figure 19–8). Ampullary carcinomas are mainly intestinal in type. About one-fifth of the tumors are poorly differentiated, sometimes exhibiting signet-ring cell differentiation.

NEUROENDOCRINE TUMORS

Endocrine tumors account for about one-third of small-bowel tumors.[3] There is a histologic spectrum of neuroendocrine tumors, ranging from classic carcinoid tumors (Figures 19–9 and 19–10) to neuroendocrine carcinomas with varying degrees of differentiation (Figure 19–11), including small cell carcinomas that are histologically similar to their more common pulmonary counterparts. Carcinoid tumors are likely derived from isolated neuroendocrine cells located in the lamina propria whereas neuroendocrine carcinomas probably arise from neuroendocrine cells dispersed within the small-bowel epithelium.

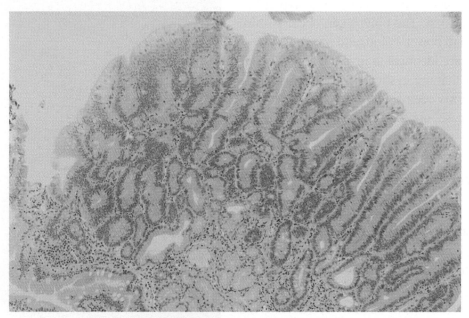

Figure 19–6.   Duodenal adenoma. This is a polypoid lesion with dysplastic changes in the lining epithelium (lack of goblet cells, enlarged and elongated nuclei, and cell crowding). Note the Brunner's glands at the bottom and the normal-appearing small-bowel mucosa at the lower left corner of the field, along with scattered goblet cells.

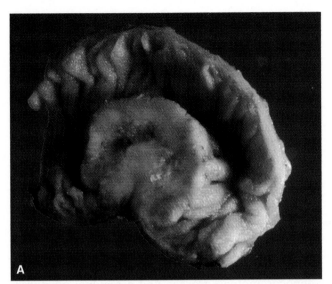
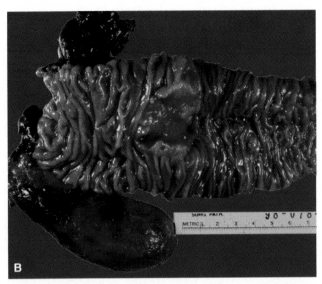

Figure 19–7. *A*, Small-bowel adenocarcinoma: a solid mass infiltrates the wall of the small bowel, causing flattening of the mucosal surface as compared to the delicate circular folds (plicae circulares) in the surrounding uninvolved mucosa. *B*, Adenocarcinoma arising at the ampulla of Vater. The tumor has elevated edges and a central ulcer.

Small-bowel carcinoid tumors most commonly arise from the ileum (Figure 19–12) and the duodenum (see Figure 19–11). They grow slowly and have an indolent natural history even when metastatic disease is present at diagnosis. Metastases are quite rare for tumors < 1 cm in size but are common in tumors of 1 to 2 cm and very likely in tumors > 2 cm³. Metas-

tases most often occur to mesenteric lymph nodes and the liver. Secretion of 5-hydroxytryptamine (5-HT) by liver metastases can cause carcinoid syndrome (diarrhea, facial flushing, and stenosis of the pulmonary and tricuspid valves). Duodenal neuroendocrine tumors that secrete gastrin (ie, gastrinomas) are associated with Zollinger-Ellison syndrome.

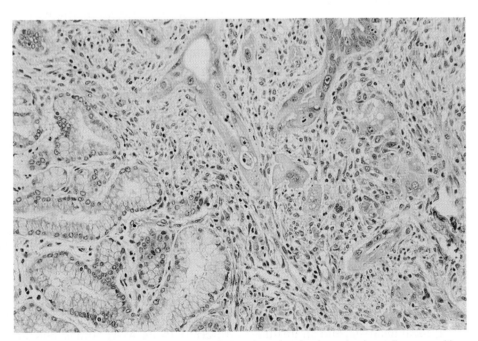

Figure 19–8. Adenocarcinoma of the duodenum. Irregular glands are haphazardly arranged in a reactive stroma that is infiltrated by some mononuclear inflammatory cells. Many of the tumor glands are lined by cells with large vesicular nuclei and other dysplastic features.

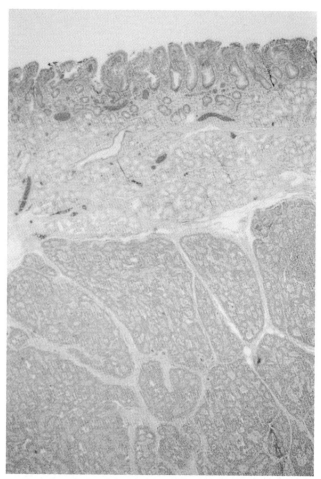

Figure 19–9. Duodenal carcinoid tumor. A well-circumscribed submucosal tumor mass is arranged in lobules separated by fibrous septa. The tumor is located beneath normal duodenal mucosa with Brunner's glands.

microscopic features are of little prognostic value.[3] When differentiation is poor, ancillary studies may be necessary for diagnosis. The tumor cells may be immunohistochemically reactive with various markers of neuroendocrine differentiation, including neuron-specific enolase, chromogranin A, and synaptophysin antibodies. Occasionally, specific hormone products (such as gastrin vasoactive intestinal polypeptide [VIP] or bombesin) are also produced. Somatostatin-producing tumors have a predilection for the region of the ampulla of Vater and are also peculiar in that psammoma body–like calcifications are often present microscopically.[3,5]

Neuroendocrine carcinomas resemble regular adenocarcinomas grossly, and a residual adenomatous mucosa often can be identified at the edges of the mass. Microscopically, they sometimes display a semblance of the architectural arrangements typical of carcinoid tumors, but they always exhibit more cytologic atypia and pleomorphism and a greater mitotic rate than do carcinoid tumors.

LYMPHOMAS AND HODGKIN'S DISEASE INVOLVING THE SMALL BOWEL

Primary lymphomas make up about 17 to 30 percent of primary small-bowel malignancies. Two groups of patients are particularly prone to develop small-bowel lymphomas: patients with acquired immunodeficiency syndrome (AIDS) and patients with celiac disease. In addition, post-organ-transplantation patients are prone to develop post-transplant lymphoproliferative disorder (PTLD), which can involve the small bowel (Figure 19–13). The classification of small-bowel lymphomas follows that of node-based lymphomas, but only a few types are common enough to warrant discussion here. In general, primary lymphomas present as mucosal nodules or masses, which can lead to obstruction, gastrointestinal hemorrhage, or perforation (Figures 19–14 and 19–15; also see Figure 19–13). The cut surface of most lymphomas is soft and usually has the color of fish flesh. Lymphomas arising from the mucosa-associated lymphoid tissue (MALT) are referred to as MALTomas and are thought to be caused by chronic antigen exposure (similar to the gastric MALTomas associated with *Helicobacter*

Grossly, carcinoids form intramural nodules or masses, usually with intact and normal overlying mucosa. An adenomatous mucosa is never seen in association with a carcinoid. Carcinoid tumors sometimes cause marked mesenteric fibrosis, producing kinking of the bowel loops and strictures. The cut surface of carcinoid tumors is yellow tan and may have focal areas of hemorrhage or necrosis. Microscopically, carcinoid tumors consist of uniform and cytologically bland cells forming islands, with peripheral palisading (see Figure 19–10), cords, thick trabeculae, diffuse sheets, glandular structures, and various mixed forms. The cells usually have granular nuclei, with inconspicuous nucleoli. Cytologic atypia, focal necrosis, and an infiltrative growth pattern may be seen in tumors of higher malignant potential (see Figure 19–11) although

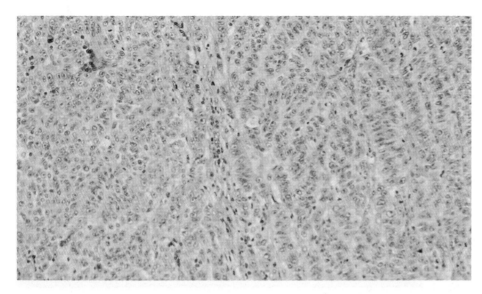

Figure 19–10. Small-bowel carcinoid tumor. This tumor has a trabecular growth pattern.

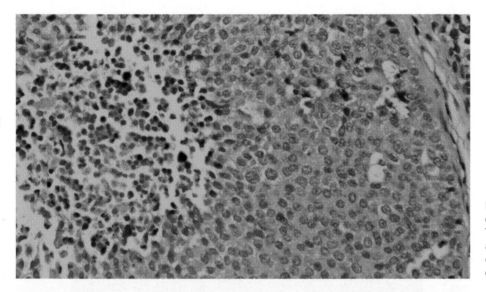

Figure 19–11. Neuroendocrine carcinoma arising at the ampulla of Vater. There is more prominent nuclear atypia in the tumor cells. Other areas of the tumor showed necrosis and vascular invasion.

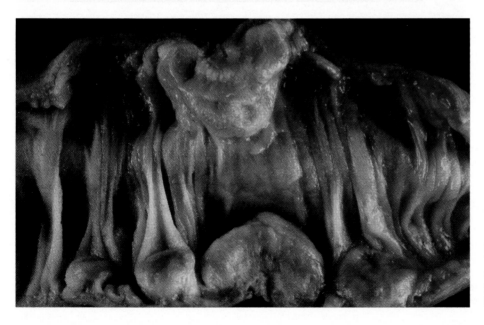

Figure 19–12. Ileal carcinoid tumor. The well-circumscribed mass has a uniform homogeneous tan cut surface, protrudes into the lumen, but does not involve the overlying mucosa.

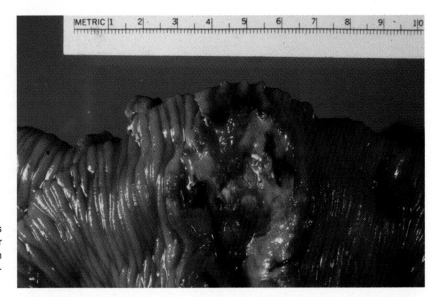

Figure 19–13.   Small-bowel lymphoma. This is a post-transplant lymphoproliferative disorder (PTLD) presenting as discrete mass lesions in the small bowel, after orthotopic liver transplantation.

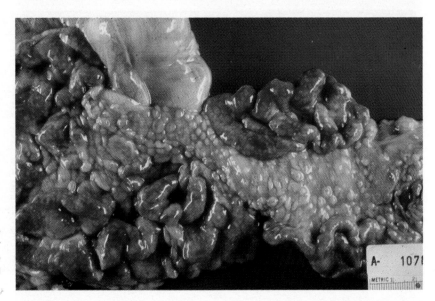

Figure 19–14.   B-cell lymphoma involving the ileum. This is from a patient with a primary nasopharyngeal diffuse B-cell lymphoma. The involved mucosal surface exhibits numerous small nodules and areas of markedly thickened folds.

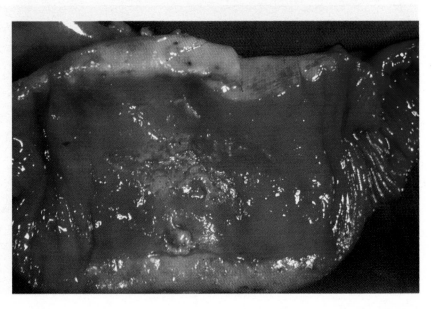

Figure 19–15.   B-cell lymphoma. There is diffuse involvement of the small-bowel mucosa.

pylori infection) (Figure 19–16). By convention, only low-grade B-cell lymphomas are included in this category although the possibility exists that high-grade large B-cell lymphomas may evolve from a pre-existing MALToma.[9] High-grade lymphomas typically protrude into the bowel lumen as bulky ulcerated masses (Figure 19–17). Burkitt's lymphoma (the most common childhood gastrointestinal lymphoma) has a predilection for the ileocecal region and consists of large B cells that resemble lymphoblasts. About 15 percent of Burkitt's lymphomas are associated with Epstein-Barr virus (EBV) infection. Microscopically, there is a high mitotic rate and a "starry-sky" appearance due to scattered tingible body macrophages containing phagocytosed cellular and nuclear debris.[9] Mediterranean lymphoma more often involves the proximal small bowel and usually exists as a diffuse infiltration of the bowel wall.[5] T-cell lymphomas, which occur as a complication of celiac disease, usually present as multiple ulcers in the proximal small bowel and rarely as a mass lesion. Some patients with celiac disease develop widespread denudation of the small-bowel mucosa (ulcerative jejunoileitis), most often as a result of a diffuse form of T-cell lymphoma.[5,9] The diagnosis is quite difficult to make from biopsy specimens, however, because the dispersed neoplastic cells are difficult to recognize within the intense reactive inflammatory cell reaction caused by the ulceration. Molecular gene re-arrangement studies to document the presence of a clonal T-cell population are often required in this setting.[5,9]

Hodgkin's disease very rarely disseminates to the small intestine, which is virtually unheard of as the primary site of disease.[5] Microscopically, it is characterized by focal mucosal ulceration, with a mixed

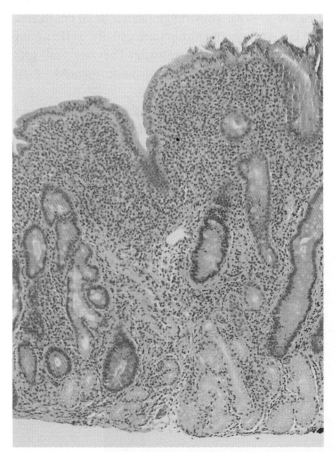

Figure 19–16. Duodenal B-cell lymphoma arising from mucosa-associated lymphoid tissue (MALT), called MALToma. A monotonous population of small lymphocytes is in the lamina propria, widely separating the crypts and causing flattening of the villi. Note the Brunner's glands at the bottom of the field.

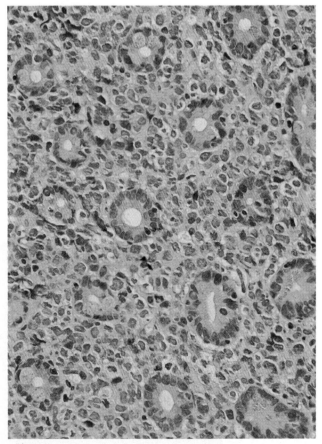

Figure 19–17. B-cell lymphoma of the large cell type involving the duodenum, occurring in an acquired immunodeficiency syndrome (AIDS) patient. Note the tumor cells containing monotonous nuclei that are larger than the nuclei of the epithelial cells in the glands. Some glands are infiltrated by the large lymphocytes.

inflammatory cell background consisting of eosinophils and plasma cells in addition to many small lymphocytes. The scattered large Hodgkin's cells with bizarre irregular vesicular nuclei and prominent nucleoli may be very inconspicuous, making diagnosis from a biopsy specimen extremely challenging. These large cells express CD15 and CD30, a unique combination of markers not shared by any other types of malignant cells.

GASTROINTESTINAL STROMAL TUMORS

In the past, it was assumed that most mesenchymal tumors of the gastrointestinal tract were of smooth-muscle origin. This assumption was based on the observations that (a) most of these tumors appeared to arise from the muscularis propria and that (b) the light-microscopic appearance of this tumor resembled that of leiomyoma or leiomyosarcoma more than that of any other soft-tissue mesenchymal tumor. However, smooth-muscle differentiation could never be demonstrated by electron microscopy or immunohistochemistry in a large majority of these tumors despite the introduction of increasingly sophisticated methodologies over a period of several decades. Evidence of neural differentiation was even more rare. Since no definite cell of origin could be assigned to the vast majority of these mesenchymal tumors, the noncommittal name "gastrointestinal stromal tumor" (GIST) became accepted.[5] Recently, it has been demonstrated that GISTs uniformly exhibit strong and diffuse immunoreactivity for c-kit (CD117) antibody. It is likely that these tumors derive from the interstitial cells of Cajal as these are the only cells (other than mast cells) in the gastrointestinal tract that normally express c-kit protein. The interstitial cells of Cajal, which are located within the myenteric plexus, serve as the gastrointestinal peristaltic pacemaker by connecting the autonomic nervous system to the muscularis propria. The strong immunoreactivity of these tumors with the c-kit antibody often reflects the presence of activating mutations (usually deletions) in the KIT gene.[2,10,11]

The small bowel is the second most common site of origin of GISTs (20 to 25%) after the stomach (60 to 70%). Clinically, no sex or racial predisposition is described for these tumors, and adults of all ages can be affected. Multiple tumors may develop in patients with Carney's syndrome. Grossly, the tumors present as masses protruding from either the serosa or mucosa or creating a dumbbell shape (Figure 19–18). They range from 2 to 20 cm in size. On cut surface, the tumors are usually well circumscribed but lack a true capsule. They are pink-gray or light tan in color. Lymph node metastases are exceedingly rare.[5,11]

Microscopically, the tumor consists of either spindle (Figures 19–19 and 19–20) or epithelioid cells (Figure 19–21), with eosinophilic cytoplasm. Although usually well circumscribed, the tumor often infiltrates insidiously into the surrounding tissue. Areas of apparent smooth-muscle differentiation

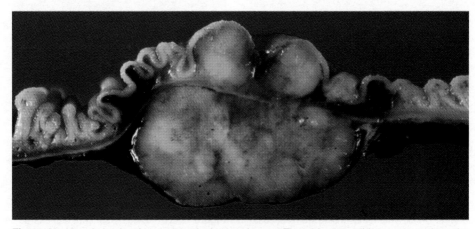

Figure 19–18.   A duodenal gastrointestinal stromal tumor. The white-tan solid mass arose from the muscularis propria of the small bowel and protrudes from both the mucosal and serosal surfaces, forming a "dumbbell" configuration. Note that the mucosal layer overlying the tumor is relatively uninvolved by the tumor.

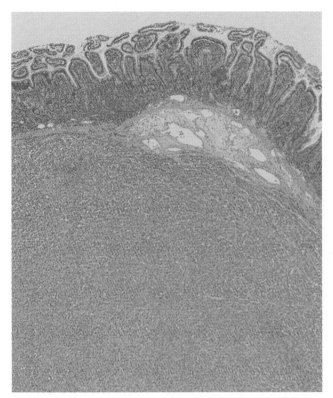

Figure 19–19. A jejunal gastrointestinal stromal tumor. This is a well-circumscribed spindle cell tumor. The overlying mucosa is normal.

(cigar-shaped nuclei with blunt ends and perinuclear vacuoles) and neural differentiation (nuclear palisading, with a plexiform appearance) are frequently seen in the same tumor. Distinctive extracellular bundles of collagen fibers known as skienoid fibers appear to be unique to small-bowel GISTs but are encountered infrequently.[2,5,10,11]

Local recurrence can be expected if complete surgical resection is not achieved. Other than the presence of metastasis, there are no absolute histologic criteria for malignancy. Small-bowel GISTs are generally considered to behave more aggressively than GISTs arising from the stomach. A mitotic rate greater than 5 per 50 high-power fields (hpf) is generally considered to indicate a significant risk of malignant behavior, and a mitotic rate greater than 10 per 50 hpf suggests behavior similar to that of a high-grade soft-tissue sarcoma. The malignant potential also increases with tumor size although a distinct size cut-off separating benign from malignant tumors has not been determined.[2,10,11]

As described above, nearly all the GISTs are immunohistochemically strongly and diffusely reactive with the CD117 (c-kit) antibody (Figure 19–22); the majority are also reactive with the CD34 antibody. In contrast, schwannomas and malignant peripheral nerve sheath tumors are reactive with the S-100 antibody, and leiomyomas and leiomyosarcomas exhibit desmin expression, but all of these tumors lack reactivity with the CD117 (c-kit) antibody.[10,11]

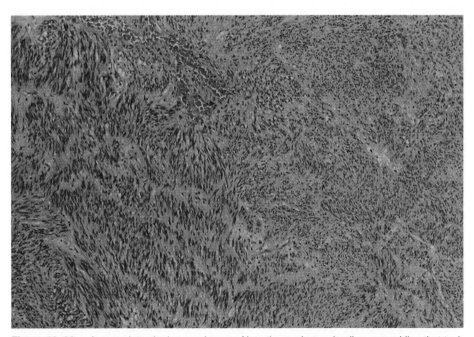

Figure 19–20. A gastrointestinal stromal tumor. Note the nuclear palsading, resembling that typically seen in a schwannoma.

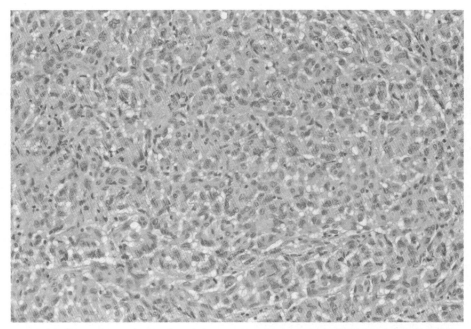

Figure 19–21. A gastrointestinal stromal tumor. Focally, the tumor exhibits epithelioid cell differentiation, with abundant pink cytoplasm.

NEUROGENIC TUMORS

Neurogenic tumors include benign schwannoma (neurolemmoma), neurofibroma, gangliocytic paraganglioma, and malignant peripheral nerve sheath tumors.[2-5] Schwannomas are rarely encountered in the small bowel and have been discussed briefly above. Neurofibroma and malignant peripheral nerve-sheath tumors involving the small bowel usually occur in patients with neurofibromatosis (von Recklinghausen's disease). Most gangliocytic paragangliomas arise in the duodenum. Patients

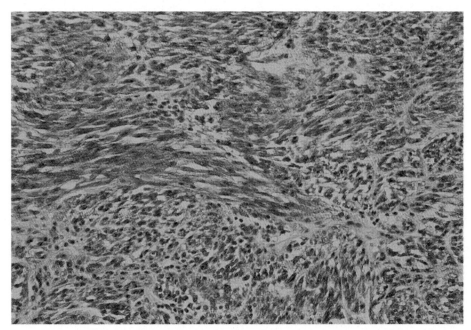

Figure 19–22. An immunohistochemical section, using an anti-CD117 (c-kit) antibody. Most of the tumor cells exhibit strong cytoplasmic reactivity.

are generally in their fifth to sixth decade and present with abdominal pain and gastrointestinal (GI) bleeding. The lesion has a polypoid gross appearance and consists of an admixture of spindle cells positive for S-100 protein, neuroendocrine cells, and typical ganglion cells. Gastrointestinal autonomic nerve tumors (GANTs), which were once recognized by their distinctive ultrastructural features (complex cell processes and neuroendocrine secretory granules), are now considered to be variants of GISTs since they uniformly express c-kit protein.[11,12]

OTHER BENIGN AND MALIGNANT MESENCHYMAL TUMORS

Neoplasms can derive from any component of the small-intestinal wall, such as smooth muscle (leiomyosarcoma), blood vessel (hemangioma, Kaposi's sarcoma, angiosarcoma), and adipose tissue (lipoma). Leiomyomas are virtually unheard of in the small bowel. With the exception of hemangiomas, vascular tumors are also quite rare. Hemangiomas may be diffuse and infiltrating or well circumscribed and can consist of cavernous or capillary vessels.[3]

Although three forms of Kaposi's sarcoma have been described, most of the cases involving the GI tract occur in AIDS or post-transplant patients. Involvement of the small bowel usually is in the form of multiple mucosal erythematous plaques or dome-shaped nodules, sometimes with hemorrhage or central ulceration (Figure 19–23). Although early lesions are limited to the submucosa, the mucosa can be focally infiltrated. Microscopically, the lesions consist of proliferating spindle cells and poorly developed vascular spaces, with extravasation of red blood cells.[2,3,5]

Benign mature teratomas can rarely occur in the mesentery or in the wall of the small bowel. They present as an intra-abdominal mass or produce obstructive symptoms. They are usually well circumscribed dark red to yellow masses that are adherent to the bowel loops (Figure 19–24). The cut surface of the tumor usually shows various elements, including yellow lobulated fat, cartilage, bone, portions of GI tract, and hairs (Figure 19–25).

Lipomas are less common in the small bowel than the colon. They usually present as an asymptomatic mass that protrudes into the lumen. They arise from the submucosa and are covered by normal mucosa (Figure 19–26). Like lipomas from other sites, they consist of mature adipose tissue.[3,5]

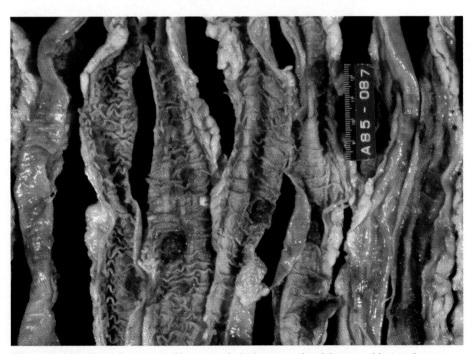

Figure 19–23.   Kaposi's sarcoma. Numerous dark plaques and nodules are evident on the mucosa of the entire small bowel.

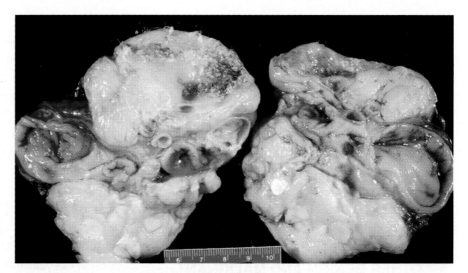

Figure 19–24. Teratoma. This mature teratoma arose in the wall of jejunum, compressing the lumen of the small bowel and causing severe obstruction. The tumor was composed of multiple tissue types, including skin, gastrointestinal tract (stomach and small intestine), bone, cartilage, and respiratory mucosa.

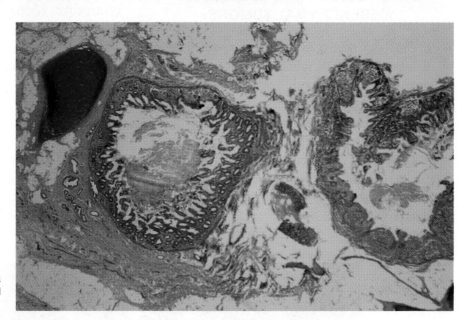

Figure 19–25. Teratoma. This area shows spaces lined by gastric mucosa and small-bowel mucosa, cartilage, and fat.

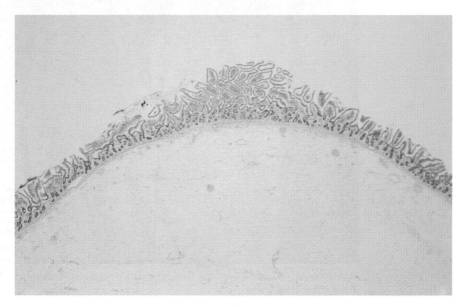

Figure 19–26. Lipoma. This duodenal mass has a soft yellow cut surface and is well circumscribed. It consists entirely of mature fat.

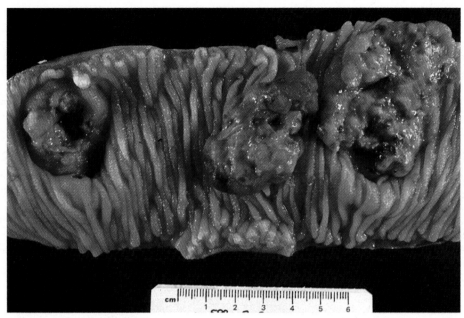

Figure 19–27. Metastatic melanoma to the small bowel. There are multiple mucosal nodules with irregular surfaces and dark pigmentation. (Courtesy of Richard A. Pucci.)

MALIGNANT MELANOMA AND OTHER METASTATIC TUMORS

Metastatic deposits of melanoma, which are often multiple, can cause obstruction, hemorrhage, and intussusception (Figure 19–27). Grossly, they appear as rounded or irregular nodules protruding into the lumen, and they are sometimes pigmented. Microscopically, the tumor cells are epithelioid, with abundant eosinophilic cytoplasm and large vesicular nuclei containing prominent nucleoli (Figure 19–28). Immunohistochemically, these cells express S-100 protein and HMB-45 and are not reactive with keratin antibodies (in contrast to carcinomas).[3,5]

Metastatic carcinoma from virtually every organ can involve the small intestine, but colon, pancreas, stomach, ovary, uterus, and kidney involvements are most common. Metastasis from lung and breast are the most common extra-abdominal sites of origin. Involvement by tumors originating in other segments of the GI tract and pancreas is often a result of direct invasion rather than metastasis, sometimes with the formation of a malignant fistula. True metastases are often in the form of multiple small serosal nodules or plaques although mucosa-based deposits may also occur in patients with disease that is widely disseminated via hematogenous spread.[5]

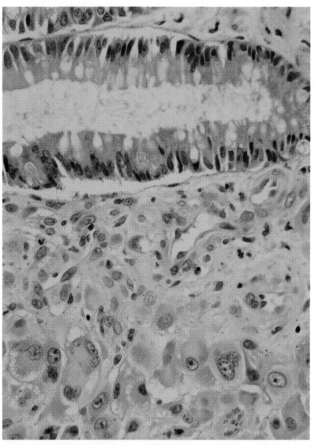

Figure 19–28. Metastatic melanoma to the small bowel. This is a microscopic view of the same tumor shown in Figure 19–25. There are large tumor cells infiltrating between the crypts. The tumor cells have abundant cytoplasm and large vesicular nuclei with prominent nucleoli. (Courtesy of Richard A. Pucci.)

REFERENCES

1. Cooper H. Benign epithelial polyps of the intestines. In: Ming SC, Goldman H, editors. Pathology of the gastrointestinal tract. 2nd ed. Baltimore: Williams & Williams; 1998. p. 819–53.

2. Jass JR. Tumors of the small and large intestines (including the anal region). In: Fletcher CDM, editor. Diagnostic histopathology of tumors. 2nd ed. London: Churchill-Livingstone; 2000. p. 369–409.

3. Fenoglio-Preiser CM, Pascal RR, Perzin KH. Tumors of the intestine. In: Atlas of tumor pathology. Second series. Vol. 27. Bethesda (MD): Armed Forces Institute of Pathology; 1990.

4. Owen DA, Kelly JK. Atlas of gastrointestinal pathology. Philadelphia: WB Saunders Company; 1994. p. 61–122.

5. Lewin KJ, Riddell RH, Weinstein WM, editors. Gastrointestinal pathology and its clinical implications. New York: Igaku-Shoin; 1992. p. 1167–97.

6. Walk L. Nodular hyperplasia of duodenal Brunner's glands—does it exist? Endoscopy 1982;14:162–5.

7. McGarrity TJ, Kulin HE, Zaino RJ. Peutz-Jeghers syndrome. Am J Gastroenterol 2000;95:596–604.

8. Assarian GS, Sundareson A. Inflammatory fibroid polyp of the ileum. Human Pathol 1985;16:11–2.

9. Isaacson PG. Gastrointestinal lymphomas and lymphoid hyperplasia. In: Knowles DM, editor. Neoplastic hematopathology. Baltimore: William & Wilkins; 1992. p. 953–78.

10. Miettinen M, Lasota J. Gastrointestinal stromal tumors—definition, clinical, histological, immunohistochemical, and molecular genetic features and differential diagnosis. Virchows Arch 2001;438:1–12.

11. Berman J, O'Leary J. Gastrointestinal stromal tumor workshop. Hum Pathol 2001;32:578–82.

12. Lauwers GY, Erlandson RA, Casper ES, et al. Gastrointestinal autonomic nerve tumors. Am J Surg Pathol 1993;17:889–97.

20

Diagnosis of Small-Bowel Tumors

PETER M. MACENEANEY, MB, FRCR
ARUNAS E. GASPARAITIS, MD

The mucosa of the small bowel accounts for over 90 percent of the surface of the gastrointestinal (GI) tract; however, it is a rare site of tumors and accounts for less than 2 percent of all GI neoplasms[1] and 1 percent of GI carcinomas.[2] Details regarding the rate and distribution of tumors of the small bowel vary among published series, and exact figures are difficult to determine. Some series include tumors arising in the duodenum.

Tumors may develop in all tissue components of the small-bowel wall. Mucosa-originating adenocarcinomas and submucosal carcinoid tumors are the most common primary malignancies. Adenocarcinomas are concentrated in the duodenum and jejunum. Per square centimeter, the duodenum, especially the periampullary region, has the highest rate of small-bowel adenocarcinoma. Relatively few adenocarcinomas originate in the ileum.[2] Conversely, small-bowel carcinoid tumors are most frequent in the ileum whereas small-bowel lymphoma and leiomyosarcoma favor the jejunum and ileum, respectively. These observations have important implications for diagnosis and imaging.

Survival from primary malignances of the small intestine has not improved in parallel with significant advances in diagnostic imaging over the last four decades.[3] Curative treatment depends on early diagnosis and surgical resection.[4,5] Unfortunately, many cancers of the small bowel are diagnosed at an advanced stage, after the window of opportunity afforded by local disease has elapsed. Maglinte and colleagues showed that there was an average delay of almost 9 months between onset of symptoms and diagnosis.[6] Several factors contributed to this delay;

however, almost 8 months of this delay occurred while the patient was under the care of a physician. This was due to delayed ordering of appropriate investigations by the clinician and/or misinterpretation of investigations by radiologists.

Apart from metastatic carcinoid tumors and Peutz-Jehgers syndrome, the presenting features of tumors of the small bowel are vague.[5] Metastatic carcinoid has characteristic features that are manifest in a minority of patients with the disease. Peutz-Jehgers syndrome produces typical buccal pigmentation (Figure 20–1).[7] Apart from these, the commonest clinical features associated with tumors of the small bowel are abdominal pain, gastrointestinal bleeding, nausea and vomiting, and weight loss.[6] Obstructive features occur relatively late. These nonspecific clinical features, coupled with the low incidence of small-bowel tumors, result in a low index of suspicion (or low pretest probability[8]) on the part of the physician and the radiologist and contribute to the slow diagnosis of such tumors. Only by consideration of the small bowel as a potential cause of vague symptoms will diagnosis be expedited and (it is hoped) outcomes be improved.

IMAGING TECHNIQUES

Depending on local availability and expertise, endoscopy and imaging are the primary tools for investigation of the upper and lower gastrointestinal tracts. Ultrasonography has a limited role.[9] Enteroscopes were introduced in the 1980s. Peroral push enteroscopy, sonde (withdrawal) enteroscopy, and intraoperative enteroscopy are used in specialized

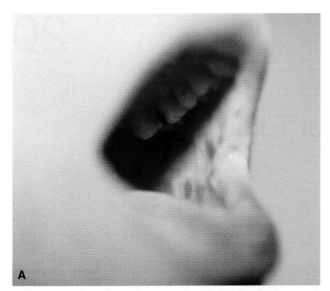
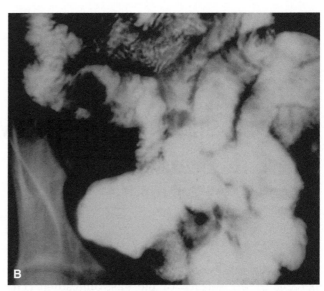

Figure 20–1. *A,* Photograph of the buccal mucosa of a patient with Peutz-Jeghers syndrome, demonstrating characteristic pigmentation. *B,* Study of the small bowel of the same patient. Numerous polyps, ranging in size from a few millimeters to almost 2 cm, are distributed throughout the small bowel.

centers. However, the diagnosis of small-bowel tumors remains largely the domain of the radiologist. To date, computed tomography (CT) and magnetic resonance imaging (MRI) are used for staging cancers and not for the primary detection of small-bowel tumors. Promising new techniques for examining the small bowel with these modalities (CT and MRI enteroclysis) are being developed.[10–16] These may eventually replace barium studies, which are currently the most sensitive modality for the early detection of small-bowel tumors.

Detailed barium evaluation of the small bowel is difficult due to the presence of multiple peristalsing intestinal loops overlapped in a limited area. This results in lower sensitivity and specificity of barium studies in the small bowel, compared to the equivalent study of the stomach and colon. The reported sensitivity of the conventional (non-enteroclysis) small-bowel study (SBS) varies widely.[17–19] An abnormality demonstrated by SBS was present in up to 83 percent of cases of primary small-bowel malignancies, but the tumor was directly visualized in less than 50 percent of cases. This suboptimal diagnostic performance of the conventional barium SBS inevitably leads to false-negative results and diagnostic delays. Enteroclysis is the preferred method for detecting small (resectable) small-bowel tumors.[20]

Enteroclysis involves passing a catheter under fluoroscopic control to the proximal jejunum. The catheters used have a balloon at the tip. This is inflated prior to the infusion of contrast material, to prevent reflux and to therefore maintain enough pressure in the small-bowel lumen to actively distend it. The superior performance of enteroclysis (relative to the SBS) is partly due to this distention of the small bowel by the active infusion of contrast material.

Enteroclysis and SBS were compared in a population of patients with mesenteric small-bowel tumors. In that study, enteroclysis had a sensitivity of 95 percent, compared to 61 percent for SBS.[21] Using long-term follow-up, Barloon and colleagues determined the specificity of enteroclysis to be 92 percent.[22] It is important to note that most adenocarcinomas of the small intestine occur in the duodenum, a site not evaluated routinely by enteroclysis. The duodenum should be evaluated endoscopically or by hypotonic duodenography in all patients with suspected pathology of the small bowel (Figure 20–2).

Computed tomography has been employed in the assessment of small-bowel pathology in two settings: (1) in patients with bowel obstruction and in whom barium studies are unpleasant, difficult, and risky and (2) when staging tumors. Computed tomography evaluates the level, grade, and (frequently) the cause of the obstruction.[23–25] In patients with intestinal obstruction secondary to a small-bowel tumor, the tumor is relatively large and may therefore be identified by CT. However, diagnosis of early non-obstructive tumors of the small bowel by standard CT is usually serendipitous.[26] Neoplastic disease should be suspected on CT if the thickness of the wall of the small bowel is > 1.5 cm or if there are discreet mesenteric masses larger than 1.5 cm.[27] When a small bowel mass was identified by CT in one series, radiologic features led to the correct specific diagnosis in 69 percent of cases.[28] Lipomas, leiomyomas, leiomyosarcomas, and carcinoid tumors were easily recognized, but adenocarcinomas and lymphomas were often mistaken for each other.[28]

Computed tomography plays a prominent role in the diagnosis of periampullary tumors. Barium studies may indicate the site of a mass but may not be able to differentiate between a primary duodenal malignancy and a secondary invasion of the duodenum by a pancreatic or biliary tumor. These may be distinguished by CT, with important prognostic implications.[26]

Computed tomography is the imaging modality of choice for clinical staging of small-bowel tumors. Due to the rarity of these neoplasms, large series describing the accuracy of CT in this role are scarce. Reported accuracy ranges from 47 to 61 percent.[28,29] Computed tomography tends to be very sensitive but not specific for the detection of mesenteric infiltration, regional lymphadenopathy, and distant metastases.

Recently, CT enteroclysis has been reported in the literature in the investigation of low-grade small-bowel obstruction and inflammatory bowel disease.[30,31] This technique combines the benefits of enteroclysis and CT. Moderate distention of the mesenteric small bowel with dilute contrast is achieved by placing a catheter beyond the ligament of Treitz and administering dilute contrast by pump. When the small bowel is completely opacified, the patient is scanned by CT. The images acquired overcome the problem of overlapping bowel loops encountered in conventional barium studies, and there is the potential of performing multiplanar reformatting.[32] This is a very promising new application of CT; to date, however, there are no data on its diagnostic performance in the setting of small-bowel tumors. As with standard enteroclysis, the

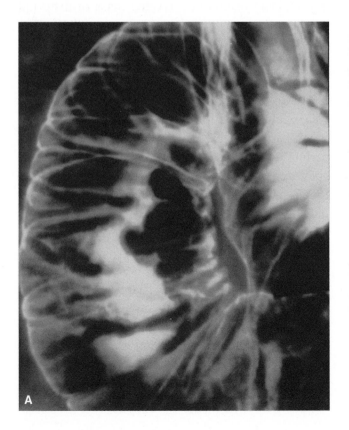

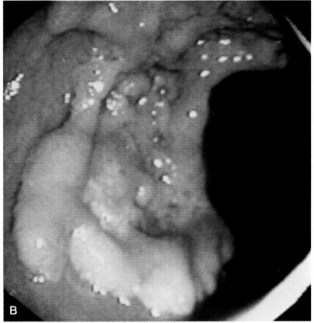

Figure 20–2. Duodenography (*A*) and an endoscopic image (*B*) demonstrate a villous adenoma at the ampulla of Vater. This lesion could easily be missed on enteroclysis as it would not impede intubation of the jejunum.

duodenum is not well demonstrated on CT enteroclysis and should be examined separately.

There have been parallel developments in MRI of the small bowel. Development of contrast agents, coils, and rapid pulse sequences have improved MRI of the GI tract.[33] Fast pulse sequences allow for imaging during a breath-hold and minimize the motion artifact associated with peristalsis and respiration. Magnetic resonance (MR) has been used to evaluate small-bowel obstruction, and MR enteroclysis has been reported.[10,11,16] Small-bowel tumors have been demonstrated in a small series; however, many of these tumors were advanced cases (a mean tumor size of 4 cm).[34] Bowel contrast is important in MR to avoid mistaking bowel loops for adenopathy or mesenteric masses. Positive-contrast agents such as gadolinium, manganese, or ferric ammonium citrate reduce T1 relaxation times. These agents can accentuate "ghosting" artifacts from peristalsis. Rapid imaging techniques and antiperistaltic agents minimize these effects. Gadolinium-based positive contrast agents have proven valuable in the assessment of small-bowel Crohn's disease.[12] Negative contrast agents may be classed as diamagnetic preparations (eg, barium) and superparamagnetic iron oxides. These negative agents represent the major options for radiologists.[35] As more contrast preparations are developed and approved, it is likely that oral contrast administration will become routine and that the role of MRI in small-bowel pathology will evolve. Magnetic resonance enteroscopy has the potential to become the method of choice for evaluating the entire small bowel.[36]

Angiography may be used to evaluate and embolize bleeding from ulcerated and vascular tumors. Angiography is occasionally used as an aid to surgical planning.

PRIMARY MALIGNANCIES

Carcinoid Tumors

The distal 60 cm of ileum is the second most common site of carcinoid tumors (after the appendix). Carcinoids account for 25 percent of all small-bowel tumors,[37] and multiple primary sites occur in 15 to 35 percent of patients with small-bowel carcinoid.[28] Embryologically, the cells from which carcinoids arise are from the neural crest. However, the proximal duodenum does not contain the classic argentaffin-positive enterochromaffin cell found in the midgut; as a result, proximal duodenal carcinoids are not associated with carcinoid syndrome.[26] Carcinoid tumors arise in the submucosa and grow slowly, but all have malignant potential (Figure 20–3). Malignancy is determined by the presence of local invasion or metastatic spread, rather than histologically.[38] Tumors smaller than 1 cm are rarely invasive whereas those larger than 2 cm have usually metastasized by the time of diagnosis.[37] Presenting features vary with the growth pattern of the tumor and with its ability to release serotonin. If growth is predominantly toward the lumen, the tumor may become the lead point of an intussusception or the overlying mucosa may ulcerate, with subsequent GI bleeding. Alternatively, if enlargement is predominantly serosal or exophytic, then the patient may present with features attributable to the local effects of serotonin. Serotonin generates a profound fibrotic reaction when released into the mesentery (Figure 20–4). This desmoplasia results in a fixated mass of distorted bowel loops and mesentery that may calcify. The associated retraction may cause bowel obstruction, and involvement of mesenteric vessels may result in ischemia.

Radiographic findings depend on the stage of disease at presentation and on the pattern of growth. Small carcinoids are usually incidental findings on barium studies (see Figure 20–3) (as discussed above, enteroclysis is the more sensitive technique). Small carcinoids have no specific features and are indistinguishable from other small lesions such as leiomyomas. Cross-sectional imaging is not usually helpful at this stage of disease.

The desmoplastic reaction is seen as a stellate mass on CT (Figure 20–5). There is angulation of involved bowel loops, with crowding of valvulae conniventes at their apices. Intestinal obstruction may be associated. Calcification is demonstrated on CT in approximately 50 percent of cases. Mesenteric lymphadenopathy and vascular involvement are also established by cross-sectional imaging.

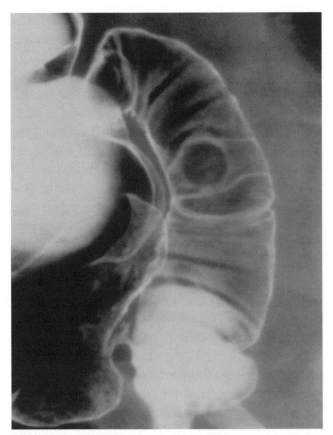

Figure 20–3. A 1-cm carcinoid tumor in the terminal ileum. The radiologic features are those of a submucosal lesion although otherwise nonspecific.

There are extensive hepatic metastases in 95 percent of patients with carcinoid syndrome.[37] Typically, hepatic metastases show enhancement in the arterial phase of contrast enhancement and are hypointense in the portal venous phase of CT and MRI, relative to

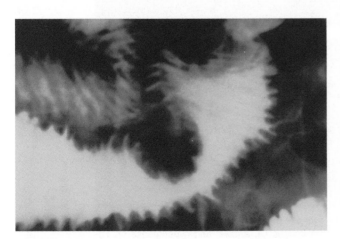

Figure 20–4. A carcinoid tumor, with typical tethering of adjacent bowel due to the desmoplastic reaction generated by the local effects of serotonin.

normal hepatic parenchyma (Figure 20–6). Rarely, nuclear medicine is required to distinguish carcinoid from other causes of mesenteric fibrosis. The somatostatin analogue octreotide may be used in the diagnosis of carcinoid tumors. Radionuclide scanning with radiolabeled octreotide is a sensitive method of localizing somatostatin-positive tumors. The technique may also be used to identify patients who may respond to octreotide therapy.[39]

ADENOCARCINOMA

Small-bowel adenomas are among the most common benign lesions, accounting for 20 percent of all small-bowel tumors.[26] They occur most frequently in the duodenum and proximal jejunum, especially the peri-

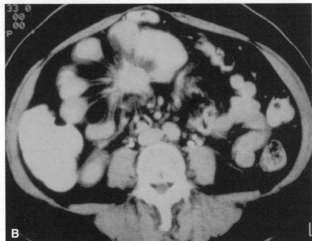

Figure 20–5. Consecutive images from a computed tomography study with oral and intravenous contrast. The desmoplastic response is seen as a stellate mesenteric mass although the primary carcinoid tumor is not identified.

ampullary region (see Figure 20–2). Most are asymptomatic. Rarely, they may bleed or intussuscept.

Small-bowel adenocarcinoma, like other small-bowel tumors, has nonspecific symptoms and signs. Since most of these lesions occur within 25 cm of the duodenojejunal junction, patients with pain, vomiting, and anemia should have assessment of the proximal jejunum as part of an extended upper-GI investigation.[40] Most (70%) duodenal carcinomas are polypoid, larger lesions tend to ulcerate, and infiltrative duodenal carcinomas are relatively rare.[3] Depending on location, these may be identified by upper-GI endoscopy or barium studies. Carcinomas of the mesenteric small bowel are commonly constricting "apple core" lesions at the time of diagnosis. These display the typical features of GI malignancies on barium studies: shouldering; mucosal destruction; irregular luminal narrowing; and rigidity of a short segment, with variable degrees of intestinal obstruction (Figures 20–7, 20–8, and 20–9). The main differential diagnoses for these appearances are Crohn's disease, lymphoma, and leiomyosarcoma of the small bowel. Crohn's disease usually involves longer segments than carcinoma, and the mucosa has a "cobblestone" appearance; lymphoma and leiomyosarcoma tend to be larger and softer tumors.

Small-bowel adenocarcinomas have various manifestations on CT, depending on their growth patterns. Polypoid tumors may be identified as luminal filling defects, depending on their size and the presence of oral contrast material. Small lesions are easily missed on CT and may be identified only if they cause a degree of obstruction or act as the lead point of an intussusception. Infiltrative lesions are seen as areas of bowel-wall thickening. Computed tomography is more helpful in staging the carcinoma than in primary diagnosis.

However, CT is also used to show extraluminal features that help narrow down differential diagnoses in difficult cases. Mesenteric lymphadenopathy is associated with lymphoma and metastatic small-bowel carcinoma; however, lymph node metastases in small-bowel carcinoma are smaller than those encountered in lymphoma.[26] Leiomyosarcoma is often more easily identified on CT than on barium studies due to the predominantly exophytic

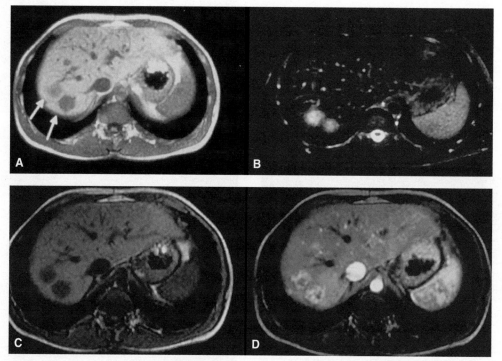

Figure 20–6.   Magnetic resonance images through the liver of a patient with a metastatic carcinoid tumor. These lesions are hypointense on T1-weighted spin echo images (*A, arrows*) and hyperintense on T2-weighted fast spin echo sequences (*B*). Spoiled-gradient echo sequences performed prior to contrast enhancement (*C*) and in the arterial phase of contrast enhancement (*D*) demonstrate the typical arterial-phase enhancement of carcinoid metastases.

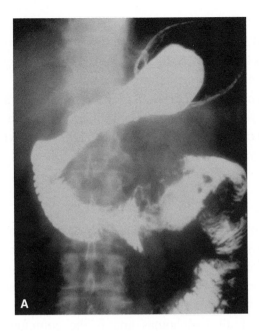

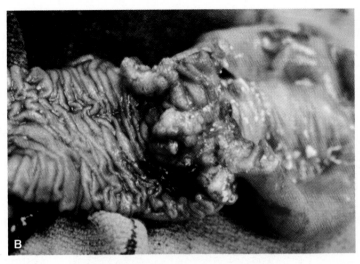

Figure 20–7. Barium study (*A*) and corresponding surgical specimen (*B*) demonstrate a constricting carcinoma of the third part of the duodenum. The proximal shouldering is typical of a carcinoma.

nature of the tumor, which frequently cavitates (vide infra). Strictures of Crohn's disease are associated with the "creeping fat" in the adjacent mesentery, identifying the inflammatory rather than neoplastic nature of the stricture.

Leiomyosarcoma

Leiomyosarcomas account for 9 percent of all small-bowel malignancies. Some authors report that they are most prevalent in the ileum[1] whereas others have found them most commonly in the jejunum.[41] They are rare in the duodenum. They occur most frequently in men in their sixth and seventh decades.

The relationship between leiomyoma and leiomyosarcoma is not clear. These entities can be difficult to differentiate histologically if there is little necrosis.[42,43] Even histologically benign-appearing leiomyomas may metastasize.[43]

Clinically, leiomyosarcoma presents with a long history of pain (since the tumor is slow growing) and bleeding. These are very vascular tumors, and bleeding, intraperitoneal or intraluminal, may be brisk. The growth of leiomyosarcoma is predominantly extraluminal; therefore, obstruction is rare unless the tumor grows to a size such that it can compress the bowel. Several cases of large leiomyosarcomas have been misdiagnosed as ovarian tumors.[44]

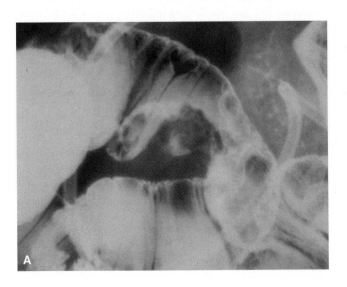

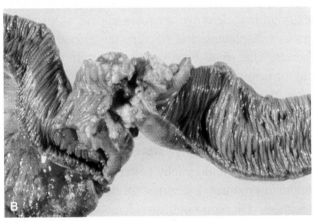

Figure 20–8. Images of an enteroclysis study (*A*) and the corresponding surgical specimen (*B*) of an ulcerated jejunal carcinoma.

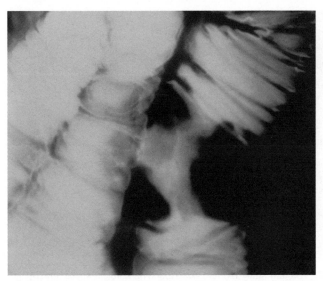

Figure 20–9. An "apple core" carcinoma of the jejunum with central ulceration.

Large leiomyosarcomas tend to outgrow their blood supply and become necrotic centrally. These tumors then cavitate via their connection with the intestinal lumen. As a result, plain radiography may demonstrate abnormal collections of air in a cavitary leiomyosarcoma and thus confuse it with bezoars or large abscess cavities.

Leiomyomas and small leiomyosarcomas are also difficult to differentiate radiologically. However, larger lesions with significant ulceration or cavitation are more likely malignant.[37] In a series of 29 cases, sarcomas were generally larger (12 cm on average) than leiomyomas (4 cm on average).[45] As with other small-bowel malignancies, the appearance of leiomyosarcomas on barium study depends on their growth pattern. Since their growth is mainly extraluminal, leiomyosarcomas appear as extrinsic masses displacing and (if very large) compressing bowel. The small-bowel segment from which the tumor originated is frequently ulcerated and draped over the mass. Barium may fill the cavity of a necrotic leiomyosarcoma communicating with the bowel lumen. Like lymphomas, leiomyosarcomas are soft and may change shape on compression.

Computed tomography better demonstrates most leiomyosarcomas by virtue of their extraluminal location. On non-contrast-enhanced scans, small lesions appear as nonspecific soft-tissue densities intimately related to small bowel. After administration of intravenous contrast, there is rapid enhancement of the lesion. Larger lesions, lesions with necrosis and cavitation, and lesions with heterogeneous enhancement patterns are more likely to be malignant[45] (Figure 20–10). Hepatic metastases are hypodense relative to normal liver on contrast-enhanced scans and may be heterogeneous, with mixed cystic and solid components.

Lymphoma

The GI tract may be the primary site of lymphoma or become secondarily involved as a manifestation of systemic disease. In recent series, lymphoma accounted for 12 percent of small-bowel malignancies.[4,5] The GI tract is the site of approximately 15 percent of all lymphomas and is the commonest extranodal site. Within the GI tract, the stomach is the most frequent location of lymphomas (51%), followed by the small bowel (33%), the colon (16%), and, rarely, the esophagus (< 1%).[46] The ileum and jejunum are equally involved.[47] Non-Hodgkin's lymphoma (NHL) is the commonest variety that involves the GI tract. Almost 90 percent of primary NHLs of the small bowel are of the B-cell type.[48] Apart from cases related to celiac disease, T-cell lymphomas are rare, as are Burkitt's lymphoma and Hodgkin's disease of the small bowel. Burkitt's lymphoma of the bowel is usually confined to the ileocecal region.

Most GI lymphomas occur in middle-aged people. Males and females are equally affected. Symptoms are nonspecific. In two series of GI lymphoma cases, abdominal pain was the most common symptom, followed by nausea. Fever and bleeding occurred in 20 to 30 percent of patients.[49,50] Compared to other small-bowel malignancies, obstruction and perforation occur relatively frequently, and up to 40 percent of patients present with an acute abdomen.[49] A palpable mass is present in approximately one-quarter of cases.[50]

Radiologically, diagnosis and staging are performed with a combination of CT and barium studies. Computed tomography may also be used to guide percutaneous biopsy of the bowel or a nodal mass. On barium studies, small-bowel lymphoma has diverse appearances that depend on the gross morphology of the tumor. Several patterns of involvement are described, as follows:[26,40,51–56]

1. Circumferential segmental infiltration. This typically involves one or more well-defined lengths of bowel. Folds may be thickened or effaced and have shallow ulcers. The wall is thickened up to several centimeters. The lumen is more frequently dilatated than stenosed. Calcification of untreated small-bowel NHL has been reported.

2. Endoexoenteric disease with cavitation. Localized perforation may follow transmural infiltration into the mesentery. This and the above form are typical of primary small-bowel lymphoma (Figure 20–11).

3. Aneurysmal dilatation. This form occurs when the unsupported antimesenteric wall of the small bowel is infiltrated and the muscularis is replaced by tumor (Figure 20–12).

4. Multiple polypoid lesions. This is a relatively rare manifestation of small-bowel lymphoma and may represent disease originating in mantle cells or mucosa-associated lymphoid tissue (MALT) (Figure 20–13).

5. Mesenteric nodal lymphoma with secondary infiltration of the small bowel. This first displaces then invades the small bowel. Computed tomography best demonstrates the mesenteric lymphadenopathy. These nodes coalesce to encase adjacent bowel loops to produce a typical "sandwich" pattern seen on CT and ultrasonography.

6. Possible transformation of diffuse nodular hyperplasia into lymphoma. Changes in enteropathy-related T-cell lymphoma, seen in celiac disease, range from subtle irregular nodular fold thicken-

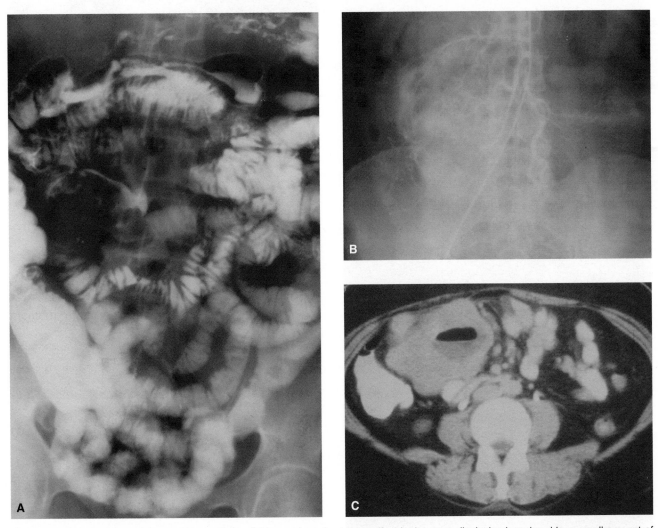

Figure 20–10. *A,* A large leiomyosarcoma in the right upper quadrant is manifest by its mass displacing bowel and by a small amount of barium tracking into its cavity. *B,* The corresponding angiogram demonstrates a large heterogeneous hypervascular mass perfused by branches of the superior mesenteric artery. *C,* Computed tomography depicts an air-fluid level in the central cavity of the thick-walled tumor.

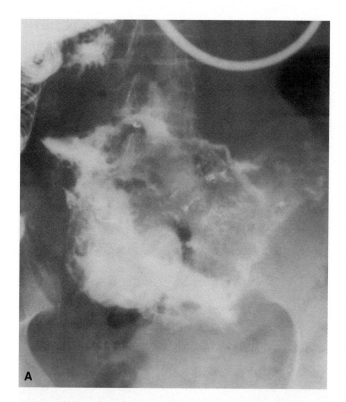

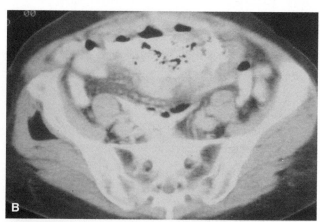

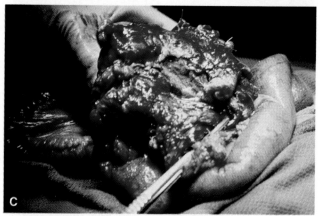

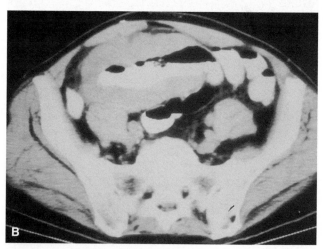

Figure 20–11. Enteroclysis study (*A*) and computed tomography (*B*) demonstrate enteric contrast material filling a large cavity in a small-bowel lymphoma. Surgical resection (*C*) of the lymphoma also demonstrates the cavity.

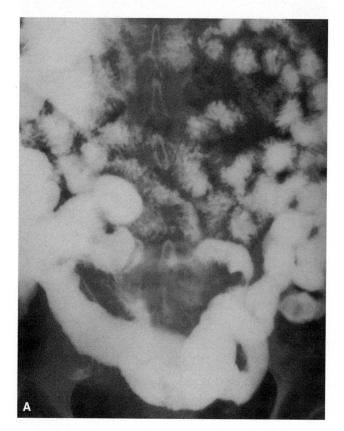

Figure 20–12. Small-bowel series (*A*) and computed tomography (*B*) depict aneurysmal dilatation of a segment of ileum; CT shows marked thickening of small-bowel wall due to infiltration by the lymphoma.

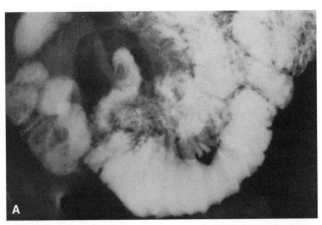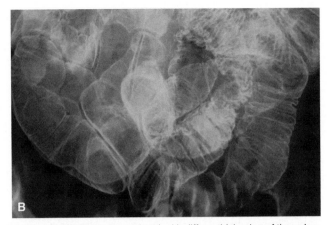

Figure 20–13. Two images from an enteroclysis study demonstrate a short segment (left lowermost loop) with diffuse thickening of the valvulae conniventes and a subtle background nodular pattern consistent with "maltoma."

ing to extensive ulceration and (occasionally) mass lesions. Widespread disease is common at presentation. Enteroclysis is needed for early diagnosis, and definitive diagnosis is based on full-thickness biopsy specimens obtained surgically.

The diagnosis of small-bowel lymphoma is usually reached with a combination of CT and enteroclysis. Lymphoma tends to involve longer segments of bowel than adenocarcinoma, and "apple core" lesions are rare in lymphoma. Cavities associated with leiomyosarcoma are intralesional whereas those in lymphoma are often between the leaves of the mesentery. Bulky mesenteric adenopathy favors a diagnosis of lymphoma although metastatic disease, mesenteric lymphadenitis, and lipodystrophy may mimic the disease.[26] Mesenteric panniculitis is associated with lymphoma and with carcinomas of the breast and lung[57] (Figure 20–14).

Metastatic Disease

Tumors may metastasize to the bowel by hematogenous or lymphatic spread, by intraperitoneal seeding, or by direct invasion.[58] Three of these mechanisms account for roughly equal proportions of metastatic spread to the bowel; lymphatic spread has a relatively minor role. The mechanism of spread influences the radiologic appearance and may help identify the lesion(s) as secondary and direct further investigations toward the most likely primary neoplasms.[58]

Metastatic disease to the small bowel is manifest (broadly) in patients with and without known primary malignancies. In those with known treated tumors, the development of GI symptoms, especially obstructive features, may represent adhesions, metastatic spread, or radiation enteropathy[59] and careful investigation is warranted. Obstructive symptoms and occult GI bleeding are the commonest manifestations of small-bowel metastases in patients without a known primary malignancy.

Malignant melanoma and bronchogenic and breast carcinomas are the most frequent bloodborne metastases that involve the small bowel. The vasa recta supply the rich submucosal plexus on the antimesenteric border of the small bowel.[60] Most hematogenous metastases are found at this site.[61] Transperitoneal seeding of metastases follows the pathways of the circulation of ascitic fluid.[60] In the midabdomen, fluid cascades over mesenteric recesses between small-bowel loops and eventually settles at the termination of the small-bowel mesentery at the ileocecal region. Fluid lodges against the mesenteric side of the bowel wall. Therefore, transcoelomic metastases grow on the mesenteric aspect of the small bowel, in contrast to bloodborne metastases, and most are found in the right lower quadrant.

On barium studies, melanoma metastases are seen as submucosal smooth polypoid filling defects (Figure 20–15). As they grow, they may ulcerate centrally, attaining a typical "target" or "bull's-eye" appearance; however, this occurs more frequently in the stomach than in the small bowel. Melanoma metastases are very cellular and soft and tend not to cause obstruction,[37] although intussusception is com-

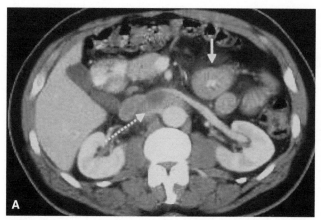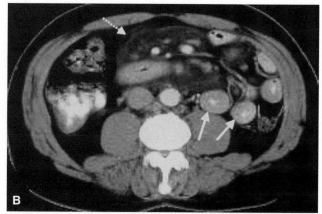

Figure 20–14.   Abdominal computed tomography (CT) in a patient with lymphoma and mesenteric panniculitis. *A,* Pathologic circumferential thickening of a loop of jejunum (*solid arrow*), and pathologic lymphadenopathy between the left renal vein and the aorta (*dashed arrow*). *B,* Panniculitis is identified as well-defined infiltration of the mesenteric fat (*dashed arrow*). Thickened loops of jejunum are again identified (*solid arrows*).

mon. Metastases from bronchogenic carcinoma also ulcerate. Lung cancer metastases to the small bowel often present as intestinal perforation and indicate a poor prognosis; however, most are clinically silent. Eleven percent of patients with lung cancer were found to have small-bowel metastases at autopsy.[62]

Metastases from primary breast carcinomas are more common in the stomach than in the small bowel.

Renal cell carcinoma is the commonest tumor to spread by direct invasion (Figure 20–16). The descending duodenum (on the right) and the jejunum (on the left) are the most frequently involved sites.

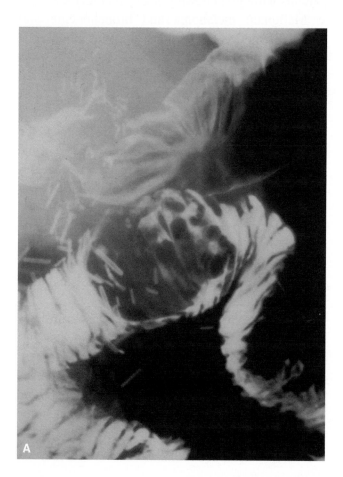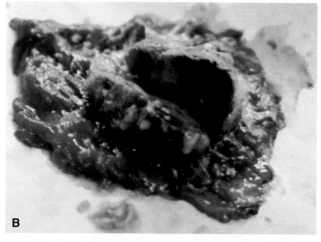

Figure 20–15.   *A,* Small-bowel series reveals a large single polypoid lesion in the small bowel. *B,* The cut surgical specimen shows pigmentation typical of melanotic melanoma.

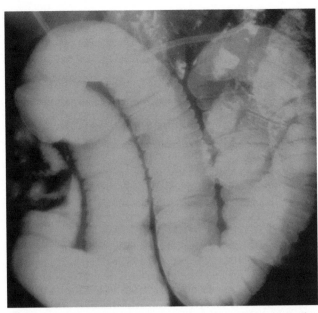

Figure 20–16. An image from an enteroclysis study demonstrating obstructing small-bowel lesion in a patient with a history of renal cell carcinoma. The location and position of the lesion suggest blood-borne spread rather than direct invasion.

Cross-sectional imaging is useful for demonstrating the full extent of metastatic disease and may help identify the primary tumor. Small serosal and peritoneal metastases may not be visualized on CT; however, mesenteric adenopathy and visceral metastases are well demonstrated.

SUMMARY

Early diagnosis of small-bowel malignancies is necessary to allow curative surgery. Maintaining a degree of clinical suspicion disproportionate to the rarity of the tumor may accelerate diagnosis and improve outcome. Enteroclysis is the most accurate diagnostic test available for small-bowel tumors, and its use should be encouraged. CT enteroclysis and MR enteroclysis are promising developments, but their respective roles in the setting of small-bowel tumors have not been thoroughly evaluated.

REFERENCES

1. Barclay THC, Shapira DV. Malignant tumors of the small intestine. Cancer 1983;51:878–81.
2. Gore RM. Small bowel cancer. Clinical and pathological features. Radiol Clin North Am 1997;35:351–60.
3. Maglinte DT, Reyes BL. Small bowel cancer; radiologic diagnosis. Radiol Clin North Am 1997;35:361–80.
4. North JH, Pack MS. Malignant tumors of the small intestine: a review of 144 cases. Am Surg 2000;66:46–51.
5. Ojha A, Zacherl J, Scheuba C, et al. Primary small bowel malignancies: single-center results of three decades. J Clin Gastroenterol 2000;30:289–93.
6. Maglinte DD, O'Connor K, Bessette J, et al. The role of the physician in the late diagnosis of primary malignant tumors of the small intestine. Am J Gastroenterol 1991; 86:304–8.
7. Linos DA, Dozois RR, Dahlin DC, Bartholomew LG. Does Peutz-Jeghers syndrome predispose to gastrointestinal malignancy? A later look. Arch Surg 1981;116:1182–4.
8. MacEneaney PM, Malone DE. The meaning of diagnostic test results: a spreadsheet for swift data analysis. Clin Radiol 2000;55:227–35.
9. Nolan DJ. Imaging of the small intestine. Schweiz Med Wochenschr 1998;128:109–14.
10. Maglinte DD, Siegelman ES, Kelvin FM. MR enteroclysis: the future of small-bowel imaging? [editorial]. Radiology 2000;215:639–41.
11. Umschaden HW, Szolar D, Gasser J, et al. Small-bowel disease: comparison of MR enteroclysis images with conventional enteroclysis and surgical findings. Radiology 2000;215:717–25.
12. Rieber A, Wruk D, Nussle K, et al. [Current imaging in Crohn's disease: value of MRI compared with conventional proceedings]. Rontgenpraxis 2000;52:378–83.
13. Orjollet-Lecoanet C, Menard Y, Martins A, et al. [CT enteroclysis for detection of small bowel tumors]. J Radiol 2000;81:618–27.
14. Marcos HB, Semelka RC. Evaluation of Crohn's disease using half-fourier RARE and gadolinium-enhanced SGE sequences: initial results. Magn Reson Imaging 2000; 18:263–8.
15. Lomas DJ, Graves MJ. Small bowel MRI using water as a contrast medium. Br J Radiol 1999;72:994–7.
16. Gollub MJ, DeCorato D, Schwartz LH. MR enteroclysis: evaluation of small-bowel obstruction in a patient with pseudomyxoma peritonei. AJR Am J Roentgenol 2000; 174:688–90.
17. Vuori JV, Vuorio MK. Radiological findings in primary malignant tumours of the small intestine. Ann Clin Res 1971;3:16–21.
18. Zollinger RM Jr. Primary neoplasms of the small intestine. Am J Surg 1986;151:654–8.
19. Ekberg O, Ekholm S. Radiology in primary small bowel adenocarcinoma. Gastrointest Radiol 1980;5:49–53.
20. Maglinte DDT, Kelvin FM, O'Connor K, et al. Current status of small bowel radiography. Abdom Imaging 1996; 21:247–57.
21. Bessette JR, Maglinte DD, Kelvin FM, Chernish SM. Primary malignant tumors in the small bowel: a comparison of the small-bowel enema and conventional follow-through examination. AJR Am J Roentgenol 1989;153:741–4.
22. Barloon TJ, Lu CC, Honda H, Berbaum KS. Does a normal small-bowel enteroclysis exclude small-bowel disease? A long-term follow-up of consecutive normal studies. Abdom Imaging 1994;19:113–5.
23. Fukuya T, Hawes DR, Lu CC, et al. CT diagnosis of small-bowel obstruction: efficacy in 60 patients. AJR Am J Roentgenol 1992;158:765–9.

24. Taourel PG, Fabre JM, Pradel JA, et al. Value of CT in the diagnosis and management of patients with suspected acute small-bowel obstruction. AJR Am J Roentgenol 1995;165:1187–92.

25. Megibow AJ, Balthazar EJ, Cho KC, et al. Bowel obstruction: evaluation with CT. Radiology 1991;180:313–8.

26. Buckley JA, Jones B, Fishman EK. Small bowel cancer. Imaging features and staging. Radiol Clin North Am 1997;35:381–402.

27. James S, Balfe DM, Lee JK, Picus D. Small-bowel disease: categorization by CT examination. AJR Am J Roentgenol 1987;148:863–8.

28. Laurent F, Raynaud M, Biset JM, et al. Diagnosis and categorization of small bowel neoplasms: role of computed tomography. Gastrointest Radiol 1991;16:115–9.

29. Buckley JA, Siegelman SS, Jones B, Fishman EK. The accuracy of CT staging of small bowel adenocarcinoma: CT/pathologic correlation. J Comput Assist Tomogr 1997;21:986–91.

30. Bender GN, Timmons JH, Williard WC, Carter J. Computed tomographic enteroclysis: one methodology. Invest Radiol 1996;31:43–9.

31. Kloppel R, Thiele J, Bosse J. [The Sellink CT method]. Rofo Fortschr Geb Rontgenstr Neuen Bildgeb Verfahr 1992;156:291–2.

32. Raptopoulos V, Schwartz RK, McNicholas MM, et al. Multiplanar helical CT enterography in patients with Crohn's disease. AJR Am J Roentgenol 1997;169:1545–50.

33. Hahn PF. Biliary system, pancreas, spleen and alimentary tract. 3rd ed. St Louis: Mosby; 1999.

34. Semelka RC, John G, Kelekis NL, et al. Small bowel neoplastic disease: demonstration by MRI. J Magn Reson Imaging 1996;6:855–60.

35. Siegelman ES, Ros PR. Magnetic resonance imaging for small bowel related diagnosis. In: Clinical imaging of the small intestine. New York: Springer-Verlag; 1999.

36. Adamek HE, Breer H, Karschkes T, et al. Magnetic resonance imaging in gastroenterology: time to say good-bye to all that endoscopy? Endoscopy 2000;32:406–10.

37. Maglinte DDT, Kelvin KM, Herlinger H. Malignant tumors of the small bowel. In: Textbook of gastrointestinal radiology. 2nd ed. WB Saunders Co.; 2000.

38. Wallace S, Ajani JA, Charnsangavej C, et al. Carcinoid tumors: imaging procedures and interventional radiology. World J Surg 1996;20:147–56.

39. Critchley M. Octreotide scanning for carcinoid tumours. Postgrad Med J 1997;73:399–402.

40. Maglinte DDT, Helinger H. Small bowel neoplasms. In: Clinical imaging of the small intestine. 2nd ed. New York: Springer-Verlag; 1999.

41. Shiu MH, Farr GH, Egeli RA, et al. Myosarcomas of the small and large intestine: a clinicopathologic study. J Surg Oncol 1983;24:67–72.

42. Ranchod M, Kempson RL. Smooth muscle tumors of the gastrointestinal tract and retroperitoneum: a pathologic analysis of 100 cases. Cancer 1977;39:255–62.

43. Salari GR, Peny MO, Van de Stadt J, et al. Late liver metastases of small bowel leiomyoma. The difficulty in assessing malignancy in gastro-intestinal smooth muscle tumours. Acta Chir Belg 1998;98:107–9.

44. Vincenzoni C, Mariani L, Iacovelli A, et al. Leiomyosarcomas of the small intestine misdiagnosed as ovarian masses: report of three cases. Eur J Gynaecol Oncol 1998;19:271–4.

45. Megibow AJ, Balthazar EJ, Hulnick DH, et al. CT evaluation of gastrointestinal leiomyomas and leiomyosarcomas. AJR Am J Roentgenol 1985;144:727–31.

46. Berg JW. Primary lymphomas of the human gastrointestinal tract. Natl Cancer Inst Monogr 1969;32:211–20.

47. Rubesin SE, Gilchrist AM, Bronner M, et al. Non-Hodgkin lymphoma of the small intestine. Radiographics 1990; 10:985–98.

48. Kojima M, Nakamura S, Kurabayashi Y, et al. Primary malignant lymphoma of the intestine: clinicopathologic and immunohistochemical studies of 39 cases. Pathol Int 1995;45:123–30.

49. Back H, Gustavsson B, Ridell B, et al. Primary gastrointestinal lymphoma incidence, clinical presentation, and surgical approach. J Surg Oncol 1986;33:234–8.

50. Jaser N. Primary gastrointestinal non-Hodgkin's lymphomas. Clinical presentation and results of treatment. Ann Chir Gynaecol 1993;82:7–16.

51. Breslin NP, Urbanski SJ, Shaffer EA. Mucosa-associated lymphoid tissue (MALT) lymphoma manifesting as multiple lymphomatosis polyposis of the gastrointestinal tract. Am J Gastroenterol 1999;94:2540–5.

52. Balthazar EJ, Noordhoorn M, Megibow AJ, Gordon RB. CT of small-bowel lymphoma in immunocompetent patients and patients with AIDS: comparison of findings. AJR Am J Roentgenol 1997;168:675–80.

53. Gourtsoyiannis NC, Nolan DJ. Lymphoma of the small intestine: radiological appearances. Clin Radiol 1988;39: 639–45.

54. Mueller PR, Ferrucci JT Jr, Harbin WP, et al. Appearance of lymphomatous involvement of the mesentery by ultrasonography and body computed tomography: the 'sandwich sign.' Radiology 1980;134:467–73.

55. Ishikawa T, Kobayashi Y, Omoto A, et al. Calcification in untreated non-Hodgkin's lymphoma of the jejunum. Acta Haematol 1999;102:185–9.

56. Helinger H, Metz DC. Malabsorption states. In: Clinical imaging of the small intestine. 2nd ed. New York: Springer-Verlag; 1999.

57. Daskalogiannaki M, Voloudaki A, Prassopoulos P, et al. CT evaluation of mesenteric panniculitis: prevalence and associated diseases. AJR Am J Roentgenol 2000;174:427–31.

58. Meyers MA. Intraperitoneal spread of malignancies. In: Dynamic radiology of the abdomen. 4th ed. New York: Springer-Verlag; 1994.

59. Caroline DF, Herlinger H, Laufer I, et al. Small-bowel enema in the diagnosis of adhesive obstructions. AJR Am J Roentgenol 1984;142:1133–9.

60. Meyers MA. The small bowel: normal and pathological anatomy. In: Dynamic radiology of the abdomen. 4th ed. New York: Springer-Verlag; 1994.

61. Meyers MA. Clinical involvement of mesenteric and antimesenteric borders of small bowel loops. II. Radiologic interpretation of pathologic alterations. Gastrointest Radiol 1976;1:49–58.

62. McNeill PM, Wagman LD, Neifeld JP. Small bowel metastases from primary carcinoma of the lung. Cancer 1987;59:1486–9.

21

Management of Benign and Malignant Small-Bowel Neoplasms

FABRIZIO MICHELASSI, MD

DANNY M. TAKANISHI JR, MD

Neoplasms of the small bowel are rare entities. This feature alone has provided the greatest obstacle to the study of the natural history of these lesions. To further compound this issue, small-bowel tumors represent a group of histologically distinct *heterogeneous* neoplasms. Much of what is currently understood about their biology and behavior is derived from population-based tumor registries. Approximately one-third of these tumors are benign, and the remaining two-thirds are malignant. The malignant tumors comprise about 2 percent of all gastrointestinal cancers, and they account for approximately 5,300 new cases of small-bowel cancers per year in the United States.[1,2] This statistic has slowly but gradually increased over the past two decades, primarily due to a slow rise in the incidence of lymphomas. The estimated total new cancer cases (in all sites) in the United States for the year 2001 is 1,268,000.[1] Therefore, small-bowel malignancies contribute less than 0.4 percent of all cancers. This has been attributed to a number of factors: a relatively rapid transit time, decreasing the contact between epithelium and carcinogenic agents; high amounts of secretory immunoglobulin A (IgA), which may contribute to the local immune response; a low population of anaerobic bacteria, resulting in less conversion and production of carcinogenic agents from precursor procarcinogens; and the presence of enzyme systems that detoxify carcinogens.[3,4] Epidemiologic studies have identified certain conditions that have a significant association with small-bowel malignancies. The blind loop syndrome, familial polyposis syndromes, Gardner's syndrome, Crohn's disease, celiac sprue, neurofibromatosis, and IgA deficiency have all been reported to be risk factors in this regard.[3-8]

This chapter provides a general overview of the characteristics of these cancers, including clinical presentation, and reviews the current strategies to the diagnostic evaluation and management of these tumors. Although even less common, a concomitant review of the basic principles of management of benign neoplasms is also warranted in this context, not only because the majority of benign neoplasms have malignant potential but also because the natural history of benign lesions may be characterized by pain, bleeding, perforation, and obstruction, symptoms and signs indistinguishable from those of their malignant counterparts.[3] Lastly, this chapter also touches upon metastatic tumors to the small bowel.

CLINICAL PRESENTATION

Similar to other benign and malignant neoplasms of the gastrointestinal tract, small-bowel tumors do not elicit specific pathognomonic symptoms or signs. Symptoms, when they do occur, tend to be vague and nonspecific. In general, most symptoms can be attributed to the location of the tumor, its rate of growth, and its size.[3,4,9-11] For example, tumors in the duodenum tend to be asymptomatic whereas those in the jejunum or ileum may present with obstructive symptoms, as discussed below. The vast majority of patients with benign neoplasms are asymptomatic whereas the vast majority of those with malignancies are symptomatic prior to diagnosis. Malignant tumors have a male predominance, and most appear during the fifth to sixth decades of life. Delay in the establishment of a diagnosis is common; this often reflects an unfamiliarity on the part of physicians as a high index of suspicion is necessary, given the rarity of these lesions and their nonspecific symptomatology. Many of these tumors are discovered unexpectedly at laparotomy.[12]

The most common presentation of benign tumors is pain associated with obstruction, followed by chronic bleeding with iron deficiency anemia in up to 50 percent of patients. Malignant lesions are generally associated with pain and weight loss, particularly because patients tend to present late, with advanced disease. Obstruction in this setting tends to be progressive, compared to benign lesions, whose obstructive symptoms tend to be intermittent as they relate to episodes of intussusception. Bleeding and perforation (in up to 10%) may also occur, predominantly in lymphomatous lesions, but this can also be a feature of any malignant tumor because of ulceration or necrosis. A palpable mass may be noted in about one-fifth of these patients, but in general, a mass lesion or perforation is not characteristic of benign tumors.

PATHOLOGY

Approximately one-third of primary small-bowel neoplasms are benign, and two-thirds are malignant. The most common benign tumors, in descending order, are leiomyomas, adenomas, lipomas, and hemangiomas.[3,4,9–11] These tumors can occur throughout the small bowel but tend to increase in frequency from proximal to distal, with the exception of adenomas, which have been reported with highest frequency in the duodenum. A similar pattern is seen with malignant tumors, which overall tend to increase in frequency from proximal to distal, again with one exception: adenocarcinomas are reported as being in highest frequency in the duodenum. The most common primary malignant neoplasms (based on the National Cancer Institute Surveillance, Epidemiology, and End Results program) are adenocarcinomas (45.3%), carcinoids (29.3%), lymphomas (14.8%), and sarcomas (10.4%).[13] Pathologic staging

is performed according to the American Joint Committee on Cancer (AJCC) tumor-node-metastasis (TNM) system (Table 21–1). Metastatic malignancies are discussed later in this chapter.

DIAGNOSTIC EVALUATION: GENERAL PRINCIPLES

A high index of suspicion is required due to nonspecific symptoms and signs. A correct preoperative diagnosis is made in up to only 50 percent of patients. Biochemical and hematologic studies are often not helpful. Iron deficiency anemia may be detected with chronic blood loss; elevated hepatobiliary-tract enzymes may be noted with periampullary lesions or hepatic metastases. The exception is the detection of elevated 24-hour urinary 5-hydroxyindoleacetic acid in more than 50 percent of patients with carcinoid tumors, even when asymptomatic.

Radiographic-contrast imaging modalities tend to be the most useful in the establishment of the diagnosis. Plain films of the abdomen are generally not helpful and at best may demonstrate nonspecific signs of obstruction or a mass effect with displacement of bowel gas (with large tumors). Contrast stud-

Table 21–1. PATHOLOGIC STAGING OF SMALL-BOWEL MALIGNANCIES*

Primary tumor (T)
- T1 Invades lamina propria or submucosa
- T2 Invades muscularis propria
- T3 Invades into subserosa or into nonperitonealized perimuscular tissue (mesentery or retroperitoneum), with extension ≤ 2 cm
- T4 Perforates visceral peritoneum *or* directly invades other organs or structures (includes other loops of small intestine, mesentery, *or* retroperitoneum > 2 cm, *and* the abdominal wall by way of the serosa; for the duodenum *only*, includes invasion of the pancreas)

Regional lymph nodes (N)
- N0 No regional node involvement
- N1 Regional node metastasis

Distant metastasis (M)
- M0 No distant metastasis
- M1 Distant metastasis

TNM stages
- I   T1–2 N0 M0
- II   T3–4 N0 M0
- III Any T N1 M0
- IV   Any T Any N M1

*According to the American Joint Committee on Cancer (AJCC) tumor-lymph node-metastasis (TNM) system.

ies such as a small-bowel follow-through can detect approximately 50 percent of small bowel-tumors; if enteroclysis is performed, the sensitivity can be increased up to 90 percent.[3,4] Abdominal computed tomography (CT) has a sensitivity of 50 to 80 percent and generally does not add to other contrast studies in terms of detecting primary lesions, with the exception of extraluminal tumors such as leiomyomas and sarcomas. Yet, CT is valuable in providing additional and important staging information related to local extent of the tumor and the presence or absence of lymph node or hepatic metastases. Demonstration of mesenteric metastases may be helpful with carcinoids that may have small primary tumors that are not often detectable with conventional imaging modalities. Angiography, although helpful in diagnosing and localizing neoplasms of vascular origin, is rarely helpful in establishing or refining a diagnosis of small-bowel malignancy. This study is often not beneficial in localizing bleeding tumors since the vast majority bleed at a rate considerably below the limit of detection for this technique.

Enteroscopy has become a welcome addition to the currently available endoscopic armamentarium. Enteroscopy has allowed nonsurgical access to the small bowel and can usually be performed on an outpatient basis. Two types of small-bowel enteroscopy are available. The first, called push enteroscopy, initially made use of a pediatric or adult colonoscope that was advanced orally.[14] Specialized scopes that can be used to visualize distal jejunum 100 cm or farther from the ligament of Treitz are now available. The bowel is evaluated as the endoscope is both advanced and withdrawn, and biopsy or cauterization can be done concomitantly through an accessory channel. The second type of enteroscopy, called sonde enteroscopy, is a less used method.[15] The procedure involves a thin endoscope with a balloon tip that is inserted transnasally. Peristalsis moves the scope distally. Evaluation of the bowel occurs as the scope is withdrawn. This scope does not allow for biopsy or therapeutic intervention, the entire bowel lumen is often not visualized, and the duration of the procedure is on the order of 6 hours. This modality is useful in the diagnostic work-up of those individuals who have had nondiagnostic contrast studies and upper and lower endoscopies (Figure 21–1).[16]

Limited information is available regarding the efficacy of diagnostic laparoscopy in the diagnosis and work-up of small-bowel neoplasms. At present, its usefulness may reside (1) in obtaining staging information and determining resectability prior to formal laparotomy in the case of adenocarcinomas, particularly of the duodenum, and (2) in obtaining tissue diagnoses in equivocal instances when other imaging studies have failed to suggest an etiology.

It is clear, however, that despite the currently available technology, the diagnosis of these tumors is difficult to establish preoperatively in a significant group of individuals. Laparotomy is often required for definitive diagnosis.

MANAGEMENT OF BENIGN TUMORS

Leiomyoma

Leiomyomas are the most common tumor of the small bowel. These neoplasms arise from smooth muscle and can occur both intra- and extraluminally. They can often grow to become very large before causing symptoms. On gross inspection, it is sometimes difficult to distinguish these lesions from their malignant counterparts. This distinction is made histologically with standard criteria including nuclear pleomorphism, increased mitosis, and the presence of necrosis. The treatment is strictly surgical and requires segmental resection with negative surgical margins (Figure 21–2).[3] At times, it may be difficult to unequivocally distinguish between the benign and malignant tumor, despite careful pathologic evaluation; thus, *all* smooth-muscle tumors of the small bowel require resection with negative surgical margins.

Adenoma

Adenomas are the next most common benign tumor of the small intestine. The duodenum is the most common site of involvement, and the lesion most commonly noted is the villous adenoma. These lesions tend to involve the region of the ampulla of Vater. They present with stigmas of obstructive jaundice and are all easily amenable to diagnosis by endoscopy and biopsy. Of concern is the risk of

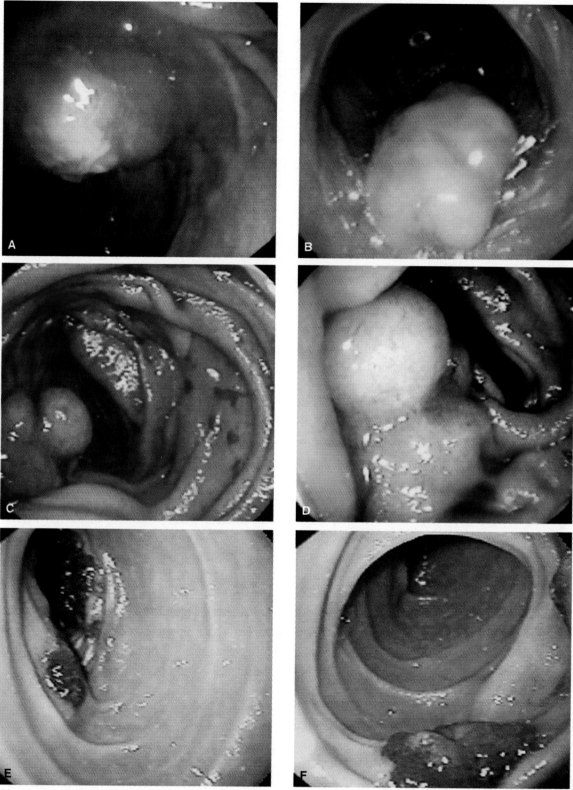

Figure 21–1.   The use of enteroscopy techniques to establish the diagnosis of small-bowel neoplasms. *A*, Benign mucous cyst adjacent to the ampulla of Vater. *B*, Jejunal lipoma. Note the well-circumscribed, glistening, yellow, and fatty-appearing tumor resembling its benign counterparts in other organs. *C* and *D*, Two views of a polypoid lesion that biopsy proved to be adenocarcinoma of the jejunum, which was subsequently resected en bloc. *E* and *F*, Kaposi's sarcoma of the small bowel (jejunum) in an individual with acquired immune deficiency syndrome who presented with occult intermittent gastrointestinal hemorrhage. Upper and lower endoscopic evaluation (with esophagogastroduodenoscopy and colonoscopy), tagged red cell scans, and angiography did not reveal the source of bleeding.

malignant degeneration in a significant proportion (up to 30%) of these tumors. This feature poses challenges to treatment planning. Simple local excision (endoscopically or via transduodenal excision) (Figure 21–3) with negative surgical margins is feasible; a wide range of local recurrence rates is reported.[3] Thus, inherent in this approach is the mandate for close endoscopic surveillance. If complete histologic evaluation of the specimen demonstrates adenocarcinoma or if there is any suspicion of carcinoma, all lesions in the first or second portion of the duodenum are best treated by a pancreaticoduodenectomy (Whipple procedure) (Figure 21–4). For tumors that are more distal, in the third or fourth portion of the duodenum, or in the distal small bowel, treatment is wedge or segmental resection with histologic control of margins. Chemoprevention with sulindac or newer cyclooxygenase-2 (COX-2) inhibitors may be necessary in patients with familial polyposis syndromes (ie, Gardner's syndrome).

Other Benign Tumors

There are other benign tumors, of extremely low incidence, that involve the small bowel. The more common entities include inflammatory polyps, hemangiomas, lipomas, hamartomas (Peutz-Jeghers syndrome), and fibromas.[3] Patients require intervention generally secondary to bleeding or obstructive symptoms due to intermittent intussusception. The approach is either polypectomy or simple excision of the culprit lesion, or segmental resection of the small bowel (for larger tumors). The guiding principle is the same in all instances: preservation of as much normal intestine as possible, given the benign nature of these neoplasms.

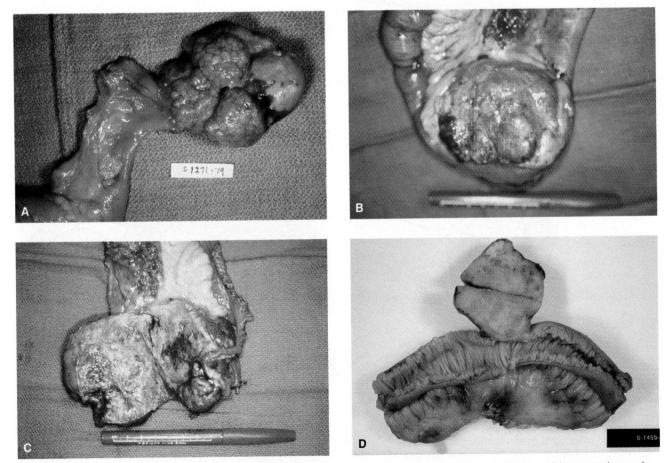

Figure 21–2. Small-bowel leiomyoma, demonstrating an exophytic extraluminal growth pattern. As a result, many of these neoplasms characteristically grow to large size before rendering patients symptomatic from obstructive symptoms. *A,* Tumor present on the antimesenteric border of the small bowel. *B* and *C,* Another example of a leiomyoma, present on the mesenteric border of the small intestine in this instance, as de novo lesion (*B*) and cut section (*C*). *D,* A formalinized cut specimen, demonstrating the absence of mechanical obstruction.

MANAGEMENT OF MALIGNANT TUMORS

Adenocarcinoma

Adenocarcinoma is the most common primary malignant neoplasm of the small bowel and the most common proximal small-bowel neoplasm.[3,4,9–11,17–21] It comprises approximately 45 percent of all small-bowel malignancies. These tumors are most commonly found in the duodenum, followed by the jejunum and ileum. In the duodenum, the vast majority occur in the second portion of the duodenum. Pain related to partial obstruction is the most common symptom, followed by anemia (due to chronic bleeding) and jaundice. Further distally, in the jejunum and ileum, pain and weight loss from progressive intestinal obstruction occur in nearly all patients. Upper-gastrointestinal endoscopy with biopsy establishes the diagnosis for proximal tumors. In the jejunum and ileum, the diagnosis may be made presumptively, by small-bowel follow-through (circumferential lesion with mucosal ulceration is the pattern most commonly seen) or by CT; however, many patients may require laparotomy for diagnosis. The recent availability of enteroscopy may alter these statistics.[14–16] Surgical extirpation is the therapeutic modality of choice. Tumors in the first and second portions of the duodenum are treated by pancreatico-duodenectomy whereas those in the third and fourth portions are treated by segmental resection, including regional lymphadenectomy.[3,4,17–20] In the jejunum and ileum, wide excision (including areas of con-

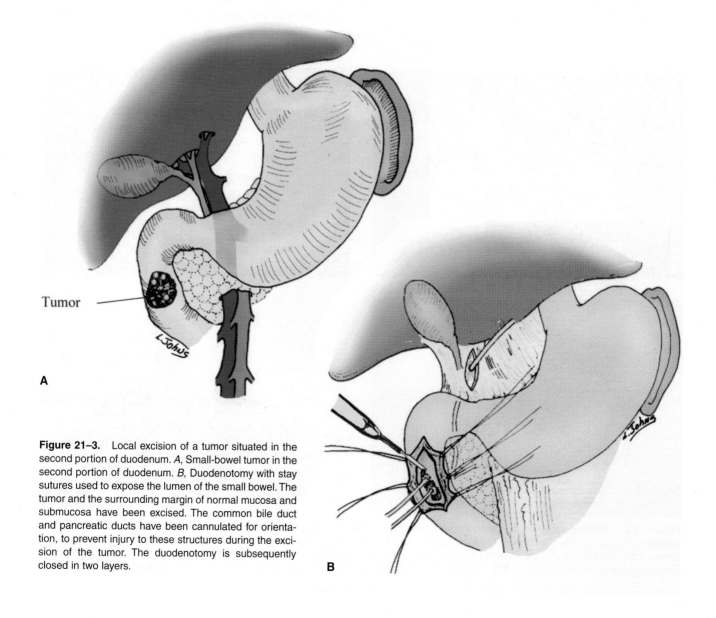

Tumor

A

Figure 21–3. Local excision of a tumor situated in the second portion of duodenum. *A*, Small-bowel tumor in the second portion of duodenum. *B*, Duodenotomy with stay sutures used to expose the lumen of the small bowel. The tumor and the surrounding margin of normal mucosa and submucosa have been excised. The common bile duct and pancreatic ducts have been cannulated for orientation, to prevent injury to these structures during the excision of the tumor. The duodenotomy is subsequently closed in two layers.

B

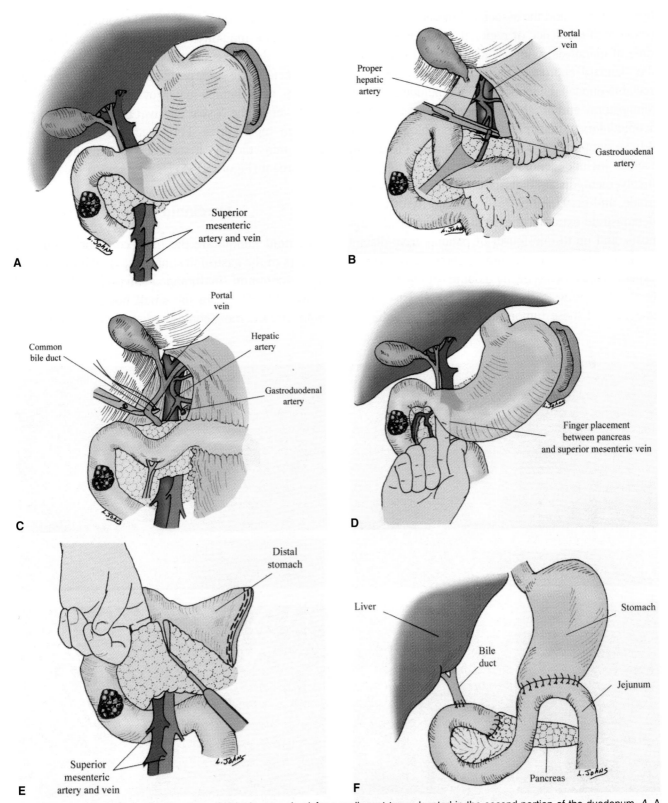

Figure 21–4. Pancreaticoduodenectomy (Whipple procedure) for a malignant tumor located in the second portion of the duodenum. *A*, A malignant neoplasm in the second portion of the duodenum. *B*, Once distant disease is ruled out, the porta hepatis is dissected out and exposed, then the gastroduodenal artery is divided. *C*, The common bile duct is divided proximal to the pancreatic head. *D*, Gentle blunt dissection is performed to separate the head and neck of the pancreas from the mesenteric vessels; distal gastrectomy and cholecystectomy are performed. *E*, The pancreas is divided anterior to mesenteric vessels, and the vascular tributaries to the pancreatic head are ligated and divided. The proximal jejunum is then divided to complete the pancreaticoduodenectomy. *F*, The restoration of gastrointestinal continuity is completed with pancreaticojejunostomy, choledochojejunostomy, and gastrojejunostomy.

tiguous spread and the associated mesentery, in view of the high incidence of regional involvement at the time of diagnosis) with negative surgical margins is the standard approach. Palliative options for unresectable duodenal adenocarcinoma include a gastrojejunostomy and/or a biliary enteric bypass or endoscopic/interventional placement of radiologic stent to relieve symptoms of obstructive jaundice. Prognostic factors include depth of penetration, lymph node involvement, distant metastases, perineural invasion, grade, and resectability.[10,17–19] A majority of tumors demonstrate extramural extension of tumor at diagnosis, and up to one-fourth of patients have distant organ disease. Although most centers have limited experience, there has been no demonstrable response to chemotherapy (5-fluorouracil [5-FU]–based protocols), and these tumors also tend to be radiation

dose limited due to small-bowel toxicity, limiting the use of this modality for therapy. For palliation of chronic blood loss in patients with locally advanced unresectable disease, particularly involving the duodenum, radiotherapy may provide a short-term benefit. Overall, the 5-year survival rate is 20 to 30 percent in most series. For resectable disease of the duodenum, the 5-year survival rate approaches 50 to 60 percent (Figure 21–5).[10,11,17–21]

Carcinoid Tumors

Carcinoid tumors are the most common endocrine tumors of the gastrointestinal system and the second most common malignancy involving the small bowel.[3,4,9,11,13,22,23] In the small bowel itself, carcinoids are the most common distal small-bowel neo-

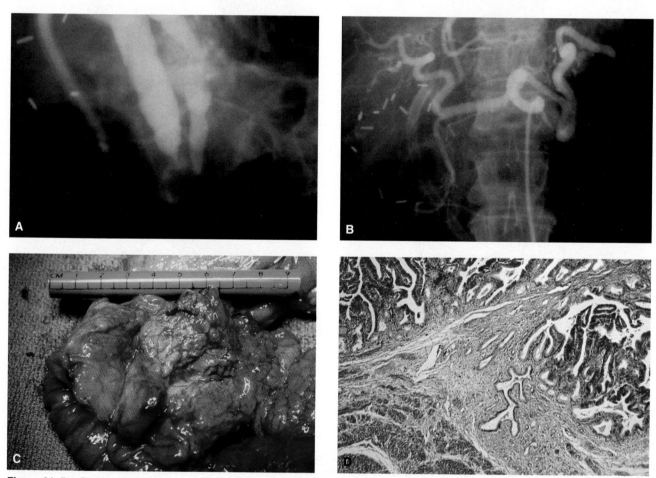

Figure 21–5. Duodenal adenocarcinoma in a patient who presented with painless jaundice. *A*, Endoscopic retrograde cholangiopancreatography, demonstrating dilated proximal and distal biliary tree. Biopsy is indicated if the periampullary tumor is consistent with adenocarcinoma. *B*, Angiography demonstrates no evidence of vascular involvement. *C*, Pancreaticoduodenectomy (Whipple procedure) is performed; the gross specimen reveals the cancer upon the opening of the duodenum. *D*, Light microscopy findings of glandular patterns and invasion of surrounding tissue by adenocarcinoma (hematoxylin and eosin; ×100 original magnification).

plasm (Figure 21–6). These neoplasms arise from enterochromaffin cells and are characterized by the ability to secrete many biologically active substances (Table 21–2). They tend to be small (< 2 cm) and submucosal in location, with a propensity for multicentricity. The most common classification scheme for these tumors is based on embryologic derivation: foregut (stomach and pancreas), midgut (small bowel), and hindgut (colon and rectum). The presentation depends largely on the hormones elaborated and on the site of origin.[22,23] Many patients with carcinoids present late in their course, and lymph node and hepatic metastases are not uncommon at the time of diagnosis. Midgut lesions produce symptoms of hormone excess (carcinoid syndrome) when either bulky disease or hepatic metastases are present. Foregut and hindgut tumors tend to be asymptomatic although hindgut tumors rarely produce serotonin. The most common presentation of hindgut tumors is bleeding. The majority demonstrate an indolent growth pattern and consequently tend to be asymptomatic until later stages. Mesenteric fibrosis can result from a desmoplastic response that is associated with these tumors, resulting in progressive intestinal ischemia or obstruction.

Carcinoid tumors are probably best known for their ability to cause carcinoid syndrome.[3,22,23] The syndrome itself is uncommon, occurring in only approximately 10 percent of patients. Manifestations occur when hepatic metabolism is bypassed. Examples include hepatic metastases, tumors outside of the gastrointestinal tract (bronchogenic, ovarian, or testicular), and extensive retroperitoneal disease. The majority of tumors (90% or more) are midgut primaries. Presenting symptoms vary and may consist of vasomotor instability and flushing (which can be precipitated by red wine, blue cheese, alcohol, chocolate, or exercise), watery diarrhea, sweating, wheezing (bronchospasm) and dyspnea, abdominal pain, and hypotension and right heart failure (generally due to endocardial fibrosis with tricuspid regurgitation or pulmonic stenosis that occurs in 50% of patients with carcinoid syndrome). It is commonly held that many amine mediators may be responsible for these manifestations, including serotonin, prostaglandins, bradykinin, histamine, substance P, and vasoactive intestinal polypeptide.[3,22,23] Further

along the spectrum of severity, a small subgroup of these patients may present with "carcinoid crisis," which is life threatening and often precipitated by a specific trigger event such as anesthesia, surgery, or chemotherapy. Symptoms are very intense in nature and are often refractory to treatment with intravenous fluids and vasopressors. This feature has important ramifications in the preoperative evaluation and management of these patients. Consideration for octreotide blockade preoperatively is therefore important, particularly for the patient with a large tumor burden (eg, hepatic metastases, extensive metastatic involvement), to prevent the potential life-threatening consequences of carcinoid crisis.

The diagnostic evaluation of these tumors is based on the biochemical confirmation of elaborated hormones and/or their metabolites, combined with localization studies. Measurement of 24-hour urinary excretion of 5-hydroxyindoleacetic acid (5-HIAA), a metabolite of serotonin, is found to be elevated in at least 50 percent of patients, regardless of the presence of symptoms. If this assay is negative and the diagnosis is still suspected, additional diagnostic measurements to consider include urinary 5-hydroxytryptamine (serotonin), urinary and plasma 5-hydroxytryptophan, platelet serotonin, serum chromogranin A, substance P, neuron-specific enolase, and neuropeptide K levels.[22,23] These additional studies are not mandatory before proceeding with treatment because many patients present with symptoms that require operative intervention regardless of the results of biochemical testing, and in many sympto-

Table 21–2. ACTIVE SUBSTANCES SECRETED BY CARCINOID TUMORS

Serotonin (5-hydroxytryptamine)
5-Hydroxytryptophan
5-Hydroxyindoleacetic acid (5-HIAA)
Bradykinin
Histamine
Kallikrein
Dopamine
Substance P
Neuropeptide K
Neurotensin
Prostaglandins
Chromogranin
Human chorionic gonadotropin (HCG)
Vasoactive intestinal polypeptide (VIP)
Pancreatic polypeptide

matic patients, the diagnosis is often suspected on the basis of clinical findings. Localization and imaging studies follow a presumptive biochemical diagnosis. Contrast studies such as small-bowel follow-through and enteroclysis may demonstrate mucosal abnormalities although small lesions (< 1 cm) may be missed. Computed tomography likewise has limited ability to detect small tumors (< 1 cm); however, it is a useful modality for evaluating retroperitoneal and mesenteric involvement and for detecting hepatic metastases. Radionuclide imaging with radiolabeled metaiodobenzylguanidine (MIBG)[24,25] or tyrosine = 3-octreotide (labeled with iodine-123 [^{123}I])[24] is able to detect tumors in up to 50 percent and 70 to 80 percent of cases, respectively. In equivocal cases, mesenteric angiography may demonstrate a tumor "blush," reflecting the high vascularity of these lesions. Localization studies are helpful but are not mandatory prior to operative exploration. These studies may be beneficial in the rare situation in which the primary tumor cannot be found at the time of surgery (a situation more likely with foregut lesions).

The mainstay of therapy is surgical extirpation. The anesthesiologist should be aware of the diagnosis of carcinoid tumor and should be prepared to treat these patients with octreotide either before or during surgery, to prevent carcinoid crisis. Wide en bloc resection is the standard approach, including the draining mesentery.[3,4,22,23] This is based partly on the propensity of these lesions to metastasize even when very small (< 1 cm). The cure rates are high for patients in whom all visible gross disease can be resected. In patients operated on for obstruction or bleeding and subsequently found to have a carcinoid on pathologic review only if there was no other gross disease, it is not mandatory to re-explore and to perform a regional lymphadenectomy. Large lesions near the ampulla may require pancreaticoduodenectomy for resection (however, small lesions may be amenable to local excision with close postoperative endoscopic surveillance for recurrence); likewise, lesions in the terminal ileum may require a right colectomy for oncologic clearance of disease. An important caveat is that up to 40 percent of midgut carcinoids are associated with a second gastrointestinal malignancy, and 30 percent may be multicentric, warranting careful assessment of the entire small bowel and large bowel.[3,22,23] The prognosis for localized disease is excellent after resection and approaches a 100 percent 5-year survival rate. In the vast majority (> 90%) of symptomatic patients, metastatic disease is present at the time of surgical exploration. The likelihood of distant disease correlates closely with both the size of the primary lesion and the depth of invasion. For tumors < 1 cm in size, the risk of lymph node metastases is on the order of 2 percent; for 1- to 2-cm lesions, there is an approximate 50 percent incidence of lymph node metastases; and for tumors > 2 cm, the incidence of lymph node metastases rises to 80 percent. The most common sites of organ involvement are the liver, the lungs, and bone.

Treatment for advanced locoregional and distant disease comprises both medical and surgical modalities. Medical therapy may suffice for mild symptoms as these tumors tend to have an indolent natural history. Diarrhea may be controlled with antispasmodics and antidiarrheal agents such as loperamide, diphenoxylate, or cyproheptadine (a serotonin antagonist). Flushing and vasomotor symptoms are amenable to therapy with clonidine, phenoxybenzamine, or a combination of H_1 and H_2 receptor antagonists. Bronchodilators, such as albuterol and theophylline, are helpful in controlling bronchospastic manifestations. Octreotide may also be useful for symptom control; it provides additional benefits in terms of slowing tumor growth in more than 50 percent of cases, and it has been demonstrated to effect tumor regression for variable periods of time in 10 to 20 percent of patients.[26] Provided that a patient's performance status and physiologic reserve permits all patients should be considered candidates for an attempt at complete extirpation, for this approach has resulted in prolonged disease-free and symptom-free survival. The duration of relief is generally less than 1 year, and there is no documented survival benefit although 5-year survival rates of up to 68 percent have been reported when all gross metastatic disease, including hepatic metastases, is resected. All of these patients should receive octreotide preoperatively to prevent the carcinoid crisis.

For those unfortunate individuals with extensive unresectable disease, the indications for surgical intervention include obstruction, perforation, and severe symptoms intractable to medical therapy. Debulking in this setting has proven to be of some benefit in terms of palliation of symptoms. Chemotherapy is of extremely limited value; response rates are generally < 30 percent, with no complete responses, and are characterized by a duration of response of a few months. The agents that have demonstrated the most activity include 5-FU, streptozocin, and doxorubicin (Adriamycin), in single- and multidrug regimens. Likewise, regional therapy with hepatic artery chemoembolization, cryotherapy or radiofrequency ablation for hepatic metastases and carcinoid syndrome achieves limited and temporary success.[27] Radiation therapy has not proven to be effective for this disease, in either the adjuvant or palliative setting. The 5-year survival for unresectable disease is approximately 35 to 40 percent, reflecting the relatively indolent growth characteristic of these tumors.

Lymphoma

Small-bowel lymphomas parallel the distribution of lymphoid follicles, resulting in the ileum being the most common site of involvement.[3,4,9,11,13,28,29] These tumors may be multifocal in up to 15 percent of patients. The disease may be primary or secondary, a manifestation of generalized involvement by disease originating outside the small bowel. The development of this tumor is associated with immunodeficiency diseases (eg, acquired immunodeficiency syndrome [AIDS], rheumatoid arthritis, and immune disorders in transplant recipients), Crohn's disease, and celiac disease.[3,6–8,10,29] Most lymphomas of the small bowel are diffuse, high-grade, non-Hodgkin's B-cell lymphomas. Bulky disease is characteristic at the time of diagnosis, and up to 70 percent of patients have tumors > 5 cm in size. Typical clinical presentations include malaise and

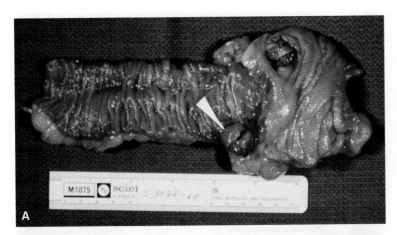
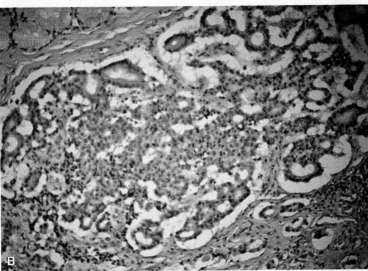

Figure 21–6. Carcinoid of the distal ileum. This was an incidental finding at the time of laparotomy in a patient who presented for elective resection for complications of recurrent colonic diverticular disease. *A*, The opened ileum, demonstrating the tumor. *B*, Light microscopy revealed a low-grade fairly well-circumscribed tumor with neuroendocrine features. Special stains later confirmed the cytoplasmic presence of serotonin (hematoxylin and eosin; ×100 original magnification).

Stage	Criteria
I	Involvement of a single nodal group (I) or single extralymphatic organ or site (IE)
II	Involvement of more than one nodal group on the same side of the diaphragm (II) or involvement of a single extralymphatic site with one or more nodal groups on the same side of the diaphragm (IIE)
III	Involvement of nodes on both sides of the diaphragm (III), with or without involvement of extralymphatic sites (IIIE), spleen (IIIS), or both (IIIES)
IV	Diffuse involvement of viscera or bone marrow

Table 21–3. ANN ARBOR STAGING SYSTEM FOR SMALL-BOWEL LYMPHOMA

fatigue, weight loss, ulceration and bleeding, an obstructing mass (with crampy abdominal pain), and perforation in up to 25 percent of cases. Contrary to other types of lymphomas (particularly Hodgkin's lymphomas), small-bowel lymphomas do not typically present with fever or night sweats. The most commonly used staging system is the Ann Arbor system (Table 21–3). The diagnostic evaluation is aided by radiographic studies. Loss of mucosal definition with thickened folds and mucosal ulcerations on contrast studies, combined with CT findings of large and sometimes bulky mesenteric lymph nodes and a bowel-wall mass or a transmurally thickened small bowel, provides presumptive evidence for a diagnosis of lymphoma. Treatment requires extended en bloc resection of the primary and regional lymph nodes (Figure 21–7).[3,4,10,11,28,29] The traditional approach was to obtain frozen-section control of the margins of resection due to the submucosal spread of the tumor, to prevent recurrence. Para-aortic and mesenteric lymph node sampling, liver biopsy, and bone marrow biopsy are performed for staging. For low-grade localized tumors, resection alone suffices. For intermediate- and high-grade lesions, resection is combined with

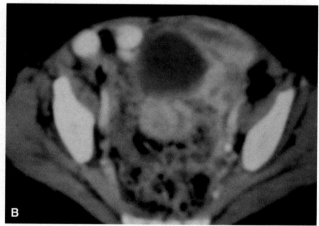

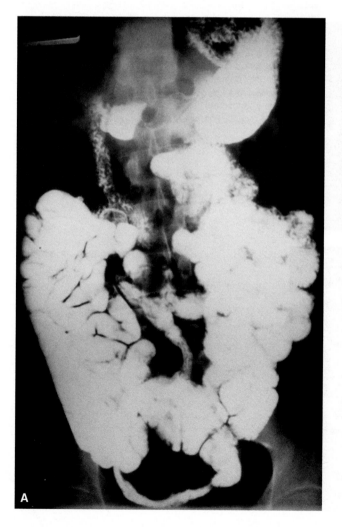

Figure 21–7. Lymphoma of the small bowel. The two patients represented both presented with obstructive symptoms. *A*, A small-bowel follow-through, revealing the loss of mucosal outline and narrowing of the lumen in the ileum of a 66-year-old patient with progressive crampy abdominal pain. *B*, Computed tomography (CT) demonstrates a mass lesion in the pelvis corresponding to the site of partial obstruction, posterior to the bladder.

chemotherapy. This represents the only primary small-bowel malignancy for which adjuvant therapy appears to play a role in treatment. In fact, although surgery was considered the primary treatment modality in the past, it is now more frequently used as a diagnostic modality, with a shift toward chemotherapy being the primary treatment modality. No appreciable survival benefit has been achieved with the addition of radiation. However, the use of radia-

tion as a single modality may be considered in patients with poor performance status who are unable to tolerate surgical exploration or the side effects related to chemotherapy.[28] This modality is not without risks, the most devastating of which are significant necrosis, bleeding, and bowel perforation, all of which have been associated with radiotherapy. Poor prognostic factors that have been identified include higher grade, greater depth of

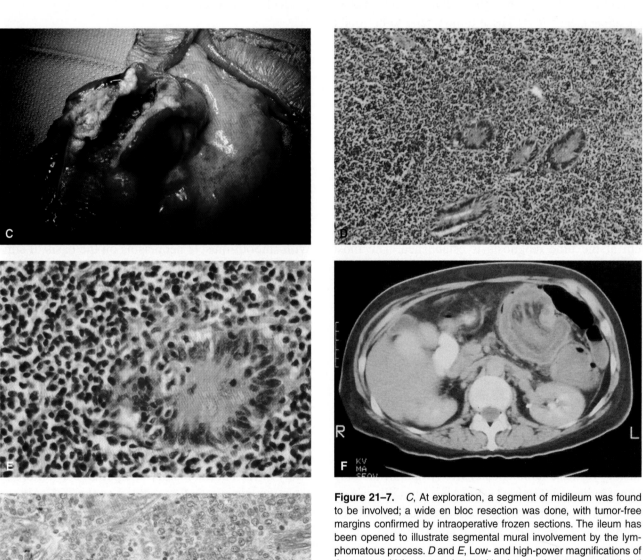

Figure 21–7. *C,* At exploration, a segment of midileum was found to be involved; a wide en bloc resection was done, with tumor-free margins confirmed by intraoperative frozen sections. The ileum has been opened to illustrate segmental mural involvement by the lymphomatous process. *D* and *E,* Low- and high-power magnifications of the tumor, which was consistent with a low-grade mucosa-associated lymphoid tissue (MALT)–type lymphoma (hematoxylin and eosin; ×100 original magnification). *F,* Computed tomography scan of a different but similar patient, demonstrating a mass of small bowel with mural thickening. *G,* This patient (the same as represented in *F*) also underwent resection, and light microscopy reveals a large-cell lymphoma (hematoxylin and eosin; ×100 original magnification).

tumor penetration, lymph node involvement, peritoneal disease, and distant metastases.[10,28,29] Overall 5-year survival rates range from 20 to 40 percent for all stages. Five-year survivals of up to 60 percent have been reported for patients in whom localized low-grade tumors have been curatively resected.[4]

Sarcomas

Sarcomas make up only 10 percent of small-bowel malignancies.[3,4,9,11,13] These tumors tend to be found in the jejunum and ileum, are relatively slow growing, and are locally invasive. Their growth pattern is most commonly extramural; therefore, they rarely result in obstruction. The most common clinical presentation includes pain (65%), a palpable mass (50%), and bleeding that results from necrosis as the tumor outgrows its blood supply. Of significance is that the bleeding may occur either intraluminally or extraluminally, directly into the peritoneal cavity. Due to their insidious nature and growth pattern, greater than three-fourths of these tumors exceed 5 cm at the time diagnosis is established. The most common histologic subtypes (in descending order of frequency) are leiomyosarcomas (approximately 75%), fibrosarcomas, liposarcomas, and malignant schwannomas and angiosarcomas.[3] Computed tomography is often used during a work-up for abdominal pain in the setting of a palpable mass without obstructive symptoms. An extraluminal large heterogeneous mass lesion with central necrosis is generally identifiable in this setting. Treatment consists of en bloc segmental resection with tumor-free margins. Based on the understanding of the natural history of these tumors, extensive lymphadenectomy is not indicated (Figure 21–8).[3,4,30,31] Similarly to sarcomas from other anatomic regions, small-bowel sarcomas rarely metastasize to regional lymph nodes. Hematogenous dissemination tends to be the preferred route of distant spread, primarily to the liver, lungs, and bone. Peritoneal sarcomatosis is also commonly noted in later stages of the disease. Up to 50 percent of these tumors are unresectable for cure at the time of diagnosis. Local resection may be considered for palliative purposes (even with associated distant disease) to ameliorate or prevent symptoms of bleeding or obstruction.[31] There is no clear benefit

from chemotherapy or radiation therapy in the adjuvant setting. Radiation doses are limited due to small-bowel toxicity. In the presence of recurrent or metastatic disease, partial response rates of 10 to 40 percent have been reported, with minimal improvement in survival at best. Prognosis correlates most closely with grade, followed by stage.[30,31] Five-year survival after curative resection ranges from 60 to 80 percent for low-grade lesions and is no more than 20 percent for high-grade lesions.

Gastrointestinal Stromal Tumors

Gastrointestinal stromal tumors (GISTs) are complex and rare entities of mesenchymal origin that account for approximately 0.1 to 3.0 percent of all gastrointestinal tumors. They represent a heterogeneous group of neoplasms, which partly accounts for the confusing debate in the literature over their cell of origin, their pathologic classification and nomenclature, and their clinical behavior and natural history.[32–39] These tumors were previously classified with smooth-muscle neoplasms on the basis of similarities on light microscopy. Immunohistochemical and electron-microscopic studies have demonstrated that these neoplasms also have neural differentiation, which relegates them to another distinct class of tumors. The cell of origin is thought to be an intestinal pacemaker cell, the interstitial cell of Cajal.[32–39] Most published reports are composed of small retrospective series, with some reporting on tumors scattered throughout the gastrointestinal tract and with others evaluating both benign and malignant lesions together. This has confounded the study of the natural history and patterns of failure of these neoplasms and has added to the difficulty of treatment planning. Additionally, many prognostic variables have been reported, with no consistent pattern, and there is no standard universally accepted staging system. A few generalities do exist, however.

Gastrointestinal stromal tumors have been reported to occur throughout the gastrointestinal tract. They tend to occur during the sixth and seventh decades of life, but a few isolated case reports of GISTs in infants exist in the literature.[32,39] Their presentation parallels that of other small-bowel neoplasms in that most result in nonspecific signs, most frequently a palpable mass, pain or discomfort, and bleeding. The diagnosis is frequently not made prior to surgery in more than one-half of cases. The mainstay of therapy is complete surgical resection, and an aggressive approach is advocated even for recurrent or metastatic disease that is amenable to surgical resection. Poor prognostic factors include not only the inability to achieve a complete resection but also tumor size (> 5 cm), tumor grade (high), gender

(male), and extent of disease at presentation (metastatic disease).[32–39] Lymph node metastases are rare; the most common sites of failure are the peritoneal surfaces and the liver. An extended lymphadenectomy is therefore not advocated. These patients are at high risk for recurrence, and close follow-up surveillance is imperative. Late recurrences are not uncommon, necessitating a follow-up of beyond 5 years. There has been no proven benefit

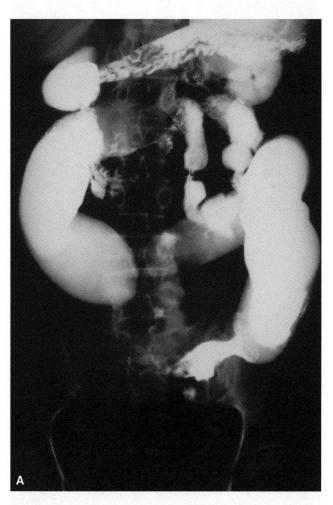

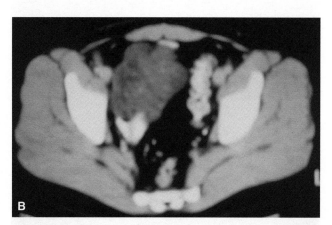

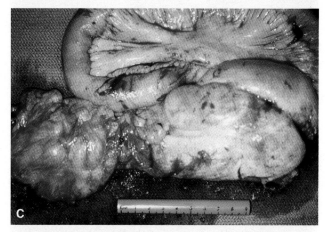

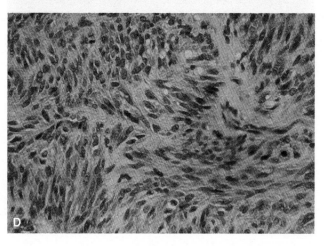

Figure 21–8. A 68-year-old male who was eventually diagnosed with a leiomyosarcoma presented with vague lower abdominal pain, cramping, and bloating. *A,* A small-bowel follow-through reveals a high-grade near-obstructing lesion in the right lower quadrant. *B,* Computed tomography scan demonstrates an irregular, large, and heterogeneous-appearing mass in the right lower quadrant, corresponding to the site of obstruction. *C,* At exploration, a large extraluminal exophytic lobulated tumor was found impinging on the small bowel. It was resected, and a primary anastomosis was done. There was no evidence of regional node involvement, and there was no peritoneal or hepatic disease. *D,* Histologic examination shows a spindle cell tumor of smooth-muscle origin with nuclear pleomorphism and increased scattered mitotic figures, consistent with an intermediate-grade leiomyosarcoma (hematoxylin and eosin; ×100 original magnification).

from radiotherapy or chemotherapy, but promising strategies do exist, based partly on the current understanding of the molecular mechanisms governing the biologic behavior of these tumors.

A mutation of the c-kit proto-oncogene, localized to chromosome 4q, which encodes for a growth factor receptor with tyrosine kinase activity, has been identified in these neoplasms.[32–36] The product of

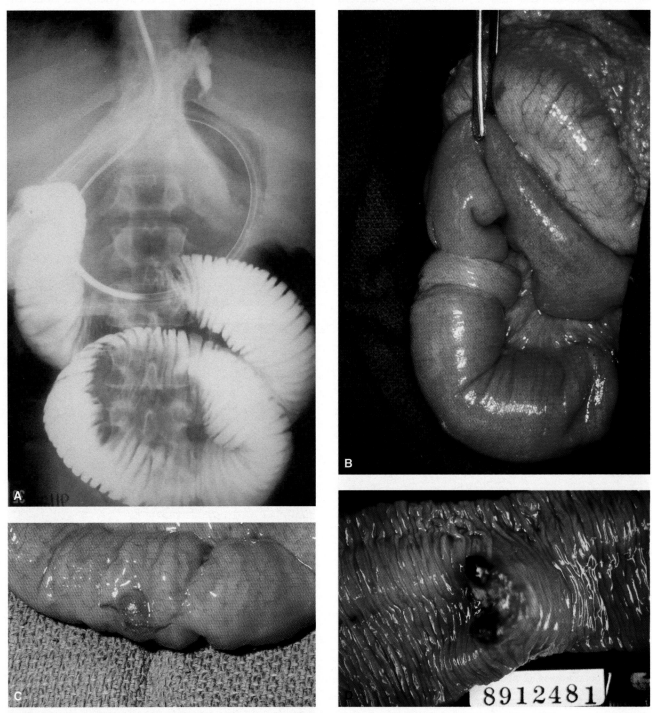

Figure 21–9.   A patient with metastatic melanoma to the small intestine acutely presented with near-complete obstruction as a result of intussusception. *A,* A small-bowel follow-through confirms the clinical suspicion of a high-grade obstruction at the midjejunum. *B,* At exploration, the site of intussusception is shown. *C,* Operative reduction was performed, at which time the lead point for the intussusception was revealed to be a metastatic tumor implant. *D,* A segmental bowel resection including the draining regional node basin was done. The opened segment of small bowel clearly demonstrates the nature of the culprit lesion.

this gene (CD117) can be detected by immunohisto-chemistry, and this is the most specific diagnostic test for this group of tumors. In addition, this feature also provides a specific target for directed therapeutic intervention. A phenylaminopyrimidine derivative inhibitor of the tyrosine kinase activity of this mutated c-kit gene product, STI571 (Novartis, Basel, Switzerland), has demonstrated promise in a recent case report and in early clinical trials. Significant early-response rates have been noted over short-interval follow-up, and reported toxicity thus far has been minimal.[40,41]

Metastatic Malignancy

Metastatic malignancies represent collectively the most common tumors of the small bowel.[3,4] The most common primary cancers are ovarian, colon, lung cancers renal cell carcinoma, and melanoma (which may also involve mesentery and draining regional lymph nodes). Most metastatic malignancies result from hematogenous or lymphatic spread. The vast majority remain confined to the bowel wall and may subsequently result in obstruction or perforation. Treatment consists of segmental resection, generally for palliation; regional lymphadenectomy is not recommended except for melanoma, to effect improved local control.[42] This approach is taken provided that the patient's physiologic reserve is adequate and that the disease is not diffuse and widespread. For both metastatic and locally advanced unresectable disease, palliative approaches may also include enteric bypass, intra-arterial embolization (although there is a risk of bowel ischemia and perforation), and chemoradiotherapy. As would be intuitively expected, however, the outcome in this group of patients is dismal despite therapeutic intervention (Figure 21–9).

SUMMARY

Small-intestinal neoplasms are unusual entities that pose a significant challenge in terms of early diagnosis and management. Symptoms are uniformly vague and nonspecific, which contributes to the delay in diagnosis. Most institutional series are small and heterogeneous, so that much of our pre-sent understanding of the behavior of these tumors has been derived from population-based registries. At the time of diagnosis, only 50 percent of patients at best are amenable to resection for cure. An aggressive surgical approach with resection still remains the modality of choice for the optimum treatment of these neoplasms. For those unfortunate patients whose tumors are deemed unresectable, improvements in the application of chemotherapy and radiotherapy are needed for any impact on their long-term survival. Until this occurs, coupled with earlier diagnoses, the outcome for patients with small-bowel malignancies will remain poor.

REFERENCES

1. Greenlee RT, Murray T, Thun MB, Hill-Harmon MB. Cancer statistics, 2001. CA Cancer J Clin 2001;51:15–36.
2. Landis SH, Murray T, Bolden S, Wingo PA. Cancer statistics, 1999. CA Cancer J Clin 1999;49:8–31.
3. Ashley SW, Wells SA Jr. Tumors of the small intestine. Semin Oncol 1988;15:116–28.
4. Martin RG. Malignant tumors of the small intestine. Surg Clin North Am 1986;66:779–85.
5. Giardiello FM, Welsh SB, Hamilton SR, et al. Increased risk of cancer in the Peutz-Jeghers syndrome. N Engl J Med 1987;316:1511–4.
6. Collier PE, Turowski P, Diamond DL. Small intestinal adenocarcinoma complicating regional enteritis. Cancer 1985;55:516–21.
7. Ribeiro MB, Greenstein AJ, Heimann TM, et al. Adenocarcinoma of the small intestine in Crohn's disease. Surg Gynecol Obstet 1991;173:343–9.
8. Trier JS. Celiac sprue. N Engl J Med 1991;325:1709–19.
9. Weiss NS, Yang C. Incidence of histologic types of cancer of the small intestine. J Natl Cancer Inst 1987;78:653–6.
10. Cunningham JD, Aleali R, Aleali M, et al. Malignant small bowel neoplasms: histopathologic determinants of recurrence and survival. Ann Surg 1997;225:300–6.
11. North JH, Pack MS. Malignant tumors of the small intestine: a review of 144 cases. Am Surg 2000;66:46–51.
12. Maglinte DD, O'Connor K, Bessette J, et al. The role of the physician in the late diagnosis of primary malignant tumors of the small intestine. Am J Gastroenterol 1991;86:304–8.
13. Chow JS, Chen CC, Ahsan H, Neugut A. A population-based study of the incidence of malignant small bowel tumours: SEER, 1973-1990. Int J Epidemiol 1996;25:722–8.
14. Chong J, Tagle M, Barkin JS, Reiner DK. Small bowel push-type fiberoptic enteroscopy for patients with occult gastrointestinal bleeding or suspected small bowel pathology. Am J Gastroenterol 1994;89:2143–6.
15. Berner JS, Mauer K, Lewis BS. Push and sonde enteroscopy for the diagnosis of obscure gastrointestinal bleeding. Am J Gastroenterol 1994;89:2139–42.
16. Lewis BS, Kornbluth A, Waye JD. Small bowel tumours: yield of enteroscopy. Gut 1991;32:763–5.

17. Ouriel K, Adams JT. Adenocarcinoma of the small intestine. Am J Surg 1984;147:66–71.

18. van Ooijen B, Kalsbeek HL. Carcinoma of the duodenum. Surg Gynecol Obstet 1988;166:343–7.

19. Lowell JA, Rossi RL, Munson JL, Braasch JW. Primary adenocarcinoma of third and fourth portions of duodenum: favorable prognosis after resection. Arch Surg 1992;127:557–60.

20. Barnes G Jr, Romero L, Hess KR, Curley SA. Primary adenocarcinoma of the duodenum: management and survival in 67 patients. Ann Surg Oncol 1994;1:73–8.

21. Howe JR, Karnell LH, Menck HR, Scott-Conner C. Adenocarcinoma of the small bowel: review of the national cancer data base, 1985-1995. Cancer 1999;86:2693–706.

22. Moertel CG. An odyssey in the land of small tumors. J Clin Oncol 1987;5:1503–22.

23. Thompson GB, van Heerden JA, Martin JK Jr, et al. Carcinoid tumors of the gastrointestinal tract: presentation, management, and prognosis. Surgery 1985;98:1054–63.

24. Bomanji J, Mather EUS, Moyes J, et al. A scintigraphic comparison of iodine-123-metaiodobenzylguanidine and an iodine-labeled somatostatin analog (tyr-3-octreotide) in metastatic carcinoid tumors. J Nucl Med 1992;33:1121–4.

25. Hanson MW, Feldman JM, Blinder RA, et al. Carcinoid tumors: iodine-131 MIBG scintigraphy. Radiology 1989;172:699–703.

26. Kvols LK, Moertel CG, O'Connell MJ, et al. Treatment of the malignant carcinoid syndrome: evaluation of a long-acting somatostatin analogue. N Engl J Med 1986;315:663–6.

27. Carrasco CH, Charnsangavej C, Ajani J, et al. The carcinoid syndrome: palliation by hepatic artery embolization. AJR Am J Roentgenol 1986;147:149–54.

28. Contreary K, Nance FC, Becker WF. Primary lymphoma of the gastrointestinal tract. Ann Surg 1980;191:593–8.

29. Cooper BT, Read AE. Small intestinal lymphoma. World J Surg 1985;9:930–7.

30. Ng E-H, Pollack RE, Romsdahl MM. Prognostic implications of patterns of failure for gastrointestinal leiomyosarcomas. Cancer 1992;69:1334–41.

31. Ng E-H, Pollack RE, Munsell MF, et al. Prognostic factors influencing survival in gastrointestinal leiomyosarcomas: implications for surgical management and staging. Ann Surg 1992;215:68–77.

32. Pidhorecky I, Cheney RT, Kraybill WG, Gibbs JF. Gastrointestinal stromal tumors: current diagnosis, biologic behavior and management. Ann Surg Oncology 2000;7:705–12.

33. Crosby JA, Catton CN, Davis A, et al. Malignant gastrointestinal stromal tumors of the small intestine: a review of 50 cases from a prospective database. Ann Surg Oncol 2001;8:50–9.

34. Graadt van Roggen JR, van Velthuysen ML, Hogendoorn PC. The histopathologic differential diagnosis of gastrointestinal stromal tumours. J Clin Pathol 2001;54:96–102.

35. Berman J, O'Leary TJ. Gastrointestinal stromal tumor workshop. Hum Pathol 2001;32:578–82.

36. Miettinen M, Lasota J. Gastrointestinal stromal tumors-definition, clinical, histological, immunohistochemical, and molecular genetic features and differential diagnosis. Virchows Arch 2001;438:1–12.

37. Kim CJ, Day S, Yeh KA. Gastrointestinal stromal tumors: analysis of clinical and pathologic factors. Am Surg 2001; 67:135–7.

38. Clary BM, DeMatteo RP, Lewis JJ, et al. Gastrointestinal stromal tumors and leiomyosarcoma of the abdomen and retroperitoneum: a clinical comparison. Ann Surg Oncol 2001;8:290–9.

39. Pierie JPEN, Choudry U, Muzikansky A, et al. The effect of surgery and grade on outcome of gastrointestinal stromal tumors. Arch Surg 2001;136:383–9.

40. Joensuu H, Roberts PJ, Sarlomo-Rikala M, et al. Effect of the tyrosine kinase inhibitor sti571 in a patient with a metastatic gastrointestinal stromal tumor. N Engl J Med 2001;344:1052–6.

41. Goldman JM, Melo JV. Targeting the bcr-abl tyrosine kinase in chronic myeloid leukemia. N Engl J Med 2001;344: 1084–6.

42. Blecker D, Abraham S, Furth EE, Kochman ML. Melanoma in the gastrointestinal tract. Am J Gastroenterol 1999;94: 3427–33.

Index

Page numbers followed by f indicate figure. Page numbers followed by t indicate table.
Note: GIST stands for gastrointestinal stromal tumor